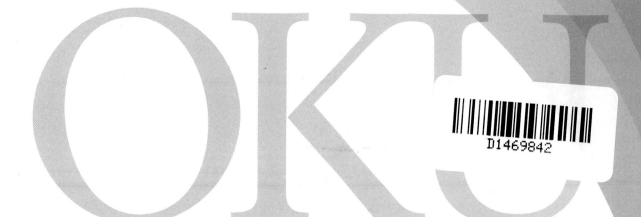

Orthopaedic Knowledge Update:
Sports Medicine

AAOS
AMERICAN ACADEMY OF
ORTHOPAEDIC SURGEONS

OKU

4

Orthopaedic Knowledge Update: Sports Medicine

EDITOR:
W. Ben Kibler, MD
Medical Director
Shoulder Center of Kentucky
Lexington, Kentucky

Developed by the
American Orthopaedic Society for Sports Medicine

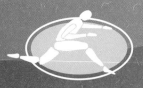

The American Orthopaedic
Society for Sports Medicine

AAOS
AMERICAN ACADEMY OF
ORTHOPAEDIC SURGEONS

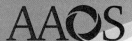

AMERICAN ACADEMY OF ORTHOPAEDIC SURGEONS

The material presented in the **Orthopaedic Knowledge Update: Sports Medicine 4** has been made available by the American Academy of Orthopaedic Surgeons for educational purposes only. This material is not intended to present the only, or necessarily best, methods or procedures for the medical situations discussed, but rather is intended to represent an approach, view, statement, or opinion of the author(s) or producer(s), which may be helpful to others who face similar situations.

Some drugs or medical devices demonstrated in Academy courses or described in Academy print or electronic publications have not been cleared by the Food and Drug Administration (FDA) or have been cleared for specific uses only. The FDA has stated that it is the responsibility of the physician to determine the FDA clearance status of each drug or device he or she wishes to use in clinical practice.

Furthermore, any statements about commercial products are solely the opinion(s) of the author(s) and do not represent an Academy endorsement or evaluation of these products. These statements may not be used in advertising or for any commercial purpose.

Published 2009 by the
American Academy of Orthopaedic Surgeons
6300 North River Road
Rosemont, IL 60018

Fourth Edition
Copyright 2009
by the American Academy of Orthopaedic Surgeons

ISBN 978-0-89203-575-5
Printed in the USA
Library of Congress Cataloging-in-Publication Data

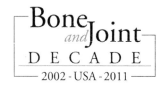

Acknowledgments

Editorial Board, Orthopaedic Knowledge Update: Sports Medicine 4

W. Ben Kibler, MD
Medical Director
Shoulder Center of Kentucky
Lexington, Kentucky

Timothy Averion-Mahloch, MD
Musculoskeletal Radiologist
Department of Radiology
Lexington Clinic
Lexington, Kentucky

Todd S. Ellenbecker, DPT, MS, SCS, OCS, CSCS
Clinical Director
Physiotherapy Associates
Scottsdale Sports Clinic
Scottsdale, Arizona

Andrew Gregory, MD, FAAP, FACSM
Assistant Professor, Orthopedics and Pediatrics
Program Director, Pediatric Sports Medicine
   Fellowship
Vanderbilt Sports Medicine
Vanderbilt University
Nashville, Tennessee

Stanley A. Herring, MD
Medical Director for Spine Care
Clinical Professor
Departments of Rehabilitation Medicine,
   Orthopaedics and Sports Medicine,
   and Neurological Surgery
University of Washington
Seattle, Washington

Darren L. Johnson, MD
Professor and Chairman
Department of Orthopaedic Surgery
University of Kentucky
Lexington, Kentucky

Karim Khan, MD, PhD
Associate Professor
Department of Family Practice and School of
   Human Kinetics
University of British Columbia
Vancouver, British Columbia, Canada

John E. Kuhn, MD
Associate Professor
Chief of Shoulder Surgery
Vanderbilt University Medical Center
Nashville, Tennessee

Margot Putukian, MD, FACSM
Director of Athletic Medicine
Head Team Physician
Princeton University
Associate Clinical Professor
Robert Wood Johnson University of Medicine
   and Dentistry of New Jersey
Princeton University Health Services
Princeton, New Jersey

Marc R. Safran, MD
Professor, Orthopaedic Surgery
Department of Orthopaedic Surgery
Stanford University
Stanford, California

American Orthopaedic Society for Sports Medicine Board of Directors and Council Chairs, 2008-2009

Freddie H. Fu, MD
President

James R. Andrews, MD
President-Elect

Robert A. Stanton, MD
Vice President

Jo A. Hannafin, MD, PhD
Secretary

Robert A. Arciero, MD
Treasurer

Bernard R. Bach Jr, MD
Past President

Champ L. Baker Jr, MD
Past President

Col. Thomas M. DeBerardino, MD
Member at Large

William N. Levine, MD
Member at Large

Allen F. Anderson, MD
Member at Large

Patricial A. Kolowich, MD
Council of Delegates Chair (Ex Officio)

Bruce Reider, MD
Executive Editor, Medical Publishing and
   Editor, AJSM

Barry P. Boden, MD
Communications Chair

Michael G. Ciccotti, MD
Education Chair

Scott A. Rodeo, MD
Research Chair

Contributors

Håkan Alfredson, MD, PhD
Professor
Sports Medicine Unit
University of Umeå
Umeå, Sweden

Annunziato Amendola, MD
Professor and Director, University of Iowa
  Sports Medicine
Department of Orthopaedic Surgery and
  Rehabilitation
University of Iowa
Iowa City, Iowa

Brett Andres, MD
Orthopedic Surgeon
Orthopedic and Fracture Clinic
Portland, Oregon

Michael J. Angel, MD
Kerlan-Jobe Orthopaedic Clinic
Los Angeles, California

Timothy Averion-Mahloch, MD
Musculoskeletal Radiologist
Department of Radiology
Lexington Clinic
Lexington, Kentucky

Roald Bahr, MD, PhD
Professor and Chair
Oslo Sports Trauma Research Center
Norwegian School of Sport Sciences
Oslo, Norway

John P. Batson, MD, FAAP
The Sport and Spine Center of the Low Country
Hilton Head Island, South Carolina

Michael F. Bergeron, PhD, FACSM
Director, National Institute for Athletic Health
  and Performance
Professor, Department of Pediatrics
Sanford School of Medicine
The University of South Dakota
Sioux Falls, South Dakota

David T. Bernhardt, MD
Professor
Department of Pediatrics, Orthopedics and
  Rehabilitation
Division of Sports Medicine
University of Wisconsin School of Medicine and
  Public Health
Madison, Wisconsin

Julie Y. Bishop, MD
Assistant Professor of Orthopaedics
Department of Orthopaedics
The Ohio State University
Columbus, Ohio

Brian L. Bixler, MD
Pediatric Orthopedic Surgeon
Orthopedic and Spine Specialists
York, Pennsylvania

Karen K. Briggs, MPH
Director of Clinical Research
Steadman Hawkins Research Foundation
Vail, Colorado

Robert H. Brophy, MD
Assistant Professor
Department of Orthopaedic Surgery
Washington University School of Medicine
St. Louis, Missouri

Robert C. Cantu, MD, FACS, FACSM
Clinical Professor of Neurosurgery
Boston University School of Medicine
Co-Director, Center for the Study of Traumatic
  Encephalopathy
Boston University Medical Center
Boston, Massachusetts
Co-Founder and Chairman of the Medical
  Advisory Board
Sports Legacy Institute
Waltham, Massachusetts

Akin Cil, MD
Clinical Fellow
Division of Sports Medicine
Department of Orthopedics
Children's Hospital Boston
Boston, Massachusetts

Mandy Clark-Gruner, MS, RD, CSSD
Sports Dietitian and Nutrition Therapist
The Chirofit Wellness Center
East Grand Rapids, Michigan
Comprehensive Treatment for Eating Disorders,
  LLC
Grand Rapids, Michigan

Jill L. Cook, PhD
Associate Professor
Centre for Physical Activity and Nutrition
  Research
Deakin University
Melbourne, Victoria, Australia

David B. Coppel, PhD
Clinical Professor
Department of Psychiatry and Behavioral
  Sciences
University of Washington
Seattle, Washington

Charles L. Cox, MD
Assistant Professor
Department of Orthopaedics and Rehabilitation
Vanderbilt University Medical Center
Nashville, Tennessee

George J. Davies, DPT, MEd, PT, SCS, ATC
Professor
Department of Physical Therapy
Armstrong Atlantic State University
Savannah, Georgia

Mark S. DeCarlo, PT, MHS, SCS, ATC
Vice President, Clinical Operations
Methodist Sports Medicine/The Orthopaedic
  Specialists
Indianapolis, Indiana

Carl DeRosa, PT, PhD
Professor of Physical Therapy
Northern Arizona University
Flagstaff, Arizona

Brian G. Donley, MD
Director, Center for Foot and Ankle
Department of Orthopaedic Surgery
Cleveland Clinic
Cleveland, Ohio

Ruben J. Echemendia, PhD
Clinical Neuropsychologist
Psychological and Neurobehavioral
  Associates, Inc.
State College, Pennsylvania

Todd S. Ellenbecker, DPT, MS, SCS, OCS, CSCS
Clinical Director
Physiotherapy Associates
Scottsdale Sports Clinic
Scottsdale, Arizona

Kenneth J. Faber, MD, MHPE, FRCSC
Associate Professor
Hand and Upper Limb Centre
University of Western Ontario
London, Ontario, Canada

Gregory C. Fanelli, MD
Orthopaedic Surgeon
Danville, Pennsylvania

Jonathan B. Feibel, MD
Director, Foor and Ankle Surgery
Assistant Program Director
Mount Carmel Health Orthopaedic Residency
  Program
The Cardinal Orthopaedic Institute
Columbus, Ohio

Ronald A. Feinstein, MD
Professor of Clinical Pediatrics
Department of Pediatrics
Louisiana State University New Orleans School
  of Medicine
New Orleans, Louisiana

Karl B. Fields, MD, CAQSM
Chief of Family Medicine Education
Director of Sports Medicine Fellowship
Moses Cone Hospital
Greensboro, North Carolina

Donald C. Fithian, MD
Department of Orthopedics and Podiatry
Southern California Permanente Medical Group
San Diego, California

Freddie H. Fu, MD
David Silver Professor and Chairman
Department of Orthopaedic Surgery
University of Pittsburgh School of Medicine
Pittsburgh, Pennsylvania

Aimee E. Gibbs, MPH
Research Assistant
MedSport
Department of Orthopaedic Surgery
University of Michigan
Ann Arbor, Michigan

Eric Giza, MD
Assistant Professor of Orthopaedic Surgery
Chief, Foot and Ankle Surgery
Department of Orthopaedics
University of California Davis Medical Center
Sacramento, California

Mark Glazebrook, MSc, PhD, MD, FRCSC
Assistant Professor of Orthopedic Surgery
Department of Surgery, Division of Orthopedics
Dalhousie University
Halifax, Nova Scotia, Canada

Thomas J. Graham, MD
Chief, Curtis National Hand Center
Vice-Chairman, Department of Orthopaedic
    Surgery
Union Memorial Hospital
Baltimore, Maryland

Ruby Grewal, MD, MSc, FRCSC
Assistant Professor
Hand and Upper Limb Centre
University of Western Ontario
London, Ontario, Canada

Kevin M. Guskiewicz, PhD, ATC
Professor and Chair
Department of Exercise and Sport Science
University of North Carolina
Chapel Hill, North Carolina

Mark A. Harrast, MD
Clinical Associate Professor
Department of Rehabilitation Medicine
University of Washington
Seattle, Washington

William Hennrikus, MD
Medical Director, Orthopaedics and
    Sports Medicine
Associate Clinical Professor, UCSF
Children's Hospital
Madera, California

James J. Irrgang, PhD, PT, ATC
Associate Professor and Director of Clinical
    Research
Department of Orthopedic Surgery
University of Pittsburgh
Pittsburgh, Pennsylvania

Walter L. Jenkins, PT, DHS, ATC
Associate Professor and Associate Chair
Department of Physical Therapy
College of Allied Health Sciences
East Carolina University
Greensville, North Carolina

Christopher Johnson, MPT, MCMT
Senor Physical Therapist, Research Assistant
Nicholas Institute of Sports Medicine and
    Athletic Trauma
Lenox Hill Hospital
New York, New York

Darren L. Johnson, MD
Professor and Chairman
Department of Orthopaedic Surgery
University of Kentucky
Lexington, Kentucky

Susan M. Joy, MD
Director, Women's Sports Health
Orthopaedic and Rheumatologic Institute
Cleveland Clinic
Cleveland, Ohio

David M. Junkin Jr, MD
Orthopaedic Specialty Center
Willow Grove, Pennsylvania

Bryan T. Kelly, MD
Assistant Attending, Sports Medicine and
    Hip Injuries
Department of Orthopaedic Surgery
Hospital for Special Surgery
New York Presbyterian Hospital
Weill Cornell
New York, New York

Karim Khan, MD, PhD
Associate Professor
Department of Family Practice and School of
*   Human Kinetics*
University of British Columbia
Vancouver, British Columbia, Canada

W. Ben Kibler, MD
Medical Director
Shoulder Center of Kentucky
Lexington, Kentucky

John E. Kuhn, MD
Associate Professor
Chief of Shoulder Surgery
Vanderbilt University Medical Center
Nashville, Tennessee

Jennifer C. Laine, MD
Department of Orthopaedic Surgery
University of California, San Francisco
San Francisco, California

L. Daniel Latt, MD, PhD
Fellow, Sports Medicine
Kaiser Permanente San Diego
El Cajon, California

Christian Lattermann, MD
Assistant Professor
Director, Center for Cartilage Repair and
*   Restoration*
Department of Orthopaedic Surgery
University of Kentucky
Lexington, Kentucky

Umile Giuseppe Longo, MD
Department of Trauma and
*   Orthopaedic Surgery*
University Campus Biomedico
Rome, Italy

C. Benjamin Ma, MD
Chief, Sports Medicine and Shoulder
Department of Orthopaedic Surgery
University of California, San Francisco
San Francisco, California

Nicola Maffulli, MD, PhD, FRCS(Orth)
Professor of Trauma and Orthopaedic Surgery
Department of Orthopaedic and
*   Trauma Surgery*
Keele University
Stoke-on-Trent, England

Scott D. Mair, MD
Associate Professor
Department of Orthopaedic Surgery and
*   Sports Medicine*
University of Kentucky
Lexington, Kentucky

Robert C. Manske, PT, DPT, MED, SCS, ATC
Associate Professor
Department of Physical Therapy
Wichita State University
Wichita, Kansas

Cory Manton, PT, DPT, OCS, CSCS
Physical Therapist
DeRosa Physical Therapy
Flagstaff, Arizona

Teri M. McCambridge, MD
Department of Pediatrics
Johns Hopkins School of Medicine
Baltimore, Maryland

Eric C. McCarty, MD
Chief of Sports Medicine and Shoulder Surgery
Associate Professor
Department of Orthopaedics
University of Colorado Denver
*   School of Medicine*
Denver, Colorado

Lyle J. Micheli, MD
Clinical Professor of Orthopedic Surgery
Harvard Medical School
Department of Orthopedics
Division of Sports Medicine
Children's Hospital Boston
Boston, Massachusetts

Mark D. Miller, MD
Professor, Department of Orthopaedic Surgery
Head, Division of Sports Medicine
University of Virginia
Charlottesville, Virginia

George A.C. Murrell, MD, DPhil
Professor
Department of Orthopaedic Surgery
St. George Public Hospital
Kogarah, New South Wales, Australia

Mark V. Paterno, PT, MS, MBA, SCS, ATC
Coordinator of Orthopaedic and
*   Sports Physical Therapy*
Assistant Professor, Department of Pediatrics
Sports Medicine Biodynamics Center
Cincinnati Children's Hospital Medical Center
Cincinnati, Ohio

Marc J. Philippon, MD
Steadman Hawkins Clinic
Steadman Hawkins Research Foundation
Vail, Colorado

Kian Raiszadeh, MD
Department of Sports Medicine
Kaiser Permanente
San Diego, California

Matthew A. Rappé Jr, MD
Knoxville Orthopedic Clinic
Knoxville, Tennessee

Marty E. Reed, MD
Sports Fellow
Department of Orthopedic Surgery
Santa Monica Orthopedic Group
Santa Monica, California

Michael M. Reinold, PT, DPT, ATC, CSCS
Coordinator of Rehabilitation Research
*   and Education*
Department of Orthopedic Surgery
Division of Sports Medicine
Massachusetts General Hospital
Boston, Massachusetts

Lance A. Rettig, MD
Volunteer Clinical Assistant Professor
Department of Orthopaedic Surgery
Methodist Sports Medicine/The Orthopaedic
*   Specialists*
Indiana University School of Medicine
Indianapolis, Indiana

M. Brennan Royalty, MD
Department of Family Medicine
University of Kentucky
Lexington, Kentucky

Mark Rowand, MD
Family Medicine Resident
Department of Family Medicine
Moses Cone Hospital
Greensboro, North Carolina

Marc R. Safran, MD
Professor, Orthopaedic Surgery
Department of Orthopaedic Surgery
Stanford University
Stanford, California

Kristen Samuhel, MD
Family Medicine Resident
Department of Family Medicine
Moses Cone Hospital
Greensboro, North Carolina

Aaron Sciascia, MS, ATC, NASM-PES, NS
Program Coordinator
Shoulder Center of Kentucky
Lexington, Kentucky

Alexander Scott, PhD
Research Fellow
Centre for Hip Health
Vancouver Coastal Health Research Institute
Vancouver, British Columbia, Canada

Jon K. Sekiya, MD
Associate Professor
MedSport
Department of Orthopaedic Surgery
University of Michigan
Ann Arbor, Michigan

Nicholas A. Sgaglione, MD
Program Director and Associate Chairman
Department of Orthopaedics
Long Island Jewish Medical Center
New Hyde Park, New York

Edwin E. Spencer Jr, MD
Attending Orthopaedic Surgeon
Department of Shoulder/Sports Medicine
Knoxville Orthopaedic Clinic
Knoxville, Tennessee

Kurt P. Spindler, MD
Professor and Vice Chairman
Director of Sports Medicine
Department of Orthopaedics and Rehabilitation
Nashville, Tennessee

Timothy F. Tyler, MS, PT, ATC
Clinical Research Associate
The Nicholas Institute of Sports Medicine and
*   Athletic Trauma*
Lenox Hill Hospital
New York, New York

Bill Vicenzino, BPhty, Grad Dip Sports Phty,
**   MSc, PhD**
Chair in Sports Physiotherapy, Head of Division
Division of Physiotherapy
School of Health and Rehabilitation Science
The University of Queensland
Brisbane, Queensland, Australia

Michael Wahoff, PT
Director, Hip Rehabilitation
Department of Physical Therapy
Howard Head Sports Medicine
Vail, Colorado

Bryan A. Warme, MD
Department of Orthopaedics and Rehabilitation
University of Iowa Hospitals and Clinics
Iowa City, Iowa

Daniel C. Wascher, MD
Professor
Department of Orthopaedics
University of New Mexico
Albuquerque, New Mexico

Stuart M. Weinstein, MD
Clinical Professor
Department of Rehabilitation Medicine
University of Washington
Seattle, Washington

Robin Vereeke West, MD
Assistant Professor
Department of Orthopaedics
University of Pittsburgh
Pittsburgh, Pennsylvania

Kevin E. Wilk, PT, DPT
National Director of Education
Champion Sports Medicine
Birmingham, Alabama

Brian R. Wolf, MD, MS
Assistant Professor
Department of Orthopaedics and Rehabilitation
University of Iowa Hospitals and Clinics
Iowa City, Iowa

Rick W. Wright, MD
Associate Professor
Department of Orthopaedic Surgery
Washington University
St. Louis, Missouri

Melissa Willenborg, MD
Department of Orthopaedics
University of Virginia
Charlottesville, Virginia

Eva Zeisig, MD
Sports Medicine Unit
University of Umeå
Umeå, Sweden

Preface

The Orthopaedic Knowledge Update series has become a valuable resource that provides a selective review of key information on many specific topics in orthopaedic surgery, but more importantly provides an update on recent advances in these topical areas. The goal of this approach is to enable readers to stay anchored in the basic principles, but also to keep abreast of the most current research, advances in knowledge, and techniques.

OKU Sports Medicine 4, in keeping with its predecessors, has taken a comprehensive look at many aspects of sports medicine. Its foundation continues to be delivering in-depth updates and significant bibliographic commentary regarding sports injuries to all aspects of the musculoskeletal system—upper extremity, hip, knee/leg, and head/neck. In addition, key areas including rehabilitation, tendinopathy, medical issues, the youth athlete, and imaging are included, with information geared toward orthopaedic applications. This balance will provide the broad base of information upon which the reader can deliver current evaluation and treatment.

Sports medicine is a very broad discipline, encompassing basic science research, pathophysiology, examination and evaluation, medical illnesses and conditions, nonsurgical and surgical orthopaedic conditions, rehabilitation, conditioning, and prevention. This broad base is reflected in this fourth edition of *OKU Sports Medicine* in the topics and put in force by the section editors and chapter authors. Six section editors and 23 senior chapter authors are nonorthopaedic surgeons, and 3 section editors and 17 senior chapter authors are orthopaedic surgeons. I would like to thank the section editors, Drs. Kuhn, Safran, Johnson, Ellenbecker, Herring, Khan, Putukian, Gregory, and Averion-Mahloch for their dedication to this project and to sports medicine. They developed the topics and authors, and provided editorial review so that the best and most comprehensive information was presented in the most concise manner. Each section editor and senior chapter author is a recognized leader in that field of sports medicine. Their expertise is reflected in the uniformly high quality of the material.

I have been honored to have been a chapter writer, section editor, and now editor, and continue to be a consumer of the OKU series. I have personally found it to be a valuable resource and a key component of my continuing medical education. I am grateful for the Academy's efforts in this essential series. This volume could not be produced without the critical facilitation and direction by the AAOS publications staff under the leadership of Marilyn L. Fox, PhD. My sincerest appreciation goes out to Lisa Claxton Moore, Managing Editor, Kathleen Anderson, Senior Editor, and Courtney Astle, Assistant Production Manager, for all their hard work.

W. Ben Kibler, MD
Editor

Table of Contents

Upper Extremity

SECTION EDITOR:
JOHN E. KUHN, MD

Chapter 1

Acute Shoulder Injuries

Rick W. Wright, MD   Robert H. Brophy, MD   Eric C. McCarty, MD   Julie Y. Bishop, MD

Traumatic Instability

Anterior Instability

The most common pattern of acute shoulder traumatic instability is anterior or anteroinferior, which represents more than 90% of dislocations. The instability events typically occur following trauma during participation in contact sports such as hockey or football. The mechanism of injury is most commonly a force applied to an abducted and externally rotated arm.

Pathophysiology

The shoulder, while allowing the most motion of any joint in the body, is normally very stable with minimal translation of the humeral head on the glenoid during routine motion. Dynamic and static restraints contribute to the normal stability of the shoulder. Dynamic restraints include the rotator cuff muscles, the scapula stabilizer muscles, and other large muscles surrounding the shoulder. Static restraints include the labrum, the glenohumeral capsule, and ligamentous structures. The inferior glenohumeral ligament consists of an anterior and a posterior band and is the most important structure preventing traumatic anterior instability. This structure tightens in the vulnerable abducted externally rotated position to prevent anterior translation. The labrum also has some role in resisting instability. At some level it acts as a block by doubling the depth of the glenoid surface.

The Bankart lesion and avulsion of the inferior glenohumeral ligament and labrum complex from the glenoid is the single most common structural injury noted with traumatic anterior shoulder instability, occurring more than 90% of the time. Humeral avulsion of the glenohumeral ligament (HAGL) occurs less than 10% of the time and is referred to as the HAGL lesion. The Bankart lesion was originally believed to be critically important for anterior instability. Further studies have shown it to be one of several factors that can contribute to instability.[1]

Presentation

Initial management of acute traumatic anterior shoulder instability depends on the situation and timing of presentation. Reduction of the injury on the field by a physician covering the event frequently can be performed when the physical examination and history are indicative of injury. Often, reduction is most easily ob-

tained before the onset of muscle spasm and pain. Postreduction radiographs and additional examination are necessary once the player is stabilized. When reduction is delayed and the patient presents to the emergency department, intravenous analgesia and sedation in addition to reduction maneuvers may be necessary. The technique of intra-articular lidocaine injection combined with the minimally traumatic Stimson method of reduction has gained popularity. This was recently supported by a systematic review that demonstrated decreased emergency room time and complications for intra-articular lidocaine compared with intravenous sedation.[2]

Postreduction radiographic views should be obtained and include, at a minimum, a true AP view of the glenoid and an axillary lateral. Additional views that may be helpful include West Point and Stryker notch views, which will improve the ability to assess potential Hill-Sachs lesions or glenoid rim fractures. Loss of greater than 25% of the glenoid surface or 30% of the humeral head surface may increase the likelihood of recurrent instability and thus require bone grafting at the time of reconstruction. If recurrent stability is suspected on plain radiographs, a CT scan may provide information about pathology.

Natural History

A large number of studies have been performed that demonstrate a high risk for recurrence following acute traumatic anterior shoulder instability. For the patient younger than 20 years, recurrence rates reportedly have been as high as 90%. Recurrence rates dropped dramatically for each decade of life after age 20 years. Beyond age 40 years, the risk of concomitant rotator cuff tear with dislocation significantly increases with a risk of 40% for people older than 60 years. Recent studies have demonstrated that in addition to younger age, males and patients returning to contact or collision sports have an increased risk of recurrence.[3,4] A recent study evaluated the 25-year follow-up of a prospective cohort of anterior instability. After 25 years, 50% of patients treated nonsurgically at ages 12 to 25 years had no recurrence or achieved stability.[5]

Treatment

A variety of issues regarding all aspects of management of traumatic shoulder instability have been studied over the past few years. Initial management of the patient with a first-time shoulder dislocation remains debatable. Nonsurgical treatment is designed to allow possible healing of the static restraints of glenohumeral instability followed by maximizing the dynamic restraints to glenohumeral instability. Immobilization of the initial shoulder dislocation has been evaluated. A recent study demonstrated decreased rates of redislocation following immobilization of the shoulder in external rotation compared with internal rotation, although the rate of redislocation remains fairly high.[6] Recent cadaver studies demonstrated increased contact force between a Bankart lesion and the anterior glenoid rim with the arm in external rotation, which may influence healing.[7] Immobilization in internal rotation for either a short or prolonged period does not significantly decrease the risk of recurrence.

One of the challenges for team physicians is management of the athlete with an in-season dislocation. According to a recent study, 87% of athletes were able to return to their sport in season following rehabilitation and indicated bracing. The athletes sustained an average of 1.4 incidents of recurrent dislocation. More than 50% of the athletes studied underwent surgical stabilization in the following off-season.[8]

Surgical stabilization is designed to correct an injury to the static restraints to glenohumeral instability. Arthroscopic stabilization continues to gain credence with orthopaedic surgeons. Improved methods have allowed surgeons to obtain results following arthroscopic stabilization approaching or equal to previous open stabilization results. Surgical management does decrease the likelihood of recurrent instability in the patient with a first-time shoulder dislocation; it may be indicated in the patient who will definitely return to high-risk activities.[9] The question remains which patients should receive this treatment, as recent evidence suggests many of these patients would not opt for surgery if initially managed nonsurgically.[4] In recent studies of arthroscopic stabilization of traumatic anterior shoulder instability, rates of postoperative recurrent dislocations have been consistent with previous open procedures, including a Level I randomized clinical trial demonstrating no difference in results between arthroscopic and open stabilization.[10,11]

Despite the successful results of arthroscopic stabilization, surgical treatment of the contact or collision athlete remains a point of debate among sports medicine surgeons. This high-risk subset of traumatic anterior shoulder instability may warrant careful consideration in choosing a technique for stabilization. Studies evaluating this question have been of low level of evidence. While suggesting either technique may be amenable to successful outcome, no definitive answer has yet been achieved by a Level I study. A recent study evaluating the results of open stabilization in American football players demonstrated no recurrent dislocations in 57 players, 52 of whom had returned to a least 1 year of organized football.[12]

Posterior Instability

Frank posterior dislocations are rare, making up 4% of all glenohumeral dislocations. These rarely occur in the absence of high-energy trauma, seizure, or electrical shock. In contrast to anterior dislocations, most posterior dislocations reduce spontaneously, unless there is an associated fracture. Diagnosis of these injuries can be difficult; 50% to 80% of posterior dislocations are missed at initial presentation. If the diagnosis is made within 6 weeks of injury, the injury is considered acute, whereas posterior dislocations diagnosed more than 6 weeks after injury are considered chronic. Athletes are more likely to suffer from isolated or repetitive posterior subluxation, which is believed to result from shear forces on the posterior labrum resulting from posterior loading of the shoulder. Approximately half of all posterior subluxation is traumatic, typically occurring after a direct blow to the anterior shoulder or a posterior directed force on an adducted, flexed, and internally rotated upper extremity.

Presentation

Patients with an acute posterior dislocation typically will present with an adducted, internally rotated arm. Patients with chronic dislocation often lack external rotation and have limited forearm supination. A posterior prominence in the shoulder may be noted. Plain films are necessary to confirm the diagnosis. An axillary view is essential because it will demonstrate an empty glenoid with the humeral head posterior. An AP view and even the transscapular Y view may be equivocal with a posterior shoulder dislocation. A CT scan may help assess bone stock after a posterior dislocation. Increased chondrolabral and osseous retroversion were reported in athletes with posterior instability based on magnetic resonance arthrography in a recent study.[13]

Posterior subluxation may be associated with pain, instability, or both, particularly if the arm is placed in the provocative position of flexion, internal rotation, and adduction. Posterior shoulder instability may be voluntary, in approximately 50% of patients, or involuntary. A small subset of voluntary shoulder instability patients are habitual dislocators, who intentionally dislocate their shoulder for personal gain. Physical examination may demonstrate posterior joint line tenderness, and scapular winging is common. The apprehension sign for posterior instability is assessed by placing a posterior-directed force on an upper extremity in 90° of flexion and 90° of internal rotation. The posterior drawer, load and shift, and jerk tests also can be performed to assess posterior instability. Patients very often report pain, even in the absence of measurable subluxation or dislocation. The shoulder also should be tested for anterior and inferior stability because patients may have a multidirectional pattern of instability. MRI is useful to evaluate posterior labral injury; a recent study reported that football players are 15 times more likely than nonfootball players to have a posterior labral injury on a magnetic resonance arthrogram of the shoulder.[14] Athletes with posterior instability have increased chondrolabral and osseous retroversion based on magnetic resonance arthrography in comparison with control subjects.

Treatment

Acute dislocations with an impression fracture involving less than 20% of the articular surface should be reduced as soon as possible, typically with traction, external rotation, and abduction. After successful closed reduction, the upper extremity should be immobilized in neutral rotation for 4 to 6 weeks. Chronic dislocations, humeral head impression fractures involving greater than 20% of the articular surface, large glenoid rim fractures, and displaced lesser tuberosity fractures are likely to need surgical treatment. Dislocations more than 6 months old and fractures involving greater than 50% of the humeral head are probably best treated with humeral head replacement.

Recurrent posterior shoulder subluxation is treated initially with physical therapy, emphasizing strengthening of the shoulder external rotators and scapula stabilizers. Patients in whom 6 months of therapy has been unsuccessful and those who have involuntary posterior shoulder instability are candidates for surgical treatment. Although open soft-tissue posterior shoulder stabilization has been shown to have good results in 80% to 95% of patients,[15] arthroscopy may be preferred for isolated posterior Bankart lesions because of the morbidity associated with the open posterior approach.

Several recent studies have demonstrated good results with arthroscopic treatment of posterior instability. A study of 27 shoulders with posterior instability treated with a bioabsorbable tack reported 92% good and excellent results with two reoperations at an average follow-up of 5.1 years.[16] In two recent studies of outcomes after arthroscopic posterior stabilization using suture anchors, recurrent instability was reportedly 4% to 12%, with previous surgery, particularly thermal capsulorrhaphy, identified as a risk factor for failure.[17,18] In another study of 41 arthroscopic posterior stabilizations, including 9 revisions, approximately 15% of patients had recurrent instability. Workers' compensation also has been associated with a higher risk of failure after arthroscopic posterior shoulder stabilization. Although there is not as much evidence on outcome after arthroscopic stabilization of isolated posterior capsular laxity, a recent study of posterior arthroscopic stabilization in athletes reported an overall 89% rate of return to sport, even though 43% of the patients had isolated capsular laxity without labral tear treated with capsular plication.[13] Although bony procedures for posterior stabilization have not traditionally had as much success as the open and arthroscopic soft-tissue stabilizations, a recent series of 21 posterior bone block procedures for posterior stabilization reported a failure rate of 14% at a mean follow-up of 6 years.[19] Radiographic evidence of glenohumeral osteoarthritis was noted in two shoulders.

Acromioclavicular Joint

The acromioclavicular (AC) joint is commonly injured during sports activity. Injury typically occurs from direct impact from a collision during football or hockey or from a fall onto the shoulder with the arm in the adducted position. The forces across the joint disrupt the AC ligaments first; then the coracoclavicular (CC) ligaments are disrupted. Injuries occur less often from an indirect force to the AC joint than when an athlete lands on an outstretched hand. The energy transmitted through the upper extremity in these indirect injuries typically affect AC ligaments only, and the CC ligaments are not injured.

Anatomy

The AC ligaments help control horizontal (anterior and posterior) stability, with the superior and posterior part of the capsule/ligament providing the strongest stabilizers. The CC ligaments control vertical stability and comprise the larger conoid ligament, which attaches posterior and medial on the clavicle, and the trapezoid ligament, which attaches more anterior and lateral. A recent anatomic study has defined the average location of the attachments of each of the CC ligaments.[20] The ratio of the distance from the lateral edge of the clavicle to the medial edge of the conoid tuberosity divided by clavicle length was 0.31 in both males and females, which resulted in a longer distance in males (47.2 mm) than in females (42.8 mm) because the clavicle is longer in males. This ratio to the center of the trapezoid from the lateral end of the clavicle was 0.17 in both sexes, with average distance of 25.4 mm in males and 22.9 mm in females. The average distance from the coracoid to the clavicle is 1.3 cm. Biomechanical testing on cadavers has shown that after the AC ligaments are disrupted, the conoid ligament is the next to fail.[21] This incomplete injury to the CC ligaments can still result in significant changes in both radiographic and mechanical measures of AC stability and functional deficits.

Classification

The original 1963 classification of these injuries described types I, II, and III. Rockwood later modified this classification by adding types IV through VI. Types I through III and V are progressive degrees of injury to the AC ligaments and the CC ligaments. Type I involves stretching of the AC ligaments. Type II involves disruption to the AC ligaments and injury to the CC ligaments without a change of position of the clavicle relative to the acromion. In type III injuries, both the AC and CC ligaments are disrupted, and there is displacement of the clavicle (up to 100% above the acromion). Further severity of the injury and progression of the displacement is evident in type V injuries, in which the clavicle is more than 100% displaced. There is often a gray area of distinguishing type III and type V injuries. Type IV injuries are uncommon and occur as the clavicle is displaced posteriorly (with the head of the clavicle poking through the trapezius muscle), and type VI injuries occur when the clavicle displaces inferiorly.[22]

Treatment

In the management of high-grade AC injuries, it has been shown that concomitant injuries do occur and are often masked by the more painful AC joint injury. In a series of 77 patients, more than 18% (14 patients) had intra-articular pathology, with most of these being superior labrum anterior and posterior (SLAP) lesions.[23]

The treatment of type I and type II injuries is nonsurgical. These injuries heal but with some potential residual pain, inflammation, and possibly long-term degenerative changes. A 2008 study of the long-term effects of a type I or a type II injury found 52% of patients had at least residual symptoms and significant difference in shoulder outcomes scores when compared with the normal contralateral shoulder.[24]

The acute treatment of type III injuries is more controversial, with most surgeons choosing nonsurgical treatment for the athlete. Some exceptions to this might be the heavy laborer or the throwing athlete. A lack of clinical studies evaluating the competitive throwing athlete makes it difficult to draw conclusions in this specialized population. A 2007 systematic review determined that nonsurgical treatment was more appropriate than surgery because the results of surgical management were associated with higher complication rates, longer convalescence, and longer time away from work and sport.[25] A 1998 meta-analysis had similar conclusions and found that, overall, 88% of surgically treated patients and 87% of nonsurgically treated patients had a satisfactory outcome.[26] In a study of 20 patients with a type III AC injury who were followed prospectively over the course of 1 year, no difference in motion or rotational shoulder strength was noted in comparison with the contralateral uninjured shoulder.[27] Results from a recent survey of 577 American Orthopaedic Society for Sports Medicine members indicated that 81% of members preferred nonsurgical treatment for uncomplicated type III injuries.[28]

Acute Repair

If an acute type III or V injury occurs, there are several methods of fixation. Biomechanical testing of different constructs has demonstrated the CC screw to have the greatest stiffness with repetitive loading, and a CC sling of 5-mm tape around the coracoid demonstrated the least amount of stiffness, with less stiffness than that of the normal AC joint.[29] The hook plate demonstrated a degree of stiffness similar to that of the native AC joint. Other methods of fixation include suture anchor fixation with an anchor placed in the coracoid process or small metallic flip button fixation through the coracoid process with sutures to the clavicle. A flip button repair or a polydioxanone cerclage around the coracoid were found to be similar in biomechanical testing, and both were found to have higher ultimate loads to failure (approximately 650 N) than suture anchor repair (approximately 300 N) with heavy-duty nonabsorbable suture.[30] One biomechanical study demonstrated that the use of two flip button devices placed under the coracoids after being placed through transcoracoid tunnels and tied to the clavicle with suture in the orientation of CC ligaments represented a construct as strong or stronger than the native ligaments.[31] Clinically, retrospective studies have demonstrated positive results for acute treatment of higher grade AC injuries. In a series of 34 patients, the use of two loops of No. 5 nonabsorbable suture passed around the coracoid through the clavicle was found to have good outcomes at 2-year follow-up.[32] Fifty patients treated with heavy absorbable polydioxane sulfate suture around the coracoid and clavicle demonstrated mostly good to excellent clinical results; however, later follow-up revealed a high incidence of osteoarthritis at the AC joint.[33] The hook plate has significantly better results than nonsurgical treatment in the acute treatment of type III AC injuries in a series of 24 patients treated surgically compared with 17 treated nonsurgically.[34]

There are various techniques and methods for the fixation of an acute type III AC injury with arthroscopic assistance, including transcoracoid placement of a flip button for distal fixation with absorbable or nonabsorbable sutures tied to the clavicle, arthroscopic placement of a cannulated screw from the clavicle to the coracoid, placement of a suture anchor into the base of the coracoid and placement of sutures into the clavicle, and placement of a ligament augmentation arthroscopically around the coracoid. Although these techniques appear to be promising, the literature describing them involves small series of patients with limited follow-up.[31]

Acute Nonsurgical Management

If the acute AC separation is treated nonsurgically, the shoulder typically is placed in a sling for comfort, and movement is allowed as the pain and acute symptoms decrease. A specific AC joint sling (Kenny Howard sling), which consists of a sling with a strap that goes around the top of shoulder over the clavicle, has been used to encourage better anatomic healing of the AC injury. However, the literature does not indicate that using this type of device makes a long-term clinical difference; because this sling has been associated with skin breakdown, it is not commonly used.[35]

The time it takes to return to sports activity after an acute type I, II, or III AC injury is variable. Many factors contribute to the ability to return or a delayed return to play. Athletes with lower grades of injury likely have a faster return to activity. The type of sport will often dictate return to play; athletes involved in contact sports usually take longer to return to activity than other athletes because reinjury is more likely. Use of the involved extremity in the sport also will have an impact on the ability to return to activity. For example, a throwing athlete with an injured throwing arm will

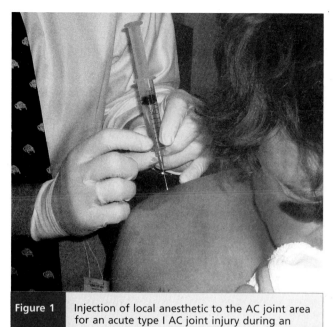

Figure 1 Injection of local anesthetic to the AC joint area for an acute type I AC joint injury during an American football game.

likely take longer to return to activity than if the nondominant arm were injured. Any associated soft-tissue injury will also potentially delay return to activity. An athlete's level of motivation and tolerance of pain also are factors. In an acute type I, II, or III injury, there are no set guidelines for the length of time in a sling and return to sports activity. Typically, an athlete is allowed to return to play when pain has diminished and there is full or near-full strength and range of motion of the affected shoulder. It is also accepted practice among team physicians that an athlete with a type I or II injury can be safely administered an injection of a long-acting local anesthetic into and around the AC joint (**Figure 1**) to allow for return to play in the acute or semi-acute time period.

In the event a type III AC injury is treated nonsurgically, there are also no guidelines for how long to wait before determining if nonsurgical treatment is going to be successful. Typically, from 3 to 6 months or as long as 1 to 2 years is recommended to overcome the symptoms from the acute injury and undergo rehabilitation to allow strengthening of the shoulder girdle musculature.

Late Reconstruction

If symptoms of pain, weakness, and/or dysfunction persist after several months of nonsurgical treatment for a type III or greater AC injury, then the late reconstruction of the CC ligaments may be done. Traditionally, a Weaver-Dunn procedure has been used for a late stabilization of the AC joint, which involves the transfer of the proximal portion of the AC ligament to the distal end of the clavicle. Cadaver testing has shown that augmentation of the traditional Weaver-Dunn reconstruction with some type of CC fixation (for example, suture cerclage or suture anchors) results in greater stability and strength than the Weaver-Dunn procedure alone.[36] Additionally, the use of a free tendon graft for an anatomic reconstruction of the conoid and trapezoid ligaments has been shown to result in significantly less anterior and posterior translation than the modified Weaver-Dunn procedure.[37] Biomechanical testing has demonstrated that a semitendinosus ligament autograft placed in the direction and orientation of the trapezoid and conoid ligaments has minimal elongation after cyclical loading, yet the stiffness and ultimate load (560 N compared with 406 N) remains greater in the native CC ligaments.[38] In addition to reconstructing the CC ligaments, it has been demonstrated that the anatomic reconstruction of the AC ligaments with a flexor carpi radialis tendon graft re-creates the tensile strength of the native AC joint complex and is superior to a modified Weaver-Dunn repair.[39]

Clinical outcomes after late reconstruction of the AC joint have traditionally been mixed. Most previous studies have been on patients using older techniques such as the Weaver-Dunn repair. More recent studies have demonstrated more positive results. In one recent study, a modified Weaver-Dunn procedure with Mersilene tape augmentation was done in a series of 15 patients at an average of 21 months after injury. Satisfactory results were obtained in all patients, and no correlation was found between the delay in surgery or functional outcome.[40] Semitendinosus allograft was used with Mersilene tape around the coracoid and through the clavicle with positive results after delayed reconstruction.[41] Revision surgery using an autogenous semitendinosus anatomic construct after a failed Weaver-Dunn procedure yielded positive results in 12 patients.[42] Instead of the traditional Weaver-Dunn transfer of the coracoacromial ligament, the biomechanical and clinical data support the use of graft around the coracoid and through the clavicle or an augmented (suture, tape, graft) Weaver-Dunn reconstruction for late AC joint reconstruction.

Postoperative Rehabilitation

After acute repair or chronic reconstruction, the shoulder is placed in a sling to allow the tissues to heal. Gentle, passive range-of-motion activities in the supine position can begin after 1 to 3 weeks. Unsupported arm range of motion at the shoulder should be delayed for approximately 6 weeks to allow for biologic healing.[22] The sling can be discontinued after 6 to 8 weeks. Strengthening can begin with isometrics in the sling after the fourth week and then later once the sling is discontinued, with emphasis on strengthening the scapula stabilizers. Progression to full strengthening can begin at approximately 12 weeks following the procedure. The patient can return to play 4 to 6 months after surgery.

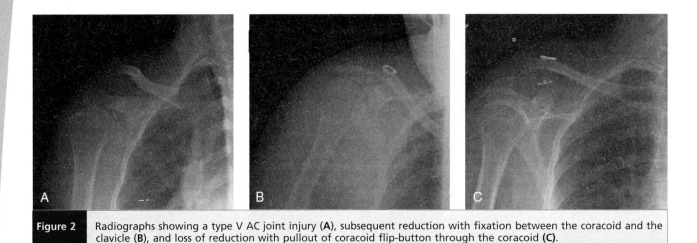

Figure 2 Radiographs showing a type V AC joint injury (**A**), subsequent reduction with fixation between the coracoid and the clavicle (**B**), and loss of reduction with pullout of coracoid flip-button through the coracoid (**C**).

Complications

Complications can occur with nonsurgical as well as surgical treatment of an AC joint injury. Skin breakdown can occur from a harness-type device, as mentioned earlier, or with tenting of the skin from a significant type IV or V injury. Late osteolysis at the distal clavicle or degenerative changes at the AC joint can occur later with nonsurgical treatment of type I and II injuries.[43]

Complications with potentially more significance can occur after surgical treatment. Postoperatively, the incidence of loss of reduction reportedly has been as high as 44%.[44] This complication has occurred after all types of initially successful reduction (**Figure 2**). Loss of reduction can occur as a result of loss of fixation, a fracture in the coracoid or clavicle, biologic failure as the graft construct gradually stretches, and failure of the hardware device. Erosions through the clavicle and fractures through the coracoid have been reported with nonabsorbable tape or suture used as augmentation for stabilization of the repair or reconstruction.[44] Issues related to bone quality and increased patient activity during early postoperative recovery are some of the causes of failure. Another complication is the migration of pins and wires used to transfix across the AC joint in acute injuries. Migration of broken pins into the lung, spinal canal, and blood vessels (including the aorta) has been reported.[43] Infection is the other complication reported by many authors using absorbable or nonabsorbable suture or tape in ligament reconstruction. Ossification of the CC or AC ligaments has been reported with both surgical and nonsurgical management of the AC injury. Degenerative changes have been reported after AC joint stabilization when the distal clavicle has not been resected as part of the index procedure.[43]

Proximal Humeral Fractures

Most proximal humeral fractures occur in elderly patients with thin, brittle, osteoporotic bone. Therefore, much of the recent research involving techniques and implant choice has been aimed at the treatment of displaced fractures in this difficult population. Proximal humeral fractures in younger, athletic patients are always the result of high-energy trauma. Given the excellent quality of cortical and cancellous bone in these patients, treatment of these fractures is often much lower risk and more straightforward. The mechanism of injury for the younger population is typically a direct blow or fall (**Figure 3**). However, indirect forces are often a factor, in particular for greater tuberosity fractures in which a strong contraction of the rotator cuff can avulse the tuberosity. This is often evidenced by the very medial position of the tuberosity in these injuries (**Figure 4**). Clear delineation of the fracture pattern is best accomplished with the radiographic trauma series, consisting of AP, lateral Y, and axillary views of the scapula. Recent reports have shown that the best profile of the greater tuberosity can be obtained with an AP view in 20° of external rotation.[45] This view, along with an AP 15° caudad projection, allows the most accurate view of the level of displacement of the greater tuberosity to assist with surgical decision making.

Stable, nondisplaced fractures are treated nonsurgically with a sling, and passive range of motion is resumed when the proximal and distal humerus "move as a unit." Recent studies show that delaying rehabilitation for more than 3 weeks will produce a slower recovery, which can continue for up to 2 years after the time of injury.[46] If radiographs are unchanged, gentle assistive exercises are begun at 3 weeks. At 6 weeks, the sling is discarded, and there is a rapid progression to active range of motion, terminal stretches, and light resistive exercises.

Displaced surgical neck fractures require realignment for optimal function. A closed reduction can often be attempted and can usually be performed if there is an unimpacted fracture without any bone contact. If the fracture is reducible and stable, initial treatment as outlined for minimally displaced fractures is continued for 4 weeks rather than 7 to 10 days. If the fracture is reducible but unstable, fixation is necessary. Percutaneous osteosynthesis is an excellent option in these cases

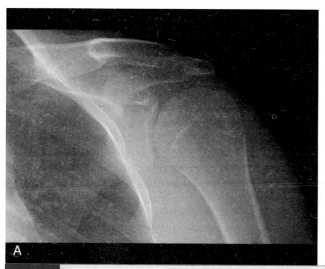

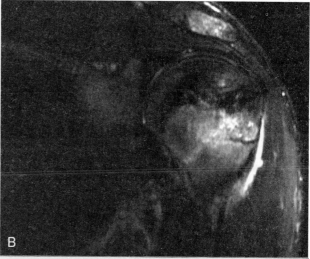

Figure 3 **A,** AP radiograph of the shoulder of a 16-year-old boy after a direct fall onto the lateral aspect of his left upper arm while snowboarding. The fracture line is very subtle and difficult to see. **B,** Coronal view on MRI scan clearly shows the fracture line and surrounding bone edema from this direct blow.

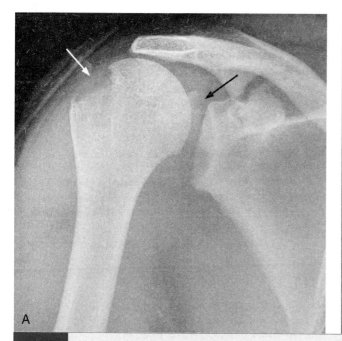

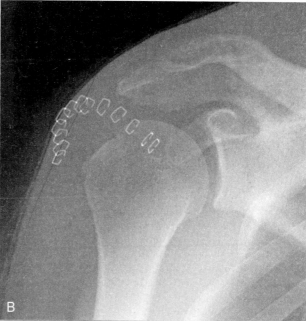

Figure 4 **A,** Radiograph of the shoulder of a 27-year-old involved in a high-speed motocross racing crash. The light arrow points to the bony bed of the greater tuberosity, and the dark arrow points to the greater tuberosity fragment that has avulsed into the joint. **B,** The fragment was very comminuted; thus anatomic fixation was obtained through an open superior approach with transosseous tunnels.

because it minimizes additional soft-tissue damage and reduces the risk of osteonecrosis of the humeral head. In older patients with osteoporotic bone, pin perforation of the head, pin migration, and stability of fixation are major concerns. However, minimally invasive techniques in the younger population with strong cortical bone may be ideal. It has been shown that the clinical result depends on the quality of the reduction obtained.[47] An incomplete reduction may yield satisfac-

tory results in elderly patients; however, an anatomic result is indicated in the younger, athletic population.

In the three-part displaced proximal humeral fracture, where reduction of tuberosity displacement can be more difficult, an anatomic result is important in the young athletic population. Great controversy exists in the management of these fractures in elderly patients; most issues pertain to failure of fixation in osteoporotic bone. Because these issues do not exist for the athletic, young population, anatomic reduction is the goal, without violation of the rotator cuff. Transosseous suture fixation with tension band constructs is an option, but it is more often reserved for osteoporotic bone.[48,49] Plate fixation as the treatment method of choice is appropriate in this population, contingent on the medial hinge being intact. If there is medial comminution, locking plate fixation may be more appropriate. Reconstitution of the inferomedial support is paramount in avoiding failure of fixation, whatever the patient's age.[50] Varus malreduction correlates significantly with failure of fixation, again, regardless of age.[50] When reduction is difficult or impossible, soft-tissue interposition must be assessed. An open approach usually is necessary. Most often the long head of the biceps is interposed at the junction of the humeral shaft and head. Distally, the biceps can be located just medial to the pectoralis major insertion on the humeral shaft. By following the biceps tendon proximally in the bicipital groove, the area of interposition can be located and the biceps freed. Comminuted cortical fragments also can block an anatomic reduction, but this can often be anticipated from the preoperative radiographs.

The incidence of isolated greater tuberosity fractures has been reported to be approximately 14% to 21%; they are reported to be associated with approximately 10% to 30% of shoulder dislocations. With an anterior dislocation, the fracture typically reduces with reduction of the glenohumeral joint. Good to excellent results with nonsurgical treatment of isolated greater tuberosity fractures with less than 5 mm of displacement have been reported. Thus, fixation is currently advocated for fractures with more than 5 mm of displacement.[48] However, in manual laborers and athletes, surgery is often recommended for displacement as little as 3 mm. When shoulder pain persists after fracture healing and adequate rehabilitation, associated injuries may be responsible. Particularly in patients with a nondisplaced greater tuberosity fracture, concomitant soft-tissue injuries, including an associated partial/full rotator cuff tear or SLAP lesion/labral pathology, do occur. Although these associated injuries have been reported most often as case reports, they should be included in the differential diagnosis when symptoms persist.

When the greater tuberosity is displaced and in need of fixation, several options exist. Arthroscopically assisted fixation is gaining popularity, and several recent reports advocate an all-arthroscopic repair using a double row technique.[51,52] However, these techniques may be more appropriate for the minimally displaced fracture. In patients with severe medial displacement of the greater tuberosity, as is often seen in with high-energy injuries, traditional approaches may be better suited. Comminuted fractures are well served by fixation with transosseous sutures performed through a superior deltoid splitting approach.[49,53] A solid tuberosity fragment can be well fixed with open or percutaneous screws, depending on the degree of fracture displacement.

Scapular Fractures

The incidence of scapular fractures is low, accounting for only 3% to 5% of fractures to the shoulder girdle. Most of these fractures are extra-articular and are the result of high-energy trauma. Because of the high-energy mechanism of injury, 90% of patients have associated injuries, including ipsilateral rib fractures, clavicular fractures, shoulder dislocations, pulmonary injuries, and brachial plexus injuries.

Most scapular fractures can be evaluated with plain radiographs, obtaining the standard shoulder trauma series, and a CT scan. According to a recent prospective study, axial and three-dimensional tomographic studies were the most useful modalities in assessing fractures in all anatomic regions of the scapula[54] (**Figure 5**). Most of these injuries can be appropriately managed nonsurgically with immobilization and early range of motion to tolerance. Injuries requiring surgical intervention often include displaced acromion fractures, displaced coracoid fractures associated with disruption of the CC ligaments, displaced glenoid neck fractures with either 1 cm of medial translation or 40% angulation, and, in particular, the intra-articular glenoid fracture.

Recently, a systematic review of 520 scapula fractures from a 22 case series was performed.[55] All studies were Level IV evidence studies with no control subjects, making drawing conclusions difficult. However, 99% of all scapular body fractures were treated nonsurgically, with 86% good to excellent results; 107 patients had fractures involving the glenoid, and 80% of these were treated surgically. Good to excellent results were reported in 82% of the patients. The most common scenario in the athlete is the displaced fracture of the anteroinferior glenoid rim subsequent to an anterior shoulder dislocation. Substantial articular step-off greater than 5 mm or a depression-impaction type fracture can lead to a nonconcentric glenohumeral joint reduction, recurrent instability, and the potential for long-term arthrosis. This type of fracture requires fixation. Traditionally, this is performed via an open anterior approach, and fixation is obtained with cannulated screws (**Figure 6**). However, recent reports have shown good outcomes with arthroscopic fixation in cases in which the glenoid fragment was a substantial size, about one fifth of the glenoid length.

Clavicular Fractures

Clavicular fractures account for 2.6% to 5% of all fractures. Many are caused by direct trauma, as is often seen in the athletic injuries obtained during contact sports. Although many of these fractures are caused by high-energy injuries, they are rarely open. However, careful evaluation will help avoid missing associated trauma, such as acromioclavicular/sternoclavicular fracture-dislocations, ipsilateral scapular and rib fractures, a pneumothorax, and neurovascular injury. Standard ra-

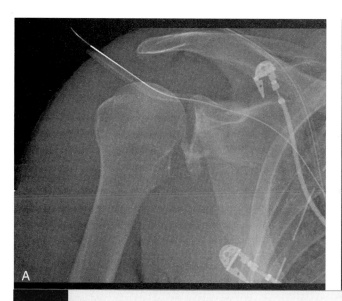
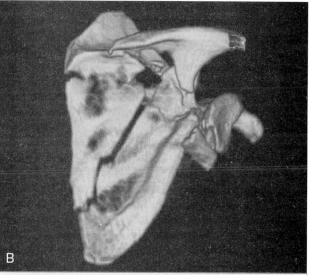

Figure 5 **A,** AP radiograph of a scapular fracture in a 32-year-old man involved in an all-terrain vehicle rollover. The fracture pattern is difficult to understand. **B,** CT scan with three-dimensional reconstructions was performed, allowing rotation of the reconstructed views in all planes. A more thorough understanding of the anatomy was obtained from this view.

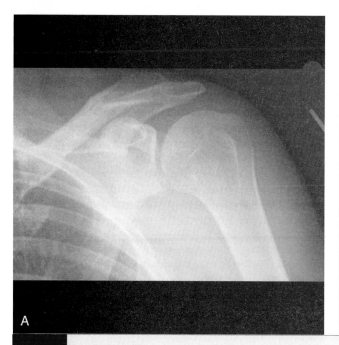
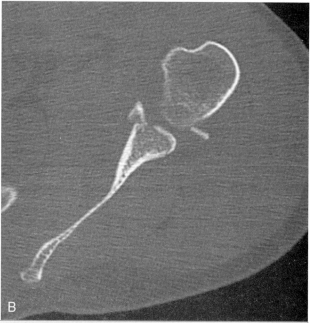

Figure 6 **A,** AP radiograph of the shoulder of a 20-year-old man who dislocated his shoulder during a football game. A bony Bankart lesion is seen, but it is difficult to assess the full extent of the size of the fragment. **B,** Axial cuts on the CT scan show the fragment is at least 30% of the anteroinferior glenoid.

diographs should include an AP view and a 45° cephalic tilt view because the degree of displacement is often difficult to assess on a single radiograph. A CT scan may be of value in assessing intra-articular fractures/dislocations of the medial clavicle.

Medial fractures are uncommon and typically do not require any surgical intervention. The medial growth plate accounts for up to 80% of longitudinal growth and is the last physis to close, generally at age 22 to 25 years. Thus, for most skeletally immature athletes, medial injuries are fractures through the growth plate near the sternoclavicular joint, rather than sternoclavicular dislocations, and inherently have great healing potential. Surgery is primarily indicated for those posteriorly displaced fractures that compromise the airway or underlying neurovascular structures.

Middle third fractures are the most common and account for 69% to 82% of all clavicular fractures. Most of these fractures can be treated successfully with nonsurgical management (which includes rest, ice, and pain medication as needed), a sling, and return to play when there is radiographic and clinical evidence of healing. However, when midshaft fractures are shortened, comminuted, or completely displaced, as is often seen in high-energy athletic injuries, the risk of nonunion, deformity, and poor outcome may be higher than once believed. Early studies classically have used surgeon-based or radiographic outcome measures that equate union with a successful outcome. However, recent studies using patient-based outcome measures have raised the question of whether these high-energy, displaced fractures should be reduced and internally fixed or not. According to results from a recent prospective, randomized clinical trial of 100 patients, 100% displacement without bony contact, especially with a transversely displaced fragment, is a risk factor strongly predictive of long-term sequelae.[56]

According to another recent study, final clavicular shortening of more than 18 mm in male patients and 14 mm in female patients was significantly associated with an unsatisfactory result.[57] Functional outcomes following displaced midshaft clavicular fractures were assessed in yet another recent study, and it was concluded that fractures with more than 2 cm of shortening tended to be associated with decreased abduction strength, greater patient dissatisfaction, and substantial residual disability.[58]

The Canadian Orthopaedic Trauma Society published a multicenter, prospective, randomized clinical trial of 132 patients with midshaft clavicular fractures.[59] Those patients with 100% displacement and no cortical contact between the proximal and distal fragments were included. Plate fixation and nonsurgical treatment were compared, and it was concluded that surgical treatment resulted in improved functional outcomes and a lower rate of nonunion and malunion at 1-year follow-up. The patients in the surgical group were more likely than those in the nonsurgical group to be satisfied with their shoulder, in general. In addition, early surgical intervention in the athlete may allow an earlier return to play because the average time to union was significantly shorter in the surgical group. If surgical stabilization is deemed appropriate, it can be obtained with either traditional plate and screw constructs or intramedullary devices. Recent innovations in the design of the intramedullary devices have led to a resurgence of interest in this fixation technique because there are many potential benefits, such as less soft-tissue stripping, better cosmesis, and easier hardware removal. However, prospective, randomized studies are needed to determine the optimal fixation technique.

A recently published systematic review of the literature of 2,144 acute midshaft clavicle fractures found an overall nonunion rate of 5.9%.[60] However, the nonunion rate for displaced fractures was 15.1%. Fracture comminution, female gender, and advancing age also were associated with nonunion. The nonunion rates in surgically treated displaced fractures were much lower: 2.2% for surgically plated fractures and 2.0% for fractures treated with intramedullary fixation. However, the authors warn that the results should be interpreted with caution because most of the studies were retrospective, had no control group, and did not use any randomization if there was a control group.[60]

Fractures of the distal part of the clavicle are classified on the basis of the integrity of the CC ligaments. Type I fractures occur lateral to the CC ligaments; the medial clavicle is stable, and these have a successful union rate. Type III fractures have intra-articular extension into the AC joint, potentially predisposing to later posttraumatic AC arthritis. However, the fracture pattern is stable and is accompanied by a high union rate. Type IV fractures are physeal injuries in which the distal end of the clavicle is essentially ruptured superiorly out of the thick periosteal sleeve. The AC and CC ligaments are usually intact and these fractures are stable and respond well to nonsurgical treatment. Return to sports participation for patients with these stable fracture patterns is typically allowed when there is clinical and radiographic evidence of healing and the patient is asymptomatic. However, contact sports are often avoided for at least 2 to 3 months after injury.

In type II distal clavicle fractures, the fracture occurs near the CC ligaments. In type IIA fractures, both CC ligaments are attached to the lateral fragment; in type IIB, the trapezoid is attached to the lateral fragment, but the conoid is torn. Both scenarios render the CC ligaments incompetent and unable to maintain the CC interval, which leads to instability of the medial fragment. The distal clavicular fragment with the attached scapula (through the AC/CC ligaments) will droop inferiorly and medially under the weight of the attached upper extremity as the medial clavicle elevates away from the distal fragment. This instability leads to a higher rate of symptomatic nonunion in active patients. Although nonunion may be well tolerated in the elderly population, it is less likely to be tolerated in the younger, athletic population.[61] Therefore, immediate surgical options are typically considered in this demographic for this fracture pattern. Because this fracture pattern is by nature complex and unstable, the optimal surgical technique has yet to be determined. All current fixation options are fraught with their own set of pitfalls and difficulties. Much attention has recently been paid to using the clavicular hook plate. Although results with various case series have been good, this technique requires plate removal, and more prospective, controlled clinical trials are necessary. Other options include distal clavicular plates, suture fixation with or without tension band fixation, Bosworth screws, and Knowles pins.

Summary

Shoulder instability continues to be a common athletic injury. Young age and increased activity levels continue to be risk factors for recurrent instability. An arthroscopic approach to surgical management of instability continues to gain popularity.

Injuries to the AC joint are one of the most common shoulder injuries in the contact athlete. Treatment of type II AC separations remains chiefly nonsurgical, with the throwing athlete a possible exception. Newer techniques are available for repair and reconstruction of the AC joint. Biomechanically, a ligament reconstruction consisting of a ligament re-creating the CC ligaments is favorable over other techniques, including the traditional Weaver-Dunn procedure.

Most fractures of the shoulder girdle in the young athletic population are the result of high-energy trauma. Appropriate studies allow a clear understanding of the fracture pattern, which is necessary for surgical decision making. Displaced, unstable, and intra-articular fractures require an anatomic reconstruction to provide the athlete with the best chance for return to full function. Fixation techniques vary based on the fracture pattern. However, the strong cortical bone of younger patients allows more fixation options than for elderly, osteoporotic patients with similar fractures.

Annotated References

1. Bui-Mansfield LT, Banks KP, Taylor DC: Humeral avulsion of the glenohumeral ligament: The HAGL lesion. *Am J Sports Med* 2007;35:1960-1966.

   The HAGL lesion was evaluated during a systematic review, which demonstrated that the West Point nomenclature is practical, easy to understand, and assists in communication about these lesions.

2. Fitch RW, Kuhn KE: Intraarticular lidocaine versus intravenous procedural sedation with narcotics and benzodiazepines for reduction of the dislocated shoulder: A systematic review. *Acad Emerg Med* 2008;15:703-708.

   The authors present a systematic review of six Level I randomized trials and demonstrate that the use of intraarticular lidocaine led to fewer complications and decreased emergency department time. This method should be considered as the first option for reducing shoulder dislocations.

3. Robinson CM, Howes J, Murdoch H, Will E, Graham C: Functional outcome and risk of recurrent instability after primary traumatic anterior shoulder dislocation in young patients. *J Bone Joint Surg* 2006;88:2326-2336.

   A prospective cohort study evaluating 252 patients age 15 to 35 years was performed to evaluate risk factors of recurrent instability. At two years, 55.7% had sustained recurrent dislocation. Risk factors included younger males. Level of evidence: I.

4. Sachs RA, Lin D, Stone ML, Paxton E, Kuney M: Can the need for future surgery for acute traumatic anterior shoulder dislocation be predicted? *J Bone Joint Surg* 2007;89:1665-1674.

   One hundred thirty-one patients were followed following traumatic anterior shoulder instability. Forty-three patients had at least one recurrent dislocation episode; 88 (67%) never had further instability. Twenty patients underwent Bankart reconstruction. Risk factors for future instability included younger age and participation in contact or collision sports. Level of evidence: I.

5. Hovelius L, Olofsson A, Sandstrom B, et al: Nonoperative treatment of primary anterior shoulder dislocation in patients forty years of age and younger: A prospective twenty-five-year follow-up. *J Bone Joint Surg* 2008; 90:945-952.

   At 25-year follow-up, the authors evaluated 257 patients who had received nonsurgical treatment for anterior shoulder dislocation when they were 12 to 40 years of age. Half of the patients treated nonsurgically achieved shoulder stability and did not have recurrent instability.

6. Itoi E, Hatakeyama Y, Kido T, et al: A new method of immobilization after traumatic anterior dislocation of the shoulder: A preliminary study. *J Shoulder Elbow Surg* 2003;12:413-415.

   Forty patients were randomly assigned to either immobilization in internal versus external rotation for 3 weeks. Recurrence rates at 1 year or 30% for the internal rotation group versus 0% for the external rotation group.

7. Miller BS, Sonnabend DH, Hatrick C, et al: Should acute anterior dislocations of the shoulder be immobilized in external rotation? A cadaveric study. *J Shoulder Elbow Surg* 2004;13:589-592.

   A cadaveric study evaluating contact force between the anterior labrum and glenoid rim in external rotation demonstrated a rise in contact force from 0 g at neutral rotation to 83.5 g at 45° external rotation.

8. Buss DD, Lynch GP, Meyer CP, Huber SM, Freehill MQ: Nonoperative management for in-season athletes with anterior shoulder instability. *Am J Sports Med* 2004;32:1430-1433.

   Thirty athletes with in-season anterior shoulder instability were treated with physical therapy and functional bracing if indicated. Of these athletes, 87% were able to return to their sports participation but averaged 1.4 recurrent instability episodes per season. Fifty-three percent pursued surgical stabilization in the ensuing off-season.

9. Bottoni CR, Wilckens JH, DeBerardino TM, et al: A prospective, randomized evaluation of arthroscopic stabilization versus nonoperative treatment in patients with acute, traumatic, first-time shoulder dislocations. *Am J Sports Med* 2002;30:576-580.

10. Bottoni CR, Smith EL, Berkowitz MJ, Towle RB, Moore JH: Arthroscopic versus open shoulder stabilization for recurrent anterior instability: A prospective

randomized clinical trial. *Am J Sports Med* 2006;34: 1730-1737.·

A randomized trial comparing open versus arthroscopic stabilization was performed with 61 patients, of whom 60 were males. Twenty-nine underwent open stabilization with two subsequent clinical failures. Thirty-two underwent arthroscopic stabilization with one clinical failure at a minimum of 2-year follow-up (range, 24 to 48 months). Level of evidence: I.

11. Kim SH, Ha KI, Cho YB, Ryu BD, Oh I: Arthroscopic anterior stabilization of the shoulder: Two to six-year follow-up. *J Bone Joint Surg Am* 2003;85:1511-1518.

One hundred sixty-seven patients underwent arthroscopic stabilization for recurrent traumatic anterior shoulder instability in this therapeutic study. Postoperatively, 4% sustained recurrent instability at a mean of 44 months follow-up (range, 2 to 6 years). Level of evidence: IV.

12. Pagnani MJ, Dome DC: Surgical treatment of traumatic anterior shoulder instability in American football players. *J Bone Joint Surg Am* 2002;84:711-715.

13. Bradley JP, Baker CL III, Kline AJ, Armfield DR, Chhabra A: Arthroscopic capsulolabral reconstruction for posterior instability of the shoulder: A prospective study of 100 shoulders. *Am J Sports Med* 2006;34: 1061-1071.

A prospective cohort of 100 shoulders in 91 athletes were treated with arthroscopic posterior stabilization and evaluated at a mean follow-up of 27 months. There was significant improvement in stability, pain, and function, with no difference between contact and non-contact athletes. Only eight shoulders (8%) required revision surgery, and 89% returned to sports participation, with 67% at the same level. Level of evidence: II.

14. Escobedo EM, Richardson ML, Schulz YB, Hunter JC, Green JR III, Messick KJ: Increased risk of posterior glenoid labrum tears in football players. *AJR Am J Roentgenol* 2007;188:193-197.

A retrospective review of 166 shoulder arthrograms in 157 patients revealed posterior labral tears in 11 of 20 football players (55%) compared to 10 of 137 other patients (7%). Based on the commons odd ratio, football players were 15.0 times more likely to have a posterior labral tear than nonfootball players.

15. Wolf BR, Strickland S, Williams RJ, Allen AA, Altchek DW, Warren RF: Open posterior stabilization for recurrent posterior glenohumeral instability. *J Shoulder Elbow Surg* 2005;14:157-164.

The results of open posterior stabilization of 44 shoulders in 41 patients were reviewed at 1.8 to 22.5 years after surgery. Only eight shoulders (19%) had recurrent instability, and 84% of the patients were satisfied with their shoulders. Worse patient satisfaction and outcomes were seen in patients with a chondral defect at the time of surgery and in patients older than age 37 years at the time of surgery.

16. Williams RJ III, Strickland S, Cohen M, Altchek DW, Warren RF: Arthroscopic repair for traumatic posterior shoulder instability. *Am J Sports Med* 2003;31:203-209.

A retrospective review of 27 shoulders in 26 patients treated with bioabsorbable tack fixation is presented. At a mean follow-up of 5.1 years, no patients had loss of motion or instability greater than 1+ in the anterior, posterior, or inferior directions, and only two patients (8%) required additional surgery.

17. Kim SH, Ha KI, Park JH, et al: Arthroscopic posterior labral repair and capsular shift for traumatic unidirectional recurrent posterior subluxation of the shoulder. *J Bone Joint Surg Am* 2003;85:1479-1487.

In this therapeutic study, 27 patients with unidirectional posterior instability treated with arthroscopic labral repair and capsular shift were evaluated at a mean follow-up of 39 months. All patients had improved shoulder function and scores, and only one patient had recurrent subluxation and could not return to sports participation. Level of evidence: IV.

18. Provencher MT, Bell SJ, Menzel KA, Mologne TS: Arthroscopic treatment of posterior shoulder instability: Results in 33 patients. *Am J Sports Med* 2005;33:1463-1471.

Thirty-three patients with unidirectional posterior instability treated with arthroscopic labral repair and capsular shift were evaluated at a mean follow-up of 39 months. Failures were due to recurrent instability in four patients (12%) and pain in three patients (9%). Worse outcomes were associated with voluntary instability and prior shoulder surgery. Level of evidence: IV.

19. Servien E, Walch G, Cortes ZE, Edwards TB, O'Connor DP: Posterior bone block procedure for posterior shoulder instability. *Knee Surg Sports Traumatol Arthrosc* 2007;15:1130-1136.

In a retrospective review, 21 shoulders treated with posterior bone block for posterior shoulder instability were evaluated at an average follow-up of 6 years. All patients reported their outcomes as good or excellent, even though three patients were considered clinical failures (one recurrent posterior dislocation and two with substantial posterior apprehension on follow-up examination).

20. Rios CG, Arciero RA, Mazzocca AD: Anatomy of the clavicle and coracoid process for reconstruction of the coracoclavicular ligaments. *Am J Sports Med* 2007;35: 811-817.

The anatomy of the CC ligaments and relationship on the clavicle was studied in 120 cadaveric clavicles. Findings included absolute differences in the origin of the CC ligaments existing between men and women, but with a constant ratio of these origins to total clavicle length.

21. Mazzocca AD, Spang JT, Rodriguez RR, et al: Biomechanical and radiographic analysis of partial coracoclavicular ligament injuries. *Am J Sports Med* 2008;36: 1397-1402.

Sectioning of the AC ligaments in 40 cadaveric shoulders in conjunction with partial disruption of the CC ligament complex led to significant changes in both radiographic and mechanical measures of AC stability. The conoid was found to fail first.

22. Mazzocca AD, Arciero RA, Bicos J: Evaluation and treatment of acromioclavicular joint injuries. *Am J Sports Med* 2007;35:316-329.

    The principles of the evaluation and treatment of AC injuries, including a discussion of pertinent anatomy as well as outlined summaries of biomechanical and clinical evidence for various types of research, are reviewed.

23. Tischer T, Salzmann GM, El-Azab H, Vogt S, Imhoff AB: Incidence of associated injuries with acute acromioclavicular joint dislocations types III through V. *Am J Sports Med* 2009;37:136-139.

    Concomitant injuries to the shoulder occurring during traumatic AC joint separation include a 14% occurrence of a SLAP lesion. Higher grades of AC injury correlate with a higher incidence of SLAP lesions.

24. Mikek M: Long-term shoulder function after type I and II acromioclavicular joint disruption. *Am J Sports Med* 2008;36:2147-2150.

    Twenty-three patients who were treated for type I or II AC joint disruption were evaluated at a mean of 10.2 years after injury. Impairment in long-term shoulder function was evident in approximately 50% of the patients. Level of evidence: IV.

25. Spencer EE Jr: Treatment of grade III acromioclavicular joint injuries: A systematic review. *Clin Orthop Relat Res* 2007;455:38-44.

    In this systematic review, the authors determine if grade III AC joint separations are best treated with or without surgery. Based on limited evidence (mainly Level IV), nonsurgical treatment was deemed more appropriate than traditional surgical treatment.

26. Phillips AM, Smart C, Groom AF: Acromioclavicular dislocation: Conservative or surgical therapy. *Clin Orthop Relat Res* 1998;353:10-17.

27. Schlegel TF, Burks RT, Marcus RL, Dunn HK: A prospective evaluation of untreated acute grade III acromioclavicular separations. *Am J Sports Med* 2001;29:699-703.

28. Nissen CW, Chatterjee A: Type III acromioclavicular separation: Results of a recent survey on its management. *Am J Orthop* 2007;36:89-93.

    In a survey of American Orthopaedic Society for Sports Medicine members and orthopaedic program residency directors, most respondents (86% and 81%, respectively) favored nonsurgical treatment of type III AC injuries.

29. McConnell AJ, Yoo DJ, Zdero R, Schemitsch EH, McKee MD: Methods of operative fixation of the acromioclavicular joint: A biomechanical comparison. *J Orthop Trauma* 2007;21:248-253.

    Three different methods of fixation were compared for AC fixation: the CC Bosworth screw, a CC sling of Mer-

silene 5-mm tape, and a hook plate. Hook plate fixation was mechanically the most similar to the native AC joint.

30. Wellmann M, Zantrop T, Weimann A, Raschele M, Petersen W: Biomechanical evaluation of minimally invasive repairs for complete acromioclavicular joint dislocation. *Am J Sports Med* 2007;35:955-961.

    The authors of this study evaluated four different minimally invasive techniques for CC joint repair. The flip button and polydioxanone repairs were more successful than the suture anchor repair.

31. Walz L, Salzmann GM, Fabbro T, Eichhorn S, Imhoff AB: The anatomic reconstruction of acromioclavicular joint dislocations using 2 TightRope devices: A biomechanical study. *Am J Sports Med* 2008;36:2398-2406.

    Reconstruction of the conoid and trapezoid ligaments with two TightRope devices (Arthrex; Naples, Florida) was evaluated. Results were equal or even better than native ligaments in resisting forces.

32. Dimakopoulos P, Panagopoulos A, Syggelos SA, Panagiotopoulos E, Lambiris E: Double-loop suture repair for acute acromioclavicular joint disruption. *Am J Sports Med* 2006;34:1112-1119.

    Favorable results were evident in this case series of 34 patients who underwent underwent surgical reconstruction of acute AC injury with the CC loop stabilization technique using two pairs of Ethibond No. 5 nonabsorbable sutures—one passed in front and the other behind the clavicle—through a central drill hole. Level of evidence: IV.

33. Greiner S, Braunsdorf J, Perka C, Herrmann S, Scheffler S: Mid to long-term results of open acromioclavicular-joint reconstruction using polydioxansulfate cerclage augmentation. SpringerLink Web site. http://www.springerlink.com/contents/0120W908116n7413/ Accessed January 5, 2009.

    This case series of 50 patients with follow-up of a mean of 70 months demonstrated the treatment of AC joint dislocation using polydioxane sulfate cerclage augmentation led to good to excellent clinical results. However, follow-up revealed a high incidence of radiographic signs of osteoarthritis of the AC joint. Level of evidence: IV.

34. Gstettner C, Tauber M, Hitzl W, Resch H: Rockwood type III acromioclavicular dislocation: Surgical versus conservative treatment. *J Shoulder Elbow Surg* 2008;17:220-225.

    In this retrospective study of patients with type III AC injuries, better results were achieved by surgical treatment (24 patients) with the hook plate than by conservative treatment (17 patients). Level of evidence: IV.

35. Allman FL Jr: Fractures and ligamentous injuries of the clavicle and its articulation. *J Bone Joint Surg Am* 1967;49:774-784.

36. Deshmukh AV, Wilson DR, Zilberfarb JL, Perlmutter GS: Stability of acromioclavicular joint reconstruc-

1: Upper Extremity

tion: Biomechanical testing of various surgical techniques in a cadaveric model. *Am J Sports Med* 2004;32:1492-1498.

In this study of six AC joint fixations, Weaver-Dunn, suture cerclage, and four different suture anchors, it was demonstrated that augmentative CC fixation provided better stabilization of the AC joint and an increased load to failure than the Weaver-Dunn reconstruction alone.

37. Mazzocca AD, Santangelo SA, Johnson ST, Rios CG, Dumonski ML, Arciero RA: A biomechanical evaluation of an anatomical coracoclavicular ligament reconstruction. *Am J Sports Med* 2006;34:236-246.

In this cadaver study, the anatomic CC ligament reconstruction with ultrasound and nonabsorbable suture material had less anterior and posterior translation and more closely approximates the AC joint stability than a modified Weaver-Dunn procedure.

38. Costic RS, Labriola JE, Rodosky MW, Debski RE: Biomechanical rationale for development of anatomical reconstructions of coracoclavicular ligaments after complete acromioclavicular joint dislocations. *Am J Sports Med* 2004;32:1929-1936.

In nine cadavers, an anatomic reconstruction of the CC ligaments with a semitendinosus tendon demonstrated a strong yet significantly less stiffness and load to failure (23.4 ± 5.2 N/mm and 406 ± 60 N) than the intact CC ligament complex(60.8 ± 12.2 N/mm and 560 ± 206 N).

39. Grutter PW, Petersen SA: Anatomical acromioclavicular ligament reconstruction: A biomechanical comparison of reconstructive techniques of the acromioclavicular joint. *Am J Sports Med* 2005;33:1723-1728.

In six cadavers, anatomic AC reconstruction with a flexor carpi radialis tendon graft provided a load to failure (774 N) similar to that of the native AC joint complex (815 N) and was superior to a modified Weaver-Dunn repair (483 N) or reconstruction with a palmaris longus tendon graft (326 N).

40. Kumar S, Penematsa SR, Selvan T: Surgical reconstruction for chronic painful acromioclavicular joint dislocations. *Arch Orthop Trauma Surg* 2007;127:481-484.

Fifteen patients with type III AC injury were reconstructed 21 months after injury with a modified Weaver-Dunn procedure incorporating augmentation with Mersilene tape. All patients were satisfied in follow-up, and no correlation was seen between delay in surgery and outcome. Level of evidence: IV.

41. Nicholas SJ, Lee SJ, Mullaney MJ, Tyler TF, McHugh MP: Clinical outcomes of coracoclavicular ligament reconstructions using tendon grafts. *Am J Sports Med* 2007;35:1912-1917.

Nine patients underwent CC ligament reconstruction using augmented cadaveric semitendinosus tendon allografts after a grade V AC injury. At 1 year follow-up, all patients had excellent outcomes scores, full recovery of strength, minimal range-of-motion loss, and no clinical or radiographic loss of reduction of the AC joint. Level of evidence: IV.

42. Tauber M, Eppel M, Resch H: Acromioclavicular reconstruction using autogenous semitendinosus tendon graft: Results of revision surgery in chronic cases. *J Shoulder Elbow Surg* 2007;16:429-433.

A semitendinosus tendon autograft was used in an anatomic CC reconstruction and good to excellent results were achieved in 12 revision cases of failed modified Weaver-Dunn procedures. Level of evidence: IV.

43. Lemos MJ, Tolo ET: Complications of the treatment of the acromioclavicular and sternoclavicular joint injuries, including instability. *Clin Sports Med* 2003;22:371-385.

Complications occurring during surgical and nonsurgical treatment of AC joint injuries are reviewed.

44. Guttman DP, Paksima NE, Zuckerman JD: Complications of treatment of complete acromioclavicular joint dislocations, in Ireland ML (ed): *Instructional Course Lectures Sports Medicine*. Rosemont, IL, American Academy of Orthopaedic Surgeons, 2005 pp 107-113.

This chapter discusses the complications occurring in the treatment of AC joint injuries.

45. Parsons BO, Klepps SJ, Miller S, Bird J, Gladstone J, Flatow E: Reliability and reproducibility of radiographs of greater tuberosity displacement: A cadaveric study. *J Bone Joint Surg Am* 2005;87:58-65.

The authors present a cadaveric study in which the accuracy and reliability of determining displacement of the greater tuberosity is best determined with multiple views. In particular, the AP view in external rotation profiles the greater tuberosity to allow visualization of small amounts of displacement.

46. Hodgson SA, Mawson SJ, Saxton JM, Stanley D: Rehabilitation of two-part fractures of the neck of the humerus (two-year follow-up). *J Shoulder Elbow Surg* 2007;16:143-145.

The authors present a Level I evidence study supporting early range of motion of minimally displaced proximal humerus fractures. Delayed rehabilitation by 3 weeks or greater produced a slower recovery, which continued for at least 2 years after the time of injury.

47. Calvo E, Miguel I, Cruz JJ, Lopez-Martin N: Percutaneous fixation of displaced proximal humerus fractures: Indications based on the correlation between clinical and radiographic results. *J Shoulder Elbow Surg* 2007;16:774-781.

The authors report the results of closed reduction and percutaneous pinning of 74 patients with displaced proximal humerus fractures. They found the clinical results correlated with the quality of the reduction and recommend that percutaneous pinning be reserved for two-part fractures or three-part fractures in which an anatomic reduction is possible.

48. George MS: Fractures of the greater tuberosity of the humerus. *J Am Acad Orthop Surg* 2007;15:607-613.

This article presents an overview of the mechanism of injury, associated injuries, surgical indications, treatment options and outcomes in the management of greater tuberosity fractures.

49. Dimakopoulos P, Panagopoulos A, Kasimatis G: Transosseous suture fixation of proximal humerus fractures. *J Bone Joint Surg* 2007;89:1700-1709.

This article presents the results of the largest published series of select displaced fractures of the proximal humerus treated solely with nonabsorbable sutures. Level of evidence: IV (therapeutic).

50. Agudelo J, Schurmann M, Stahel P, et al: Analysis of efficacy and failure of proximal humerus fractures treated with locking plates. *J Orthop Trauma* 2007;21:676-681.

In this retrospective review, 153 patients with a displaced proximal humeral fracture were treated with a proximal humeral locking plate. When loss of fixation occurred, it was primarily in the presence of varus malreduction. A head-shaft angle of greater than 120° was recommended to maintain fixation and the reduction.

51. Cadet ER, Ahmad CS: Arthroscopic reduction and suture anchor fixation for a displaced greater tuberosity fracture: A case report. *J Shoulder Elbow Surg* 2007;16:e6-e9.

This case report describes indications and technique for an all-arthroscopic repair via suture anchors for a displaced greater tuberosity fracture.

52. Ji JH, Kim WY, Ra RH: Arthroscopic double-row suture anchor fixation of minimally displaced greater tuberosity fractures. *Arthroscopy* 2007;23:e1131-e1134.

This case report describes the surgical technique for an arthroscopic double-row suture anchor fixation technique for a minimally displaced, comminuted greater tuberosity fracture.

53. Flatow EL, Cuomo F, Maday MG, Miller SR, McIlveen SJ, Bigliani LU: Open reduction and internal fixation of two-part displaced fractures of the greater tuberosity of the proximal part of the humerus. *J Bone Joint Surg* 1991;73:1213-1218.

54. Tadros AM, Lunsjo K, Czechowski J, Corr P, Abu-Ziden FM: Usefulness of different imaging modalities in the assessment of scapular fractures caused by blunt trauma. *Acta Radiol* 2007;48:71-75.

Forty-four patients with scapular fractures were prospectively collected, and all studies were reviewed blindly and independently by two observers. The three-dimensional reconstructed CT scan was the most useful imaging modality to define the extent of the injury.

55. Zlowodzki M, Bhandari M, Zelle BA, Kregor PJ, Cole PA: Treatment of scapula fractures: Systematic review of 520 fractures in 22 case series. *J Orthop Trauma* 2006;20:230-233.

This article presents a systematic review of 22 retrospective case series involving scapula fractures. Surgical and nonsurgical outcomes were evaluated for all categories of scapula fractures.

56. Nowak J, Holgersson M, Larsson S: Can we predict long-term sequelae after fractures of the clavicle based on initial findings? A prospective study with nine to ten years of follow-up. *J Shoulder Elbow Surg* 2004;13:479-486.

Two hundred eight patients with clavicle fractures were enrolled prospectively in this Level II evidence study and were evaluated at 9- to 10-year follow-up. Forty-six percent continued to have sequelae. Displacement with no bony contact was the greatest predictor for sequelae.

57. Lazarides S, Zafiropoulos G: Conservative treatment of fractures at the middle third of the clavicle: The relevance of shortening and clinical outcome. *J Shoulder Elbow Surg* 2006;15:191-194.

In this retrospective study of 132 patients with united fractures of the midshaft clavicle that were treated conservatively, 34 patients (25.8%) were dissatisfied with their outcome. Final clavicular shortening of more than 18 mm in males and more than 14 mm in females was significantly associated with an unsatisfactory result.

58. McKee MD, Pedersen EM, Jones C, et al: Deficits following nonoperative treatment of displaced midshaft clavicular fractures. *J Bone Joint Surg Am* 2006;88:35-40.

Thirty patients underwent nonsurgical management of a midshaft clavicle fracture. Outcomes were measured with the Constant shoulder score, the Disabilities of the Arm, Shoulder and Hand Questionnaire, and objective shoulder muscle strength testing. Residual deficits in shoulder strength and endurance were detected, which may correlate to the significant level of dysfunction detected by the patient-based outcome measures.

59. Canadian Orthopaedic Trauma Society: Nonoperative treatment compared with plate fixation of displaced midshaft clavicular fractures: A multicenter, randomized clinical trial. *J Bone Joint Surg Am* 2007;89:1-10.

In this study of 132 displaced, midshaft clavicle fractures that were randomized to either surgical treatment with plate fixation or nonsurgical treatment in a sling, there was a significantly lower nonunion rate, an overall faster time to union, and a better functional outcome in the surgical group. Hardware removal was the most common reason for repeat intervention in the surgical group. Level of evidence: I.

60. Zlowodzki M, Zelle BA, Cole PA, Jeray K, McKee MD, Evidence-Based Orthopaedic Trauma Working Group: Treatment of acute midshaft clavicle fractures: Systematic review of 2144 fractures: On behalf of the Evidence-Based Orthopaedic Trauma Working Group. *J Orthop Trauma* 2005;19:504-507.

This article is a systematic review of 2,144 midshaft clavicle fractures from a total of 22 studies.

61. Robinson CM, Cairns DA: Primary nonoperative treatment of displaced lateral fractures of the clavicle. *J Bone Joint Surg Am* 2004;86:778-782.

The authors determine that nonsurgical treatment of most displaced lateral fractures of the clavicle leads to good results in middle-aged and elderly patients.

1: Upper Extremity

Chapter 2
Nonacute Shoulder Injuries

W. Ben Kibler, MD   Aaron Sciascia, MS, ATC, NASM-PES, NS   Brian R. Wolf, MD, MS
Bryan Warme, MD   John E. Kuhn, MD

Roles of the Scapula in Shoulder Function

The scapula is a key component of normal shoulder function. It is the "A" of the acromioclavicular (AC) joint, the "G" of glenohumeral function, and the "S" of scapulohumeral rhythm (SHR), which is the basis of normal shoulder kinematics. SHR, the coordinated movement of the scapula and humerus to achieve shoulder motion, is the key to efficient shoulder function. Scapular position and motion are closely integrated with arm motion to accomplish most shoulder functions. Scapular movement is a composite of three motions: upward/downward rotation around a horizontal axis perpendicular to the plane of the scapula, internal/external rotation around a vertical axis through the plane of the scapula, and anterior/ posterior tilt around a horizontal axis in the plane of the scapula[1] (**Figure 1**). The clavicle acts as a strut for the shoulder complex, connecting the scapula to the central portion of the body. This allows two translations to occur: upward/downward translation on the thoracic wall and retraction/protraction around the rounded thorax.

The scapula has several roles in normal shoulder function. Control of static position, motions, and translations allows the scapula to fulfill these roles. In addition to upward rotation, the scapula must also posteriorly tilt and externally rotate to clear the acromion from the moving arm in forward elevation or abduction. Also, the scapula must synchronously internally/ externally rotate and posteriorly tilt to maintain the glenoid as a congruent socket for the moving arm and maximize concavity compression and ball and socket kinematics. The scapula must be dynamically stabilized in a position of relative retraction during arm use to maximize activation of all the muscles that originate on the scapula. Finally, it is a link in the kinetic chain of integrated segment motions that starts from the ground and ends at the hand. Because of the minimal bony stabilization of the scapula, dynamic muscle function is the major method by which the scapula is stabilized and purposefully moved to accomplish its roles. Muscle activation is coordinated in task-specific force couple patterns to allow stabilization of position and control of dynamic coupled motion.

Roles of the Scapula in Muscle Function

Primary scapular stabilization and motion on the thorax involves coupling of the upper and lower fibers of the trapezius muscle with the serratus anterior and rhomboid muscles. Other muscles, such as the pectoralis minor, also play roles. Elevation of the scapula with arm elevation is accomplished through activation and coupling of the serratus anterior and lower trapezius with the upper trapezius and rhomboids[2,3] (**Figure 2**). During this motion, the lower trapezius helps maintain the instant center of rotation of the scapula through its attachment to the medial scapular spine. Its attachment to the scapular spine allows for a straight line of pull as the arm elevates and the scapula upwardly rotates, and creates a mechanical advantage to maintain this position. The lower trapezius often has been identified as an upward rotator of the scapula because it maintains its long moment arm during the full range of upward rotation.[3] However, it also has a role as a scapular stabilizer when the arm is lowered from an elevated position. During the descent or return from upward elevation, the well-positioned lower trapezius, when operating efficiently, helps maintain the scapula against the thorax.

The serratus anterior also has a role as a stabilizer of the scapula. This muscle has been historically identified as a protractor of the scapula because of high elec-

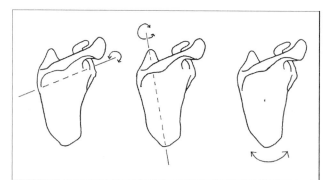

| Figure 1 | Depiction of three-dimensional scapular motions. **A,** Upward/downward rotation around a horizontal axis perpendicular to the plane of the scapula. **B,** Internal/external rotation around a vertical axis through the plane of the scapula. **C,** Anterior/posterior tilt around a horizontal axis in the plane of the scapula. |

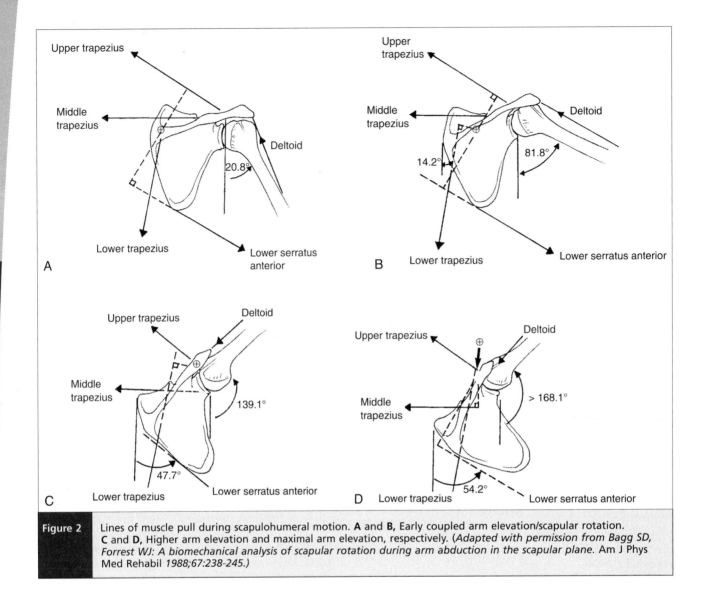

Figure 2 Lines of muscle pull during scapulohumeral motion. **A** and **B,** Early coupled arm elevation/scapular rotation. **C** and **D,** Higher arm elevation and maximal arm elevation, respectively. (*Adapted with permission from Bagg SD, Forrest WJ: A biomechanical analysis of scapular rotation during arm abduction in the scapular plane. Am J Phys Med Rehabil 1988;67:238-245.*)

tromyographic activity elicited during various push-up maneuvers.[4] Other evidence suggests that the serratus anterior helps upwardly rotate the scapula. The serratus anterior is actually multifaceted in that it contributes to all components of three-dimensional motion of the scapula during arm elevation. The serratus anterior helps produce scapular upward rotation, posterior tilt, and external rotation while stabilizing the medial border and the inferior angle, which prevents scapular winging. These actions of the serratus anterior are most likely the result of variable fiber orientation of the serratus anterior on the scapula and thorax. The highest level of serratus anterior activation occurs in the cocking phase of the throwing motion, and serratus anterior activation occurs in the earliest stages of arm elevation. It would appear that a prime role of the serratus anterior in these activities is as an external rotator/stabilizer of the scapula with arm motion.

The scapular position that allows optimal muscle activation of the shoulder joint muscles to occur is retraction and external rotation. Scapular retraction is an obligatory and integral part of normal SHR in coupled shoulder motions and functions. It results from synergistic muscle activations in patterns from the hip and trunk through the scapula to the arm, which then facilitates maximal muscle activation of the muscles attached to the scapula. The retracted scapula then can act as a stable base for the origin of all the rotator cuff muscles.

Because these roles are key components of normal shoulder function, alterations in these roles may play a part in shoulder dysfunction. Research has demonstrated alterations of scapular motion and position in association with a wide variety of shoulder injuries.[5-9]

Roles of the Scapula in Shoulder Pathology

Scapular dyskinesis can be defined as abnormal static scapular position or dynamic scapular motion characterized by medial border prominence or inferior angle prominence, early scapular elevation or shrugging on arm elevation, or rapid downward rotation during arm lowering. Scapular dyskinesis is a nonspecific response to a painful condition in the shoulder rather than a specific response to certain glenohumeral pathology. Scapular dyskinesis has multiple causative factors, both proximally (muscle weakness/imbalance, nerve injury) and distally (AC joint injury, superior labral tears, rotator cuff injury) based. This dyskinesis can alter the roles of the scapula in SHR. It can be caused by alterations in the bony stabilizers or alterations in activation patterns or strength in the dynamic muscle stabilizers.

AC Joint

The bony components of the shoulder must be intact for optimal function to occur. Arthrosis in the AC joint with instability or high-grade AC separations alter the strut function of the clavicle on the scapula and change the biomechanical screw axis of SHR, allowing excessive scapular protraction and decreased dynamic acromial elevation when the arm is elevated. This change in scapular position is known as the third translation of the scapula and allows the scapula to move in an inferior-medial manner, in relation to the clavicle. This scapular movement is most often seen when high-grade separations (type III-V AC injuries) occur. The protracted scapular position creates many of the dysfunctional conditions associated with chronic AC separations, including impingement and decreased demonstrated rotator cuff strength. One of the clinical examination findings that may help to determine surgical treatment of type III AC injuries is the presence of scapular dyskinesis, showing the third translation with arm elevation or forward flexion.

Clavicle Fractures

Fractures of the clavicle, with either nonunion or shortened, rotated malunion, also alter the strut function and result in poor functional patient outcomes. The functional deficiencies most often seen in association with low scores on the outcomes measures in malunion and/or nonunion of clavicle fractures are muscle weakness or loss of range of motion.[10] The altered strut function of the clavicle allows excessive protraction of the scapula, which has been shown to be a position that limits rotator cuff function and prevents full elevation of the humerus. Assessment of scapular position in patients with an acute or chronic fracture of the clavicle can help determine if surgery is indicated to realign the clavicular body and restore the ability of the clavicle to serve as a strut.

Impingement

Impingement is the most commonly diagnosed disorder around the shoulder. There are at least nine specific diagnoses that may be associated with impingement; each contains a component that may either affect the width of the subacromial space or be the driving factor of pain. Scapular dyskinesis is associated with impingement by altering scapular position at rest and in dy-

namic motion. Scapular dyskinesis in injured patients is characterized by a loss of acromial upward rotation, excessive scapular internal rotation, and excessive scapular anterior tilt. These positions create scapular protraction, which decreases the subacromial space and decreases demonstrated rotator cuff strength.

Activation sequencing patterns and the strength of the muscles that stabilize the scapula are altered in patients with impingement and scapular dyskinesis. Although each muscle attaching to the scapula makes a specific contribution to scapular function, the lower trapezius and serratus anterior appear to play the major role in stabilizing the scapula during arm movement. Weakness, fatigue, or injury in either of these muscles may cause a disruption of dynamic stability, which can lead to abnormal kinematics and cause symptoms of impingement. Injury to the spinal accessory nerve can alter function of the trapezius, and injury to the long thoracic nerve can alter muscle function of the serratus anterior muscle, which can cause abnormal stabilization and control. Scapular muscle inhibition or weakness has been seen in patients with impingement, with the lower trapezius and serratus anterior being most susceptible to the effect of inhibition and fatigue. Inhibition is seen as a decreased ability of the muscles to exert torque and stabilize the scapula as well as disorganization of normal muscle firing patterns. The exact nature of the inhibition is unclear. The nonspecific response and the altered motor patterns suggest a proprioceptively based mechanism.

Increased upper trapezius activity, imbalance of upper trapezius/lower trapezius activation, and decreased serratus anterior activity have been reported in patients with impingement. Increased upper trapezius activity is clinically observed as a shrug maneuver, resulting in a type III (upper medial border prominence) dyskinesis pattern. This causes impingement because of a lack of acromial elevation. Frequently, lower trapezius activation is inhibited or delayed. This results in a type III/ type II (entire medial border prominence) dyskinesis pattern, with impingement caused by a loss of acromial elevation and posterior tilt. Serratus anterior activation has been decreased in patients with impingement, creating a lack of external rotation.

The pectoralis minor has been frequently shortened in length in patients with impingement. This tight muscle creates a position of scapular protraction at rest and does not allow scapular posterior tilt or external rotation during arm motion, predisposing patients to impingement symptoms.

Rotator Cuff

There may be several reasons that muscles demonstrate weakness. Some factors, such as actual injury, disuse atrophy, and inhibition caused by pain, are intrinsic to the muscle and create an absolute weakness. Other factors, such as lack of a stable base of origin or decreased facilitation by proximal muscle activation patterns, are extrinsic to the muscle and create an apparent weak-

1: Upper Extremity

ness even though the muscle itself may be capable of developing strength.

Positions of scapular protraction have been shown to be limiting to maximal rotator cuff strength. One study showed that excessive scapular protraction, a posture that is frequently seen in injured patients as part of scapular dyskinesis, decreased maximum rotator cuff strength by 23%.[11] Maximal rotator cuff strength was achieved in association with a position of "neutral scapular protraction/retraction" and the positions of excessive protraction or retraction demonstrated decreased rotator cuff abduction strength.[12,13] According to a 2006 study, supraspinatus strength increased up to 24% in a position of scapular retraction in subjects with shoulder pain and 11% in subjects without shoulder pain.[14]

The clinically observable finding in scapular dyskinesis, prominence of the medial scapular border, is associated with the biomechanical position of scapular internal rotation and protraction. The protracted scapula is a less than optimal base for muscle strength. One-time evaluation or test-retest follow-up of rotator cuff strength should be performed with a stabilized scapula to measure true rotator cuff activation.

Multidirectional Instability

Scapular dyskinesis is often associated with an unstable glenohumeral joint. It is more often seen in microtraumatic types of instability, such as multidirectional instability (MDI), but can also be seen in recurrent types of instability with traumatic origins. The lax capsular tissue is only one component of the unstable shoulder. Altered biomechanics and muscle activations also increase the dysfunction. Studies have demonstrated that many patients with MDI have altered SHR, increased protraction of the scapula, and simultaneous humeral head migration away from the center of the joint.[7,15]

Muscle activation studies have shown that increased protraction is caused by a combination of increased pectoralis minor and latissimus dorsi activation and decreased lower trapezius and serratus anterior activation. Rotator cuff activation and biceps activation increases in an effort to compensate for the altered SHR that tends to allow the humeral head to migrate away from the joint center.

Correction of the altered scapular position by increasing scapular retraction and maximizing humeral head centering in the glenoid can be achieved in many instances with appropriate rehabilitation. This restoration of normal muscle activation patterns and strength is why rehabilitation is more frequently successful in MDI than in posttraumatic instability.

Labrum

Scapular dyskinesis is part of the pathologic cascade of labral injury.[8] Higher incidences of labral lesions in throwing athletes who had scapular dyskinesis were reported.[16] The altered scapular positioning and/or movement allow undue stress to occur to the anterior shoul-

der structures and increases the posterior peel-back of the biceps on the glenoid labrum.

Another component of the pathologic cascade is glenohumeral internal rotation deficit (GIRD), in comparison with the opposite shoulder and as an alteration in total rotation (internal plus external rotation) in comparison to the opposite shoulder. In addition to the known alteration of glenohumeral kinematics, GIRD affects normal SHR by creating a "wind-up" effect, where the glenoid and scapula are pulled in a forward inferior direction by the moving arm. This dyskinetic pattern can create an excessive amount of protraction of the scapula on the thorax as the arm continues into an adducted position in follow-through during throwing or into forward elevation in working. The ellipsoid shape of the thorax allows the scapula to move disproportionately anteriorly and inferiorly with more scapular protraction. These motions subsequently decrease the subacromial space during active motion, which allows impingement type symptoms to occur. With labral pathology, excessive scapular protraction creates glenoid antetilt, which increases the compression and shear forces on the posterior superior labrum.

Evaluation of the Scapula

The goals of the physical examination of the scapula are to establish the presence or absence of scapular dyskinesis, to evaluate proximal and distal causative factors, and to use dynamic maneuvers to assess the effect of correction of dyskinesis on impingement symptoms. The results of the physical examination will aid in establishing the complete diagnosis of all the elements of the dysfunction and will help guide treatment and rehabilitation.

The scapular examination should largely be accomplished from the posterior aspect. The scapula should be exposed for complete visualization. The patient should wear a gown or a tank top, or the shirt should be removed. The resting posture should be checked for side-to-side asymmetry but especially for evidence of inferior medial or medial border prominence. If there is difficulty with determining the positions, marking the superior and inferior medial borders may help ascertain the position.

Dynamic scapular motions may be evaluated by having the patient move the arms in ascent and descent three to five times. This will usually reveal any weakness in the muscles and display the dyskinetic patterns. If necessary, more repetitions, up to 10, or the addition of 3- to 5-lb weights will further highlight the muscle weakness. Alteration in medial scapular border motion in any plane, singly or in combination, is recorded as yes (present) or no (absent). This evaluation system allows a higher degree of reliability between the clinical examination and the biomechanical findings. Evaluation based solely on the single patterns was correlated with biomechanical findings (r = 0.49-0.54). The clinically observed yes/no evaluation correlates with biomechanically determined abnormalities in symptomatic patients (r = 0.64-

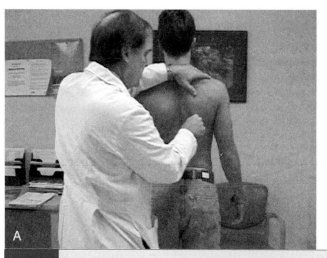
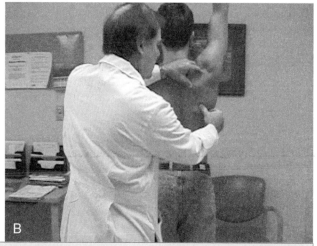

Figure 3 Scapular assistance test. **A,** Examiner's right hand position at the start of the test. **B,** Assisted scapular rotation with arm elevation. (*Reproduced with permission from Kibler WB, MCMullen J: Scapular dyskinesis and its relation to shoulder pain. J Am Acad Orthop Surg 2003;11:142-151.*)

0.84) and has a clinically useful predictive value.

The scapular assistance test (SAT) and the scapular retraction test (SRT) are corrective maneuvers that may alter the injury symptoms and provide information about the role of scapular dyskinesis in the total picture of dysfunction that accompanies shoulder injury and the restoration of function. The SAT helps evaluate scapular contributions to impingement and rotator cuff strength, and the SRT evaluates contributions to rotator cuff strength and labral symptoms. In the SAT, the examiner applies gentle pressure to assist scapular upward rotation and posterior tilt as the patient elevates the arm (**Figure 3**). A positive result occurs when the painful arc of impingement symptoms is relieved and the arc of motion is increased. In the SRT, the examiner grades supraspinatus muscle strength following standard manual muscle testing procedures or evaluates labral injury with the dynamic external rotation shear test. The clinician then places and stabilizes the scapula in a retracted position (**Figure 4**). A positive test occurs when the demonstrated supraspinatus strength is increased or the symptoms of internal impingement in the labral injury are relieved in the retracted position. Although these tests are not capable of diagnosing a specific form of shoulder pathology, a positive SAT or SRT shows that scapular dyskinesis is directly involved in producing the symptoms and indicates the need for including early scapular rehabilitation exercises to improve scapular control.

Coracoid-based inflexibility can be assessed by palpation of the pectoralis minor and the short head of the biceps brachii at their insertion on the coracoid tip. They will usually be tender to palpation, even if they are not symptomatic in use; can be traced to their insertions as taut bands; and will create symptoms of soreness and stiffness when the scapulae are manually maximally retracted and the arm is slightly abducted to approximately 40° to 50°. A rough measurement of

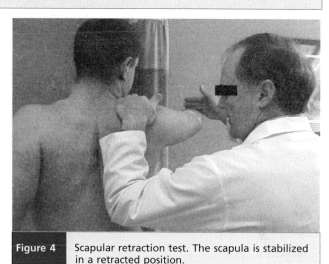

Figure 4 Scapular retraction test. The scapula is stabilized in a retracted position.

pectoralis minor tightness may be obtained when the patient stands against the wall and the distance from the wall to the anterior acromial tip is measured. This measurement can be done using a "double square" device (this instrument is the combination of two sliding squares, where two of the sliding components are connected to a single ruler). The clinician positions the patient standing with the back against a wall. The flat edge of one of the sliding components is placed flush to the wall and the other is positioned on the tip of the anterior acromion process (**Figure 5**). A bilateral measurement is taken (in inches or centimeters) to determine if there is a notable difference between the involved and noninvolved shoulders.

Treatment of Scapular Dyskinesis

Treatment of scapular dyskinesis must start with optimized anatomy. Local conditions such as nerve injury

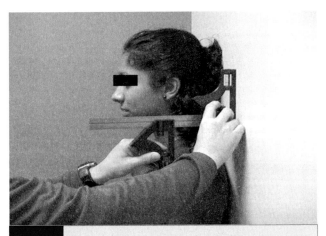

Figure 5   Double square method of measuring posture.

or scapular stabilizer muscle detachment must be treated with repair or muscle transfer. Bony or tissue derangement issues, such as AC joint or clavicle injury, labral injury, rotator cuff disease, or glenohumeral instability, must be stabilized. Rehabilitation can then proceed on the optimized anatomy.

Rehabilitation emphasis for scapular dyskinesis should start proximally and end distally. Proximal control of core stability leads to control of three-dimensional scapular motion. The goal of this phase is to achieve the position of optimal scapular function (posterior tilt, external rotation, and upward elevation). The serratus anterior is most important as an external rotator of the scapula, and the lower trapezius acts as a stabilizer of the acquired scapular position. Maximal rotator cuff strength is achieved from a stabilized, retracted scapula. Rotator cuff emphasis in rehabilitation should occur after scapular control is achieved and should emphasize closed chain, humeral head co-contractions. An increase in impingement pain when doing open chain rotator cuff exercises indicates the wrong emphasis at the wrong stage of the rehabilitation protocol.

The most common clinical findings in scapular dyskinesis are an inferior angle or medial border dyskinetic pattern with serratus anterior and lower trapezius weakness and alteration of activation sequencing and with increased upper trapezius activation. Several studies have evaluated optimal methods of activating those muscles.[17,18] For this clinical scenario, the isometric low row (**Figure 6**) and inferior glide (**Figure 7**) exercises should be done first, to activate the serratus anterior and lower trapezius in safe positions and minimize upper trapezius activation. Dynamic lawnmower (**Figure 8**) and robbery (**Figure 9**) exercises, which have been shown to activate the serratus anterior and lower trapezius but also the upper trapezius to a greater extent than isometric exercises, can be used later in the therapeutic progression, when clinically indicated to maximize early dynamic control of scapular motion. If there is minimal dyskinesis and low-grade anatomic injury around the glenohumeral joint, which is fre-

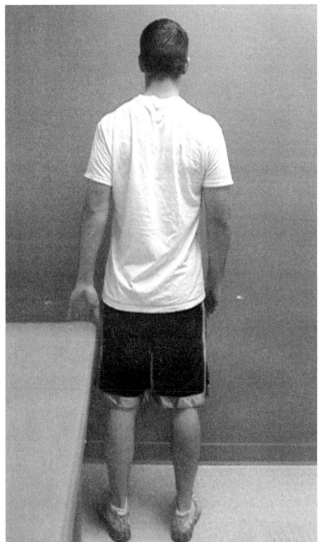

Figure 6   Low row exercise. This early phase isometric exercise is designed to strengthen the serratus anterior and lower trapezius muscles.

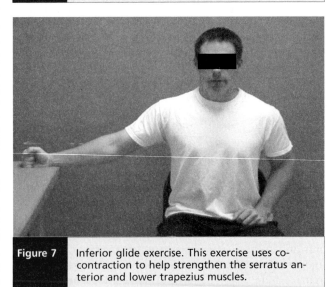

Figure 7   Inferior glide exercise. This exercise uses co-contraction to help strengthen the serratus anterior and lower trapezius muscles.

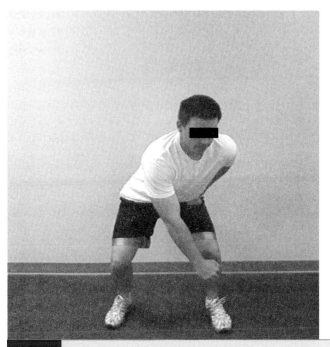
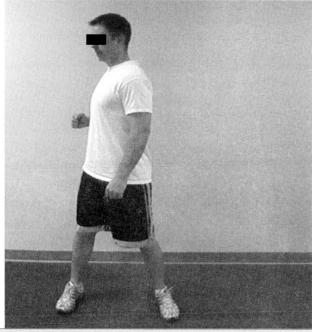

Figure 8 Lawnmower exercise. This dynamic maneuver strengthens the scapular stabilizers by using multiple kinetic chain segments.

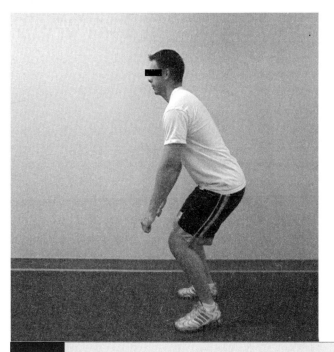
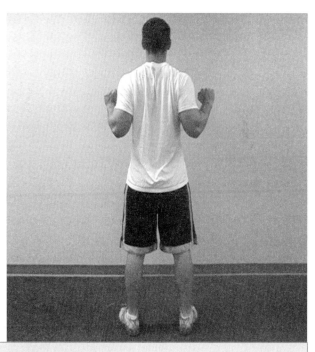

Figure 9 Robbery exercise. This midphase exercise helps initiate scapular retraction and depression.

quently seen in rotator cuff tendinopathy or impingement, and general scapular control is the goal, then all of the exercises may be introduced early in the rehabilitation protocol. If there is a need to protect the anatomy, such as after labral or rotator cuff repair, the dynamic exercises can be started later and progressed as healing allows. Similarly, all of the exercises may be implemented in a preoperative therapy protocol designed to correct deficits and prepare for postoperative rehabilitation, although clinical studies have shown that these patients tolerate the low row and lawnmower exercises better than others.[19]

Rotator Cuff Tears

Rotator cuff tears are common, potentially debilitating, and challenging to treat. Multiple studies have shown that chronic rotator cuff tears are common, and the incidence of new tears continues to rise with the aging population. Advanced imaging studies have shown a very low incidence of tears in asymptomatic individuals younger than 40 years. However, more than 50% of individuals older than 60 years have at least a partial-thickness rotator cuff tear; full-thickness tears are found in nearly half of individuals older than 80 years.[20] Procedures done to treat rotator cuff disease are already among the most common of all orthopaedic surgeries.

Impact on Society

Work-related injuries to the rotator cuff rank second in clinical frequency only to low back and neck pain. In addition to the economic cost to society from lost productivity, rotator cuff injuries ultimately preclude sports participation, professional work, and even requisite activities of daily living. Moreover, full-thickness rotator cuff tears not only can produce profound shoulder disability, but overall mental and physical health is also worse in affected patients, as determined by subjective outcome measures such as the Medical Outcomes Study 36-Item Short Form.[21]

Biomechanics

The rotator cuff muscles have roles in both mobility and stability of the glenohumeral joint. Of these two roles, stability likely is the more important function. At the midranges of motion, the lines of pull of the rotator cuff muscles are biomechanically optimized, and the rotator cuff contributes substantial stability to the glenohumeral joint. It is at these midranges of motion that the other contributors to stability are weakest. The contour of the joint itself provides little inherent stability at glenohumeral flexion angles of -30° to 30°, and other soft-tissue stabilizers, including the capsule and associated ligaments, are most relaxed in this range.[22] To maintain a ball-and-socket articulation during motion, the humeral head must be compressed into the glenoid socket by the rotator cuff. Without such compression, excessive translation of the humeral head would occur secondary to the action of the larger peripheral muscles acting on the shoulder. Synergistic coactivation of the surrounding, larger muscles with the rotator cuff also influence shoulder kinematics. Electromyographic studies show that firing of the rotator cuff muscles precedes and then is concurrent with that of other shoulder muscles, including the deltoid and pectoralis major.[23] This preceding and concurrent activation of the rotator cuff muscles likely prepares and then maintains the glenohumeral joint geometry for dynamic stability during larger muscle contractions.

How chronic tears can sometimes remain functionally asymptomatic and how rerupture after repair does not necessarily correlate with loss of function is unclear. A cadaver model was used to biomechanically examine muscle forces generated by the rotator cuff muscles during glenohumeral abduction in control specimens and in cadavers with cuff lesions of varying sizes in a recent study.[24] Results show that increasing the size of a cuff tear caused a proportionate increase in the forces generated by the remaining intact cuff. Once the remaining intact cuff cannot increase its output to account for forces lost by the torn muscles, the tear may then become functionally symptomatic. Additional recent biomechanical work suggests that partial tears involving at least 50% of the tendon thickness result in greater strain on the remaining rotator cuff.[25] Additional mechanisms for adapting to a torn cuff likely include coactivation of the larger muscles crossing the shoulder, including the deltoid. It is possible that firing patterns of such muscles are relearned through proprioceptive and neuromuscular mechanisms to maintain normal shoulder kinematics in the presence of rotator cuff tears.

Chronic Tear Characteristics
Etiology
Both extrinsic and intrinsic etiologies of rotator cuff pathology have been described. Extrinsic mechanisms are generally considered the result of impingement of the rotator cuff by the surrounding anatomic structures, most commonly the coracoacromial arch. For extrinsic mechanisms, the anatomic variation of the acromion has been extensively studied as a contributor to impingement. Three different acromion morphologies have been described: flat, curved, and hooked. The likelihood of a rotator cuff tear increases with a progressively more hooked acromion (Figure 10). Another acromion variation that is reported to influence the occurrence of rotator cuff lesions is the presence or absence of os acromiale. Os acromiale results from an unfused epiphysis of one or more of the acromial ossification centers (Figure 11). The presence of an os acromiale alone does not predispose to rotator cuff lesions. However, an os acromiale with step-off deformities was associated with a significant increase in the presence of rotator cuff disease.[26] Intrinsic mechanisms refer to qualities of the tendon itself that predispose to degeneration and tendinopathy, including the quality of tendon perfusion, the strength of muscle and collagen fibrils, and direct tendon fatigue from either overload or repetitive use. In studies of animal models, supraspinatus lesions can be caused by overuse with intrinsic etiologic factors, overuse with extrinsic etiologic factors, and with overuse alone but not secondary to extrinsic factors alone.[27]

Classification of Rotator Cuff Disease
Rotator cuff pathology can be classified by clinical examination, advanced imaging (MRI, ultrasound, CT arthrogram) and arthroscopy. Pain and disability of the rotator cuff, without a tear present, can result from external impingement of the rotator cuff and subacromial

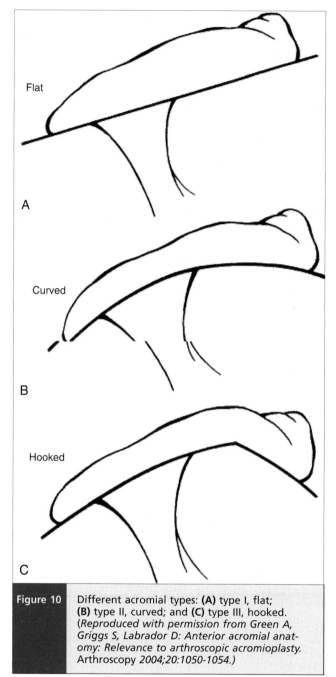

Figure 10 Different acromial types: **(A)** type I, flat; **(B)** type II, curved; and **(C)** type III, hooked. (*Reproduced with permission from Green A, Griggs S, Labrador D: Anterior acromial anatomy: Relevance to arthroscopic acromioplasty. Arthroscopy 2004;20:1050-1054.*)

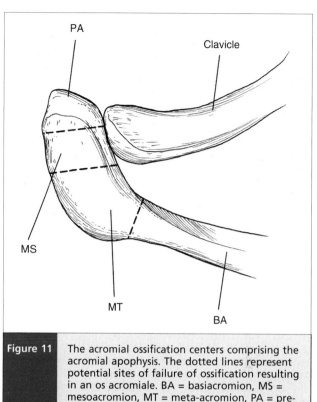

Figure 11 The acromial ossification centers comprising the acromial apophysis. The dotted lines represent potential sites of failure of ossification resulting in an os acromiale. BA = basiacromion, MS = mesoacromion, MT = meta-acromion, PA = pre-acromion. (*Reproduced from Kurtz CA, Humble BJ, Rodosky MW, and Sekiya JK: Symptomatic os acromiale. J Am Acad Orthop Surg 2006;14:12-19.*)

bursa by the acromion, coracoacromial ligament, or both. In addition, the subacromial bursa, the rotator cuff, or both can become thickened and inflamed, resulting in pain often referred to as subacromial bursitis, impingement, or rotator cuff tendinitis. A partial-thickness tear is classified in terms of location (articular, bursal, interstitial), grade (grade 1, less than 3 mm deep; grade 2, 3 to 6 mm deep; grade 3, greater than 6 mm deep), and tear area (in mm²). The insertional anatomy of the rotator cuff has been defined. The medial-to-lateral insertion widths of the supraspinatus, the infraspinatus, the teres minor, and the subscapularis are approximately 13 mm, 13 mm, 11 mm, and 18 mm, re-

spectively. This information is crucial in the classification and treatment of partial tears. Recent research shows there is good interobserver reliability among surgeons distinguishing partial-thickness tears from full-thickness tears and in identifying if the partial-thickness tear was articular or bursal sided using both arthroscopy and MRI.[28]

Full-thickness tears often are described in terms of shape and tear size in the anteroposterior and mediolateral dimensions. Full-thickness tears have been classified using multiple systems; however, intersurgeon agreement on classification was best when the tear was classified by the degree of retraction in the frontal plane[29] (**Figure 12**).

Natural History
The demographics of symptomatic and asymptomatic rotator cuff tears were recently studied in an attempt to better decipher their natural history and identify those factors that may influence the progression of lesions to become symptomatic.[30] The presence of a rotator cuff tear was highly correlated with age. Moreover, patients with symptomatic full-thickness tears in one shoulder had a 35.5% chance of full-thickness tears in the contralateral shoulder, suggesting a high prevalence of asymptomatic lesions. Furthermore, in patients with bilateral tears of which only one was symptomatic, the symptomatic shoulder's tear was on average 30%

1: Upper Extremity

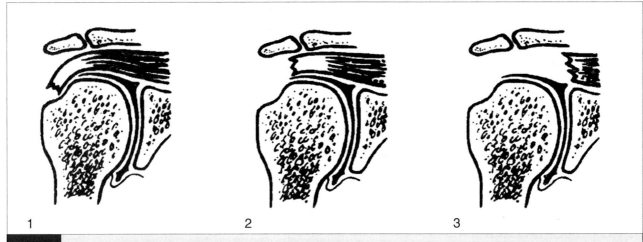

Figure 12 Patte's classification of full-thickness rotator cuff tears in the frontal plane: Stage 1, little retraction. Stage 2, tendon stump lies at the level of the humeral head. Stage 3, tendon stump at the level of the glenoid. (*Reproduced with permission from Patte D: Classification of rotator cuff lesions. Clin Orthop Relat Res 1990;254:81-86.*)

larger. A previous longitudinal study found that many patients had an increase in tear size over time.[31] It was concluded that tear size progression is likely a factor in the development of symptoms.

Long-term tears can be characterized by resultant rotator muscle atrophy[32] and fatty degeneration that may occur. It has been shown that fatty degeneration of one or more of the rotator muscles that accompanies massive tears can contribute to persistent shoulder disability following satisfactory repair.[33,34] Infraspinatus fatty infiltration has been correlated with both preoperative and postoperative function of the shoulder. Fatty degeneration of the infraspinatus actually impacts the response to repair of the supraspinatus muscle. Recent research found that successful repair did not lead to significant reversal of muscle degeneration.[35] These factors must be considered when contemplating surgical intervention and when counseling patients with rotator cuff tears.

Clinical Examination

A thorough physical examination significantly aids in the diagnosis and management of rotator cuff lesions. Specific physical examination techniques include the Neer impingement sign, the Hawkins-Kennedy impingement sign, the painful arc sign, the drop-arm sign, the supraspinatus muscle strength test, and the infraspinatus muscle strength test. The diagnostic accuracy of some of these examination techniques in identifying the extent of rotator cuff disease has been reported. The combination of a positive Hawkins-Kennedy impingement sign, the painful arc sign, and the infraspinatus muscle strength test best predicted the presence of impingement syndrome.[36] For full-thickness rotator cuff tears, the combination of a positive drop-arm sign, painful arc sign, and infraspinatus muscle strength test was most predictive.[36]

Treatment of Rotator Cuff Disease

Nonsurgical Treatment

Accurate diagnosis of any pathologic or biomechanical alterations in the shoulder is imperative if nonsurgical treatment is to be successful. Physical therapy and shoulder rehabilitation should focus on restoration of appropriate range of motion, flexibility, and strength.[37] This includes not only the shoulder but also the core musculature and the periscapular muscles. In the athlete with rotator cuff symptoms, throwing, stroke, or other overhead sport mechanics must be analyzed for conditions that may have contributed to shoulder disability. An appropriate rehabilitation program will ultimately lead to improved core stability, scapular stabilization, maximized rotator cuff function, and improved power. The pace at which these goals are achieved is often dependent on the patient's age, physical demands, and individual social situation. Nonsurgical treatment also may include pain medication and anti-inflammatory drugs and subacromial injections of local anesthetic, steroid, or both. Although injections are common, a recent systematic review suggests that long-term benefits are limited.[38] Multiple corticosteroid injections should be avoided in patients who may be best served with surgical intervention. Successful nonsurgical treatment of rotator cuff disease has been correlated with symptom duration of less than 3 months before treatment. However, factors found to predict the failure of nonsurgical treatment are a full-thickness tear greater than or equal to 1 cm^2, symptoms persisting more than 1 year, and functional impairment and weakness.[39] Nonsurgical treatment often is attempted for a minimum of 6 to 12 weeks before surgery is considered. Rehabilitation guidelines presented by the Reading Shoulder Unit have provided good results for patients with massive rotator cuff tears.[40] The Reading Protocol focuses on anterior deltoid reeducation to improve active shoulder motion and function.

Surgical Treatment

Surgical treatment for external impingement consists of a subacromial bursectomy. In the presence of physical impingement on the coracoacromial arch from hypertrophy of the coracoacromial ligament or spurring on the acromion, an acromioplasty can be performed to decompress the underlying rotator cuff and create a type I flat acromion. Care must be taken to avoid removing too much anterior acromion because deltoid compromise or detachment can occur.

Surgical intervention for partial-thickness rotator cuff tears continues to evolve, mainly because of advances with arthroscopic techniques. Partial articular-sided tears often have avulsed off the tuberosity adjacent to the articular margin and are best seen and evaluated surgically using arthroscopy of the glenohumeral joint. Similarly, the bursal aspect of the cuff can be inspected with arthroscopy in the subacromial space after removal of the bursa. The current consensus on treatment leads to débridement of partial tears that involve less than 50% of the tendon's thickness and repair of higher grade lesions.[41] During débridement, frayed and degenerative tissue is removed with an arthroscopic shaver to eliminate catching and mechanical symptoms. Repair of higher grade partial-thickness tears may involve completion of the tear followed by repair using either an arthroscopic or open approach. Alternatively, partial tendon repair can be performed, leaving the intact portion of the tendon in situ. For articular-sided tears, this involves transtendinous or other arthroscopic techniques to reattach the avulsed tendon to bone using suture anchors, suture passers, or spinal needles. Likewise, bursal-sided tears can be repaired using either open or arthroscopic techniques similar to those for full-thickness tears, repairing the lateral aspect of the tendon to the lateral tuberosity. Bursal-sided tears are more frequently associated with subacromial impingement. Repair usually is accompanied by subacromial decompression, including acromioplasty.

There are multiple factors to be considered when indicating patients for rotator cuff surgery for a full-thickness tear.[42,43] Repair is more readily advocated for acute tears and chronologically (younger than 50 years) and physiologically young and active patients. Significant weakness, functional impairment, and the failure of nonsurgical measures also are important factors. Successful repair of full-thickness tears requires recognition of the tear pattern, secure fixation to bone, and restoration of the anatomic cuff footprint. Complete tears usually fall into one of three configurations: crescent shaped, U-shaped, or L-shaped, although other variations exist. The tuberosity and the torn tendon edge should be débrided of fibrinous and degenerative tissue before repair. Subacromial and intra-articular adhesions that limit tendon mobility should be released to allow anatomic repair. Crescent-shaped tears usually involve less tendon retraction and have their largest dimension in the anteroposterior plane. These tears are usually relatively mobile and more easily reduced to the tuberosity. U-shaped tears have a large medial to lateral tear dimension. These tears are often best repaired by margin convergence tendon-to-tendon suturing that converts the U-shape tear to a crescent shape. This suturing also progressively lowers strain on the lateral margin of the torn tendon(s), which are then secured to the tuberosity using suture anchors or bone tunnels[44] (**Figure 13**).

When arthroscopic techniques are used, cyclic biomechanical testing has shown that knot security is enhanced by using braided sutures, alternating suture post limbs and past-point tensioning to minimize slack within the knot. Modern suture anchors now are available with up to three sutures each, allowing increased suture fixation on the rotator cuff tendon and decreased loading on individual sutures. Simple, mattress, and combination (Mason-Allen variants) sutures have been described and advocated in various studies. Suture anchors should be entered into the tuberosity at a 45° angle to maximize the anchor's resistance to pullout. Anchor and suture configurations used for repair continue to evolve. When a single row of suture anchors is used, the anchors should be placed approximately 5 mm from the articular surface. Double-row repairs use anchors placed just lateral to the articular margin, with these sutures being passed through the tendon 3 to 4 mm lateral to the musculotendinous junction. The second more lateral "row" of repair can use bone tunnels or a variety of different anchor types that repair the lateral edge of the tendon to the lateral aspect of the tuberosity. Various suture bridging and transosseous equivalent techniques can be used to not only repair the lateral edge but also compress the tendon footprint onto the prepared bony tuberosity when sutures from the medial row of anchors are tied and then tensioned across the tendon laterally to the second row of fixation[45] (**Figure 14**). Theoretically, this type of configuration enhances the healing potential of tendon to bone by increasing the tendon to bone contact area. Comparative studies to date have shown no significant difference in subjective outcomes, with only a small trend toward slightly improved cuff integrity and healing rates with double row techniques.[46,47] The role of acromioplasty in conjunction with rotator cuff repair continues to be a subject of debate. Recent studies have shown no significant differences with or without an acromioplasty in the absence of a large acromial spur or type III acromion.[48]

Patient subjective and functional outcomes after rotator cuff repair have been found to correlate strongly with the integrity of the repair on follow-up.[49] Tendon healing and functional outcome after surgery seems to correlate with initial tear size and the quality of the tissue as gauged by fatty infiltration and muscle atrophy.[50] Larger tear size and poorer quality tissue has correlated with increased re-tear and/or failure to heal rates and lower functional levels. Comparative studies have shown comparable outcomes using both open and arthroscopic techniques.[51]

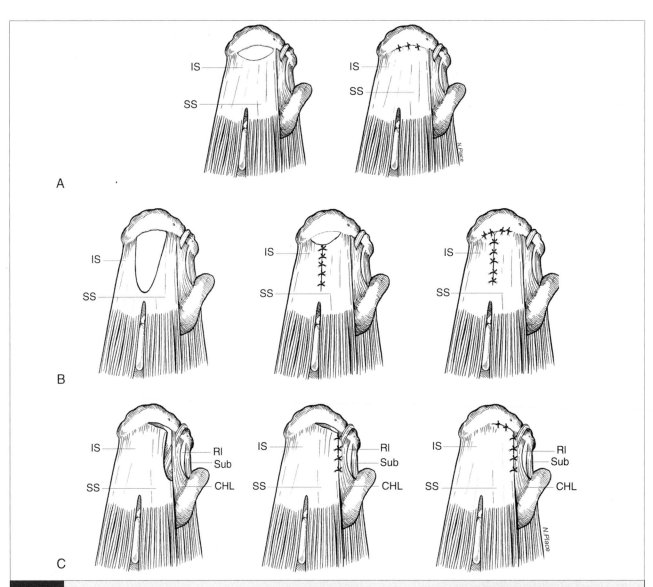

Figure 13 **A,** A crescent-shaped tear of the supraspinatus (SS) and infraspinatus (IS) tendons (left). Direct repair of the crescent-shaped tear to bone (right). (Reproduced from Burkhart SS, Lo IK:. Arthroscopic rotator cuff repair. *J Am Acad Orthop Surg* 2006;14:333-346.) **B,** A U-shaped tear of the supraspinatus and infraspinatus tendons (left). Repair is performed with side-to-side margin convergence suturing (center). The lateral edge of the tendon is sutured to bone (right). **C,** Appearance of an L-shaped tear of the supraspinatus and rotator interval (RI) (left). The longitudinal split is repaired first (center). the converged margin is repaired to bone (right). CHL = coracohumeral ligament, Sub = subscapularis.

The Disabled Throwing Shoulder

Pathomechanics

The understanding of the origin and treatment of shoulder disorders in the throwing athlete has evolved over the past few decades. In the 1950s, the thrower's shoulder involved reports of either anterior or posterior shoulder pain. In the 1970s, it was believed that throwers with shoulder pain had rotator cuff impingement, until studies of throwers who underwent a decompression yielded poorer than expected results. In the 1980s, it was suggested that throwers had "subtle instability,"

and the thrower had better success with an instability operation.[52,53] More recently, it has been recognized that shoulders in some throwers are too tight, particularly in the posterior capsule, which leads to a reduction in the total arc of glenohumeral rotation, or GIRD.[8,54,55] Additionally, the role of the scapula and dyskinesis has been recognized, often accompanied by weakness in the legs, hips, and core stability.

One way of synthesizing this collection of findings begins with weakness in core stability. At least 50% of the total force required to produce the velocity of the thrown ball is generated in the lower extremities.[56] If

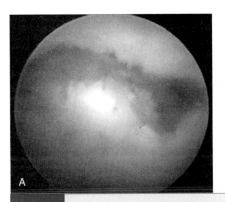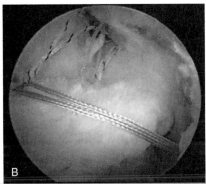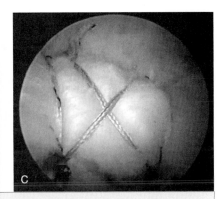

Figure 14 **A,** Arthroscopic view of a crescent shape rotator cuff tear. **B,** After placement of medial row of sutures through the rotator cuff. **C,** Completion of the transosseous equivalent repair by tensioning sutures over the lateral margin of the tear.

the lower extremities are weak, the mechanics of the pitch suffer, such that the pitcher's lead leg is directed away from home plate (which is an alteration of a critical node for pitching with proper mechanics).[57] With the lead leg drifting away from home plate, the torso "opens up" to catch up. The serratus anterior, which is an important structure in the late cocking and acceleration phases of throwing,[58] is affected as stretch on the long thoracic nerve and dysfunction of the serratus anterior are created, a common finding in dysfunctional throwers.[59]

When the serratus anterior is weak, the pectoralis minor, which has its origin and insertion very close to the serratus anterior, may be recruited to compensate. As a result, an insertional tendinopathy occurs on the medial border of the coracoid, and the muscle-tendon unit becomes tight. Serratus anterior (and lower trapezius) weakness and pectoralis minor tension moves the scapula to a position that can lead to glenohumeral joint pathology. This position of the scapula at rest is known as the SICK (Scapular malposition, Inferior medial scapular winging, Coracoid tenderness, and scapular dysKinesis) scapula, and as scapular dyskinesis when in motion.[19,55] The altered position is characterized by anterior tilt, lateral tilt, and internal rotation.

Internal rotation of the scapula then leads to stress on the anterior capsule of the shoulder in the cocking phase of throwing as the glenohumeral joint is forced into hyperextension. The anterior tilt of the scapula results in a relative overrotation of the humerus in external rotation during the cocking phase of throwing. The effect of both of these positions may lead to anterior capsule laxity,[1] increased contact of the greater tuberosity to the posterior labrum (internal impingement), and the production of superior labral tears and internal impingement by overrotation.[60-62]

The cocking phase of throwing has been described as a critical moment because of the large forces in the shoulder.[63] It is easy to see why alterations in scapular position could induce complications with mechanics and the development of pathology. Similarly, the decel-

eration phase of throwing also is associated with large forces and is a critical moment thought to be responsible for the development of pathology.[63] Again, alterations in scapular position and strength of the scapular stabilizers could lead to pathology.

During deceleration, the serratus anterior has a pivotal role in decelerating the upper extremity.[59] When this muscle is not functioning well, the scapula loosens its tether to the chest wall, which could place undue stress on the other decelerators of the humerus, particularly the supraspinatus and the infraspinatus muscles, which do show increased activity during acceleration and follow-through in throwers with shoulder pain.[59] This increased activity could causing microinjury to the external rotators of the rotator cuff and capsule. Muscle damage may produce viscosity changes, also known as thixotropy, which may be responsible for the posterior tightness seen in many throwers with pain. The association between posterior shoulder tightness in throwers and abnormal scapula position is well documented.[64]

The tight posterior shoulder is detected clinically by examining internal rotation of the abducted arm, although the tight posterior shoulder likely has kinematic effects throughout all positions of the arm during throwing. This pathologic tightness is believed to induce further rotator cuff pain and possibly contribute to superior labral tear formation[65] and internal impingement symptoms.[16]

Evaluation of the Dysfunctional Thrower

The evaluation begins with a patient history with regard to the amount of pitching because injuries, especially in adolescent throwers, are closely related to this factor.[66] The physical examination of shoulder range of motion should be done supine because of better reliability.[67] In habitual throwers, the humerus undergoes remodeling such that it is expected that the dominant arm will have approximately 15° more external rotation accompanied by a corresponding 15° loss of inter-

Table 1

MRI Findings in Asymptomatic Throwing Athletes

Author	Population	Supraspinatus Signal/Partial Tears	Full Tears	Labral Abnormal	Abnormal Fluid	Acromioclavicular Arthritis
Connor et al 2003[71]	N = 40 Throwing athletes (mean age, 26.5 years)	40% of dominant arms had partial- or full-thickness rotator cuff tears	7.5%	90%	NR	NR
Jost et al 2005[72]	N = 30 Throwing athletes	83%	0%	40%	NR	40%
Miniaci et al 2002[73]	N = 28 Professional pitchers (age 18 to 22 years, mean 20.1 years)	86%	0%	79%	79%	36%

NR = not reported

nal rotation than the contralateral arm. The arc of motion between the two sides should be the same. If there is a loss in the complete range affecting internal rotation, the examiner can surmise that there is tightness in the posterior structures. It is important to note that labral tears are very difficult to detect by physical examination,[68-70] and MRI may be required; however, clinicians should realize that asymptomatic throwers have a significant amount of MRI-documented shoulder pathology[71-73] (**Table 1**). This pathology may be adaptive and allow the thrower to perform.

Treatment

Little has been written about the nonsurgical treatment of the dysfunctional thrower's shoulder. The essence of nonsurgical treatment includes improving core stability, strengthening the serratus anterior and low trapezius, and stretching the pectoralis minor and tight posterior capsule. Several techniques to improve core stability and strengthen the serratus anterior and low trapezius have been suggested,[55] but to date no trials have been performed to identify the best method of accomplishing these goals.

Treating a tight posterior capsule can be done with effective stretching. The most effective method in a randomized controlled trial appeared to be the cross-body adduction stretch,[74] although the sleeper stretch also is recommended. In a recent case control study, pitchers who engage in regular posterior capsule stretching have better internal rotation and total arc of motion than those who do not.[75] The tight pectoralis minor tendon is best stretched using the unilateral self-stretch technique.[76]

When appropriate nonsurgical treatment fails, surgical treatment of pathology is often recommended; however, surgical treatment is not free of complications. The treatment of partial-thickness tears of the rotator cuff by arthroscopic débridement has limited success (< 65%) at returning athletes to their sport.[77-79] When done with additional procedures (treatment of labrum and biceps lesions), the success rate may reach 85%.[80] Repairing partial-thickness tears to bone has poor results, with only approximately 33% of throwing athletes able to return to their previous level of throwing.[81] Repairing delaminations of the rotator cuff without suture anchors to bone may be one option for treatment with early success of returning to play; however, the durability of this repair is unknown.[82]

Full-thickness tears of the rotator cuff can be repaired to bone with reasonable success in amateur athletes,[83] but dismal results are expected in professional pitchers, with a return rate of less than 10%.[84]

Repair of superior labral anterior and posterior (SLAP) lesions in throwers shows 75% return-to-play rates.[85] One recently published systematic review suggested the outcomes worsen with time; 69% of pitchers returned for some time, but only 28.6% were able to return for more than three seasons.[86]

There is debate regarding the role of the capsule and its treatment in the dysfunctional thrower's shoulder. There are no case series of posterior capsule releases for a tight posterior capsule in throwing athletes. The lack of studies may be related to the high effectiveness of a stretching program. There are data in the literature to support surgical treatment of a loose anterior capsule. In one study, 68% of dysfunctional throwers returned to their former level of throwing after an open anterior capsulolabral reconstruction.[53] The use of isolated thermal capsulorrhaphy was not as successful as open repair, with only 50% of throwing athletes returning to their former level of play.[87] This information contrasts that from a 2003 study in which the return to play rate after thermal capsulorrhaphy was 87%; however, 95% of the athletes in this study had concomitant procedures to treat additional pathology.[88] In a retrospective case control series, the return to play rate at 30 months follow-up was better if thermal capsulorrhaphy was performed (67% for those without thermal capsulorrhaphy compared with 90% for those with thermal capsulorrhaphy).[89] Although there are many confounders in these studies that limit comparison, it may be suggested that the treatment of laxity is possibly an important part of the management of the dysfunctional thrower's shoulder.

Prevention

Injured pitchers are likely to have pitched more months per year, more games per year, more innings per game, more pitches per game, more pitches per year, and more warm-up pitches before a game.[66] In youth pitchers, injury prevention begins with limiting play.

Summary

The scapula is the critical link within the kinetic chain, connecting the segments of the arm to the trunk. It is a proximal segmental link that allows normal arm function to occur by allowing the energy generated from the larger trunk muscles to be transferred to the shoulder, and it serves as the stable platform for the rotator cuff muscles. However, when these roles become altered, shoulder dysfunction may occur. Scapular dyskinesis has many causative factors, ranging from muscle imbalance and weakness of the scapular stabilizers and pelvis/core muscles to bony alterations, internal derangement (labral and rotator cuff pathology), and nerve injury.

Rotator cuff disease involves a spectrum of pathology. A careful clinical examination and advanced imaging are essential in diagnosis. Nonsurgical treatment should focus on restoration of biomechanical alterations in shoulder function. Surgical treatment continues to evolve with regard to rotator cuff impingement and partial- and full-thickness tears.

The understanding of the dysfunctional thrower's shoulder continues to evolve. Throwing is a skill that requires coordinated function of the kinetic chain with proximal to distal concentration of force and kinetic energy. It is now recognized that core stability is a critical component of the throwing motion and is often abnormal in the thrower with shoulder pain. The findings of scapular dyskinesis with the associated tight pectoralis minor and posterior capsule accompany the core stability deficit. These issues are the hallmark of nonsurgical treatment. Surgeons must be careful because the accumulation of rotator cuff, labral, and other abnormalities in throwers may not be pathologic. Furthermore, the results of surgery in this population are not great. Prevention is focused on limiting the number of pitches youth throwers perform, and guidelines are available from many sources. As more research is conducted, the knowledge of the approach and treatment of the dysfunctional thrower's shoulder will continue to evolve.

Annotated References

1. McClure PW, Michener LA, Sennett BJ, Karduna AR: Direct 3-dimensional measurement of scapular kinematics during dynamic movements in vivo. *J Shoulder Elbow Surg* 2001;10:269-277.

2. Bagg SD, Forrest WJ: Electromyographic study of the scapular rotators during arm abduction in the scapular plane. *Am J Phys Med* 1986;65:111-124.

3. Bagg SD, Forrest WJ: A biomechanical analysis of scapular rotation during arm abduction in the scapular plane. *Am J Phys Med Rehabil* 1988;67:238-245.

4. Decker MJ, Hintermeister RA, Faber KJ, Hawkins RJ: Serratus anterior muscle activity during selected rehabilitation exercises. *Am J Sports Med* 1999;27:784-791.

5. Lukasiewicz AC, McClure P, Michener L, Pratt N, Sennett B: Comparison of three dimensional scapular position and orientation between subjects with and without shoulder impingement. *J Orthop Sports Phys Ther* 1999;29:574-586.

6. Ludewig PM, Cook TM: Alterations in shoulder kinematics and associated muscle activity in people with symptoms of shoulder impingement. *Phys Ther* 2000; 80:276-291.

7. Ogston JB, Ludewig PM: Differences in 3-dimensional shoulder kinematics between persons with multidirectional instability and asymptomatic controls. *Am J Sports Med* 2007;35:1361-1370.

   This study evaluated trunk, scapular, and humeral kinematics at varying degrees of scaption and abduction in subjects with MDI and healthy controls. Significant abnormal kinematics were seen in the MDI subjects, demonstrating the need for addressing scapular motion and strength in rehabilitation protocols for patients with MDI. Level of evidence: I.

8. Burkhart SS, Morgan CD, Kibler WB: The disabled throwing shoulder: Spectrum of pathology. Part I: Pathoanatomy and biomechanics. *Arthroscopy* 2003; 19:404-420.

   This comprehensive review article discusses the different mechanisms that can cause pathology in the thrower's shoulder. It encompasses biomechanics and pathoanatomy that have been proven on a clinical basis. It presents the victim versus culprit approach to evaluating a painful throwing shoulder and disseminates the various causes of injury, which helps direct treatment toward the cause rather than the symptoms. Level of evidence: V.

9. Cools AM, Witvrouw EE, DeClercq GA, Danneels LA, Cambier DC: Scapular muscle recruitment pattern: Trapezius muscle latency with and without impingement symptoms. *Am J Sports Med* 2003;31:542-549.

   This study examined the muscle activation onsets in subjects with and without shoulder impingement. Those who had impingement experienced delayed activation of the middle and lower trapezius muscle. The results of this study indicate that overhead athletes with impingement symptoms show abnormal muscle recruitment timing in the trapezius muscle. Level of evidence: II.

10. McKee MD, Pedersen EM, Jones C, et al: Deficits following nonoperative treatment of displaced midshaft clavicular fractures. *J Bone Joint Surg Am* 2006;88: 35-40.

    This article used functional upper extremity outcome measures to demonstrate that shoulder dysfunction is related to the presence of malunion and/or nonunion in clavicle fractures. This shows that when the clavicle is compromised, the functional capability of the arm is negatively affected. Level of evidence: II.

11. Kebaetse M, McClure PW, Pratt NA: Thoracic position effect on shoulder range of motion, strength, and three-dimensional scapular kinematics. *Arch Phys Med Rehabil* 1999;80:945-950.

12. Smith J, Kotajarvi BR, Padgett DJ, Eischen JJ: Effect of scapular protraction and retraction on isometric shoulder elevation strength. *Arch Phys Med Rehabil* 2002;83: 367-370.

13. Smith J, Dietrich CT, Kotajarvi BR, Kaufman KR: The effect of scapular protraction on isometric shoulder rotation strength in normal subjects. *J Shoulder Elbow Surg* 2006;15:339-343.

    This study demonstrated that protracted and/or internally rotated positions of the scapula negatively affect the strength-generating capabilities of the arm. Level of evidence: I.

14. Kibler WB, Sciascia AD, Dome DC: Evaluation of apparent and absolute supraspinatus strength in patients with shoulder injury using the scapular retraction test. *Am J Sports Med* 2006;34:1643-1647.

    This study showed that demonstrated rotator cuff weakness is dependent on the position of the scapula during the testing procedure. Both injured and noninjured subjects elicited significant increases in active elevation strength with the scapula in a position of retraction in comparison to a position of resting posture. Level of evidence: I.

15. Illyés A, Kiss RM: Kinematic and muscle activity characteristics of multidirectional shoulder joint instability during elevation. *Knee Surg Sports Traumatol Arthrosc* 2006;14:673-685.

    This research study examined the kinematics and electromyographic activity of multiple shoulder muscles in MDI patients. The authors found that patients with MDI have increased durations of rotator cuff activation and decreased durations of larger global shoulder muscles throughout arm elevation. Level of evidence: I.

16. Myers JB, Laudner KG, Pasquale MR, Bradley JP, Lephart SM: Glenohumeral range of motion deficits and posterior shoulder tightness in throwers with pathologic internal impingement. *Am J Sports Med* 2006;34:385-391.

    This study measured humeral rotation and posterior shoulder tightness in baseball pitchers who had shoulder pain. The authors found that those with increased tightness and deficits in rotation had a higher correlation of experiencing shoulder pain. These findings could indicate that a tightening of the posterior structures of the shoulder may contribute to impingement. Level of evidence: III.

17. Kibler WB, Sciascia AD, Uhl TL, Tambay N, Cunningham T: Electromyographic analysis of specific exercises for scapular control in early phases of shoulder rehabilitation. *Am J Sports Med* 2008;36:1789-1798.

    This scientific article used a surface electromyogram (EMG) to analyze two isometric and two dynamic scapular strengthening exercises. No differences were found in EMG amplitude between injured and noninjured subjects. Muscle activity for the scapular muscles ranged between 15% to 30%, indicating that these exercises can be implemented in the early phases of shoulder rehabilitation. Level of evidence: I.

18. Cools AM, Declercq G, Cagnie B, Cambier D, Witvrouw E: Internal impingement in the tennis player: Rehabilitation guidelines. *Br J Sports Med* 2008;42: 165-171.

    This current concepts review discusses the importance of using the kinetic chain during shoulder rehabilitation in all phases of therapy. Useful guidelines are provided for treating overhead athletes with shoulder pain, with specific recommendations for strengthening and education on the serratus anterior and lower trapezius as retractors of the scapula. Level of evidence: V.

19. Kibler WB, McMullen J: Scapular dyskinesis and its relation to shoulder pain. *J Am Acad Orthop Surg* 2003; 11:142-151.

    This current concepts article discusses the normal biomechanics of the scapula and the definition and etiology of scapular dyskinesis and provides evaluation and treatment recommendations for scapular dysfunction. Level of evidence: V.

20. Reilly P, Macleod I, Macfarlane R, Windley J, Emery RJ: Dead men and radiologists don't lie: A review of cadaveric and radiological studies of rotator cuff tear prevalence. *Ann R Coll Surg Engl* 2006;88:116-121.

    This article reviews prior literature on the prevalence of rotator cuff tears reported in prior imaging or cadaveric studies.

21. McKee MD, Yoo DJ: The effect of surgery for rotator cuff disease on general health status: Results of a prospective trial. *J Bone Joint Surg Am* 2000;82:970-979.

22. Labriola JE, Lee TQ, Debski RE, McMahon PJ: Stability and instability of the glenohumeral joint: The role of shoulder muscles. *J Shoulder Elbow Surg* 2005;14: 32S-38S.

    The authors used computational and cadaveric models to examine the contributions of the shoulder muscles to glenohumeral stability at various joint positions.

23. David G, Magarey ME, Jones MA, Dvir Z, Turker KS, Sharpe M: EMG and strength correlates of selected shoulder muscles during rotations of the glenohumeral joint. *Clin Biomech (Bristol, Avon)* 2000;15:95-102.

24. Hansen ML, Otis JC, Johnson JS, Cordasco FA, Craig EV, Warren RF: Biomechanics of massive rotator cuff tears: Implications for treatment. *J Bone Joint Surg Am* 2008;90:316-325.

    The authors used cadaveric biomechanical testing to evaluate shoulder function in the presence of a massive rotator cuff tear.

25. Mazzocca AD, Rincon LM, O'Connor RW, et al: Intra-articular partial-thickness rotator cuff tears: Analysis of injured and repaired strain behavior. *Am J Sports Med* 2008;36:110-116.

    This biomechanical study demonstrated greater tendon strain with articular-sided, partial-thickness rotator cuff tears of increasing depth. Tendon repair restored near normal tendon strain.

26. Ouellette H, Thomas BJ, Kassarjian A, et al: Re-examining the association of os acromiale with supraspinatus and infraspinatus tears. *Skeletal Radiol* 2007;36:835-839.

    The authors retrospectively reviewed 42 shoulder MRIs of patients with an os acromiale and compared them to a case-matched set of MRIs. The presence of an os acromiale did not significantly predispose to a rotator cuff tear. However, an os acromiale with a step-off deformity is significantly more likely to be associated with a tear than an os acromiale without a step-off deformity.

27. Carpenter JE, Flanagan CL, Thomopoulos S, Yian EH, Soslowsky LJ: The effects of overuse combined with intrinsic or extrinsic alterations in an animal model of rotator cuff tendinosis. *Am J Sports Med* 1998;26:801-807.

28. Kuhn JE, Dunn WR, Ma B, et al: Interobserver agreement in the classification of rotator cuff tears. *Am J Sports Med* 2007;35:437-441.

    This study examined interobserver agreement among experienced shoulder surgeons when using currently described classifications systems for rotator cuff tears.

29. Patte D: Classification of rotator cuff lesions. *Clin Orthop Relat Res* 1990;254:81-86.

30. Yamaguchi K, Ditsios K, Middleton WD, Hildebolt CF, Galatz LM, Teefey SA: The demographic and morphological features of rotator cuff disease: A comparison of asymptomatic and symptomatic shoulders. *J Bone Joint Surg Am* 2006;88:1699-1704.

    The authors found that rotator cuff disease was highly correlated with age and demonstrated a high prevalence of bilateral rotator cuff tears in patients with unilateral symptoms.

31. Yamaguchi K, Tetro AM, Blam O, Evanoff BA, Teefey SA, Middleton WD: Natural history of asympto-matic rotator cuff tears: A longitudinal analysis of asymptomatic tears detected sonographically. *J Shoulder Elbow Surg* 2001;10:199-203.

32. Thomazeau H, Boukobza E, Morcet N, Chaperon J, Langlais F: Prediction of rotator cuff repair results by magnetic resonance imaging. *Clin Orthop Relat Res* 1997;344:275-283.

33. Goutallier D, Postel JM, Bernageau J, Lavau L, Voisin MC: Fatty muscle degeneration in cuff ruptures: Pre- and postoperative evaluation by CT scan. *Clin Orthop Relat Res* 1994;304:78-83.

34. Goutallier D, Postel JM, Gleyze P, Leguilloux P, Van Driessche S: Influence of cuff muscle fatty degeneration on anatomic and functional outcomes after simple suture of full-thickness tears. *J Shoulder Elbow Surg* 2003;12:550-554.

    The authors demonstrate the importance of fatty degeneration in relation to the outcome of rotator cuff repair in this large series of patients who underwent postoperative imaging.

35. Gladstone JN, Bishop JY, Lo IK, Flatow EL: Fatty infiltration and atrophy of the rotator cuff do not improve after rotator cuff repair and correlate with poor functional outcome. *Am J Sports Med* 2007;35:719-728.

    This study examined the impact of fatty infiltration and muscle atrophy on functional outcome after rotator cuff surgery. The authors also examined the reversibility of muscle atrophy and fatty infiltration after tendon repair. Level of evidence: II.

36. Park HB, Yokota A, Gill HS, El Rassi G, McFarland EG: Diagnostic accuracy of clinical tests for the different degrees of subacromial impingement syndrome. *J Bone Joint Surg Am* 2005;87:1446-1455.

    The authors examined the diagnostic accuracy of common shoulder examination tests for subacromial impingement and rotator cuff tears. Level of evidence: I.

37. Kibler WB, Chandler TJ, Pace BK: Principles of rehabilitation after chronic tendon injuries. *Clin Sports Med* 1992;11:661-671.

38. Koester MC, Dunn WR, Kuhn JE, Spindler KP: The efficacy of subacromial corticosteroid injection in the treatment of rotator cuff disease: A systematic review. *J Am Acad Orthop Surg* 2007;15:3-11.

    The authors performed a systematic review of literature to determine the efficacy of subacromial injection.

39. Bartolozzi A, Andreychik D, Ahmad S: Determinants of outcome in the treatment of rotator cuff disease. *Clin Orthop Relat Res* 1994;308:90-97.

40. Levy O, Mullett H, Roberts S, Copeland S: The role of anterior deltoid reeducation in patients with massive irreparable degenerative rotator cuff tear. *J Shoulder Elbow Surg* 2008;17:863-870.

    This prospective study of 17 patients with massive irreparable rotator cuff tears and pseudoparalysis showed significant improvement in subjective scores and active forward flexion after the institution of an anterior deltoid rehabilitation program.

41. Weber SC: Arthroscopic debridement and acromioplasty versus mini-open repair in the treatment of significant partial-thickness rotator cuff tears. *Arthroscopy* 1999;15:126-131.

42. Wolf BR, Dunn WR, Wright RW: Indications for repair of full-thickness rotator cuff tears. *Am J Sports Med* 2007;35:1007-1016.

   The authors review the evidence surrounding factors that influence consideration of rotator cuff repair surgery.

43. Oh LS, Wolf BR, Hall MP, Levy BA, Marx RG: Indications for rotator cuff repair: A systematic review. *Clin Orthop Relat Res* 2007;455:52-63.

   The authors performed a systematic review of the factors influencing the decision for rotator cuff repair surgery. Level of evidence: IV.

44. Burkhart SS: A stepwise approach to arthroscopic rotator cuff repair based on biomechanical principles. *Arthroscopy* 2000;16:82-90.

45. Park MC, Elattrache NS, Ahmad CS, Tibone JE: "Transosseous-equivalent" rotator cuff repair technique. *Arthroscopy* 2006;22:1360.

   The authors present an arthroscopic technique that uses two rows of rotator cuff fixation and compresses the torn tendon to the greater tuberosity.

46. Franceschi F, Ruzzini L, Longo UG, et al: Equivalent clinical results of arthroscopic single-row and double-row suture anchor repair for rotator cuff tears: A randomized controlled trial. *Am J Sports Med* 2007;35:1254-1260.

   The authors performed a randomized clinical trial comparing single row and double row arthroscopic rotator cuff repair. They found no statistical difference in cuff integrity using postoperative MRI or in subjective outcomes in this trial of 60 patients. Level of evidence: I.

47. Park MC, Idjadi JA, ElAttrache NS, Tibone JE, McGarry MH, Lee TQ: The effect of dynamic external rotation comparing 2 footprint-restoring rotator cuff repair techniques. *Am J Sports Med* 2008;36:893-900.

   A tendon suture-bridging rotator cuff repair showed higher yield loads compared with double-row repairs with lateral row knots in this cadaver model. This study also showed that dynamic external rotation testing of repair constructs can accentuate gap formation, especially in the anterior aspect of the rotator cuff.

48. Gartsman GM, O'Connor DP: Arthroscopic rotator cuff repair with and without arthroscopic subacromial decompression: A prospective, randomized study of one-year outcomes. *J Shoulder Elbow Surg* 2004;13:424-426.

This study found randomized patients to no acromioplasty versus acromioplasty in addition to arthroscopic rotator cuff repair. No significant differences in outcomes were found.

49. Knudsen HB, Gelineck J, Sojbjerg JO, Olsen BS, Johannsen HV, Sneppen O: Functional and magnetic resonance imaging evaluation after single-tendon rotator cuff reconstruction. *J Shoulder Elbow Surg* 1999;8:242-246.

50. Gerber C, Schneeberger AG, Hoppeler H, Meyer DC: Correlation of atrophy and fatty infiltration on strength and integrity of rotator cuff repairs: A study in thirteen patients. *J Shoulder Elbow Surg* 2007;16:691-696.

   This study examined the correlation of postoperative function with preoperative and postoperative fatty infiltration and muscle atrophy.

51. Liem D, Bartl C, Lichtenberg S, Magosch P, Habermeyer P: Clinical outcome and tendon integrity of arthroscopic versus mini-open supraspinatus tendon repair: A magnetic resonance imaging-controlled matched-pair analysis. *Arthroscopy* 2007;23:514-521.

   The authors compared outcomes for open and arthroscopic rotator cuff repairs in a matched fashion and found comparable outcomes. Level of evidence: III.

52. Jobe FW, Kvitne RS, Giangarra CE: Shoulder pain in the overhand or throwing athlete: The relationship of anterior instability and rotator cuff impingement. *Orthop Rev* 1989;18:963-975.

53. Jobe FW, Giangarra CE, Kvitne RS, Glousman RE: Anterior capsulolabral reconstruction of the shoulder in athletes in overhand sports. *Am J Sports Med* 1991;19:428-434.

54. Bigliani LU, Codd TP, Connor PM, et al: Shoulder motion and laxity in the professional baseball player. *Am J Sports Med* 1997;25:609-613.

55. Burkhart SS, Morgan CD, Kibler WB: The disabled throwing shoulder: Spectrum of pathology. Part III: The SICK scapula, scapular dyskinesis, the kinetic chain, and rehabilitation. *Arthroscopy* 2003;19:641-661.

   The authors present the third part in a series of theoretic articles on the dysfunctional thrower's shoulder. A rehabilitation program for the thrower is discussed. Level of evidence: V.

56. Kibler WB: Biomechanical analysis of the shoulder during tennis activities. *Clin Sports Med* 1995;14:79-85.

57. Dillman CJ, Fleisig GS, Andrews JR: Biomechanics of pitching with emphasis upon shoulder kinematics. *J Orthop Sports Phys Ther* 1993;18:402-408.

58. Jobe FW, Moynes DR, Tibone JE, Perry J: An EMG analysis of the shoulder in pitching: A second report. *Am J Sports Med* 1984;12:218-220.

59. Glousman R, Jobe F, Tibone J, et al: Dynamic electromyographic analysis of the throwing shoulder with glenohumeral instability. *J Bone Joint Surg Am* 1988; 70:220-226.

60. Pradhan RL, Itoi E, Hatakeyama Y, Urayama M, Sato K: Superior labral strain during the throwing motion: A cadaveric study. *Am J Sports Med* 2001;29:488-492.

61. Kuhn JE, Lindholm SR, Huston LJ, Soslowsky LJ, Blasier RB: Failure of the biceps superior labral complex: A cadaveric biomechanical investigation comparing the late cocking and early deceleration positions of throwing. *Arthroscopy* 2003;19:373-379.

    In this in vitro cadaver study, SLAP lesions were created more frequently when the arm is placed in the late cocking position of throwing as opposed to the early deceleration position.

62. Shepard MF, Dugas JR, Zeng N, Andrews JR: Differences in the ultimate strength of the biceps anchor and the generation of type II superior labral anterior posterior lesions in a cadaveric model. *Am J Sports Med* 2004;32:1197-1201.

    In this in vitro cadaver study, the late cocking position was more likely to produce SLAP lesions.

63. Fleisig GS, Andrews JR, Dillman CJ, Escamilla RF: Kinetics of baseball pitching with implications about injury mechanisms. *Am J Sports Med* 1995;23:233-239.

64. Borich MR, Bright JM, Lorello DJ, et al: Scapular angular positioning at end range internal rotation in cases of glenohumeral internal rotation deficit. *J Orthop Sports Phys Ther* 2006;36:926-934.

    In this in vitro, case-controlled kinematic study, 23 athletes were divided into two groups: those with glenohumeral internal rotation deficit and those without. Three-dimensional electromagnetic tracking of the scapula demonstrated significantly greater anterior scapular tilt in the GIRD group.

65. Grossman MG, Tibone JE, McGarry MH, et al: A cadaveric model of the throwing shoulder: A possible etiology of superior labrum anterior-to-posterior lesions. *J Bone Joint Surg Am* 2005;87:824-831.

    In this in vitro cadaver study, stretching the capsule produced increased external rotation, plication of the posterior capsule changed kinematics to drive the humerus posterior and superior.

66. Olsen SJ II, Fleisig GS, Dun S, Loftice J, Andrews JR: Risk factors for shoulder and elbow injuries in adolescent baseball pitchers. *Am J Sports Med* 2006;34: 905-912.

    In this case control study, 95 adolescent pitchers who had shoulder or elbow surgery were compared with 45 who never had a pitching-related injury. The injured group pitched more months per year, more games per year, more innings per game, more pitches per game, more pitches per year, and more warm-up pitches before a game. High pitch velocity and participation in show-

cases were also associated with higher injury rates. Level of evidence: III.

67. Myers JB, Oyama S, Wassinger CA, et al: Reliability, precision, accuracy, and validity of posterior shoulder tightness assessment in overhead athletes. *Am J Sports Med* 2007;35:1922-1930.

    An agreement study of different methods to measure internal rotation of the glenohumeral joint is presented. The supine method had higher reliability and validity than the side-lying method. Level of evidence: II.

68. Dessaur WA, Magarey ME: Diagnostic accuracy of clinical tests for superior labral anterior posterior lesions: A systematic review. *J Orthop Sports Phys Ther* 2008; 38:341-352.

    A systematic review of studies evaluating the diagnosis of SLAP lesions is presented. No test is sensitive or specific. Level of evidence: II.

69. Hegedus EJ, Goode A, Campbell S, et al: Physical examination tests of the shoulder: A systematic review with meta-analysis of individual tests. *Br J Sports Med* 2008; 42:80-92.

    A comprehensive systematic review of physical examination tests for the shoulder is presented. Many studies in the literature are of poor quality. Many physical examination tests are of little value.

70. Jones GL, Galluch DB: Clinical assessment of superior glenoid labral lesions: A systematic review. *Clin Orthop Relat Res* 2007;455:45-51.

    This systematic review of SLAP physical examination tests showed that developers of physical examination tests had better success than subsequent investigators. Such examinations were of little benefit. Level of evidence: III.

71. Connor PM, Banks DM, Tyson AB, Coumas JS, D'Alessandro DF: Magnetic resonance imaging of the asymptomatic shoulder of overhead athletes: A 5-year follow-up study. *Am J Sports Med* 2003;31:724-727.

    In a prospective cohort study, 20 asymptomatic athletes who had MRI were contacted 5 years later. Pathology was common on MRI; the pathology did not relate to the development of symptoms over 5 years. Level of evidence: II.

72. Jost B, Zumstein M, Pfirrmann CW, Zanetti M, Gerber C: MRI finding in throwing shoulders: Abnormalities in professional handball players. *Clin Orthop Relat Res* 2005;434:130-137.

    MRI scans of the dominant shoulders of 30 competitive professional handball players were compared with those of 20 volunteers (50 total shoulders). Ninety-three percent of throwing shoulders showed pathology that did not correlate with symptoms. Level of evidence: III.

73. Miniaci A, Mascia AT, Salonen DC, Becker EJ: Magnetic resonance imaging of the shoulder in asymptomatic professional baseball pitchers. *Am J Sports Med* 2002;30:66-73.

1: Upper Extremity

74. McClure P, Balaicuis J, Heiland D, et al: A randomized controlled comparison of stretching procedures for posterior shoulder tightness. *J Orthop Sports Phys Ther* 2007;37:108-114.

    Fifty-four asymptomatic subjects were randomized into two methods to stretch the posterior capsule. The cross-body stretch was more effective than no stretching. The cross-body stretch improved internal rotation more than the sleeper stretch, a finding that was not statistically significant. Level of evidence: I.

75. Lintner D, Mayol M, Uzodinma O, Jones R, Labossiere D: Glenohumeral internal rotation deficits in professional pitchers enrolled in an internal rotation stretching program. *Am J Sports Med* 2007;35:617-621.

    Eighty-five professional pitchers were divided into two groups based on their length of participation in an internal rotation stretch program. Those who stretched for more than 3 years had better internal rotation and total range of motion. Level of evidence: III.

76. Borstad JD, Ludewig PM: Comparison of three stretches for the pectoralis minor muscle. *J Shoulder Elbow Surg* 2006;15:324-330.

    In this in vitro kinematic study, three stretches (unilateral self-stretch, supine manual stretch, sitting manual stretch) were compared in 50 individuals using an electromagnetic tracking device. The unilateral self-stretch showed the greatest change in length.

77. Payne LZ, Altchek DW, Craig EV, Warren RF: Arthroscopic treatment of partial rotator cuff tears in young athletes: A preliminary report. *Am J Sports Med* 1997;25:299-305.

78. Riand N, Boulahia A, Walch G: Posterosuperior impingement of the shoulder in the athlete: Results of arthroscopic debridement in 75 patients. *Rev Chir Orthop Reparatrice Appar Mot* 2002;88:19-27.

79. Reynolds SB, Dugas JR, Cain EL, McMichael CS, Andrews JR: Debridement of small partial-thickness rotator cuff tears in elite overhead throwers. *Clin Orthop Relat Res* 2008;466:614-621.

    The authors present a case series of 82 professional pitchers who underwent débridement of small, partial-thickness rotator cuff tears. Follow-up on 67 patients demonstrated that 37 patients (55%) returned to professional pitching at the same or a higher level. Level of evidence: IV.

80. Andrews JR, Broussard TS, Carson WG: Arthroscopy of the shoulder in the management of partial tears of the rotator cuff: A preliminary report. *Arthroscopy* 1985;1:117-122.

81. Ide J, Maeda S, Takagi K: Arthroscopic transtendon repair of partial thickness articular side tears of the rotator cuff: Anatomical and clinical study. *Am J Sports Med* 2005;33:1672-1679.

    A cadaver study was mixed with a case series of 17 patients who had transtendon repair of articular-sided partial-thickness tears of the rotator cuff. Of six overhead throwing athletes, two returned to the same level of throwing. Level of evidence: IV.

82. Conway JE: Arthroscopic repair of partial-thickness rotator cuff tears and SLAP lesions in professional baseball players. *Orthop Clin North Am* 2001;32:443-456.

83. Liem D, Lichtenberg S, Magosch P, Habermeyer P: Arthroscopic rotator cuff repair in overhead-throwing athletes. *Am J Sports Med* 2008;36:1317-1322.

    In this retrospective cohort study, 21 overhead throwing athletes (average age, 58 years) were evaluated after arthroscopic rotator cuff repair. The re-tear rate was 24%. All returned to preinjury levels of athletic participation. Level of evidence: III.

84. Mazoué CG, Andrews JR: Repair of full-thickness rotator cuff tears in professional baseball players. *Am J Sports Med* 2006;34:182-189.

    A case series of 16 baseball players who had mini-open repair of full-thickness rotator cuff tears to bone is presented. Only one pitcher (8%) returned to high level pitching. One of two position players returned to activity. Level of evidence: IV.

85. Ide J, Maeda S, Takagi K: Sports activity after arthroscopic superior labral repair using suture anchors in overhead-throwing athletes. *Am J Sports Med* 2005;33:507-514.

    A case series of 40 patients with SLAP lesion repair is discussed. Thirty patients (75%) returned to play at the same level. Results were better for patients with traumatic SLAP tears than overuse SLAP tears. Level of evidence: IV.

86. Cerynik DL, Ewald TJ, Sastry A, et al: Outcomes of isolated glenoid labral injuries in professional baseball pitchers. *Clin J Sport Med* 2008;18:255-258.

    Forty-two Major League baseball pitchers with isolated glenoid labral injuries were assessed retrospectively. Although the percentage of pitchers returning to activity was low (69%) and declined with time, other parameters (earned run average and walks plus hits per inning) did not change. The number of innings pitched did decline. Level of evidence: IV.

87. Enad JG, ElAttrache NS, Tibone JE, Yocum LA: Isolated electrothermal capsulorrhaphy in overhand athletes. *J Shoulder Elbow Surg* 2004;13:133-137.

    Nineteen symptomatic overhand athletes were evaluated 23 months after isolated thermal capsulorrhaphy. Ten athletes returned to prior level of sport, with recurrence requiring open stabilization in two patients. Level of evidence: IV.

88. Reinold MM, Wilk KE, Hooks TR, Dugas JR, Andrews JR: Thermal-assisted capsular shrinkage of the glenohumeral joint in overhead athletes: A 15- to 47-month follow up. *J Orthop Sports Phys Ther* 2003;33:455-467.

    One hundred thirty of 231 athletes who had thermal capsulorrhaphy were contacted by phone after 29-month follow-up; 123 of 130 patients (95%) underwent concomitant procedures. Of this group, 113 of 130 patients (87%) returned to sports, and 75 of 113 patients (66%) reported excellent results. Level of evidence: IV.

89. Levitz CL, Dugas J, Andrews JR: Use of thermal capsulorraphy to treat internal impingement in baseball players. *Arthroscopy* 2001;17:573-577.

Chapter 3

Acute Elbow Injuries

Matthew A. Rappé Jr., MD   *Edwin E. Spencer Jr, MD

Introduction

Elbow injuries are common in athletes, secondary to overuse and repetitive type injuries. Acute fractures and dislocations in athletes are most often caused by a fall on an outstretched hand. The clinical management of these injuries must be carefully undertaken to avoid long-term disability.

Anatomy

Elbow injuries occur via specific mechanisms and lead to predictable bony and ligamentous injuries. Knowledge of these patterns guides the management of these injuries. The elbow joint is a complex joint comprising flexion-extension motion as well as pronation-supination motion.[1] The elbow joint has significant stability secondary to a combination of bony and ligamentous/capsular restraints.[2] Primary bony stability of the elbow is conferred by the coronoid and olecranon that form the trochlear notch of the ulna, which provides nearly 180° capture of the trochlea. Secondarily, the radial head provides secondary bony stability by acting as a restraint to valgus stress.[3] This inherent bony stability is supported by strong capsuloligamentous connections. In extension, the anterior joint capsule provides resistance to both varus and valgus stress. In throwing and nonthrowing athletes, the anterior band of the ulnar collateral ligament (UCL) has been shown to be the main stabilizer of the elbow joint to valgus stress.[3-5] The lateral collateral ligament (LCL) is composed of the lateral UCL and the radial collateral ligament. The lateral UCL resists posterolateral rotatory instability and varus stress.[6-8] The annular ligament stabilizes the proximal radioulnar joint.[7]

Dislocations

The elbow is the second most commonly dislocated major joint in adults. The classification of elbow dislocation is based on the absence of fracture (simple dislocation) or the presence of fracture (complex dislocation) as well as the position of the radius and ulna with respect to the humerus. The most common pattern of dislocation is posterior, but lateral or medial dislocation can occur, which possibly are variants of posterior dislocations. Other rare patterns include anterior and divergent dislocation.[9-12]

In most posterior elbow dislocations, the injury proceeds from a lateral to a medial direction. When the athlete falls on an outstretched hand, a combination of valgus, supination, and axial forces applied to the elbow lead to a failure of the supporting soft tissues. This failure begins with the LCL complex, then the anterior and posterior capsule, and finally the UCL.[8,13] Posterior dislocation of the elbow can occur while the integrity of the UCL is maintained. The elbow pivots around the UCL, which is the only structure left intact. Another mechanism for failure includes a varus posteromedial rotational force that results in a fracture through the anteromedial facet of the coronoid accompanied by LCL injury, fracture of the olecranon, or both.[14,15]

Careful neurovascular assessment of the patient with acute injury is important. In a series of 110 elbow dislocations, 22% were reported to have neurologic symptoms with most involving the ulnar nerve.[16] Although less likely than a nerve injury, a vascular injury also can occur with elbow dislocations. Immediate closed reduction is the standard of care for simple posterior dislocations; however, some authors advocate infusion of local anesthetic within the joint before reduction.[17] The treatment method obviously depends on the direction of the dislocation. The patient is placed supine while the physician applies traction to the lower arm and an assistant provides countertraction to the humerus. This maneuver is best accomplished with the patient's arm in approximately 30° of flexion, first correcting the medial or lateral displacement, and then supination of the forearm and traction to reduce the posterior displacement. An alternative method of reducing a posterior dislocation requires only one arm. With this method the examiner places his or her elbow in the antecubital fossa of the patient's arm. The examiner grasps the patient's wrist with the same arm. The examiner then flexes the elbow of the patient while maintaining a good grip on the wrist to provide longitudinal traction. The examiner's elbow is used as a fulcrum to reduce the patient's elbow. Following this reduction,

Edwin E. Spencer Jr, MD or the department with which he is affiliated has received royalties from Tornier, holds stock or stock options in Tornier, and is a consultant for or an employee of Tornier.

1: Upper Extremity

1: Upper Extremity

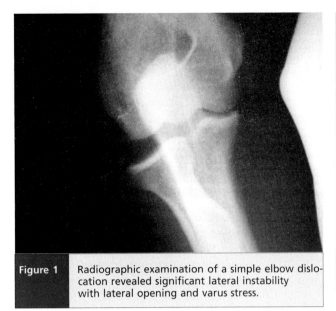

Figure 1 | Radiographic examination of a simple elbow dislocation revealed significant lateral instability with lateral opening and varus stress.

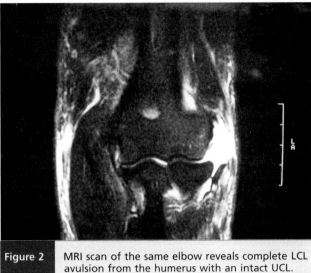

Figure 2 | MRI scan of the same elbow reveals complete LCL avulsion from the humerus with an intact UCL.

assessment of the stability of the reduction is of the utmost importance because it dictates the path of the patient's rehabilitation and treatment. Crepitus or a lack of motion may indicate an intra-articular fracture that may require surgery. Radiographs are obtained to show concentric reduction; additional radiographs may be necessary if clinical findings are indicative of profound soft-tissue instability or fracture.

Fluoroscopic examination is often more informative than MRI in assessing the severity of the soft-tissue injury; the presence of edema in the elbow makes MRI interpretation difficult. **Figure 1** is an AP radiograph demonstrating lateral instability with varus stress following a simple elbow dislocation. **Figure 2** is an MRI scan of the same elbow demonstrating a humeral avulsion of the LCL; this diagnosis is easily made via fluoroscopic examination. Fluoroscopic examination can determine the range of motion in which the elbow is stable and thus allow the physician to start early range of motion in the "safe zone," where the elbow remains reduced. The elbow is usually stable in 90° of flexion; the degree of extension in which the elbow becomes unstable is noted. Extension block splinting can be initiated to limit extension beyond the point of instability. An elbow that is stable in pronation is indicative of an intact UCL. This is a common finding because most dislocations begin on the lateral side of the joint and spare the UCL from injury. If the elbow is unstable in pronation and supination, both the LCL and UCL are injured. If more than 60° of flexion is required to maintain reduction, the elbow is considered grossly unstable and repair or reconstruction is indicated.

Associated bony injuries occur often; osteochondral fractures are most common, followed by radial head and neck fractures, coronoid fractures, and medial or lateral epicondyle fractures. Fracture-dislocations of the elbow can be difficult to treat and require particular attention to detail. These complex dislocations usually re-

quire surgery to reduce the bony fracture and restore bony stability. Posterior dislocations can be associated with coronoid and radial head fractures. These so-called terrible triad injuries require open reduction and internal fixation (ORIF) or replacement of the radial head, reconstruction of the LCL, and possibly ORIF of the coronoid fragment depending on its size and associated instability. If the elbow remains unstable in pronation, repair or reconstruction of the UCL is indicated (**Figures 3** and **4**). If osseous and ligamentous repair does not provide optimum stability, a hinged external fixator can be applied. Because prolonged immobilization has yielded poor results, stability and a concentric reduction should be obtained so that early motion is feasible.[18]

Fractures

Radial Head and Neck

The most common bony injury to the adult elbow is a radial head fracture. The Mason classification describes these fractures in terms of displacement. Nondisplaced fractures are classified as type 1, displaced fractures involving only a portion of the head are type 2, and those involving significant comminution and the entire radial head are type 3.[19] Morrey modified Mason's classification by including radial neck fractures and classifying fractures based on displacement and size.[20] Hotchkiss described a modification to the Mason classification based on treatment: type 1 are minimally displaced fractures that respond to nonsurgical treatment; type 2 are displaced partial fractures that lead to a block in motion and require surgical treatment; type 3 are irreparable fractures that require replacement or excision.[21] Controversy concerning this classification does exist; some authors have demonstrated that primary nonsurgical treatment of moderately displaced two-part fractures of the radial head has a pre-

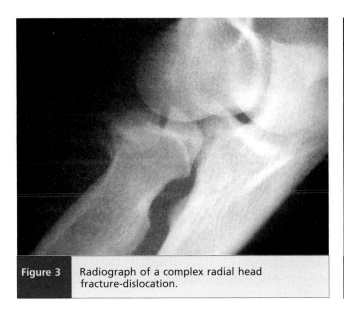

Figure 3 Radiograph of a complex radial head fracture-dislocation.

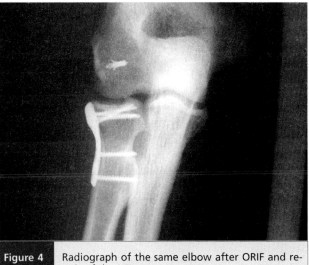

Figure 4 Radiograph of the same elbow after ORIF and repair of the LCL.

dominantly favorable outcome.[22] Furthermore, ORIF using a contoured plating system as an alternative to excision or replacement of the radial head also has been shown to have favorable results.[23] However, if more than three fragments are present, replacement has better results.

Treatment of radial head fractures also is influenced by ligamentous status and joint stability. If the patient has an intact UCL complex, excision of the comminuted radial head is a viable treatment option. When complex elbow instability involving disruption of the UCL complex is present, radial head replacement or fixation is paramount to maintain joint stability.

Coronoid Fractures

For many years, the understanding of coronoid fractures was based on the classification of Regan-Morrey: type 1, a simple fracture of the distal tip; type 2, a fracture involving approximately 50% of the coronoid; and type 3, a fracture involving greater than 50% of the coronoid.[24] Surgical treatment of type 3 fractures has consisted of suture, screw, or plate fixation according to the size of the fragment. The understanding of coronoid fractures was advanced by the classification of O'Driscoll, which focused on fracture location rather than on the size of the fracture fragment.[25] Identification of the importance of the anteromedial facet of the coronoid as a separate fracture entity that requires surgical treatment has improved patient outcomes.[26] These smaller fragments, which can be difficult to identify on standard plain films, are now known to be associated with posteromedial subluxation and instability.

Olecranon Fractures

The subcutaneous border of the ulna is at risk of injury during sports participation, especially for contact athletes and those athletes such as gymnasts or basketball players who risk falling on an outstretched hand. Most injuries occur secondary to direct trauma to the posterior elbow but can occur via indirect trauma. The classification of olecranon fractures is based on displacement, the stability of the ulnohumeral articulation, and the presence of comminution.[27] Nondisplaced fractures can be treated with simple immobilization, whereas displaced fractures require surgical intervention. Simple transverse fractures of the olecranon can be treated successfully with tension band wiring, whereas the more complex comminuted fractures are best treated with low-profile plating systems that allow multiple points of fixation within the proximal fragment. For proximal olecranon fractures, simple excision of the fragment and advancement of the triceps can be done but is not recommended in athletes. The olecranon is approached through a posterior midline incision over the olecranon, taking care to avoid the ulnar nerve medially during dissection. The medial extension of the fracture should be evaluated to ensure that it does not extend into the anteromedial facet of the coronoid; if it does, either plate or lag screw fixation can ensure postoperative stability.[28] The most common complication in the treatment of olecranon fractures is prominent hardware that requires removal. The presence of prominent hardware was as high as 82% when tension band wiring was used and as low as 20% when plate fixation was used.[29,30]

Distal Humerus

Distal humeral fractures rarely occur in athletic populations during sports participation; it is more common in patients with osteoporosis or following high-velocity trauma such as a motor vehicle crash. The overall incidence of distal humeral fractures in individuals age 12 years and older is approximately 5.7 fractures per 100,000 of the population per year.[31]

1: Upper Extremity

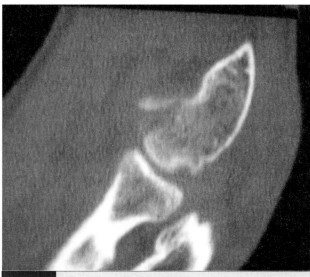

Figure 5 CT scan of a type I capitellum fracture. Note that the radial head is intact.

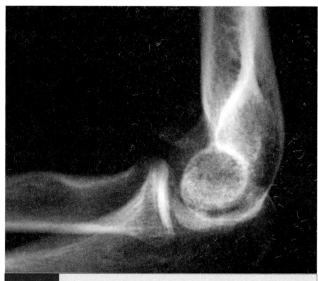

Figure 6 Lateral radiograph of the same elbow with a type I capitellum fracture.

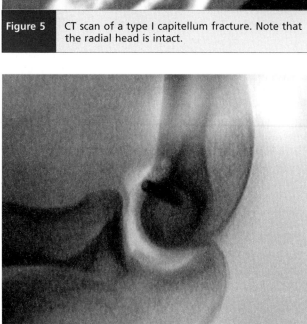

Figure 7 Intraoperative lateral radiograph of fixation of the capitellum with a headless screw. This elbow also required repair of the LCL. Note the gapping of the ulnohumeral joint, indicating LCL disruption.

Restoration of the articular surface and rigid stability to allow motion to prevent stiffness is the goal of treatment. There is no consensus regarding classifications of distal humeral fractures. Most systems describe these fractures in terms of column involvement, articular involvement, and degree of comminution. For intra-articular fractures, an osteotomy of the olecranon process is sometimes necessary to provide exposure of the articular surface. To avoid the possible complications of osteotomy, such as nonunion, a triceps-sparing approach may be feasible but does not provide the same exposure. Through either approach, standard AO technique describes articular fracture fragment reduction and column stabilization with two 3.5-mm plates for bicolumnar fractures, one along the medial column and the other posterior along the lateral column. To address poor screw purchase in distal fractures with comminution, other authors advocate dual parallel plating in which the shaft is rigidly fixed to buttress the more distal comminution where purchase is lessened.[32]

Capitellum fractures are rare but do occur in athletes.[33] A type 1 or Hahn-Steinthal capitellum fracture is a coronal shear fracture without involvement of the trochlea (**Figures 5** through 7). Type 2 or Kocher-Lorenz fractures involve very little subchondral bone and are almost entirely made of cartilage. Type 3 fractures are comminuted fractures of the capitellum and the so-called type 4 fracture is a shear fracture of the distal end of the humerus involving the capitellum, and trochlea.[34] Fixation is either anterior to posterior with headless screws or lag screw fixation combined with an antiglide plate.[35]

Summary

The surgeon should use a treatment algorithm predicated on restoring stability when addressing elbow dislocations and fracture-dislocations. Fluoroscopy can be beneficial in determining the stable range of motion and assessing posterolateral or posteromedial instability. Complex injuries such as the terrible triad epitomize the need for a cogent treatment algorithm. With these specific cases, the surgeon must repair/reconstruct the LCL and repair or replace the radial head, but the resulting stability dictates whether the coronoid (also based on size and location) and medial collateral ligament need to be surgically treated. Knowledge of the injury patterns is paramount to good decision making.

Annotated References

1. Hildebrand KA, Patterson SD, King GJ: Acute elbow dislocations: Simple and complex. *Orthop Clin North Am* 1999;30:63-79.

2. Morrey BF, An KN: Articular and ligamentous contributions to the stability of the elbow joint. *Am J Sports Med* 1983;11:315-319.

3. Morrey BF, Tanaka S, An KN: Valgus stability of the elbow: A definition of primary and secondary constraints. *Clin Orthop Relat Res* 1991;265:187-195.

4. Hotchkiss RN, Weiland AJ: Valgus stability of the elbow. *J Orthop Res* 1987;5:372-373.

5. Jobe FW, Stark H, Lombardo SJ: Reconstruction of the ulnar collateral ligament in athletes. *J Bone Joint Surg Am* 1986;68:1158-1163.

6. Cohen MS, Hastings H II: Rotatory instability of the elbow: The anatomy and role of the lateral stabilizers. *J Bone Joint Surg Am* 1997;79:225-233.

7. King GJ, Morrey BF, An KN: Stabilizers of the elbow. *J Shoulder Elbow Surg* 1993;2:165.

8. Nestor BJ, O'Driscoll SW, Morrey BF: Ligamentous reconstruction for posterolateral rotatory instability of the elbow. *J Bone Joint Surg Am* 1992;74:1235-1241.

9. Symeonides PP, Grigoriadis NC, Hatzokos IG: Anterior dislocation of the elbow. *J Shoulder Elbow Surg* 2006; 15:249-251.

   This case report describes the rare anterior dislocation of the elbow in 36-year-old man treated with reduction and a removable posterior plaster splint for 3 weeks with the elbow at approximately 130° of extension. Level of evidence: IV.

10. Torchia ME, DiGiovine NM: Anterior dislocation of the elbow in an arm wrestler. *J Shoulder Elbow Surg* 1998; 7:539-541.

11. Kazuki K, Miyamoto T, Ohzono K: A case of traumatic divergent fracture-dislocation of the elbow combined with Essex-Lopresti lesion in an adult. *J Shoulder Elbow Surg* 2005;14:224-226.

    The authors report a case of traumatic divergent elbow fracture-dislocation in combination with an ipsilateral Essex-Lopresti injury of the distal radioulnar joint in an adult. The literature regarding divergent elbow fracture-dislocations is reviewed. Level of evidence: IV.

12. Zaricznyi B: Transverse divergent dislocation of the elbow. *Clin Orthop Relat Res* 2000;373:146-152.

13. O'Driscoll SW, Morrey BF, Korinek S, An KN: Elbow subluxation and dislocation: A spectrum of instability. *Clin Orthop Relat Res* 1992;280:186-197.

14. Doornberg JN, de Jong IM, Lindenhovius AL, Ring D: The anteromedial facet of the coronoid process of the ulna. *J Shoulder Elbow Surg* 2007;16:667-670.

    The authors analyzed 21 CT scans of the elbow in patients with distal humeral fractures. On average, 58% of the anteromedial facet was found to be unsupported by the proximal ulnar metaphysis. This study demonstrates the relatively vulnerable position of the anteromedial facet of the coronoid in complex elbow dislocations.

15. Ring D: Fractures of the coronoid process of the ulna. *J Hand Surg Am* 2006;31:1679-1689.

    This article provides a comprehensive description of the coronoid process fracture morphology and treatment.

16. Linscheid RL, Wheeler DK: Elbow dislocations. *JAMA* 1965;194:1171-1176.

17. Mehta JA, Bain GI: Elbow dislocations in adults and children. *Clin Sports Med* 2004;23:609-627.

    This article presents a review of elbow dislocations, including clinical presentation, examination, and investigations and management of complex cases that require repair or reconstruction of the ligamentous complexes.

18. Mehlhoff TL, Noble PC, Bennett JB, Tullos HS: Simple dislocation of the elbow in the adult: Results after closed treatment. *J Bone Joint Surg Am* 1988;70: 244-249.

19. Mason ML: Some observations on fractures of the head of the radius with a review of one hundred cases. *Br J Surg* 1954;42:123-132.

20. Morrey BF: Radial head fractures, in *The Elbow and its Disorders*. Philadelphia, PA, WB Saunders, 1985, pp 355-381.

21. Hotchkiss RN: Displaced fractures of the radial head: Internal fixation or excision? *J Am Acad Orthop Surg* 1997;5:1-10.

22. Akesson T, Herbertsson P, Josefsson PO, Hasserius R, Besjakov J, Karlsson MK: Primary nonoperative treatment of moderately displaced two-part fractures of the radial head. *J Bone Joint Surg Am* 2006;88:1909-1914.

    In this 19-year follow-up study, results were favorable in the nonsurgical treatment of moderately displaced two-fragment fractures of the radial head. Level of evidence: III.

23. Ikeda M, Yamashina Y, Kamimoto M, Oka Y: Open reduction and internal fixation of comminuted fractures of the radial head using low-profile mini-plates. *J Bone Joint Surg Br* 2003;85:1040-1044.

    This study discusses favorable findings in 10 patients with severely comminuted fractures of the radial head using low-profile mini-plates. Level of evidence: III.

24. Regan W, Morrey B: Fractures of the coronoid process of the ulna. *J Bone Joint Surg Am* 1989;71:1348-1354.

1: Upper Extremity

25. O'Driscoll SW, Jupiter JB, Cohen MS, Ring D, Mc-Kee MD: Difficult elbow fractures: Pearls and pitfalls. *Instr Course Lect* 2003;52:113-134.

This review article identifies coronoid fracture classification based on whether the fracture involves the tip, the anteromedial facet, or the base (body) of the coronoid. It further identifies anteromedial coronoid fractures as varus posteromedial rotatory fracture subluxations, which are often serious injuries.

26. Doornberg JN, Ring DC: Fracture of the anteromedial facet of the coronoid process. *J Bone Joint Surg Am* 2006;88:2216-2224.

The authors followed 18 patients with a fracture of the anteromedial facet of the coronoid process over a 6-year period and concluded that anteromedial fractures of the coronoid are associated with either subluxation or complete dislocation of the elbow in most patients. Level of evidence: III.

27. Morrey BF: Current concepts in the treatment of fractures of the radial head, the olecranon, and the coronoid. *Instr Course Lect* 1995;44:175-185.

28. Doornberg J, Ring D, Jupiter JB: Effective treatment of fracture-dislocations of the olecranon requires a stable trochlear notch. *Clin Orthop Relat Res* 2004;429:292-300.

Twenty-six patients with coronoid/olecranon fracture-dislocations were followed for 3 years. Twenty-one patients had true coronoid fractures. All were treated surgically. The five unsatisfactory results were related to inadequate coronoid fixation. Level of evidence: III.

29. Chalidis BE, Sachinis NC, Samoladas EP, Dimitriou CG, Pournaras JD: Is tension band wiring technique the "gold standard" for the treatment of olecranon fractures? A long term functional outcome study. *J Orthop Surg* 2008;3:9.

This long-term retrospective study of patient-rated outcome after tension band treatment demonstrated good patient satisfaction; however, degenerative changes were recorded in nearly 50% of all elbows, and 82% required hardware removal. Level of evidence: III.

30. Bailey CS, MacDermid J, Patterson SD, King GJ: Outcome of plate fixation of olecranon fractures. *J Orthop Trauma* 2001;15:542-548.

31. Robinson CM, Hill RM, Jacobs N, Dall G, Court-Brown CM: Adult distal humeral metaphyseal fractures: Epidemiology and results of treatment. *J Orthop Trauma* 2003;17:38-47.

This observational cohort study of a consecutive series of 320 patients with distal humeral fractures in a well-defined catchment population revealed 5.7 cases per 100,000 in the population per year with an almost equal male to female ratio. Level of evidence: III.

32. O'Driscoll SW: Optimizing stability in distal humeral fracture fixation. *J Shoulder Elbow Surg* 2005;14:186S-194S.

The author provides eight technical pearls to address complex fractures of the distal humerus and advocates parallel plating of each column to create an arch. Level of evidence: V.

33. McKee MD, Jupiter JB: Trauma to the adult elbow and fractures of the distal humerus, in Browner BD, Jupiter JB, Levin AM, Trafton PG (eds): *Skeletal Trauma: Fractures, Dislocations, Ligamentous Injuries*. Philadelphia, PA, WB Saunders, 2002, pp 1469–1472.

34. Mehdian H, McKee MD: Fractures of capitellum and trochlea. *Orthop Clin North Am* 2000;31:115-127.

35. Sen MK, Sama N, Helfet DL: Open reduction and internal fixation of coronal fractures of the capitellum. *J Hand Surg Am* 2007;32:1462-1465.

The authors describe lag screw fixation combined with an antiglide plate to neutralize shearing forces in coronal shear fractures.

Chapter 4

Nonacute Medial Elbow Injuries

*Marc R. Safran, MD

Introduction

Because the medial elbow is subject to significant forces during sports activities, this area of the elbow is frequently injured. Appropriate diagnosis and treatment require a detailed understanding of the normal anatomy of the elbow and the pathophysiology of injuries to the medial elbow.

The anatomic structures of the elbow provide stability through a complex range of motions: flexion-extension and pronation-supination. The dynamic stability seen in the elbow depends on varying contributions from the osseous, ligamentous, and other soft-tissue structures about the elbow.

Pathophysiology and Pathomechanics

The elbow may be subjected to numerous unusual forces during sports activities. Overhead athletes subject their elbows to major valgus forces that place the elbow at risk for specific elbow injuries. Sports such as baseball, football, tennis, volleyball, golf, and water polo are most commonly associated with acute and chronic elbow pathology. Overhead throwing athletes are predisposed to overuse syndromes secondary to repetitive, high-velocity stress across the elbow. The highest stress at the elbow occurs during the late cocking and acceleration phases of the throwing cycle. Studies have indicated that the valgus stress at the elbow during the acceleration phase can be as high as 64 N-m, which exceeds the ultimate tensile strength of the ulnar collateral ligament (UCL).[1] Although the curveball has long been implicated in UCL injury in young baseball players, biomechanical analysis has not supported this claim.[2] In baseball, the number of pitches (during a game, season, and year) is considered the most important factor for elbow injury, although the type of pitches, pitching mechanics, and physical conditioning are still considered potentially important.[2-4] The stresses of throwing result in loads that produce traction or tensile forces on the medial-sided structures,

compression forces on the lateral side of the elbow, and medially-directed shear posteriorly.[5,6] The athletes commonly have chronic and acute injuries to the UCL with or without medial epicondylitis, as well as ulnar nerve symptoms. Laterally, compression leads to radiocapitellar degeneration and loose bodies, and posterior shear forces may lead to osteophyte formation, loose bodies, and olecranon stress fractures.

Medial Epicondylitis

Medial epicondylitis is a term for tendinosis at the common medial flexor-pronator origin. Specifically, the origins of the flexor carpi radialis and the pronator teres are most affected. This injury is actually a tendinosis, and thus the term epicondylitis is a misnomer. Medial epicondylitis is much less common than lateral epicondylitis in the general population. Young to middle-aged athletes involved in golf, tennis, and overhead throwing are most commonly affected. Although medial epicondylitis is also known as golfer's elbow, it is more common than lateral epicondylitis in professional tennis players. The repetitive valgus stress of these sports activities subjects these muscles to microtraumatic injury.

The peak incidence of medial epicondylitis occurs in the fourth and fifth decades of life. Patients generally report medial elbow pain that is worse with gripping, batting, hitting a serve in tennis, or throwing, and, less commonly, swelling of the inner elbow. Patients have medial elbow pain and sometimes symptoms of ulnar nerve irritation. Examination reveals tenderness over the medial epicondyle and slightly distal and lateral in the pronator teres tendon, as well as pain with resisted pronation or wrist flexion. Careful assessment for UCL laxity and ulnar nerve symptoms is required because medial epicondylitis may occur simultaneously. Radiographs are usually normal. MRI is not usually necessary for the diagnosis of medial epicondylitis, but the changes seen are consistent with a tendinosis or may be more extensive and include muscular and/or bony edema.

The treatment generally is nonsurgical, consisting of rest and anti-inflammatory medications, with a gradual return to stretching and strengthening of the involved muscles. In more than 80% of patients, symptoms resolve with conservative treatment, and the patient is able to return to the sport or activity. Cortisone

*Mark R. Safran, MD or the department with which he is affiliated has received research or institutional support from Smith & Nephew; holds stock or stock options in Cool Systems, Inc; and is a consultant for or an employee of Cool Systems, Inc.

1: Upper Extremity

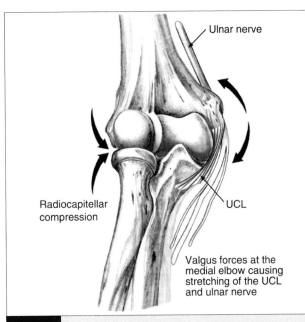

| Figure 1 | Schematic representation of the effects of valgus force as seen from the anterior elbow. Valgus forces applied to the elbow result in tensile forces medially, to the UCL and ulnar nerve, and the flexor-pronator muscle group, which may be injured during excessive eccentric contraction. Laterally, the radiocapitellar joint is a secondary restraint to valgus force, and thus compression of this joint may result in chondral injury. (*Reproduced with permission from Safran MR: Injury to the ulnar collateral ligament: Diagnosis and treatment.* Sports Med Arthrosc Rev 2003;11:17.) |

injections may be of benefit as an adjunct to rehabilitation.[7] Rehabilitation includes application of ice, anti-inflammatory medications, and stretching and strengthening of the flexor/pronator muscle group. A counterforce brace may be beneficial in patients who are rehabilitating but still involved in activites that may aggravate the symptoms.

If the condition does not respond to an appropriate trial (4 to 6 months) of nonsurgical treatment, surgery may be required. Surgical intervention involves excision of the abnormal degenerative tissue at the common flexor-pronator origin and reapproximation of the remaining healthy tissue. Unfortunately, the surgery for medial epicondylitis is not as successful as that for lateral epicondylitis. Part of the reason for decreased success is failure to recognize concomitant disease. Ulnar neuropathy is present 40% to 60% of the time. The success of medial epicondylitis débridement is significantly reduced when concomitant ulnar neuropathy is a factor.[8] According to one study, 96% of patients treated for medial epicondylitis without ulnar nerve symptoms had good to excellent results, compared with only 40% good to excellent results in patients with concomitant moderate to severe ulnar neuropathy requiring ulnar nerve decompression or transposition at the time of medial epicondylitis surgery.[8] Furthermore, UCL instability should be suspected in throwing athletes, and the appropriate work-up needs to be done in these patients.[6]

UCL Injury

Anatomy

The UCL is a ligamentous complex on the medial aspect of the elbow between the distal humerus and the proximal ulna. Its anterior portion, the anterior oblique ligament (AOL), is the primary restraint against valgus stress, especially the forces associated with throwing.[9-13] The AOL consists of an anterior band, which is taut at 0° to 60° flexion, and a posterior band, which is taut at 60° to 120° of flexion.[12] The anterior band is primarily responsible for stability against valgus stresses at 30°, 60°, and 90° of flexion, making it the most important for overhead sports activities.[13] The posterior band of the AOL begins as a secondary restraint to valgus stability at 30° and 90° and is a primary restraint to valgus force at 120° flexion.[11] The posterior oblique ligament forms the floor of the cubital tunnel and plays more of a role in restraint against valgus stress at higher degrees of flexion. The role of the transverse ligament (Cooper's ligament) in elbow stability remains unclear.

Recent studies have demonstrated that the flexor-pronator muscles, particularly the flexor carpi ulnaris, in addition to the flexor digitorum superficialis and flexor carpi radialis, play a significant role in providing valgus stability of the elbow and are activated at higher levels in patients with medial elbow pain.[14-16]

Pathomechanics

Overhead throwing athletes subject their elbows to severe and repetitive valgus stress, placing the anterior band of the AOL of the UCL complex at risk of injury. Chronic UCL insufficiency results from microscopic tears and attenuation. Patients report pain and soreness in the medial elbow with throwing, usually in the late cocking or early acceleration phases or with ball release. Specifically, such athletes are unable to throw at more than 75% of maximal effort. Acute rupture can also occur with or without chronic changes. Most acute UCL ruptures (87%) occur midsubstance.[17] Ulnar and humeral avulsions are much less common. Athletes often report the sudden onset of pain and the feeling of giving way during throwing. The most common situation is an acute exacerbation of a chronically injured ligament. Associated pathology, such as ulnar neuropathy, loose bodies, osteophytes, and a flexion contracture, also can produce symptoms.

The stresses of throwing result in a consistent pattern of potential elbow injuries: traction or tensile forces of the medial-sided structures, compression of the lateral side of the elbow, and medially directed shear posteriorly[5,6] (**Figures 1 and 2**). The tensile forces

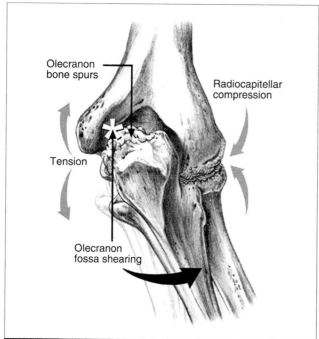

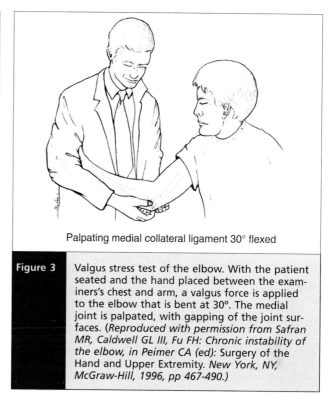

Palpating medial collateral ligament 30° flexed

| Figure 2 | Schematic representation of the effects of valgus force as seen from the posterior elbow. The olecranon is forced in the tight-fitting olecranon fossa. With valgus force, there is an additional shear force of the olecranon against the medial wall of the olecranon fossa. This may result in chondral injury, osteophyte formation, and loose bodies. (*Reproduced with permission from Safran MR: Injury to the ulnar collateral ligament: Diagnosis and treatment. Sports Med Arthrosc Rev 2003;11:17.*) |

| Figure 3 | Valgus stress test of the elbow. With the patient seated and the hand placed between the examiners's chest and arm, a valgus force is applied to the elbow that is bent at 30°. The medial joint is palpated, with gapping of the joint surfaces. (*Reproduced with permission from Safran MR, Caldwell GL III, Fu FH: Chronic instability of the elbow, in Peimer CA (ed): Surgery of the Hand and Upper Extremity. New York, NY, McGraw-Hill, 1996, pp 467-490.*) |

lead to attenuation or tearing of the UCL, either chronic or acute. Acute or overuse injury to the flexor-pronator muscle-tendon group may occur as the tensile valgus forces are dynamically resisted. Ulnar nerve symptoms also may develop in conjunction with UCL injury. An acute UCL tear may result in bleeding near the nerve, causing nerve irritation as well as compression from the swelling. A chronic UCL injury may result in ulnar nerve symptoms from several different potential causes: (1) increased tensile force as the nerve is stretched at the elbow as a result of increased medial joint gapping from the incompetent ligament and/or (2) compression from a tight cubital tunnel due to scarring or ossification of the UCL or osteophytes. Incompetence of the UCL also may result in increased compressive force at the radiocapitellar joint, a secondary stabilizer to valgus force, which leads to softening and degeneration of the articular cartilage (**Figure 1**). Osteochondral loose bodies may result and cause mechanical symptoms and pain. Eventually, degenerative arthritis of the radiocapitellar joint may develop. Posteriorly, the olecranon is repeatedly and forcefully driven into the olecranon fossa with throwing as the arm goes into extension. Further, valgus stress typically causes shearing posteriorly; this results in impingement of the posteromedial olecranon against the lateral as-

pect of the medial wall of the olecranon fossa, which results in chondromalacia, synovitis, and pain (valgus extension overload syndrome [VEOS]; **Figure 2**). According to a 2004 study, UCL injury results in contact alterations in the posterior compartment that lead to osteophyte formation.[18] Compounding this posterior impingement is the bony hypertrophic narrowing of the olecranon fossa and hypertrophy of the proximal ulna that occur in overhead athletes who have participated in sports since childhood. With persistent impaction and shear forces, the osteophytes may break off and become loose bodies within the joint.[19,20] These loose bodies can get caught in the joint surfaces and damage the articular cartilage.

Evaluation

Patients generally have point tenderness at the insertion on the ulna, 2 cm distal to the medial epicondyle. UCL deficiency should be tested with the elbow at 30° to 120° of flexion. The valgus stress test has been described with the elbow at 30° of flexion (**Figure 3**). The milking maneuver and its modification assess for valgus laxity at a higher degree of flexion.[5] In this test, the patient's arm is stabilized proximally, while the thumb is pulled laterally, imparting a valgus stress to the elbow in 70° to 90° of flexion, while the examiner palpates the medial joint line for opening (**Figure 4**). The moving valgus stress test (during which the elbow is brought from full flexion into extension with constant valgus force reproducing the patient's medial pain) has recently been described, although the pain from the UCL usually is reproducibly present between 80° and 120° of flexion[21] (**Figure 5**). It is important that the

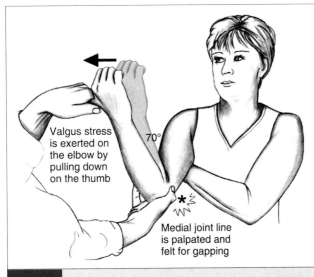

Figure 4 Modified milking maneuver. The patient's elbow is flexed 70° while the shoulder is externally rotated. The examiner palpates the medial joint with one hand while the other hand pulls distally on the patient's thumb, imparting a valgus force. The advantage of this position of examination is that external shoulder rotation, which may confound the examination, is eliminated. (*Reproduced with permission from Safran MR: Injury to the ulnar collateral ligament: Diagnosis and treatment. Sports Med Arthrosc Rev 2003;11:19.*)

Valgus stress is exerted on the elbow by pulling down on the thumb

70°

Medial joint line is palpated and felt for gapping

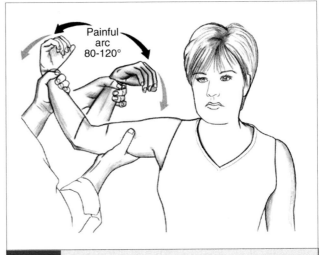

Painful arc 80-120°

Figure 5 Moving valgus stress test. With the patient's shoulder in abduction and external rotation, the elbow is flexed and extended while a valgus force is imparted on the elbow (by externally rotating the shoulder). Pain felt at a particular point within an arc of 80° and 120° is consistent with an injury to the UCL. (*Reproduced with permission from Safran MR: Injury to the ulnar collateral ligament: Diagnosis and treatment. Sports Med Arthrosc Rev 2003;11:20.*)

examiner evaluate for VEOS (posterior elbow impingement) because studies have shown that 42% of patients who undergo surgery for VEOS require a second operation, and 25% of these patients required a UCL reconstruction as a result of valgus instability.[22] Patients must also be evaluated for medial epicondylitis and ulnar neuritis, as well as for lateral elbow tenderness that is worsened by pronation and supination of the elbow because this may be indicative of radiocapitellar degeneration.

Physical examination of the throwing athlete with elbow pain, and potentially UCL injury, should also include evaluation of the shoulder, particularly the scapulothoracic joint (scapular malposition, inferior medial scapular winging, coracoid tenderness, and scapular dyskinesis [the SICK scapula]; and dyskinesis), core strength, and hip motion (rotation) and strength, as a breakdown in the kinetic chain may place the elbow at increased risk for injury and potentially play a role in the outcome of nonsurgical treatment.

Stress radiographs can be helpful for demonstrating UCL insufficiency.[6,23] With the elbow flexed approximately 20° to 45°, an AP radiograph is taken while a valgus stress is applied.[23] With UCL insufficiency, gapping at the medial joint line exceeds that of the contralateral normal side by more than 2 mm. This may be done manually or with an instrumented device. Plain radiographs may also show secondary changes of chronic UCL insufficiency, such as osteophyte forma-

tion at the medial joint, loose bodies, sclerosis, radiocapitellar degeneration, or osteophytes of the olecranon. MRI can be helpful for detecting a torn UCL and for defining associated pathology.[23] However, magnetic resonance arthrography is even more sensitive (97%) in detecting UCL injury.[24,25] Studies have shown ultrasonography to be useful in detecting UCL injury and changes in the ligament and medial joint opening with valgus stress, although it continues to be used only sparingly at this time because it is technician dependent.[26,27]

Treatment

The initial treatment of UCL injury generally is nonsurgical and consists of rest from the overhead sport, anti-inflammatory medications, and physical therapy.[5] The first goal of treatment is to establish a painless range of motion that also will allow the ligament to heal. Gradual strengthening should begin with isometric exercises of the elbow and wrist. Strengthening should focus on the flexor pronator muscles, which recently have been shown to be important local dynamic stabilizers of the medial elbow.[14-16] A shoulder program should be implemented to normalize range of motion and flexibility and improve shoulder strength. Once full motion, full strength, and dynamic stability have returned and the patient is symptom free, the patient may begin an interval throwing program. Upon satisfactory completion of the interval throwing program (pain-free throwing at full velocity), the patient may return to high-level activity.

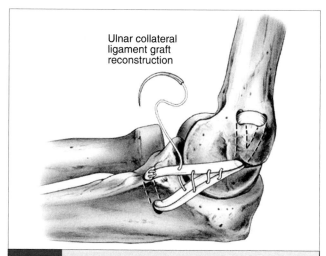

Figure 6 Classic Jobe UCL reconstruction with one tunnel in the proximal ulna at the sublime tubercle and the Y-shaped tunnels at the medial epicondyle. This results in a three-ply reconstruction of the UCL. (*Reproduced with permission from Safran MR: Injury to the ulnar collateral ligament: Diagnosis and treatment. Sports Med Arthrosc Rev 2003;11:21.*)

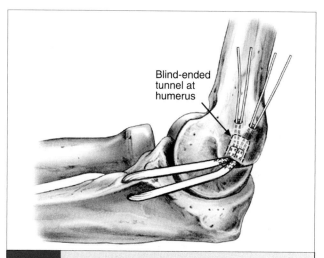

Figure 7 The docking procedure is a modification of UCL reconstruction where the ulnar tunnel is the same and there is a blind-ended tunnel in the medial epicondyle. Sutures of the graft are tied over the medial epicondyle. (*Reproduced with permission from Safran MR: Injury to the ulnar collateral ligament: Diagnosis and treatment. Sports Med Arthrosc Rev 2003;11:22.*)

One study indicated that approximately half of patients with UCL injury can be treated successfully without surgery and are able to return to the same level of athletic activity.[28] Surgery is indicated if symptoms recur after an appropriate trial of nonsurgical treatment. Surgical treatment of a UCL injury also should be considered with acute ruptures in high-level throwing athletes, with significant chronic instability, and after débridement of UCL calcification.

When nonsurgical treatment of UCL injuries fails, surgical options must be considered.[6] Surgical treatment of the UCL depends on several variables. Currently, the mainstay of surgical treatment is UCL reconstruction. Primary repair of acute ruptures of the UCL had been advocated for years; however, ligamentous reconstruction now has consistently better results overall.[5,6] The less common avulsion injury is considered by some to be amenable to suture repair.[17,29] Repair of the torn UCL was the treatment of choice until 1992, when a study reviewed the results of repair and reconstruction.[17] Those authors recommended reconstruction, citing the finding that overhead athletes performed significantly worse with repair than with reconstruction. The study also noted that repair could be considered if the tear was a proximal avulsion, if the procedure was performed soon after injury, if the rest of the ligament was undamaged, and if no ulnar nerve symptoms were present. Repair of most injuries usually involves repair of tissue that frequently is chronically injured and therefore not ideal tissue. There was not much in the literature about repair until a recent study reported a series of 60 patients with an average age of 17 years who underwent UCL repair, predominantly with proximal and distal insertional injuries.[29] A 93%

success rate at 5-year follow-up was reported, with 4 patients (7%) having failed repair (early and late repair, two patients each). Generally, however, UCL reconstruction with a free graft has become the treatment of choice for UCL deficiency.

UCL reconstruction has evolved considerably over the years.[6,30] It was reported that 81% of patients were able to return to the same level of sports activity after UCL reconstruction, compared with 63% of patients who had primary repair.[24] The rate of surgical success of reconstruction has reliably and reproducibly improved from 68% with Jobe's original report to up to 97%, with success defined as the patient returning to play at the same level or better than before the injury.[6,24,31-38]

Several graft options are available. An ipsilateral palmaris longus autograft most often is used, but other grafts, including the contralateral palmaris longus, the fourth toe extensor, the hamstring tendon, a strip of Achilles tendon, the plantaris tendon, and allograft (hamstring and posterior or anterior tibialis tendon), have been used. Palmaris longus and hamstring grafts currently are used most often.[6,30]

The technique of UCL reconstruction as first described used a tunnel in the sublime tubercle and a Y-shaped tunnel with three drill holes in the medial epicondyle to make a figure-of-8, three-ply graft configuration[33] (**Figure 6**). Because of concerns about the strength of suture fixation of the free tendon graft, adequate tensioning of the graft at the time of final fixation, and the potential for complications as a result of the multiple drill holes, the technique has been modified.[36] The variations include the docking procedure (**Figure 7**), placement of interference screws (**Figure 8**),

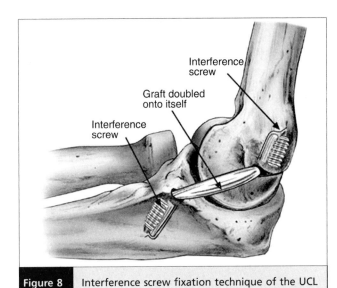

Figure 8 Interference screw fixation technique of the UCL reconstruction. (*Reproduced with permission from Safran MR: Injury to the ulnar collateral ligament: Diagnosis and treatment.* Sports Med Arthrosc Rev 2003;11:22.)

nerve transposition is performed at the same time as the reconstruction.

To achieve reproducible and successful outcomes from this surgery, all sources of pathology need to be addressed, including medial epicondylitis and loose bodies. If there is concomitant VEOS, the osteophytes on the proximal medial olecranon are débrided, but the surgeon must take care not to remove any normal olecranon. There is an association with UCL insufficiency and VEOS, although it is unclear whether removal of the osteophytes increases stress on the UCL, leading to injury.[18,45-47] If clinically present, associated ulnar neuritis, as noted previously, is addressed through nerve transposition. The optimal technique for reconstruction is unclear, as there are no prospective, randomized controlled trials, and thus research is needed.[30,38,48]

A recent series of revision UCL reconstructions has been published and reveals a lower success rate, defined as return to the same level of play (33%) and a higher complication rate (40%), including one retear of the UCL (7%).[41]

and a combination known as the DANE procedure (interference screw in the ulna and docking proximally).[31,36,39,40] This latter technique has been useful in revision UCL insufficiency, including sublime tubercle avulsions or tunnel blowout at the ulnar insertion.[40,41]

The original technique involved detachment of the flexor-pronator muscle group.[36] However, the muscle-splitting approach demonstrated that reconstruction can be performed safely without detaching the flexor-pronator muscles.[36,37]

Biomechanical studies evaluating the different techniques have had conflicting results, partly because of methodological differences. According to one study, the Jobe tunnel technique has better overall strength and initial and overall stiffness as compared with the interference screw technique.[42] According to a 2003 study, reconstruction using interference screw fixation was statistically equivalent to an intact ligament.[39] In a 2007 study, the docking procedure was compared with bioabsorbable interference screws. The interference screws provided greater stability in response to early cyclic valgus loading using a palmaris longus graft.[43] The cyclic loading strength of four UCL reconstruction techniques using palmaris longus graft—docking, interference screw, transosseous figure-of-8 Jobe technique, and hybrid Endobutton docking reconstruction—was compared.[44] The authors found that none of the techniques was equivalent to the intact ligament, but docking and the hybrid Endobutton/docking reconstructions were superior to interference screw and classic Jobe reconstruction.

Routine ulnar nerve transposition, originally recommended with UCL reconstruction,[33] generally is not performed in conjunction with UCL reconstruction because of the high rate of complications (21%).[17,24] If significant ulnar nerve symptoms are present, ulnar

Ulnar Nerve Injuries

After carpal tunnel syndrome, ulnar nerve compression at the elbow is the most common compressive neuropathy of the upper extremity. Medial elbow pathology seen in throwing athletes is associated with ulnar nerve symptoms approximately 50% of the time. The ulnar nerve is susceptible to injury because of (1) the tight path it follows, which changes its dimensions with elbow flexion and extension; (2) its subcutaneous location; and (3) the considerable excursion required to accommodate the full motion of not only the elbow but also the shoulder. Proximally, the ulnar nerve can be compressed by the intermuscular septum or by a hypertrophied medial head of the triceps. At the cubital tunnel, nerve irritation and injury can result from osteophytes, loose bodies, a thickened retinaculum, or an inflamed UCL, especially with elbow flexion. The most common site of ulnar nerve compression is distal, between the two heads of the flexor carpi ulnaris.

Both physiologic and pathologic factors contribute to irritation and compression of the ulnar nerve. Compression, either alone or in combination with other causes, can result in ulnar nerve irritation. With the elbow in full flexion, the confines of the cubital tunnel become restrictive and the retinaculum becomes taut, compressing the nerve. Flexion of the elbow and wrist extension increase the normal pressure on the ulnar nerve threefold, while overhead throwing increases the pressure on the nerve to six times greater than normal.[49] Recent research has demonstrated that the maximal strain on the ulnar nerve occurs in the acceleration phase, where the nerve moves an average of 12 mm with a strain of 13%; this measurement is close to the elastic and circulatory limits of the nerve, explaining the high incidence of nerve injury in throwing athletes.[50] The confines of the cubital tunnel may be reduced by scarring of the UCL (the floor of the cubital tunnel) or by osteophytes of the medial ulna at the olecranon or distal humerus. The cumulative effect of repeated and prolonged pressure elevations is nerve ischemia and fibrosis. This pathology can be exacerbated when it occurs in association with ulnar nerve subluxation or dislocation.

The first symptoms often are medial elbow pain and clumsiness or heaviness of the hand. Subsequently, paresthesias and more significant weakness may occur. Patients may note numbness at night in the ulnar hand if they sleep with the elbow bent. Throwers usually note loss of ball control. The results of nerve conduction tests can be normal, especially in the earlier stages of injury. Symptoms may be reproduced by a positive Tinel sign and/or by having the patient maximally flex the elbows and extend the wrists and hold that position for 1 minute. Overhead athletes may have a symptomatic subluxating ulnar nerve that may require surgery to prevent the nerve from becoming irritated as it traverses the medial epicondyle. Radiographs are usually normal, but MRI scans may reveal ulnar neuritis.

The initial treatment is nonsurgical, focusing on reducing ulnar nerve irritation, enhancing dynamic medial joint stability, and gradually returning the patient to previous levels and types of activities. Nonsteroidal anti-inflammatory drugs often are prescribed, and rehabilitation includes iontophoresis and cryotherapy (with care not to injure the nerve because of cold), although the initial goal should be pain control. This treatment may involve the use of a night splint to limit flexion and prevent recurrent compression and further damage, especially if there are also night symptoms. If stability is a concern, strengthening exercises should focus on the elbow flexors and extensors. Ulnar neuropathy may be associated with perineural scar formation, and thus nerve glides (taking the arm through a range of motion to allow improved gliding of the nerve in its native position) may be helpful in breaking scar tissue. In the athlete, ulnar neuropathy often is a sequela of some other pathology and will not improve unless the underlying pathology is treated. The patient is allowed to begin an interval throwing program when full, pain-free range of motion and muscle performance are not accompanied by neurologic symptoms, and the patient may gradually return to activity if progression through the interval throwing program does not reveal neurologic symptoms. However, throwing athletes tend to have a recurrence of symptoms when throwing resumes, particularly those athletes with subluxation of the ulnar nerve.

When nonsurgical treatment fails or is deemed inappropriate, ulnar neuropathy may be treated surgically. Decompression of the ulnar nerve at all sites of potential tightness is the primary goal. However, treating all possible sites of decompression may result in instability of the ulnar nerve and painful subluxation of the nerve out of its groove. For this reason, transposition of the nerve to a position that would prevent instability may be necessary, particularly in athletes.

Surgical treatment most often involves either anterior subcutaneous or submuscular transposition of the nerve. The disadvantage of subcutaneous transposition is that the nerve remains vulnerable to direct injury in contact sports. Submuscular transposition requires a longer rehabilitation because of detachment and reapproximation of the flexor-pronator origin, but the nerve is protected from direct trauma. With submuscular transpositions, the wrist also must be immobilized. The postoperative rehabilitation must be considered carefully because early motion is encouraged to prevent scarring about the nerve, but the flexor-pronator muscle attachment must be protected until it heals.

Simple decompression and medial epicondylectomy are thought to produce poor results in the throwing athlete because of the risk of UCL injury and subluxation of the nerve. However, simple decompression may be a reasonable alternative in nonthrowing athletes. Two recent prospective studies showed similar results for simple decompression and anterior submuscular decompression.[51,52]

Summary

The elbow is subjected to significant forces in sports, particularly in sports that require repeated gripping or throwing. Valgus forces of throwing result in medial-sided tensile forces, lateral compressive forces, and posterior compressive and shear forces. Understanding anatomy and pathophysiology allow for correct diagnosis and a coherent treatment plan.

Annotated References

1. Fleisig GS, Andrews JR, Dillman CJ, Escamilla RF: Kinetics of baseball pitching with implications about injury mechanisms. *Am J Sports Med* 1995;23:233-239.

2. Dun S, Loftice J, Fleisig GS, Kingsley D, Andrews JR: A biomechanical comparison of youth baseball pitches: Is the curveball potentially harmful? *Am J Sports Med* 2008;36:686-692.

   Twenty-nine pitchers (average age, 12 years) were studied. The greatest strain on the shoulder and elbow was with the fastball; the least strain occurred with changeup. The curveball was not believed to be a risk factor for elbow injury.

3. Olsen SJ III, Fleisig GS, Dun S, Loftice J, Andrews JR: Risk factors for shoulder and elbow injuries in adolescent baseball pitchers. *Am J Sports Med* 2006;34:905-912.

   The authors present a case-controlled study of 95 adolescent pitchers who had shoulder or elbow surgery and 45 age-matched control subjects. The factors most strongly associated with injury were overuse and fa-

1: Upper Extremity

tigue. Also associated with injury were high pitch velocity and participation in showcases.

4. Petty DH, Andrews JR, Fleisig GS, Cain EL: Ulnar collateral ligament reconstruction in high school baseball players: Clinical results and injury risk factors. *Am J Sports Med* 2004;32:1158-1164.

   The authors present a retrospective cohort study of 27 former high school baseball pitchers who underwent UCL reconstruction; 20 patients (74%) returned to baseball at the same or higher level of activity. Overuse and throwing breaking pitches at an early age were considered risk factors for injury.

5. Safran MR: Ulnar collateral ligament injury in the overhead athlete: Diagnosis and treatment. *Clin Sports Med* 2004;23:643-663.

   The diagnosis and treatment options regarding UCL injuries in throwing athletes are reviewed. Detailed physical examination techniques are presented.

6. Safran M, Ahmad CS, Elattrache NS: Ulnar collateral ligament injuries of the elbow. *Arthroscopy* 2005;21: 1381-1395.

   The authors present a current concepts review of UCL injuries, including a detailed review of surgical options and considerations.

7. Stahl S, Kaufman T: Efficacy of an injection of steroids for medial epicondylitis: A prospective study of sixty elbows. *J Bone Joint Surg Am* 1997;79:1648-1652.

8. Gabel GT, Morrey BF: Operative treatment of medial epicondylitis: Influence of concomitant ulnar neuropathy at the elbow. *J Bone Joint Surg Am* 1995;77:1065-1069.

9. Hotchkiss RN, Weiland AJ: Valgus stability of the elbow. *J Orthop Res* 1987;5:372-377.

10. Morrey BF, Tanaka S, An KN: Valgus stability of the elbow: A definition of primary and secondary constraints. *Clin Orthop Relat Res* 1991;265:187-195.

11. Callaway GH, Field LD, Deng XH, et al: Biomechanical evaluation of the medial collateral ligament of the elbow. *J Bone Joint Surg Am* 1997;79:1223-1231.

12. Regan WD, Korinek SL, Morrey BF, An KN: Biomechanical study of ligaments around the elbow joint. *Clin Orthop Relat Res* 1991;271:170-179.

13. Dugas JR, Ostrander RV, Cain EL, Kingsley D, Andrews JR: Anatomy of the anterior bundle of the ulnar collateral ligament. *J Shoulder Elbow Surg* 2007;16: 657-660.

   In a cadaver study of 13 fresh-frozen cadaver elbows using a three-dimensional electromagnetic digitizing device, quantitative data described the anterior bundle of the UCL.

14. Lin F, Kohli N, Perlmutter S, et al: Muscle contribution to elbow joint valgus stability. *J Shoulder Elbow Surg* 2007;16:795-802.

   Eight fresh-frozen cadaver elbow specimens were tested for the role of muscles on elbow stability. The flexor carpi ulnaris, flexor digitorum superficialis, and flexor carpi radialis may function as dynamic stabilizers, with the flexor carpi ulnaris being the primary stabilizer for valgus elbow stability.

15. Park MC, Ahmad CS: Dynamic contributions of the flexor-pronator mass to elbow valgus stability. *J Bone Joint Surg* 2004;86-A:2268-2274.

   Six cadaver specimens were tested and showed that the flexor-pronator mass dynamically stabilizes the elbow against valgus torque. The flexor carpi ulnaris is the primary stabilizer, and the flexor digitorum superficialis is a secondary stabilizer.

16. Seiber K, Gupta R, McGarry MH, Safran MR, Lee TQ: The role of elbow musculature, forearm rotation and elbow flexion in elbow stability: An in vitro study. *J Shoulder Elbow Surg* 2008 [published online ahead of print.]

   Fourteen cadaver elbows were tested. Medial and lateral elbow musculature affect total elbow varus-valgus stability equally, and the UCL affects stability twice as much as the muscles. The medial elbow muscles are most effective in supination.

17. Conway JE, Jobe FW, Glousman RE, Pink M: Medial instability of the elbow in throwing athletes: Treatment by repair or reconstruction of the ulnar collateral ligament. *J Bone Joint Surg Am* 1992;74:67-83.

18. Ahmad CS, Park MC, ElAttrache NS: Elbow medial ulnar collateral ligament insufficiency alters posteromedial olecranon contact. *Am J Sports Med* 2004;32:1607-1612.

   A controlled laboratory study of seven cadaver elbows showed that UCL insufficiency alters contact area and pressure between the posteromedial trochlea and olecranon, which helps explain the development of posteromedial osteophytes in throwing athletes.

19. Ahmad CS, ElAttrache NS: Valgus extension overload syndrome and stress injury of the olecranon. *Clin Sports Med* 2004;23:665-676.

   The authors review valgus extension overload in the throwing athlete and discuss the role of UCL insufficiency, evaluation, and treatment.

20. Eygendaal D, Safran MR: Posteromedial elbow problems in the adult athlete. *Br J Sports Med* 2006;40: 430-434.

   A review of UCL stress and injury and its relationship to valgus extension overload in the overhead athlete is presented, along with a discussion of the role of UCL insufficiency, evaluation, and treatment.

21. O'Driscoll SW, Lawton RL, Smith AM: The "moving valgus stress test" for medial collateral ligament tears of the elbow. *Am J Sports Med* 2005;33:231-239.

A sensitive test for UCL insufficiency was studied in 21 patients with surgically confirmed UCL insufficiency. A constant moderate valgus torque was applied to the fully flexed elbow and maintained; then the elbow was quickly extended. Level of evidence: II.

22. Andrews JR, Timmerman LA: Outcome of elbow surgery in professional baseball players. *Am J Sports Med* 1995;23:407-413.

23. Eygendaal D, Heijboer M, Obermann WR, Rozing PM: Medial instability of the elbow: Findings of valgus load radiography and MRI in 16 athletes. *Acta Orthop Scand* 2000;71:480-483.

24. Azar FM, Andrews JR, Wilk KE, Groh D: Operative treatment of ulnar collateral ligament injuries of the elbow in athletes. *Am J Sports Med* 2000;28:16-23.

25. Timmerman LA, Schwartz ML, Andrews JR: Preoperative evaluation of the ulnar collateral ligament by magnetic resonance imaging and computed tomography arthrography: Evaluation in 25 baseball players with surgical confirmation. *Am J Sports Med* 1994;22:26-31.

26. Nazarian LN, McShane JM, Ciccotti MG, O'Kane PL, Harwood MI: Dynamic US of the anterior band of the ulnar collateral ligament of the elbow in asymptomatic major league baseball pitchers. *Radiology* 2003;227:149-154.

The usefulness of dynamic ultrasound in evaluating the UCL was demonstrated in a case series of 26 asymptomatic professional baseball pitchers. In these athletes, the anterior band is thicker, is more likely to have hypoechoic foci and/or calcifications, and demonstrates laxity. Level of evidence: IV.

27. Sasaki J, Takahara M, Ogino T, et al: Ultrasonographic assessment of the ulnar collateral ligament and medial elbow laxity in college baseball players. *J Bone Joint Surg Am* 2002;84-A:525-531.

28. Rettig AC, Sherrill C, Snead DS, Mendler JC, Mieling P: Nonoperative treatment of ulnar collateral ligament injuries in throwing athletes. *Am J Sports Med* 2001;29:15-17.

29. Savoie FH III, Trenhaile SW, Roberts J, Field LD, Ramsey JR: Primary repair of ulnar collateral ligament injuries of the elbow in young athletes: A case series of injuries to the proximal and distal ends of the ligament. *Am J Sports Med* 2008;36:1066-1072.

In a case series of 60 patients who had direct repair of proximal and distal injuries of the UCL at 5-year follow-up, results were good to excellent in 93% of young patients (nonprofessional). Level of evidence: IV.

30. Langer P, Fadale P, Hulstyn M: Evolution of the treatment options of ulnar collateral ligament injuries of the elbow. *Br J Sports Med* 2006;40:499-506.

The authors reviewed the evolution of treatment options for UCL injury.

31. Dodson CC, Thomas A, Dines JS, et al: Medial ulnar collateral ligament reconstruction of the elbow in throwing athletes. *Am J Sports Med* 2006;34:1926-1932.

The authors discuss a case series of 100 consecutive overhead throwing athletes treated with UCL reconstruction using the docking technique. At 3-year follow-up, 90 patients (90%) were able to compete at the same or a higher level for at least 1 year. Level of evidence: IV.

32. Gibson BW, Webner D, Huffman GR, Sennett BJ: Ulnar collateral ligament reconstruction in major league baseball pitchers. *Am J Sports Med* 2007;35:575-581.

Sixty-eight major league pitchers who underwent UCL reconstruction were reviewed in a cohort study. Fifty-six patients (82%) returned to major league play at a mean of 18.5 months after surgery, with no statistical change in performance. Level of evidence: II.

33. Jobe FW, Stark H, Lombardo SJ: Reconstruction of the ulnar collateral ligament in athletes. *J Bone Joint Surg Am* 1986;68:1158-1163.

34. Koh JL, Schafer MF, Keuter G, Hsu JE: Ulnar collateral ligament reconstruction in elite throwing athletes. *Arthroscopy* 2006;22:1187-1191.

In a case series of 20 high-level baseball players (13 professional) treated with modified (three-bundle) docking UCL technique, 19 patients (95%) returned to play. Level of evidence: IV.

35. Paletta GA Jr, Wright RW: The modified docking procedure for elbow ulnar collateral ligament reconstruction: 2-year follow-up in elite throwers. *Am J Sports Med* 2006;34:1594-1598.

In a case series of 25 professional or collegiate baseball players with UCL reconstruction using the modified docking procedure with a minimum 2-year follow-up, 23 patients (92%) returned to their preinjury levels of competition at an average 11.5 months after surgery. Level of evidence: IV.

36. Rohrbough JT, Altchek DW, Hyman J, Williams RJ III, Botts JD: Medial collateral ligament reconstruction of the elbow using the docking technique. *Am J Sports Med* 2002;30:541-548.

37. Thompson WH, Jobe FW, Yocum LA, Pink MM: Ulnar collateral ligament reconstruction in athletes: Muscle-splitting approach without transposition of the ulnar nerve. *J Shoulder Elbow Surg* 2001;10:152-157.

38. Vitale MA, Ahmad CS: The outcome of elbow ulnar collateral ligament reconstruction in overhead athletes: A systematic review. *Am J Sports Med* 2008;36:1193-1205.

A systematic review of eight Level III studies is presented. The evolution in surgical techniques, most notably using a muscle-splitting approach to the flexor-pronator mass, decreased handling of the ulnar nerve; use of the docking technique resulted in improved outcomes and reduced complications.

1: Upper Extremity

39. Ahmad CS, Lee TQ, ElAttrache NS: Biomechanical evaluation of a new ulnar collateral ligament reconstruction technique with interference screw fixation. *Am J Sports Med* 2003;31:332-337.

    This cadaver laboratory study describes and tests the interference screw technique for UCL reconstruction using 10 matched pairs of cadaver elbows. Failure strength was comparable to that of the native ligament, and physiologic elbow kinematics were reliably restored.

40. Dines JS, ElAttrache NS, Conway JE, Smith W, Ahmad CS: Clinical outcomes of the DANE TJ technique to treat ulnar collateral ligament insufficiency of the elbow. *Am J Sports Med* 2007;35:2039-2044.

    In a case series of 22 athletes treated with UCL reconstruction using proximal docking and distal interference screw fixation, 19 patients (86%) had excellent results at mean 3-year follow-up. Of the three revision cases, one had a poor result. Level of evidence: IV.

41. Dines JS, Yocum LA, Frank JB, et al: Revision surgery for failed elbow medial collateral ligament reconstruction. *Am J Sports Med* 2008;36:1061-1065.

    A case series of 15 patients who underwent revision surgery for retear of a reconstructed UCL who were evaluated at a minimum 2 years is discussed. Time to revision was 36 months. Five patients (33%) returned to their previous level of play; 6 patients (40%) had complications. Level of evidence: IV.

42. Large TM, Coley ER, Piendl RD, Fleischli JE: A biomechanical comparison of 2 ulnar collateral reconstruction techniques. *Arthroscopy* 2007;23:141-150.

    In a cadaver study, 10 matched elbow pairs underwent UCL reconstruction with hamstring graft. The failure strength and initial and overall stiffness of a traditional Jobe technique are superior to that of the interference screw technique and reproduced the stiffness of an intact UCL.

43. McAdams TR, Lee AT, Centeno J, Giori NJ, Lindsey DP: Two ulnar collateral ligament reconstruction methods: The docking technique versus bioabsorbable interference screw fixation. A biomechanical evaluation with cyclic loading. *J Shoulder Elbow Surg* 2007;16:224-228.

    The authors performed a cadaver study of 16 UCL reconstructions using palmaris longus grafts and tested with cyclic valgus loads. Bioabsorbable interference screw fixation resulted in less valgus angle widening in response to early cyclic valgus load as compared with the docking technique.

44. Armstrong AD, Dunning CE, Ferreira LM, et al: A biomechanical comparison of four reconstruction techniques for the medial collateral ligament-deficient elbow. *J Shoulder Elbow Surg* 2005;14:207-215.

    The authors performed a cadaver study of 20 elbows testing UCL (intact and four reconstruction types). Peak load to failure of the reconstructions was inferior to the intact ligament. Docking and one-strand reconstruction using EndoButton were stronger than interference screw or Jobe technique.

45. Andrews JR, Heggland EJ, Fleisig GS, Zheng N: Relationship of ulnar collateral ligament strain to amount of medial olecranon osteotomy. *Am J Sports Med* 2001;29:716-721.

46. Kamineni S, ElAttrache NS, O'Driscoll SW, et al: Medial collateral ligament strain with partial posteromedial olecranon resection: A biomechanical study. *J Bone Joint Surg Am* 2004;86-A:2424-2430.

    In a cadaver study of seven elbows, an electromagnetic tracking device identified increased strain in the anterior bundle of the UCL with increasing flexion angle, valgus torque, and olecranon resection of 6 mm or more.

47. Kamineni S, Hirahara H, Pomianowski S, et al: Partial posteromedial olecranon resection: A kinematic study. *J Bone Joint Surg Am* 2003;85-A:1005-1011.

    Twelve cadaver elbows were studied with an electromagnetic tracking device. Sequential partial resection of the posteromedial aspect of the olecranon resulted in stepwise increases in valgus angulation with valgus torque.

48. Purcell DB, Matava MJ, Wright RW: Ulnar collateral ligament reconstruction: A systematic review. *Clin Orthop Relat Res* 2007;455:72-77.

    The authors present a systematic review of five Level III retrospective cohort studies that reported outcomes after UCL reconstruction. The Jobe and docking techniques were associated with high levels of return to sport. Transition to the muscle-splitting approach has decreased the occurrence of complications.

49. Pechan J, Julis I: The pressure measurement in the ulnar nerve: A contribution to the pathophysiology of the cubital tunnel syndrome. *J Biomech* 1975;8:75-79.

50. Aoki M, Takasaki H, Muraki T, et al: Strain on the ulnar nerve at the elbow and wrist during throwing motion. *J Bone Joint Surg* 2005;87:2508-2514.

    Seven cadaver specimens were studied and placed in the four phases of throwing. Ulnar nerve movement was increased during all throwing phases with increased elbow flexion. The average maximum movement was 12.4 mm, and the average maximum strain was 13.1%.

51. Bartels RH, Verhagen WI, van der Wilt GJ, et al: Prospective randomized controlled study comparing simple decompression versus anterior subcutaneous transposition for idiopathic neuropathy of the ulnar nerve at the elbow: Part 1. *Neurosurgery* 2005;56:522-530.

    One hundred fifty-two patients with ulnar neuropathy were assessed in a prospective randomized controlled study. No significant differences in outcome were noted in those with simple decompression compared with anterior subcutaneous transposition (65% and 70%, respectively). The complication rate was statistically lower in the decompression group (9.6% compared with 31.1%). Level of evidence: I.

52. Gervasio O, Gambardella G, Zaccone C, Branca D: Simple decompression versus anterior submuscular transposition of the ulnar nerve in severe cubital tunnel

syndrome: A prospective randomized study. *Neurosurgery* 2005;56:108-117.

In a prospective randomized controlled trial of 70 patients with severe cubital tunnel syndrome, 35 had simple decompression, and 35 had anterior submuscular transposition. At nearly 4-year follow-up, outcomes were similar (80% and 83%, respectively). There were no major complications, and electrophysiologic study results were similar. Level of evidence: I.

Chapter 5

Nonacute Injuries to the Lateral Elbow

Jennifer C. Laine, MD   C. Benjamin Ma, MD

Introduction

The lateral side of the elbow is a complex anatomic region that primarily involves the radiocapitellar joint, the lateral ligamentous complex, and the origin of the wrist extensors. Many patients repeatedly load or stress the lateral elbow during sports participation, recreation, or while at work. The three nonacute injuries to the lateral side of the elbow—osteochondritis dissecans (OCD) of the capitellum, posterolateral rotatory instability (PLRI), and lateral epicondylitis—have distinct pathophysiology; appropriate clinical evaluation, treatment options, and recent outcomes are discussed in the literature.

Osteochondritis Dissecans of the Capitellum

OCD is a symptomatic, localized lesion of the capitellum that affects the adolescent, most commonly throwing athletes and gymnasts. The late cocking and early acceleration phases of throwing create a valgus stress across the elbow, causing substantial shear and compressive forces to the capitellum. The compressive force in the lateral compartment is estimated at up to 500 N during throwing. In gymnasts, axial loading of the elbow contributes to injury. Many authors suggest that repetitive force is the key etiologic factor in OCD. It has been theorized that this repeated abnormal valgus stress on the elbow causes a change in the subchondral blood supply to the capitellum, which is primarily caused by posterior perforating vessels.

Patients typically present with an insidious onset of elbow pain and stiffness, with a history of minor trauma or overuse. They will often describe mechanical symptoms, such as locking and catching. Symptoms are usually aggravated by activity and relieved with rest. The patient history should include not only documenting the patient's age and symptoms but also the position played, the mechanism of injury, any exacerbating factors, and any family history of osteochondroses. The preadolescent with Panner disease, believed by some to be an early stage of OCD, will present with similar symptoms, with the exception of locking and catching. In contrast with OCD, Panner disease is usually a self-limiting disorder that tends to appear in children ages 5 to 12 years. The physical examination should include careful assessment of the cervical spine, shoulders, elbows, and wrists. Both elbows should be evaluated for tenderness to palpation, ligamentous stability, range of motion, and carrying angle.

Radiologic assessment should begin with AP, lateral, and oblique radiographs, as well as an AP view of the elbow in 45° of flexion. The earliest radiographic feature is subchondral bone flattening. The radiographic appearance typically involves a focal lucency in the subchondral bone of the anterior capitellum. The lesion is often surrounded by subchondral sclerosis and a characteristic crescent sign. CT, MRI, and ultrasound have been used to further characterize the lesion. Unstable lesions on T2-weighted MRI are surrounded by a rim of high signal intensity and occasionally a fluid-filled cyst, whereas stable lesions have no surrounding signal abnormality. Studies have shown good correlation between MRI and surgical findings.[1] CT and MRI can also be used to identify intra-articular loose bodies that could be missed on arthroscopic evaluation alone (Figure 1).

There are two classification systems for OCD of the elbow: (1) The International Cartilage Repair Society (ICRS) classification system uses radiographic assessment of the cartilage covering the bone. An ICRS OCD-I lesion is continuous and intact, OCD-II is in partial discontinuity, OCD-III is in complete discontinuity but not significantly displaced, and OCD-IV is dislocated or loose. OCD-I lesions, especially in the patient with an open physis, are considered stable. (2) An arthroscopic classification system was developed for OCD, based on the classification system for lesions of the talus.[2] Grade I lesions have smooth but soft, ballottable articular cartilage. Grade II lesions have fibrillations/fissuring, whereas grade III lesions have exposed bone with a fixed osteochondral fragment. Grade IV lesions have a loose but nondisplaced osteochondral fragment, and grade V lesions have a displaced fragment with a loose body (Figure 2). For both systems, the grade of the lesion corresponds to the recommended treatment.

Long-term sequelae of untreated OCD include progressive articular damage secondary to third body wear,

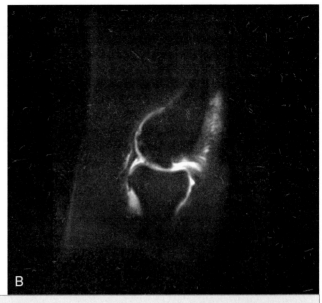
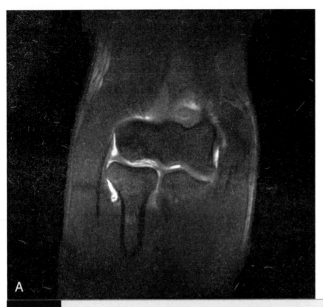

Figure 1 A and B, Magnetic resonance arthrograms of the elbow showing OCD of the capitellum. (*Courtesy of C. Benjamin Ma, MD, San Francisco, CA.*)

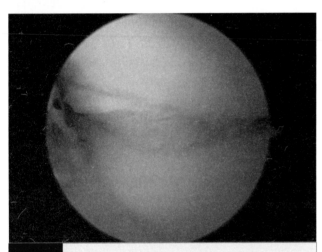

Figure 2 Arthroscopic view of the grade III OCD lesion in the same patient as in Figure 1. (*Courtesy of C. Benjamin Ma, MD, San Francisco, CA.*)

decreased range of motion, pain, and degenerative changes with osteophyte formation. Studies have shown that there are very limited indications for nonsurgical management of OCD. OCD-I or -II lesions in patients with open physes may heal spontaneously, but it has been shown that most lesions in elbows with closed physes fail to heal with nonsurgical treatment. Conservative management consists mainly of rest. Activity modification to reduce the repetitive loading of the elbow is crucial. Some authors also recommend a hinged elbow brace. In a 2008 retrospective review of 176 patients with osteochondrosis of the humeral head, a 90.5% healing rate for stage I lesions and a 52% healing rate for stage II lesions treated nonsurgically was reported. Treatment consisted of discontinuation

of heavy use of the elbow for at least 6 months. The mean period of healing was 14.9 months for stage I lesions and 12.3 months for stage II lesions.[3] Patients with open physes treated with rest showed significantly better healing, greater relief of pain, faster return to sports activity, and favorable radiographic findings than did those patients with closed physes. Also, patients with open physes treated with rest fared significantly better with respect to pain relief, radiographic findings, and healing in comparison with patients with open physes who continued their activities. Nonsurgical management has typically been described for intact, stable (grade I) lesions. Proposed indications for surgical intervention include persistent symptoms despite rest and activity modification, articular cartilage fracture (grade II or greater), symptomatic loose bodies, restricted elbow range of motion (greater than 20°), and a closed capitellar physis. A variety of surgical procedures have been described, but the choice of surgical procedure remains controversial.

In a retrospective review of 16 patients treated with arthroscopic chondroplasty and removal of loose bodies, 13 of 16 returned to their preoperative levels of activity. Half of the patients showed slight residual flattening on radiographs at an average 4 years of follow-up.[2] Another retrospective review of 10 baseball players at average 3.9-year follow-up after arthroscopic treatment reported excellent results on a standard rating scale, but only 4 of 10 returned to play and progressed with their peers.[4] Studies with longer follow-up (12 years, 23 years) reported that approximately 50% of the patients with OCD, whether treated with nonsurgical or arthroscopic treatment, have residual symptoms with activities of daily living, most commonly impaired motion or pain with effort.[5,6] More than 50% of patients had evidence of degenerative disease on radiographs. Approximately two thirds of patients had enlargement of the radial head diameter.[6]

Fragment fixation with bone graft has had satisfactory outcomes in the literature, although the case series have been small. In one study of four patients who underwent fragment fixation with bone graft and dynamic stapling, all patients achieved bony union, and three of the four returned to competitive baseball. At a mean 7.5-year follow-up, three of the four could throw a ball without pain.[7] Another study of 11 patients who underwent fragment fixation with pull-out wiring and bone grafting showed pain relief in all patients at an average 57-month follow-up; 10 of 11 returned to previous throwing levels.[8] A study of seven patients at 7- to 12-year follow-up after closing wedge osteotomy noted minimal degenerative changes on radiographs, and six of seven patients had returned to play.[9]

Reconstruction of the articular surface with osteochondral autograft pegs has been gaining popularity. The bone pegs are typically taken from the lateral femoral condyle or the proximal ulna. It is recommended that from one to three plugs be used, depending on the size of the individual defect. Reconstruction of 50% to 70% of the defect is considered sufficient. A case series of eight patients reported that all but one were pain free at a mean follow-up of 2 years; all but one had excellent or good clinical results. Radiographically, there was a normal contour of the subchondral cortex in all patients on plain radiographs, and the signal intensity had returned to normal on MRI.[10] A series of 18 baseball players at average 3.5-year follow-up showed that 6 of 9 patients with grade III lesions and 8 of 9 patients with grade IV lesions returned to playing baseball at the same level.[11] A recent study on the treatment and outcome of OCD lesions compared patients treated with fragment fixation (12 patients) and osteochondral autografts (33 patients) with those treated with fragment excision alone (55 patients). The results of fragment fixation or reconstruction were significantly better than those of fragment excision alone with respect to pain at an average of 8.2 years postoperatively.[3,12] There remains a need for randomization in the treatment of OCD lesions, as well as long-term follow-up for fragment fixation and osteochondral autograft procedures.

Posterolateral Rotatory Instability

PLRI was first described in 1991 as a distinct clinical entity, with an associated physical examination maneuver and surgical treatment.[13] The instability is often related to an injury, usually an elbow dislocation. Laxity of the lateral ulnar collateral ligament (LUCL), secondary to inadequate healing after injury, was traditionally described as the anatomic etiology for this instability. The ligamentous laxity allows a transient external rotatory subluxation of the ulna on the humerus, with a

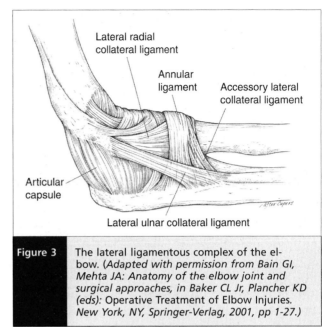

Figure 3 The lateral ligamentous complex of the elbow. (*Adapted with permission from Bain GI, Mehta JA: Anatomy of the elbow joint and surgical approaches, in Baker CL Jr, Plancher KD (eds): Operative Treatment of Elbow Injuries. New York, NY, Springer-Verlag, 2001, pp 1-27.*)

valgus displacement. There is also a subluxation or dislocation of the radiocapitellar joint, but the proximal radioulnar joint remains intact with the proximal ulna and radius moving as a unit.

The lateral collateral ligament complex, consisting of the lateral collateral ligament, the LUCL, the annular ligament, and the accessory ligament, originates from the lateral epicondyle (**Figure 3**). The humeral origin of the complex is the isometric point of the lateral elbow. The lateral ligaments insert onto the annular ligament and the ulna. The LUCL, often appearing as a thickening of the capsule, extends from the lateral epicondyle to the supinator crest, serving as a lateral stabilizer of the elbow and a posterior restraint to the radial head. PLRI was initially described as being caused by insufficiency of the LUCL, but more recent cadaver studies have challenged this belief, arguing that the entire lateral ligament complex shares the responsibility of providing posterolateral constraint. Studies have also shown that the radial head and the coronoid process are major static constraints to posterolateral laxity, and the common extensor origin contributes to stability.

PLRI is a clinical condition that is difficult to diagnose. Patients with PLRI typically have a history of elbow dislocation, recurrent sprains, or fracture of the coronoid or radial head. The injury typically occurs during a fall on an outstretched hand, causing axial compression, valgus force, and supination. Although less common, instability can occur from chronic attenuation of the lateral ligament complex secondary to chronic cubitus varus. PLRI also can be caused by iatrogenic injury following open or arthroscopic procedures on the lateral side of the elbow, such as for radial head fractures or lateral epicondylitis. Patients often report pain and discomfort in the elbow, with sensations of catching, clicking, or slipping with flexion and extension. The elbow is often most symptomatic in ap-

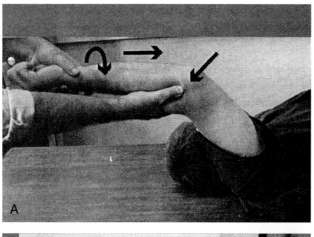
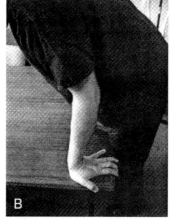
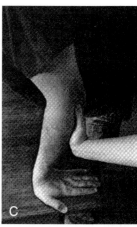
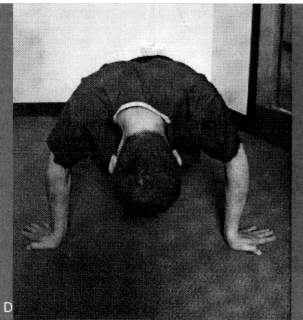
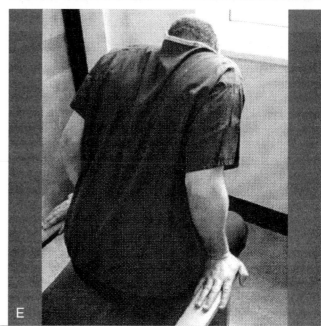

Figure 4 **A,** Lateral pivot shift test. The examiner is applying an axial load, external rotation, and valgus. **B** and **C,** The table-top relocation test. The examiner's thumb prevents displacement of the radial head and apprehension. **D,** The floor push-up test. **E,** The chair test. In the presence of instability, the patient will exhibit apprehension when pushing up from the floor or from a chair with the forearms supinated. (*Reproduced with permission from Charalambous CP, Stanley JK: Posterolateral rotatory instability of the elbow. J Bone Joint Surg Br 2008;90:272-279.*)

proximately 40° of flexion with forearm supination, such as when pushing on armrests when rising out of a chair. Patients may be asymptomatic during the activity while having frank instability.

The clinical examination is usually unremarkable unless posterolateral instability is specifically tested (**Figure 4**). Most patients have a normal-appearing, nontender elbow. The PLRI test is easiest to perform when the patient is under general anesthesia, but it can be performed on an awake patient, with apprehension signifying a positive result. The test is best performed with the patient supine, with the extremity over the patient's head and the shoulder in full external rotation. The patient's forearm is then fully supinated, and the examiner slowly flexes the elbow while applying val-

gus, supination, and axial compression. At approximately 40° of flexion, the rotatory displacement is maximized, and a dimple in the skin proximal to the radial head can be seen. As the elbow is placed into further flexion, a clunk can be felt during sudden reduction of the ulnohumeral and radiohumeral joints. This test is considered analogous to the pivot-shift test in the knee.

Another physical examination maneuver is the posterolateral rotatory drawer test, similar to the Lachman test for the knee, in which the extremity is again positioned overhead in the supine patient. The lateral side of the proximal forearm is pulled posteriorly in an attempt to subluxate the radial head. The test is considered positive if the patient becomes apprehensive during the test or if a dimple is seen in the skin proximal to the radial head. The prone push-up test, the chair push-up test, and the tabletop relocation test also have been described in the clinical evaluation for PLRI. In both the prone and chair push-up tests, the patient attempts to arise from the floor (lying prone) or from a chair with armrests by pushing up on his or her hands, first with the forearms in pronation, followed by supination. The tests are considered positive if the patient is symptomatic with the forearms in supination but not in pronation. In the tabletop relocation test, the patient performs a press-up on a table using one arm with the forearm in supination. The patient then repeats the maneuver with the examiner's thumb pressing on the radial head to prevent subluxation. If the patient is apprehensive with the first maneuver only, the test is considered positive.[14]

The elbow typically appears normal on AP radiographs, but slight widening of the ulnohumeral joint may be seen (the drop sign), which is indicative of instability. On the lateral radiograph, posterior displacement of the radial head relative to the capitellum may be identified. Performing the provocation tests under fluoroscopy or with stress radiographs can be useful in assessing the joint for PLRI, especially after an intra-articular anesthetic has been given. The radiographs should also be assessed for fractures, degenerative changes, and possible impaction defects of the capitellar articular surface. The appropriate use of MRI is controversial. There is conflicting data in the literature regarding the correlation between MRI findings and clinical instability. In some instances, when the presentation and imaging are not conclusive, the joint can be examined arthroscopically while performing the provocation tests to confirm laxity.

By definition, PLRI is a recurrent condition, and rarely does the instability resolve with time. Patients may attempt to prevent episodes of instability by avoiding the provocative maneuvers and guarding the elbow, or they may try wearing a brace, but in general, surgery is indicated in patients with symptomatic instability. The goal of surgery is to restore the integrity of the LUCL, whether through repair or reconstruction.

A Kocher approach is typically used, with a lateral Z-arthrotomy performed anteriorly to the LUCL. If adequate tissue is present, the lateral ligament complex can be reattached or advanced to the isometric point on the distal humerus, using a Bunnell transosseous suture. If repair is not possible, reconstruction is recommended. The palmaris longus, plantaris, and triceps tendons are most frequently described for LUCL reconstruction. The insertion site for the graft is prepared by creating two extra-articular, extracapsular drill holes in the ulna. The first is placed just posterior to the supinator tubercle, and the second is drilled 1.25 cm proximal to the first, at the base of the annular ligament. A suture is passed through the two drill holes and pulled toward the lateral epicondyle with a hemostat. The elbow is then flexed and extended to determine the isometric

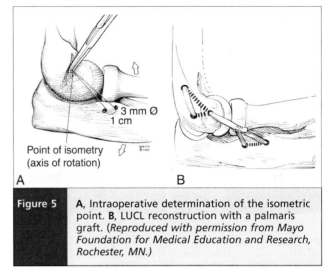

Figure 5 **A,** Intraoperative determination of the isometric point. **B,** LUCL reconstruction with a palmaris graft. *(Reproduced with permission from Mayo Foundation for Medical Education and Research, Rochester, MN.)*

ligament origin on the distal humerus, where the site of graft entry is then drilled. A Y-shaped tunnel is placed in the lateral epicondyle. The tendon graft is drawn through the ulnar and humeral tunnels and tied to itself after it recrosses the joint (**Figure 5**). The sutures are tied with the elbow flexed 30° and with the forearm in full pronation. It is important that the graft is taut in extension, because instability occurs in extension. The extremity is then placed in a long-arm splint with the elbow in 90° of flexion and the forearm in pronation.

Some authors recommend the use of arthroscopy, in addition to open reconstruction, to evaluate the degree of laxity, assess the articular surface, and débride the joint. Arthroscopic treatment of PLRI also has been reported for the use of electrothermal shrinkage of the lateral collateral ligament complex[15] and for tightening the posterolateral capsule with arthroscopic suturing.[16] If the instability is caused by fracture of the radial head, coronoid fracture or long-standing cubitus varus, then the radial head should be replaced or repaired, the coronoid process should be reconstructed, or a humeral osteotomy should be performed, respectively.

The literature reports a good outcome for most patients treated surgically with respect to pain relief, range of motion, and stability. Recent reports have shown that patients undergoing reconstruction tend to have slightly better outcomes than those undergoing repair alone. Also, outcomes are not as good in patients with generalized ligamentous laxity or degenerative changes within the joint.

An early series from the Mayo Clinic reported the outcomes of 11 patients treated surgically for PLRI at an average of 42 months. They reported excellent results with respect to pain relief, stability, and range of motion in three of three patients treated with surgical repair. In five patients treated with palmaris longus reconstruction, three had excellent and two had fair results. In the two patients in whom a synthetic ligament had been used, there was one fair and one poor result.[17]

A more recent series from the Mayo Clinic reported 12 cases of ligament repair and 33 cases of ligament reconstruction at an average of 64 months. Stability was restored in all but one patient at follow-up. Eighty-six percent of patients were subjectively satisfied. Overall, they found that patients who underwent reconstruction instead of repair, as well as those who had a traumatic etiology and subjective preoperative symptoms of instability, had better outcomes.[18] Another study reported four repairs and four reconstructions. Eighty percent of patients had good or excellent results, and there was no residual instability.[19] A series of 21 patients treated with arthroscopic electrothermal ligament shrinkage reported an average increase in the Morrey score from 40 to 77 at an average follow-up of 2.5 years. There were no complications and no episodes of recurrent instability.[15]

Relative contraindications to surgery are degenerative changes in the joint, radial head excision, generalized ligamentous laxity, and open physes. Complications of surgery include instability, persistent pain, nerve injury, fracture of the bony bridges, and flexion contracture. Multiple authors reported a mild, fixed flexion deformity on follow-up, but this was considered acceptable, for it usually did not affect function of the joint and because the most vulnerable position for the elbow is full extension.

Although PLRI is the most common chronic, symptomatic form of instability of the elbow, it remains difficult to diagnose, and the diagnosis is largely clinical. The literature supports surgical reconstruction of the lateral ligament complex, with improvement in pain and range of motion, as well as restoration of stability in most patients. In more recent years, arthroscopic techniques have been reported. Longer-term results, as well as comparative studies of arthroscopic versus open treatment, are needed to further evaluate the possible role of arthroscopy in the treatment of PLRI.

Lateral Epicondylitis

Lateral epicondylitis, also known as tennis elbow, is one of the most common causes of elbow pain in the adult general population. The dominant arm is most frequently affected. It has been attributed to overuse, especially repetitive wrist extension and/or alternating pronation and supination. A recent study from Denmark indicated that new cases of lateral epicondylitis are associated with strenuous professions, use of heavy hand-held tools, and repetitive nonneutral postures of the upper extremities. The condition was not associated with leisure activities. Also, lateral epicondylitis among women was associated with low social support in the workplace.[20]

The extensor carpi radialis brevis (ECRB) is considered the most common location of pathology, although frequent degeneration within the extensor digitorum communis has also been reported.[21] Anatomically, the common extensor tendon origin, consisting of the ECRB and the extensor digitorum communis, originates from the anterior surface of the lateral epicondyle. Histologic examination fails to reveal evidence of acute inflammation. The affected tissue instead demonstrates a noninflammatory angiofibroblastic tendinosis (not tendinitis), believed to be the result of an aborted healing response to recurrent microtears.[21] The source of pain generation is likely multifactorial. Immunohistochemical research has shown the presence of substance P receptors at the insertion of the proximal ECRB in subjects with lateral epicondylitis, suggesting a neurogenic involvement in the pathophysiology.[22]

Peak occurrence is in the fourth or fifth decade of life, with men and women being affected equally. Patients typically present with an insidious onset of lateral elbow pain in the dominant arm, exacerbated by active wrist extension and grip. On examination, patients typically have point tenderness 2 mm anterior to the tip of the lateral epicondyle, and pain can be reproduced with resisted wrist extension. The cervical spine should be examined to rule out cervical radiculopathy. The differential diagnosis also includes other sources of lateral elbow pain, such as intra-articular pathology, radial tunnel syndrome, and PLRI. The diagnosis is largely clinical. Radiographs may show radiocapitellar pathology or calcification within the extensor origin. Increased T2 signal intensity on MRI has been shown to correlate with surgical and histologic findings, although not with symptom severity.[23]

It has been shown that more than 80% of patients will have improvement in the condition at 1 year after diagnosis,[24] but more than 40% report prolonged minor discomfort with subsequent modification of their normal activities.[25] Poor improvement is associated with manual labor, dominant-side involvement, a high level of physical strain at work, and a high level of baseline pain.[24]

The nonsurgical management of lateral epicondylitis typically includes rest, nonsteroidal anti-inflammatory drugs (NSAIDs), bracing, physical therapy, and corticosteroid injections. In a multicenter, randomized, double-blind controlled trial, 129 patients were treated with either daily diclofenac or placebo for 28 days. There was a statistically significant reduction in pain in the treatment group, but there was no clinically significant difference in functional improvement or grip strength.[26] Alternatively, another multicenter randomized trial comparing a 2-week course of naproxen with placebo did not show a significant difference between the treatment group and placebo.[27] In a comparison of two NSAIDs, diflunisal and naproxen, no difference was shown.[28]

Randomized trials have shown that patients who are injected with a corticosteroid experience significant symptomatic improvement and increased satisfaction in comparison with patients treated with physiotherapy, NSAIDs, rest, and placebo at early follow-up (3 days to 6 weeks).[27,29,30] At 1 year, patients having undergone injection were no better or worse than patients receiving NSAIDs, physiotherapy, or rest.[27,29] Possible complications associated with injection are fat atrophy, skin discoloration, and rarely, tendon rupture. Botulinum toxin injection has received recent attention, with the intent of allowing the tendon to heal during partial paralysis or induced rest. Randomized trials have reported conflicting data regarding the effect of botulinum toxin on pain at 3 months, although they have consistently reported no significant improvement in grip strength.[31,32]

The classic regimen of physical therapy prescribed for lateral epicondylitis includes stretching, strengthening, and endurance training of the affected extremity. Eccentric muscle strengthening has been proposed more recently, based on the success seen in eccentric training for Achilles tendinopathy. In a randomized trial that compared stretching alone to the combination of stretching with either concentric or eccentric strengthening, there was no significant difference between the treatment groups.[33] Two types of braces are commonly prescribed: the cock-up wrist splint and the counterforce forearm band. A Cochrane review of five randomized controlled trials could not make a definitive conclusion about the effectiveness of either orthotic device.[34]

Extracorporeal shock wave therapy (ESWT) has been used to treat a variety of tendinopathies. The mechanism is not well understood, but the proposed mechanism of action includes the stimulation of a local healing response and inhibition of pain receptors. There are conflicting results in the literature regarding the efficacy of ESWT, and a Cochrane review of nine placebo-controlled trials reported little or no benefit regarding pain relief and function.[35]

It is estimated that approximately 5% of patients in a general orthopaedic practice and up to 25% in a complex referral population seen for lateral epicondylitis will need surgery.[36] Patients with persistent symptoms, despite nonsurgical management, for at least 6 months are considered candidates for surgery. Several techniques have been described. The classic surgical treatment is open excision of the degenerated tendon with subsequent repair.[37] This technique can be performed arthroscopically, and tendon release also can be made percutaneously. A 98% improvement rate after surgical release was reported, with 85% of patients returning to full activity, including sports.[37]

In a recent retrospective review of arthroscopic release compared with open release, there was no significant difference in outcomes, with 69% and 72% good or excellent results for open and arthroscopic release, respectively. The arthroscopic group required less postoperative therapy and returned to work earlier than the open group.[38] A recent large retrospective study compared open, arthroscopic, and percutaneous releases, with a minimum of 2 years of follow-up, and found no significant difference in outcomes between the groups, although each group had showed improvement since surgery.[39] In a prospective, randomized, controlled trial

of 45 patients treated with either open release or percutaneous release, the patients who underwent percutaneous release returned to work earlier and had a greater improvement in the Disabilities of the Arm, Shoulder and Hand score at a minimum of 12 months of follow-up.[40] Complications from surgical intervention include heterotopic ossification and iatrogenic PLRI.

Lateral epicondylitis is frequently encountered among middle-aged populations in both the orthopaedist's and general practitioner's offices. Most patients have good outcomes during the first year of nonsurgical management. Many nonsurgical treatment options are available, although recent studies show that the workplace environment may be more prognostic of outcome than the type of treatment itself. For the small percentage of patients who undergo surgical intervention, outcomes are generally quite good. The current literature shows that patients undergoing percutaneous or arthroscopic procedures instead of open releases tend to return to work significantly earlier.

Summary

The lateral side of the elbow contains complex anatomy and the surgeon should carefully consider the history, presentation, and examination of this particular area. It is hoped that increased focus on these injuries will enhance the ability to establish the correct diagnosis and administer appropriate treatment.

Annotated References

1. Kijowski R, De Smet AA: MRI findings of osteochondritis dissecans of the capitellum with surgical correlation. *AJR Am J Roentgenol* 2005;185:1453-1459.

   In this study, MRI findings were correlated with arthroscopic findings of OCD lesions of the capitellum. Stable and unstable OCD lesions have different appearances in the periphery of lesions on T2-weighted images. The presence of a peripheral ring of high signal intensity indicates unstable lesions.

2. Baumgarten TE, Andrews JR, Satterwhite YE: The arthroscopic classification and treatment of osteochondritis dissecans of the capitellum. *Am J Sports Med* 1998; 26:520-523.

3. Matsuura T, Kashiwaguchi S, Iwase T, Takeda Y, Yasui N: Conservative treatment for osteochondrosis of the humeral capitellum. *Am J Sports Med* 2008;36:868-872.

   In this study, 176 patients with osteochondrosis of the humeral capitellum were retrospectively reviewed. One hundred one patients had conservative treatment with discontinuation of heavy use of the elbow for 6 months. Conservative treatment led to healing of 90.5% of the stage I lesions and 52.9% of the stage II lesions. The mean period of healing was 14.9 months and 12.3 months, respectively. For the 75 patients who did not undergo conservative treatment against medical advice, 22.7% of the lesions healed.

4. Byrd JW, Jones KS: Arthroscopic surgery for isolated capitellar osteochondritis dissecans in adolescent baseball players: Minimum three-year follow-up. *Am J Sports Med* 2002;30:474-478.

5. Takahara M, Ogino T, Sasaki I, Kato H, Minami A, Kaneda K: Long term outcome of osteochondritis dissecans of the humeral capitellum. *Clin Orthop Relat Res* 1999;363:108-115.

6. Bauer M, Jonsson K, Josefsson PO, Linden B: Osteochondritis dissecans of the elbow: A long-term follow-up study. *Clin Orthop Relat Res* 1992;284:156-160.

7. Harada M, Ogino T, Takahara M, Ishigaki D, Kashiwa H, Kanauchi Y: Fragment fixation with a bone graft and dynamic staples for osteochondritis dissecans of the humeral capitellum. *J Shoulder Elbow Surg* 2002;11:368-372.

8. Takeda H, Watarai K, Matsushita T, Saito T, Terashima Y: A surgical treatment for unstable osteochondritis dissecans lesions of the humeral capitellum in adolescent baseball players. *Am J Sports Med* 2002;30:713-717.

9. Kiyoshige Y, Takagi M, Yuasa K, Hamasaki M: Closed-wedge osteotomy for osteochondritis dissecans of the capitellum: A 7 to 12 year follow-up. *Am J Sports Med* 2000;28:534-537.

10. Iwasaki N, Kato H, Ishikawa J, Saitoh S, Minami A: Autologous osteochondral mosaicplasty for capitellar osteochondritis dissecans in teenaged patients. *Am J Sports Med* 2006;34:1233-1239.

    This case series of eight patients with advanced OCD who underwent mosaicplasty reported seven of eight patients free of pain at 24-month follow-up. Radiographic incorporation of graft was seen in all patients, and the signal intensity returned to normal on MRI.

11. Yamamoto Y, Ishibashi Y, Tsuda E, Sato H, Toh S: Osteochondral autograft transplantation for osteochondritis dissecans of the elbow in juvenile baseball players: Minimum 2-year follow-up. *Am J Sports Med* 2006;34:714-720.

    This case series reports the outcomes of 18 baseball players who underwent osteochondral autograft transplant. Subjective scores improved in patients with grade III and IV lesions, but objective scores improved only in the grade IV patients.

12. Takahara M, Mura N, Sasaki J, Harada M, Ogino T: Classification, treatment, and outcome of osteochondritis dissecans of the humeral capitellum: Surgical technique. *J Bone Joint Surg Am* 2008;90:47-62.

    The authors give a clear description of their recommended preoperative assessment, surgical indications, choice of surgical procedure, and postoperative management. A thorough description of the surgical technique for arthroscopic fragment removal, fragment fixation, and articular surface reconstruction is presented.

13. O'Driscoll SW, Bell DF, Morrey BF: Posterolateral rotatory instability of the elbow. *J Bone Joint Surg Am* 1991;73:440-446.

14. Arvind CH, Hargreaves DG: Tabletop relocation test: A new clinical test for posterolateral rotatory instability of the elbow. *J Shoulder Elbow Surg* 2006;15:707-708.

    The authors describe a new clinical test for the assessment of posterolateral instability. Eight patients were assessed with this test. Six underwent surgical reconstruction, and the test was subsequently negative postoperatively in all six.

15. Spahn G, Kirschbaum S, Klinger HM, Wittig R: Arthroscopic electrothermal shrinkage of chronic posterolateral elbow instability: Good or moderate outcome in 21 patients followed for an average of 2.5 years. *Acta Orthop* 2006;77:285-289.

    Twenty-one patients with chronic PLRI underwent arthroscopic electrothermal ligament shrinkage with a bipolar probe. The Morrey score increased from 40 to 77 points: 11 patients had good results, 10 had moderate results. Manual stress radiography showed a mean lateral joint opening of 13 mm preoperatively and 2 mm postoperatively.

16. Smith JP III, Savoie FH III, Field LD: Posterolateral rotatory instability of the elbow. *Clin Sports Med* 2001;20:47-58.

17. Nestor BJ, O'Driscoll SW, Morrey BF: Ligamentous reconstruction for posterolateral rotatory instability of the elbow. *J Bone Joint Surg Am* 1992;74:1235-1241.

18. Sanchez-Sotelo J, Morrey BF, O'Driscoll SW: Ligamentous repair and reconstruction for posterolateral rotatory instability of the elbow. *J Bone Joint Surg Br* 2005;87:54-61.

    This series reports the results of 12 patients treated by lateral ligament complex repair with reattachment or imbrication and 32 by reconstruction. Stability was restored in all but 5 patients. The mean Mayo elbow performance score was 85 points: 17 excellent, 17 good, and 10 fair. The results of reconstruction were better than repair. Better results were also obtained in patients who had a traumatic cause and those with symptoms of instability on presentation.

19. Lee BP, Teo LH: Surgical reconstruction for posterolateral rotatory instability of the elbow. *J Shoulder Elbow Surg* 2003;12:476-479.

    In this series, four patients underwent ligament advancement and imbrication and six underwent reconstruction with palmaris longus or semitendinosus. There were no instances of postoperative residual instability; 80% had good or excellent result, and all reported no or mild pain.

20. Haahr JP, Andersen JH: Physical and psychosocial risk factors for lateral epicondylitis: A population based

case-referent study. *Occup Environ Med* 2003;60: 322-329.

This investigation compares questionnaire results from new cases of lateral epicondylitis to those of control subjects in general practitioner populations. New cases of lateral epicondylitis were related to physical workplace factors, such as nonneutral postures of hands and arms, the use of heavy tools, and high physical strain. It was also associated with women in an environment of low social support.

21. Nirschl RP, Ashman ES: Elbow tendinopathy: Tennis elbow. *Clin Sports Med* 2003;22:813-836.

This thorough review of lateral and medial epicondylitis includes etiology, pathology, evaluation, and nonsurgical and surgical options. The results of the senior author's surgical experience (> 1,300 cases) are briefly discussed, with 85% complete pain relief and full-strength return in the group treated for lateral epicondylitis.

22. Ljung BO, Alfredson H, Forsgren S: Neurokinin 1-receptors and sensory neuropeptides in tendon insertions at the medial and lateral epicondyles of the humerus: Studies on tennis elbow and medial epicondyalgia. *J Orthop Res* 2004;22:321-327.

Using immunohistochemistry and antibodies to NK1-R, this investigation showed the presence of the neurokinin 1-receptor in the muscle origin in patients with medial and lateral epicondylitis.

23. Potter HG, Hannafin JA, Morwessel RM, DiCarlo EF, O'Brien SF, Altchek DW: Lateral epicondylitis: Correlation or MR imaging, surgical, and histopathologic findings. *Radiology* 1995;196:43-46.

24. Haahr JP, Andersen JH: Prognostic factors in lateral epicondylitis: A randomized trial with one-year follow-up in 266 new cases treated with minimal occupational intervention or the usual approach in general practice. *Rheumatology (Oxford)* 2003;42:1216-1225.

This randomized controlled trial assessed 266 new cases of lateral epicondylitis treated nonsurgically. After 1 year, 83% showed improvement; however, poor overall improvement was associated with employment in manual jobs, dominant-side involvement, and high baseline pain.

25. Binder AI, Hazleman BL: Lateral humeral epicondylitis: A study of natural history and the effect of conservative therapy. *Br J Rheumatol* 1983;22:73-76.

26. Labelle H, Guibert R: Efficacy of diclofenac in lateral epicondylitis of the elbow also treated with immobilization: The University of Montreal Orthopaedic Research Group. *Arch Fam Med* 1997;6:257-262.

27. Hay EM, Paterson SM, Lewis M, Hosie G, Croft P: Pragmatic randomized controlled trial of local corticosteroid injection and naproxen for treatment of lateral epicondylitis of elbow in primary care. *BMJ* 1999;319: 964-968.

28. Stull PA, Jokl P: Comparison of diflunisal and naproxen in the treatment of tennis elbow. *Clin Ther* 1986; 9(suppl C):62-66.

29. Smidt N, van der Windt DA, Assendelft WJ, Deville WL, Korthals-de Bos IB, Bouter LM: Corticosteroid injections, physiotherapy, or a wait-and-see policy for lateral epicondylitis: A randomized controlled trial. *Lancet* 2002;359:657-662.

30. Lewis M, Hay EM, Paterson SM, Croft P: Local steroid injections for tennis elbow: Does the pain get worse before it gets better? Results from a randomized controlled trial. *Clin J Pain* 2005;21:330-334.

This investigation randomized 164 new cases of lateral epicondylitis to naproxen, corticosteroid injection, or placebo. Pain scores were highest in the injection group on day 1, but by day 4, pain scores were significantly lower in the injection group than the other groups.

31. Hayton MJ, Santini AJ, Hughes PH, Frostick SP, Trail IA, Stanley JK: Botulinum toxin injection in the treatment of tennis elbow: A double-blind, randomized, controlled, pilot study. *J Bone Joint Surg Am* 2005;87: 503-507.

This controlled, double-blind study randomized 40 patients with chronic tennis elbow to injection with botulinum toxin or placebo. Using the Short Form-12, the visual analog scale, and a dynamometer for grip strength, they found no significant difference between the groups at 3 months' follow-up.

32. Wong SM, Hui AC, Tong PY, Poon DW, Yu E, Wong LK: Treatment of lateral epicondylitis with botulinum toxin: A randomized, double-blind, placebo-controlled study. *Ann Intern Med* 2005;143:793-797.

In this controlled, double-blind investigation, 60 patients were randomized to a single injection of botulinum toxin versus placebo. There was significant improvement in the visual analog scale score in the treatment group at 4 and 12 weeks and no difference in grip strength. Four patients in the botulinum group reported mild paresis of the fingers at early follow-up.

33. Martinez-Silvestrini JA, Newcomer KL, Gay RE, Schaefer MP, Kortebein P, Arendt KW: Chronic lateral epicondylitis: Comparative effectiveness of a home exercise program including stretching alone versus stretching supplemented with eccentric or concentric strengthening. *J Hand Ther* 2005;18:411-419.

Ninety-four patients with chronic lateral epicondylitis were randomized to stretching or stretching with either concentric or eccentric strengthening. After performing the program for 6 weeks, significant improvements were seen in all groups, and no significant differences in outcome were seen between the groups.

34. Struijs PA, Smidt N, Arola N, Dijk CN, Buchbinder R, Assendelft WJ: Orthotic devices for the treatment of tennis elbow. *Cochrane Database Syst Rev* 2002;1: CD001821.

1: Upper Extremity

35. Buchbinder R, Green SE, Youd JM, Assendelft WJ, Barnsley L, Smidt N: Systematic review of the efficacy and safety of shock wave therapy for lateral elbow pain. *J Rheumatol* 2006;33:1351-1363.

    Using the Cochrane Database, nine placebo-controlled trials and one trial of ESWT versus steroid injection were reviewed to determine the efficacy of ESWT. The placebo-controlled trials reported conflicting results, though 11 of 13 analyses found no significant benefit over placebo.

36. Kraushaar BS, Nirschl RP: Tendinosis of the elbow (tennis elbow): Clinical features and findings of histological, immunohistochemical, and electron microscopy studies. *J Bone Joint Surg Am* 1999;81:259-278.

37. Nirschl RP, Pettrone FA: Tennis elbow: The surgical treatment of lateral epicondylitis. *J Bone Joint Surg Am* 1979;61:832-839.

38. Peart RE, Strickler SS, Schweitzer KM Jr: Lateral epicondylitis: A comparative study of open and arthroscopic lateral release. *Am J Orthop* 2004;33:565-567.

    This retrospective review evaluated 75 patients treated with either open or arthroscopic lateral release. There was no significant difference in outcome, although the arthroscopic group, on average, returned to work earlier and required less therapy postoperatively.

39. Szabo SJ, Savoie FH III, Field LD, Ramsey JR, Hosemann CD: Tendinosis of the extensor carpi radialis brevis: An evaluation of three methods of operative treatment. *J Shoulder Elbow Surg* 2006;15:721-727.

    This investigation compared 109 patients treated with either open, arthroscopic, or percutaneous procedures for lateral epicondylitis at an average follow-up of 47.8 months. There was no significant difference in outcome between the groups.

40. Dunkow PD, Jatti M, Muddu BN: A comparison of open and percutaneous techniques in the surgical treatment of tennis elbow. *J Bone Joint Surg Br* 2004;86: 701-704.

    Forty-five patients were randomized prospectively to either open release or percutaneous release for tennis elbow. At a minimum of 12 month follow-up, the percutaneous group on average had a significantly greater improvement in the Disabilities of the Arm, Shoulder and Hand score as well as an earlier return to work.

Chapter 6
Hand and Wrist Injuries

Ruby Grewal, MD, MSc, FRCSC   Kenneth J. Faber, MD, MHPE, FRCSC   Thomas J. Graham, MD
Lance A. Rettig, MD

Hand Injuries

Because the hands are instinctively used to protect the body from the initial impact of a fall or contact with another person, hand injuries are common in athletes and can occur during several types of sports activities. It is imperative that these injuries are accurately identified and promptly treated so that deformity and stiffness can be avoided.[1]

Fractures

Phalangeal tuft fractures occur when the fingertip is crushed. There may be an associated injury to the nail bed. These fractures are considered stable and require only a short period of immobilization (10 to 14 days) for symptom relief. More proximal phalangeal fractures may be extra-articular, involving the shaft (transverse, spiral, or oblique) or intra-articular, extending into the interphalangeal joint. A clinical assessment of the extent of injury and the presence of any rotational deformity is essential. Radiographs can delineate the fracture pattern and identify any displacement. Most of these fractures can be treated conservatively, but fractures with excessive displacement, rotational malalignment, or an unstable fracture pattern should be treated surgically, with either closed reduction and percutaneous pinning or open reduction and internal fixation.

Metacarpal fractures involving the neck are often called "boxer's fractures". These fractures usually involve the ring or small finger and commonly occur after a punching force, typically resulting in an apex dorsal deformity. Clinical examination should be done to rule out rotational deformity or pseudoclawing (compensatory metacarpophalangeal [MCP] hyperextension and proximal interphalangeal [PIP] flexion). Lateral radiographs help identify the degree of angular deformity. Up to 15° of angular deformity can be tolerated in the index and middle finger, 30° to 40° in the ring finger, and up to 50° to 60° in the small finger. If alignment is not acceptable, closed reduction can be attempted using the Jahss maneuver (**Figure 1**). The hand is then immobilized in an ulnar gutter cast for 2 to 3 weeks. Active range-of-motion exercises with protective splinting can follow. Some studies suggest that no immobilization is necessary, and buddy taping alone produces acceptable results.[2,3] A recent study found equivalent Disability of

Arm, Shoulder and Hand Questionnaire (DASH) scores in patients who were treated with plaster casting and follow-up compared with those whose injuries were buddy taped and had no follow-up.[2]

Intra-articular fractures involving the base of the thumb, or Bennett fractures, occur when an axial load is applied to the flexed, adducted thumb. The forces of the abductor pollicis longus cause the metacarpal shaft to displace proximally, while the Bennett fracture fragment remains nondisplaced, as it is firmly attached to the base of the second metacarpal by the anterior oblique ligament (**Figure 2**). Attempts at closed reduction and casting usually are unsuccessful because it is difficult to maintain reduction in this unstable fracture. Percutaneous pinning or open reduction and internal fixation usually are necessary to ensure that a congruous reduction is maintained at the articular surface.

Dislocations

The PIP joint commonly is dislocated after an axial load and hyperextension force, usually in a dorsal direction. Radiographs may reveal a volar plate avulsion fracture (**Figure 3**). Treatment should consist of urgent

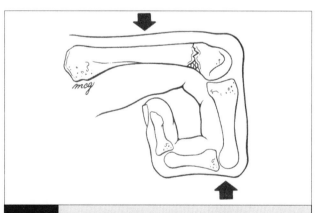

Figure 1	Drawing depicting the Jahss maneuver for reducing a boxer's fracture. Dorally directed pressure applied through the proximal phalanx helps to reduce the metacarpal neck and correct the underlying deformity. (*Reproduced with permission from Stern PJ: Fractures of the metacarpals and phalanges, in Green DP, Pederson WC, Hotchkiss RN, Wolfe SW (eds): Green's Operative Hand Surgery. Philadelphia, PA, Elsevier, 2005, p 283.*)

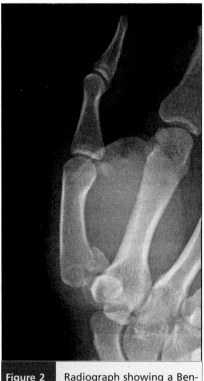

Figure 2 | Radiograph showing a Bennett fracture.

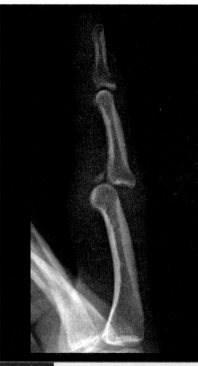

Figure 3 | Radiograph showing a dorsal PIP dislocation.

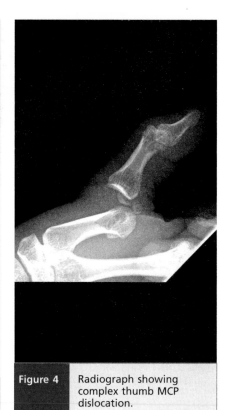

Figure 4 | Radiograph showing complex thumb MCP dislocation.

reduction, followed by extension block splinting (PIP in 20° to 30° of flexion) for 10 to 21 days, followed by an active flexion program using buddy taping.[4]

MCP joint dislocations most commonly occur in the border digits as a result of a hyperextension injury and are classified as either simple or complex. With a simple dislocation, the surfaces of the proximal phalanx and metacarpal head are still in contact, and the volar plate is draped over the metacarpal head but not entrapped in the joint. With a complex dislocation, the metacarpal head has buttonholed and become entrapped in the volar soft tissues (the metacarpal head is trapped between the lumbrical, flexor tendon, transverse bands of natatory ligaments and the superficial transverse ligament) (**Figure 4**). Although simple dislocations are easily reduced by closed means, complex dislocations can be difficult to reduce. Longitudinal traction will further tighten the soft-tissue noose around the metacarpal head, preventing a successful closed reduction. The wrist must be flexed to release tension on these tissues, and then a closed reduction can be performed by hyperextending the MCP joint, applying dorsal pressure on the proximal phalanx, firmly opposing the articular surfaces, and flexing the proximal phalanx. If attempts at closed reduction are unsuccessful, open reduction is necessary.

The fourth and fifth carpometacarpal joints also are a common source of dislocation. The mechanism of injury is usually an axial load to the two ulnar metacarpals, causing a dorsal dislocation. There may be an associated fracture of the base of the fourth or fifth metacarpal. Fractures and dislocations in this region may be difficult to identify on plain radiographs, and a CT scan may be required (**Figure 5**). Treatment consists of closed reduction (longitudinal traction and pressure on the dorsal aspect of the metacarpal base), percutaneous pinning, and immobilization for 4 to 6 weeks followed by splinting and active range-of-motion exercises.

Mallet Finger

A mallet finger (or baseball finger) occurs when there is a forced hyperflexion of the distal interphalangeal (DIP) joint and the extensor mechanism avulses from its attachment on the distal phalanx. The DIP joint rests in flexion, is and the patient is unable to actively extend this joint. If the tendon alone avulses off the bone, the injury is called a soft-tissue mallet; radiographs will demonstrate a flexed posture of the DIP joint but no skeletal abnormality. If a portion of the distal phalanx avulses with the tendon, this injury is called a bony mallet; a lateral radiograph confirms the diagnosis (**Figure 6**). Most of these injuries can be treated nonsurgically with a splint.[5] For both bony and soft-tissue mallet injuries, the splint must maintain the DIP in extension while allowing free range of motion at the PIP joint. Mallet injuries should be splinted full time for approximately 6 weeks, after which the splint can be taken off during the day but worn at night for an additional 6 weeks. Surgical treatment is indicated when there is an open injury or if there is bony avulsion with a large articular fragment causing persistent volar subluxation of the DIP joint with extension splinting.[5]

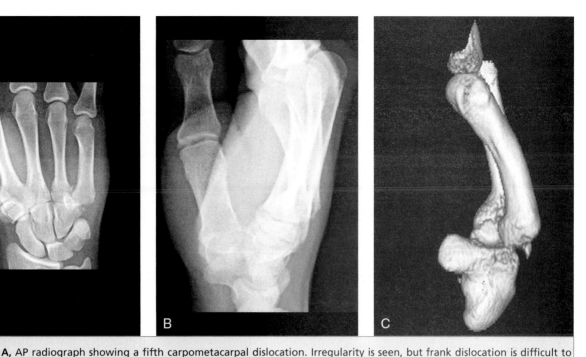
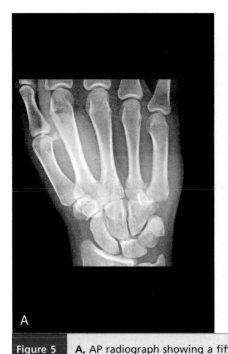
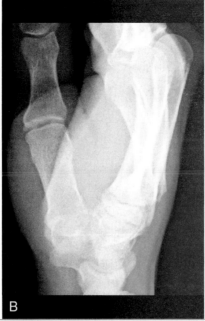

Figure 5 **A,** AP radiograph showing a fifth carpometacarpal dislocation. Irregularity is seen, but frank dislocation is difficult to appreciate. **B,** Lateral radiograph showing a further suggestion of dorsal dislocation of the fifth metacarpal. **C,** Three-dimensional CT scan clearly shows the dorsal dislocation of the fifth metacarpal.

Acute Boutonniere Deformity

An acute boutonniere deformity results from an injury to the central slip that may occur as a result of a flexion force at the PIP joint, a volar PIP joint dislocation with associated disruption of the central slip, or an acute laceration. With loss of the central slip, the patient is unable to actively extend the PIP joint, resulting in a boutonniere deformity (flexion of PIP joint and hyperextension at the DIP joint) (**Figure 7**). If untreated, this injury can progress to a fixed deformity, with contraction of the ligaments and volar plate over time. Radiographs may show a dorsal avulsion fracture at the base of the middle phalanx (avulsion of central slip) (**Figure 8**). Once the condition has been diagnosed, the patient's ability to maintain active PIP extension must be assessed. The PIP joint is passively positioned in extension. If the patient can maintain the joint in extension, the triangular ligament is intact, and treatment with splinting will likely be successful. The PIP joint should be splinted in extension (with the DIP and MCP joint left free) full time for 6 weeks, followed by an additional 6 weeks of night splinting. Surgical treatment is indicated when nonsurgical treatment fails, if there is an open injury (laceration of central slip), a large displaced avulsion fracture fragment (open reduction and internal fixation or fragment excision with repair of central slip with a suture anchor), or if there is an accompanying volar PIP dislocation.

Jersey Finger

Jersey finger is the common nomenclature given to a flexor digitorum profundus (FDP) tendon avulsion injury at the level of the distal phalanx. The mechanism

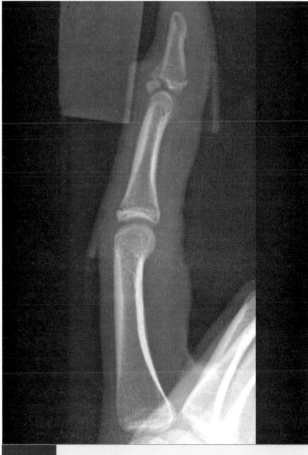

Figure 6 Radiograph showing a bony mallet injury.

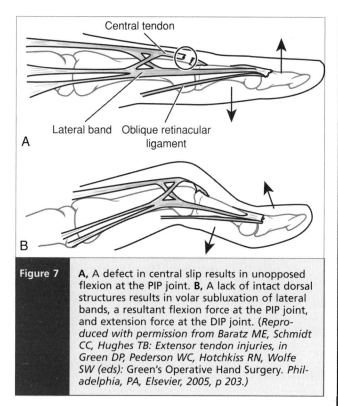

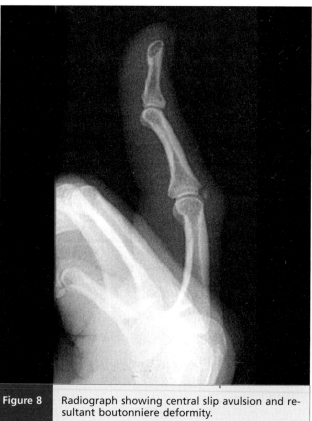

Figure 7 **A,** A defect in central slip results in unopposed flexion at the PIP joint. **B,** A lack of intact dorsal structures results in volar subluxation of lateral bands, a resultant flexion force at the PIP joint, and extension force at the DIP joint. (*Reproduced with permission from Baratz ME, Schmidt CC, Hughes TB: Extensor tendon injuries, in Green DP, Pederson WC, Hotchkiss RN, Wolfe SW (eds): Green's Operative Hand Surgery. Philadelphia, PA, Elsevier, 2005, p 203.*)

Figure 8 Radiograph showing central slip avulsion and resultant boutonniere deformity.

of injury is a hyperextension force applied to the flexed finger, such as that occurs when a player attempts to grasp an opponent's jersey. While the opponent accelerates, the player's finger is forced into extension against the active flexion force being generated. The flexor tendon avulses from the base of the distal phalanx (with or without bone) and retracts proximally. The degree of retraction is quantified according to the Leddy and Packer classification.[6] Type I injuries occur when the FDP tendon retracts to the level of the palm. With this injury, the blood supply is usually disrupted, and if treatment is delayed, the flexor sheath may not permit passage of the tendon. Type II injuries occur when the tendon retracts to the level of the PIP joint (the tendon sheath is not compromised, no significant contractures occur, and the tendon can be repaired up to 6 weeks after injury), and type III injuries occur when the tendon remains at the level of the DIP joint. When the finger is examined, the patient is unable to actively flex the DIP joint. It is difficult to predict the type of avulsion from radiographs and clinical examination. For optimal results, urgent surgery is indicated in acute cases.[5]

Pulley Rupture

Closed rupture of the flexor tendon pulleys is an injury commonly seen in rock climbers. The specific hand and finger positions required during climbing can result in significant force transmission to the pulley system. When the climber's hand or foot slips off a hold, even greater stresses are placed on the hand, and the biologic strength of the pulley can be exceeded, leading to a rupture. The middle and ring fingers are the most prone to

injury. Patients will report an acute onset of pain and may report a loud popping noise. Clinically, there will be tenderness along the palmar aspect of the injured pulley, with swelling and possible hematoma. Bowstringing will be visible only with multiple ruptures. Plain radiographs always should be obtained to rule out an associated fracture. MRI is highly accurate in identifying the dehiscence of the tendon from the bone (damage to the pulley itself cannot be detected directly). However, recent reports have shown that a dynamic ultrasound examination has similar if not better accuracy than MRI and can be considered the gold standard; only when the diagnosis is in doubt is additional imaging with MRI required.[7]

Single pulley ruptures should be immobilized for 10 to 14 days followed by supervised hand therapy and tape or rings to protect the pulleys. Multiple pulley ruptures are best treated surgically. Pulley repair has not been shown to produce adequate results, and reconstruction (with tendon graft) of the damaged pulleys is required. After surgery, the finger is immobilized for 14 days, followed by early functional motion with pulley protection as previously described. For patients treated either surgically or nonsurgically, sport-specific activities may begin at 6 to 8 weeks (with continued pulley protection) and full sports participation may begin at 3 months. Taping or the use of rings should continue for at least 6 months. Final results are usually good with near-normal recovery of motion and strength.[7]

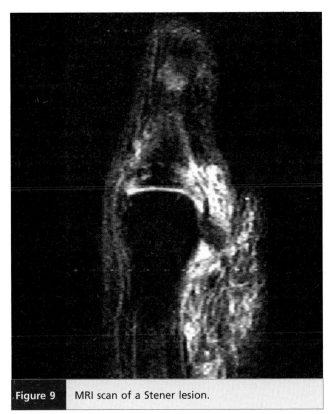

Figure 9 MRI scan of a Stener lesion.

Skier's Thumb

Acute ulnar collateral ligament (UCL) injury to the thumb is a common injury among skiers. The mechanism of injury is a sudden, forced radial deviation of the abducted thumb, which often results from a fall onto the outstretched hand while the thumb is gripping a ski pole. Patients will have tenderness and fullness along the ulnar border of the MCP joint. The thumb may be aligned in radial deviation at the MCP joint, there will be laxity of the UCL on stress testing (positive test if greater than 30° laxity is present with testing in extension and flexion or greater than 15° laxity when compared with the contralateral thumb), and there may be an appreciable ligamentous end point. In the case of a Stener lesion, a nodule of recoiled UCL may be palpable proximal to the MCP joint.[8] Radiographs may be normal or may reveal radial displacement and/or volar subluxation (suggests a significant dorsal capsular tear) of the proximal phalanx and possibly an avulsion fracture at the ulnar base of the proximal phalanx. Radiographs should be obtained before the joint is stressed to avoid displacement of a nondisplaced avulsion fracture. An MRI or ultrasound may assist in confirming the presence of an underlying Stener lesion.

Acute partial ruptures or nondisplaced avulsion fractures can be treated with 4 weeks of continuous immobilization in a thumb spica cast, followed by 2 weeks of splinting with active range-of-motion exercises. Strenuous activity should be avoided for 3 months. Large fractures with more than 2 mm displacement or with articular incongruity will require open reduction and internal fixation. Complete ruptures can be treated nonsurgically or surgically; if an associated Stener lesion (adductor aponeurosis is interposed between the distally avulsed ligament and its insertion into the base of the proximal phalanx) is present, surgery is necessary because this lesion will not heal with immobilization alone.

Ruptures that appear to be complete clinically may require additional investigation to rule out the possibility of a Stener lesion. Stress radiographs have been used to identify a complete lesion but are difficult to obtain in patients with acute injury because of pain and discomfort. With an experienced operator, ultrasonography is a noninvasive, inexpensive, accurate means of detecting a Stener lesion;[9,10] MRI is an accurate but more costly alternative[11] (**Figure 9**).

Traditionally, open reduction has been used with several fixation techniques, all resulting in uniformly good results. Recent studies describe arthroscopic techniques of reducing the Stener lesion followed by percutaneous pinning, thus avoiding violation of the joint.[12] Postoperatively, a thumb spica cast is worn for 4 weeks, followed by a protective splint and range of motion. Patients may participate in unrestricted activity at 3 months, but full athletic participation should not commence until 4 months (with continued taping or semirigid splinting as necessary).

Hook of Hamate Fractures

Hook of hamate fractures occur as a result of direct force during a fall or crush injury, or with repeated microtrauma during forceful grip while using a racket or bat during participation in sports such as golf, baseball, and hockey. Patients will have pain along the volar ulnar aspect of the hand, especially during activities requiring a tight grip. Callus may be present when examining the skin overlying the hook of hamate (suggesting repetitive trauma), along with pain during direct palpation over the hook of the hamate and possible dysesthesia involving the ulnar nerve. Standard radiographs may not reveal the fracture, making a carpal tunnel view necessary. Because diagnosis of these injuries is difficult, a CT scan should be obtained in any patient in whom fracture is suspected.

The recommended treatment for hook of hamate fractures that offers the most predictable option for pain-free results is excision of the fragment. There have been reports of success with cast immobilization; however, the risk of nonunion is high given the intrinsic forces exerted on this bone. Open reduction and internal fixation also has been described, with variable results; in the athlete, there is a risk of possible nonunion, and the mass effect created by the hardware can be bothersome. Range-of-motion and strengthening exercises may begin immediately after surgery. Patients may report scar sensitivity for 4 to 6 weeks. When an athlete returns to sports participation, a glove with a doughnut-shaped pad can be worn until the scar is no longer tender.[13]

Arthritis

The trapeziometacarpal joint is a common source of basal thumb pain commonly affecting older women but also is relatively common in younger patients. Symptoms usually consist of pain, stiffness, and difficulty with pinch and grasp. The treatment algorithm begins with conservative care, the use of nonsteroidal anti-inflammatory medications, splinting, and cortisone injections. Cortisone injections may provide temporary relief, but they also have been associated with accelerated joint damage and worsening capsular attenuation. Once nonsurgical treatment options have been exhausted, treatment for advanced disease is with trapeziectomy with or without ligament reconstruction and tendon interposition.[14] Although a viable option for the older patient who is less active, trapeziectomy is not suitable for young patients.

For young patients, surgical interventions traditionally include an extension osteotomy, which unloads the volar ulnar portion of the joint, redirects forces, and provides some pain relief in early stages of the disease. Traditionally, the other option has been fusion. Recently, there has been an increasing interest in arthroscopic management of arthritis. In younger patients, arthroscopic treatment is advantageous because it can offer significant pain relief without compromising future procedures. The arthroscope can be used to perform a joint débridement and synovectomy or to interpose a spacer (autogenous tendon, fascia lata, or synthetic material) into the degenerative joint. This technology is still evolving but may be an attractive option for the young patient with early arthritis.[15]

Ulnar Wrist Injuries

Athletes who participate in stick-and-ball sports frequently sustain acute or overuse injuries to the structures of the ulnar wrist. In addition to the ubiquitous possibility of direct trauma, all wrist structures are susceptible to the high angular velocity and torque demands resulting from striking or catching any object, accelerating or decelerating a long lever arm implement (stick, bat, club, racquet), buffering a fall, or grasping an opponent. Every tissue of the ulnar wrist may be injured, and combination trauma is not uncommon.

Osseous Pathologies

The most frequently encountered bone injuries are ulnar styloid fractures, triquetral body fractures, and pisotriquetral joint subluxations (with or without osteoarticular fracture). Additionally, ulnocarpal abutment, caused by radioulnar length discrepancy, may occur during participation in sports such as gymnastics or be a source of ulnar-sided symptomatology.

Ulnar Styloid Fracture

Ulnar styloid fractures often are associated with fractures of the distal radius and can be as different in pattern and significance as the morphology of the styloid itself. It is most important to determine whether a bony injury is stable or results in a destabilizing injury to the distal radioulnar joint.

Because the styloid is the anchor or limbi for the distal radioulnar joint ligaments, any clinical symptoms after fractures may be related more to the surrounding soft-tissue injuries. Styloid tip fractures and many styloid body fractures are not associated with significant soft-tissue disruptions. These fractures can be treated symptomatically; even nonunions of the ulnar styloid fractures that are nontender or not associated with distal radioulnar joint (DRUJ) instability can be simply acknowledged and observed.

When fractures of the styloid occur at the base or fovea, potential loss of DRUJ stability becomes an issue.[16] To determine whether the DRUJ has been rendered unstable at its bony attachment by a basistyloid fracture, examination in three positions of forearm rotation is necessary. In forearm neutral, physiologic laxity at the joint should be present. The radiocarpal unit translates rather freely in both the volar and dorsal directions; in patients with inherent physiologic laxity or a collagen vascular disorder, the magnitude of this translation may be considerable but still not reflect a pathologic condition. When the forearm is positioned in the extremes of either pronation or supination, the DRUJ relationship should be stable and resist manual translation.

When the DRUJ is stressed in pronation, excessive volar translation of the radiocarpal unit, which moves the ulnar head dorsally, may be indicative of a destabilizing injury. The converse is true in supination; if the ulna is moved to a volar position by manipulation, DRUJ instability may be present. It is often helpful to examine the contralateral extremity for asymmetry.

Advanced cross-sectional imaging (MRI or CT) will not add much diagnostic specificity to the evaluation of ulnar styloid fractures. However, evaluation of fracture behavior under live fluoroscopy, especially noting the largest degree of absolute displacement, helps to determine the severity of injury.

Triquetral Body Fracture

Isolated fractures of the triquetral body are rare, but most occur during athletic activity. When there is ulnar wrist pain distal and dorsal to the ulnar styloid, then triquetral pathology should be entertained.

Imaging of this fracture is challenging because the pisiform shadow obscures the midbody, where the fracture typically occurs. Both MRI (demonstrating edema and fracture) and a CT scan may be necessary when the diagnosis is elusive and triquetral body fracture is suspected.

Nondisplaced fractures can be treated with immobilization, and athletes may be permitted to participate in gloved sports (hockey and football). If fracture displacement occurs, variable pitch screw fixation placed through a dorsoulnar approach may be needed. Failure of the triquetrum to unite has been reported but is rare.[17]

Pisotriquetral Injury

Pisotriquetral pathology is a rare but recognizable cause of ulnar and volar pain. These injuries occur secondary to a combination of mechanisms: repeated falling onto the outstretched hand or fending off opponents with a dorsiflexed wrist posture (stiff arm), coupled with the strong activation of the flexor carpi ulnaris tendon in which the pisiform resides.

With loading and shear, there is a possibility of osteochondral fracture of the periarticular platform of the triquetrum or instability of the pisiform, in addition to crepitus, positional locking and unlocking, and pain.

Treatment of attenuation of the ligamentous investments that maintain the pisotriquetral relationship is brief immobilization, with some splinting or taping to limit flexor carpi ulnaris excursion. When a fracture has altered the articular anatomy of the pisiform or the triquetral platform, then power grasp or direct pressure on the pisiform region can be painful or manifest as perceived instability or weakness. In selected cases, the fractured fragments may cause definitive mechanical symptoms and should be removed.

Ulnocarpal Abutment

The relationship between the radius and ulna through the entire forearm axis is best thought of as a single mechanism in which the mobile radius circumscribes a "radius" around the forearm's stable unit, the ulna. In addition to rotation, there are relative length changes, as well as translations between the bones. The two critical articulations, the proximal DRUJ and the DRUJ, remain in appropriate articulation throughout the full arc of rotation. Ulnocarpal abutment is a mechanical pathology that can be either developmental or acquired as a result of chronic or acute injury to the forearm, usually to the growth centers of the radius in the skeletally immature patient (such as with gymnast's wrist). If the growth of the radius has been retarded by injury or repetitive compression (Heuter-Volkmann principle), then a radioulnar length discrepancy resulting in ulnocarpal abutment can cause ulnar-sided wrist symptoms. Although the biomechanical effects of increased ulnar variance on the ulnar wrist are well understood, few studies have been done at the microscopic level.[18] A recent study identified an increase in apoptosis within the cellular components of the triangular fibrocartilage complex (TFCC) in patients with a positive ulnar variance.[19] The study results suggest that deleterious effects at the cellular level take place as a result of increased ulnar length or ulnocarpal abutment. The spectrum of abutment and DRUJ instability are clinical conditions that can occur with positive ulnar variance. DRUJ instability results from a mismatch between the location or path of the sigmoid fossa of the radius as it accepts the articular ulna, referred to as the ulnar seat, or the portion that maintains

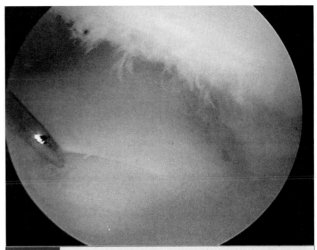

Figure 10 The arthroscopic image demonstrates a central attritional tear of the TFCC (probe palpating the defect). The findings of chondromalacia of the proximal ulnar pole of the lunate are consistent with ulnocarpal abutment.

direct articular contact with the sigmoid fossa of the radius.

Optimal treatment of recalcitrant ulnocarpal abutment has been a subject of debate. The relative success of conventional ulnar shortening and a subtotal, tangential distal articular surface resection (the wafer procedure), the two most common ways in which the ulnar column is recessed to diminish or eliminate the contact between the ulnar pole and lunate, has been studied.[20,21]

Because as many as 25% to 30% of patients undergoing TFCC débridement or radialization of TFCC tears alone had persistent symptoms, surgeons sought to decompress the ulnar column (**Figure 10**). The two options described differ in fundamental ways. Ulnar shortening osteotomy is an open procedure with substantial bony manipulation and instrumentation. The wafer procedure is a less invasive alternative that, despite technical challenges, is typically performed without substantial morbidity through standard arthroscopic portals or arthroscopy coupled with a minimally invasive approach to the distal ulna to remove the ulnar pole, the ulna's most distal portion that comes in contact with the undersurface of the TFCC articular disk, with an osteotome.

Investigators found that similar profiles of pain relief and functional restoration were obtained with both procedures. Patients undergoing the wafer procedure may have some ulnar discomfort for 3 to 4 months but ultimately achieve pain relief similar to an ulnar shortening osteotomy. However, secondary procedures (hardware removal) surrounding soft-tissue irritation (tendinitis) and more significant complication (nonunion) may occur during formal ulnar shortening.[20,21]

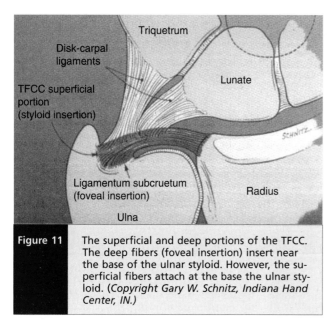

Figure 11 The superficial and deep portions of the TFCC. The deep fibers (foveal insertion) insert near the base of the ulnar styloid. However, the superficial fibers attach at the base the ulnar styloid. (*Copyright Gary W. Schnitz, Indiana Hand Center, IN.*)

Ligamentous Injury

The two most common injuries in patients with ulnar-sided wrist pain are to the TFCC-associated ligaments, including the radioulnar ligaments (or limbi) and the disk-carpal ligaments. These two separate ligament complexes represent the primary stabilizers between the radius and ulna, and the TFCC and ulnar carpus, respectively. Injuries to either or both of these soft-tissue stabilizers can cause pain or perceived instability that may prevent athletic participation.

Much has been learned about the soft tissues associated with the TFCC and volar ligaments on the ulnar side of the wrist.[22] The primary distal stabilizing ligaments anchored at both the ulna's foveal region and styloid medially and at the juxta-articular margin of the radius laterally direct forearm pronosupination and modulate joint reactive forces at the DRUJ while maintaining the stability at the forearm's distal end. On the volar aspects of the TFCC, so-called disk-carpal ligaments are the extrinsic stabilizing structures that originate from the vicinity of the volar DRUJ ligaments and insert on the ulnar carpus (**Figure 11**).

Although attritional tears and posttraumatic degeneration of the central TFCC disk are fairly common, substantial attenuation or frank rupture of the peripheral frame of the articular disk, the radioulnar ligaments or limbi, is rare. Chronic extension of a central TFCC tear that propagates into the margin, and substantial injury that causes acute rupture are two likely mechanisms by which the continuity of the limbi can be disrupted.

The frequency of diagnosis of these potentially destabilizing injuries appears to outpace their true clinical manifestation. The important role of the radioulnar ligaments for DRUJ stability was discussed in a recent kinematic study.[23] However, isolated sectioning of the radioulnar ligaments did not result in DRUJ instability because of other soft-tissue restraints.

Whether these ligaments are ruptured from the volar limbus or attenuated in their midsubstance, the patient may have a perception of instability during activities such as wrestling, setting in volleyball, or maneuvering opponents forcibly during football or hockey.

Even when ligamentous injury is appropriately diagnosed by physical examination, MRI, or wrist arthroscopy, treatment options are limited. Immobilization is the only realistic option; primary volar repair is likely not indicated unless there is concomitant volar limbus incompetence leading to DRUJ instability.

The true incidence and impact of lunotriquetral (LT) ligament ruptures is challenging to define. It is believed that isolated LT ligament sprains are fairly well tolerated, and brief immobilization or other nonsurgical modalities may be all that is needed to keep the athlete comfortable enough to continue sports participation. Although altered mechanics can result, many factors collaborate to maintain reasonable carpal alignment, even with a complete LT. Furthermore, no convincing evidence exists that long-term LT incompetence leads to an accelerated arthritis pattern, unlike scapholunate ligament rupture. Infrequently, LT tears affect overall wrist performance and perceived intercarpal instability, and the weakness that results from pain; LT arthrodesis, reconstruction, or repair may be indicated when immobilization or steroid injection is unsuccessful. A recent study indicated that the results of attempted LT arthrodesis yielded inferior results in a population of patients in whom ligament reconstruction was done.[24]

Cartilage Injuries

Injury to the TFCC is not uncommon in manual laborers or others performing hand-intensive activities; when symptomatic, these injuries affect patients in their 40s. The TFCC tears are likely to occur in athletes who perform repetitive, high force, high angular velocity actions (especially with a long stick or club).

An injury to the articular disk, the relatively avascular central component of the complex, presents as a tenderness in the ulnar wrist that is usually exacerbated by power grasp and ulnar deviation. Usually a small, radial-sided tear is suspected when tenderness is elicited by palpation through the volar portal, the region that permits access to the TFCC between the extensor carpi ulnaris and the flexor carpi ulnaris tendons. MRI can reveal a small fluid communication between the DRUJ and the ulnar aspect of the proximal wrist compartment.

Imaging studies are important in the diagnosis of ulnar wrist pain. A recent study suggests that MRI arthrography provides a higher level of accuracy in detecting TFCC injuries as compared with conventional MRI.[25] CT arthrography of the wrist is also useful in identifying pathology of the LT joint and central TFCC tears. However, a 2007 study demonstrated the limited sensitivity of CT arthrogram in identifying peripheral TFCC tears.[26]

There is no consensus regarding the actual etiology of pain in TFCC tears, specifically those of the central disk. When mechanical symptoms are present, as with large central flap tears, pain may be produced by joint dysfunction.

Pain secondary to TFCC pathology also may have a neurogenic origin. Investigators have identified a preponderance of mechanoreceptors within the dorsal and peripheral regions of the TFCC.[27] The receptors may play a role in emitting a pain response in not only TFCC tears but also DRUJ instability. In a cadaver study, the TFCC was innervated via articular branches from the dorsal ulnar nerve in all specimens.[28] The highest concentration of neural elements within the TFCC was located within the prestyloid recess, with free nerve endings extending into the meniscal homolog.

Débridement of recalcitrant central tears in the athlete with neutral or negative ulnar variance is the treatment of choice. In TFCC tears that are refractory to conservative treatment, repair is indicated. Several arthroscopic techniques continue to evolve for both ulnar detachment and the more technically demanding radial TFCC avulsion.[29]

Extensor Carpi Ulnaris

Athletes participating in stick-handling or racquet sports have the highest propensity for injuries to the extensor carpi ulnaris. Injuries vary from tendinitis to instability or subluxation of the tendon. Because of the unique anatomy of the sixth compartment, the extensor carpi ulnaris tendon is subjected to high force vectors with forearm rotation and ulnar deviation. Repetitive loading of the wrist in ulnar deviation may create inflammation within the tendon sheath. The most common mechanism is forceful supination and ulnar deviation. This maneuver, when directed acutely, may result in disruption of the extensor carpi ulnaris tendon sheath with secondary instability.

Recognition of true instability of the extensor carpi ulnaris can be challenging and is probably overdiagnosed. Additional etiologies such as TFCC, LT ligament, and osseous pathology must be considered when assessing the athlete with ulnar wrist pain. Isolated extensor carpi ulnaris instability is relatively uncommon.[30]

Increased mobility of the extensor carpi ulnaris tendon distal to the ulnar styloid that is reproduced while positioning the wrist from radial deviation/pronation to ulnar deviation/supination is suggestive of instability. Palpable dislocation or subluxation of the tendon may be possible during this maneuver in patients with complete disruption of the fibro-osseous extensor carpi ulnaris sheath (**Figure 12**). A recent article discussed the usefulness of dynamic ultrasound in the diagnosis of these injuries.[31]

The optimal management of these injuries in the acute setting remains a topic of debate. Although acute repair has been advocated, a period of immobilization with the wrist in slight pronation and radial deviation also has

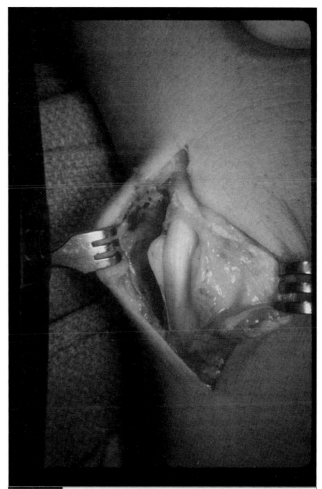

Figure 12 The intraoperative photograph demonstrates complete disruption of the extensor carpi ulnaris subsheath. Note the paucity of tissue remaining in the sixth compartment. In this particular case, retinacular reconstruction is indicated to stabilize the extensor carpi ulnaris tendon.

been recommended.[32-34] Most athletes respond well to nonsurgical treatment. The wrist is immobilized in a Muenster type cast for approximately 4 to 6 weeks, followed by a functional progression to sports participation over 3 months. This treatment approach, at all levels of competition, often results in either a stable extensor carpi ulnaris tendon or asymptomatic subluxation. In patients with recalcitrant pain and instability, retinacular reconstruction of the extensor carpi ulnaris sheath is indicated (**Figure 13**). Although direct repair is occasionally possible, the pathoanatomy is such that reconstruction of the sheath may be the only option in patients with painful, recurrent subluxation.[31,35]

Summary

Athletes can expect successful outcomes for most hand injuries, provided there has been accurate identification

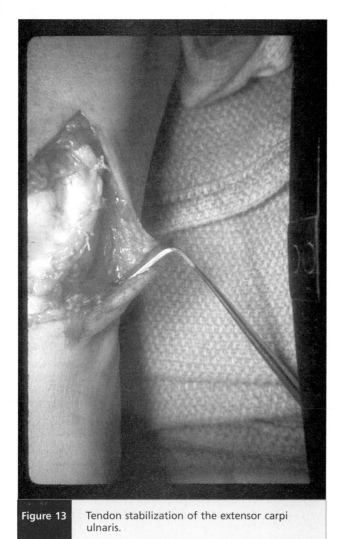

Figure 13   Tendon stabilization of the extensor carpi ulnaris.

and appropriate management of their injury. The importance of this cannot be overemphasized, even with seemingly trivial hand injuries. The specific needs of each athlete and the demands of the sport must be taken into account when planning treatment or a therapy regimen and discussed before the athlete returns to sports participation. A stable, painless wrist is almost a prerequisite for any high-performance athletic activity. The multiplanar motion requirements of this complex system are put to the test in essentially every sport, whether the demands are for great dexterity and control or for considerable strength. The complex anatomy and multiple articular relationships make injuries common and diagnosis and treatment complex. Developing a systematic, logical evaluation regimen supplemented by appropriate diagnostic imaging will serve the surgeon well. Enhancing the understanding of sophisticated treatments for wrist pathology may make the difference between returning athletes to play or limiting their participation.

Annotated References

1. Swanson AB: Fractures involving the digits of the hand. *Orthop Clin North Am* 1970;1:261-274.

2. Bansal R, Craigen MA: Fifth Metacarpal neck fractures: Is follow-up required? *J Hand Surg Eur Vol* 2007;32: 69-73.

   This study examined 78 patients with boxer's fractures: 40 received plaster casting and follow-up and 38 were treated with buddy taping and no follow-up. At 12 weeks, there was no significant difference in overall DASH scores between the two groups. The group treated with buddy taping returned to work earlier than the group that received plaster casting (2.7 weeks versus 5 weeks, *P < 0.01*).

3. Ford DJ, Ali MS, Steel WM: Fractures of the fifth metacarpal neck: Is reduction or immobilization necessary? *J Hand Surg Br* 1989;14:165-167.

4. Arora R, Lutz M, Fritz D, Zimmermann R, Gabl M, Pechlaner S: Dorsolateral dislocation of the proximal interphalangeal joint: Closed reduction and early active motion or static splinting: A retrospective study. *Arch Orthop Trauma Surg* 2004;124:486-488.

   Of 50 patients with dorsolateral PIP dislocations, 25 were treated with early active motion with a dorsal block splint and 25 were treated with static splinting in 30° of flexion. The authors concluded that early active motion produces significantly superior results when compared with static splinting.

5. Tuttle HG, Olvey SP, Stern PJ: Tendon avulsion injuries of the distal phalanx. *Clin Orthop Relat Res* 2006;445: 157-168.

   Injuries involving the distal phalanx, such as mallet finger and jersey finger, are reviewed. Level of evidence: V.

6. Leddy JP, Packer JW: Avulsion of the profundus tendon insertion in athletes. *J Hand Surg Am* 1977;2:66-69.

7. Schoffl VR, Schoffl I: Injuries to the finger flexor pulley system in rock climbers: Current concepts. *J Hand Surg Am* 2006;31:647-654.

   The authors review common pulley injuries as well as current diagnostic and therapeutic trends.

8. Stener B: Displacement of the ruptured ulnar collateral ligament of the metacarpophalangeal joint of the thumb: A clinical and anatomical study. *J Bone Joint Surg Br* 1962;44:869-879.

9. Jones MH, England SJ, Muwanga CL, Hildreth T: The use of ultrasound in the diagnosis of injuries of the ulnar collateral ligament of the thumb. *J Hand Surg Br* 2000;25:29-32.

10. Shinohara T, Horii E, Majima M, et al: Sonographic diagnosis of acute injuries of the ulnar collateral ligament of the metacarpophalangeal joint of the thumb. *J Clin Ultrasound* 2007;35:73-77.

With experienced clinicians, 100% specificity, accuracy, and sensitivity in detecting extra-aponeurotic UCL tears (Stener lesions) was reported. Although resolution is inferior to that of MRI, ultrasound offers a convenient, cost-effective, and reliable method of diagnosing displaced UCL tears.

11. Peterson JJ, Bancroft LW, Kransdorf MJ, Berquist TH, Magee TH, Murray PM: Evaluation of collateral ligament injuries of the metacarpophalangeal joints with magnetic resonance imaging and magnetic resonance arthrography. *Curr Probl Diagn Radiol* 2007;36:11-20.

MRI can be useful in detecting the severity of UCL injury and identifying retraction or displacement of the torn ligament, thereby helping to guide treatment decisions.

12. Badia A: Arthroscopy of the trapeziocarpal and metacarpophalangeal joints. *J Hand Surg Am* 2007;32: 707-724.

A review of the recent advances and indications for arthroscopy in the hand and wrist is presented.

13. Scheufler O, Andresen R, Radmer S, Erdmann D, Exner K, Germann G: Hook of hamate fractures: Critical evaluation of different therapeutic procedures. *Plast Reconstr Surg* 2005;115:488-497.

In this retrospective review of 14 patients with hook of hamate fractures, 6 patients had casts applied, and 8 underwent surgery (open reduction and internal fixation in 3 and fragment excision in 5). All surgically treated patients were asymptomatic at 3 months, whereas 5 of 6 patients in the casts had symptoms that ultimately required surgery.

14. Eaton RG, Littler JW: Ligament reconstruction for the painful thumb carpometacarpal joint. *J Bone Joint Surg Am* 1973;55:1655-1666.

15. Badia A: Arthroscopy of the trapeziometacarpal and metacarpophalangeal joints. *J Hand Surg Am* 2007;32: 707-724.

The role of arthroscopy in the small joints of the hand is reviewed.

16. Haugstvedt JR, Berger RA, Nakamura T, Neale P, Berglund L, An KN: Relative contributions of the ulnar attachments of the triangular fibrocartilage complex to the dynamic stability of the distal radioulnar joint. *J Hand Surg Am* 2006;31:445-451.

The authors performed a cadaver study evaluating the contributions of the deep and superficial TFCC insertions to the stability of the DRUJ under dynamic loading. They concluded that DRUJ instability can be produced by disruption of the TFCC foveal insertion.

17. Abboud JA, Beredijiklian PK, Bozentka DJ: Nonunion of a triquetral body fracture. A case report. *J Bone Joint Surg Am* 2003;83:2441-2444.

The authors describe a patient with an isolated fracture of the triquetrum who was surgically treated after nonunion of the fracture.

18. Werner FW, Palmer AK, Fortino MD, Short WH: Force transmission through the distal ulna: Effect of ulnar variance, lunate fossa angulation, and radial and palmar tilt of the distal radius. *J Hand Surg Am* 1992;17: 423-428.

19. Unglaub F, Wolf MB, Thome MA, Germann G, Sauerbier M, Reiter A: Correlation of ulnar length and apoptotic cell death in degenerative lesions of the triangular fibrocartilage. *Arthroscopy* 2008;24:299-304.

The authors obtained arthroscopic samples of degenerative TFCC lesions and quantified the level of necrosis and apoptosis in individuals with variable ulnar lengths. The results demonstrated a higher percentage of cell death in patients who are ulnar variance positive.

20. Bernstein MA, Nagle DJ, Martinez A, Stogin JM Jr, Wiedrich TA: A comparison of combined arthroscopic triangular fibrocartilage complex debridement and arthroscopic wafer distal ulna resection versus arthroscopic triangular fibrocartilage complex debridement and ulnar shortening osteotomy for ulnocarpal abutment syndrome. *Arthroscopy* 2004;20:392-401.

A retrospective review was performed comparing the results of ulnar shortening osteotomy versus arthroscopic wafer resection in patients with ulnocarpal abutment. Both groups (11 patients each in the osteotomy and wafer resection groups) achieved satisfactory pain relief. Five secondary procedures were required in the ulnar shortening cohort compared to one in the wafer resection group.

21. Constantine KJ, Tomaino MM, Herndon JH, Sotereanos DG: Comparison of ulnar shortening osteotomy and the wafer resection procedure as treatment for ulnar impaction syndrome. *J Hand Surg Am* 2000;25: 55-60.

22. Szabo RM: Distal radioulnar joint instability. *Instr Course Lect* 2007;56:79-89.

A comprehensive review of the pathoanatomy of acute and chronic disruptions of the DRUJ is presented.

23. Gofton WT, Gordon KD, Dunning CE, Johnson JA, King GJ: Soft-tissue stabilizers of the distal radioulnar joint: An in vitro kinematic study. *J Hand Surg Am* 2004;29:423-431.

The authors performed a cadaver study to identify the most important soft-tissue stabilizers of the DRUJ. They determined that the volar and dorsal radioulnar ligaments and the TFCC are important restraints. However, DRUJ kinematics could be maintained after sectioning the two structures if other soft-tissue stabilizers remain intact.

24. Shin AY, Weinstein LP, Berger RA, Bishop AT: Treatment of isolated injuries of the lunotriquetral ligament: A comparison of arthrodesis, ligament reconstruction and ligament repair. *J Bone Joint Surg Br* 2002; 84:1086.

25. Berná-Serna JD, Martínez F, Reus M, Alonso J, Doménech G, Campos M: Evaluation of the triangular fibrocartilage in cadaveric wrists by means of

1: Upper Extremity

arthrography, magnetic resonance (MR) imaging, and MR arthrography. *Acta Radiol* 2007;48:96-103.

The authors evaluated three methods to assess TFCC tears: conventional MRI, arthrography, and magnetic resonance arthrography. They concluded that magnetic resonance arthrography was the optimal imaging study in evaluating TFCC tears with a sensitivity of 100%, specificity of 85%, and accuracy of 95%.

26. Bille B, Harley B, Cohen H: A comparison of CT arthrography of the wrist to findings during wrist arthroscopy. *J Hand Surg Am* 2007;32:834-841.

The study compared the interpretation of CT arthrogram imaging with findings during wrist arthroscopy in 76 patients. Results revealed a sensitivity of 94% for diagnosing scapholunate ligament tears, 85% for LT pathology, and 91% for central TFCC defects. However, the study identified a sensitivity of only 30% for peripheral TFCC tears.

27. Cavalcante ML, Rodrigues CJ, Mattar R Jr: Mechanoreceptors and nerve endings of the triangular fibrocartilage in the human wrist. *J Hand Surg Br* 2004;29: 432-435.

The authors investigated the distribution of mechanoreceptors within the TFCC by using staining techniques. They identified a heterogeneous distribution of mechanoreceptors within the TFCC. Free nerve endings, believed to sense pain, predominated in the ulnar and dorsal portions of the TFCC.

28. Shigemitsu T, Tobe M, Mizutani K, Murakami K, Ishikawa Y, Sato F: Innervation of the triangular fibrocartilage complex of the human wrist: Quantitative immunohistochemical study. *Anat Sci Int* 2007;82:127-132.

Immunohistochemical staining techniques were used to assess the concentration and distribution of neural tissue within the TFCC. Articular branches from the dorsal ulnar nerve were found to innervate the TFCC.

29. Yao J, Dantular P, Osterman AL: A novel technique of all-inside arthroscopic TFCC repair. *Arthroscopy* 2007; 23:1357.

The authors describe an all-inside technique to repair peripheral tears of the TFCC. The technique evolved with the goal of avoiding painful external knots and dorsal sensory ulnar nerve injuries.

30. Allende C, Le Viet D: Extensor carpi ulnaris problems at the wrist: Classification, surgical treatment and results. *J Hand Surg Br* 2005;30:265-272.

Among the 28 patients evaluated, isolated subsheath injuries were uncommon. Concomitant pathology identified among the cohort included 11 TFCC tears, 4 LT injuries, and 4 ulnar styloid nonunions.

31. Maclennan AJ, Memechek NM, Waitayaminyu T, Trumble TE: Diagnosis and anatomic reconstruction of the extensor carpi ulnaris. *J Hand Surg Am* 2008;33: 59-64.

The authors describe a new technique for reconstruction of the extensor carpi ulnaris tendon sheath. Diagnosis in the 21 patients was confirmed with dynamic ultrasound. At an average of 31 months, improvement in pain and DASH scores wewas noted following tendon stabilization. Level of evidence: IV.

32. Rowland SA: Acute traumatic subluxation of the extensor carpi ulnaris tendon at the wrist. *J Hand Surg Am* 1986;11:809-811.

33. Burkhart SS, Wood MB, Linscheid RL: Posttraumatic recuurent subluxation of the extensor carpi ulnaris tendon. *J Hand Surg Am* 1982;7:1-3.

34. Rayan GM: Recurrent dislocation of the extensor carpi ulnaris in athletes. *Am J Sports Med* 1983;11:183-184.

35. Inoue G, Tamara Y: Surgical treatment for recurrent dislocation of the extensor carpi ulnaris tendon. *J Hand Surg Br* 2001;26:556-559.

Hip

SECTION EDITOR:
MARC R. SAFRAN, MD

Chapter 7

Groin and Pelvis Injuries

Jon K. Sekiya, MD   Aimee E. Gibbs, MPH

Introduction

Groin and pelvic pain associated with sports participation has become an increasingly common cause of both disability and impaired activity among athletes, particularly those involved in soccer, rugby, track, ice hockey, and football, where sprinting, kicking, and quick changes in direction are common.[1] In high school athletes, injuries to the hip area make up approximately 5% to 9% of all injuries.[2] In addition, groin pain can be the result of other medical conditions not related to athletic activity, including intra-abdominal disorders, genitourinary abnormalities, referred lumbosacral pain, and other hip joint disorders.[3,4] Also, there is substantial overlap of clinical signs and symptoms in the groin and pelvis region because of the complexity of the musculoskeletal anatomy, which makes the diagnosis of pelvic injuries very difficult.[1,5] In addition, as many as 27% to 90% of patients presenting with groin or pelvis pain have more than one coexisting injury. It is not clear if this is the result of one event within the region possibly causing multiple injuries because of the close proximity of anatomic structures or if it is caused by biomechanical changes resulting from the initial injury, increasing stress on other structures and leading to secondary overuse injuries.[3,4]

In response to the complexity in diagnosing groin and pelvis injuries, advances have been made in investigating and treating groin and pelvis injuries.[1,2] Recently, research on imaging tools for specific groin and pelvis conditions have shown improved diagnostic capability when used in concert with proper clinical assessment.[1] Also, new arthroscopic techniques have recently been developed to treat injuries unresponsive to nonsurgical management, with reported reduced morbidity compared to standard open techniques and the ability for the patient to return preinjury activity.[6]

Athletic Pubalgia

Athletic pubalgia or sports hernia is caused by a posterior inguinal wall weakness or tear, without a clinically recognizable hernia, leading to gradually worsening, deep groin pain of insidious onset.[4] Normally caused by overuse, athletic pubalgia occurs almost exclusively in men, particularly those who participate in sports with repetitive motions involving quick twisting and turning, such as soccer and ice hockey.[7] The gradual onset may lead to delayed diagnosis, with the patient presenting with deep groin pain that may radiate along the inguinal ligament, perineum, and rectus muscles and to the testicles in approximately 30% of men.[4] Patients may only become symptomatic with activity, coughing, or during the Valsalva maneuver.[4,7] Patients may also present with related abnormalities such as imbalance between strong adductor muscles of the thigh and weak lower abdominal muscles, causing stress on the inguinal wall muscles and leading to injury.[7]

Patients should be tested for local tenderness at the pubic tubercle, in addition to pain with resisted hip flexion, internal rotation, and abdominal muscle contraction. Also, some patients experience pain and tenderness along the adductor longus tendon with a resisted sit-up and hip adduction.[7,8] No diagnostic imaging is sensitive and specific enough to diagnose sports hernia; however, plain radiographs and MRI can be used to rule out alternative diagnoses. Ultrasound reportedly has shown findings at the superficial inguinal ring level, displaying convex anterior bulge and ballooning of the inguinal canal with active straining, potentially serving as a noninvasive modality to assess the potential benefit of surgical repair. Herniography has been reported to have a high false-positive rate or potentially overlook sports hernias. In addition, it has been associated with potentially low risks of hollow viscus perforation, vasovagal reactions, infections, abdominal wall hematomas, and reactions to contrast agents.[7]

Patients are initially treated with physical therapy (focusing on strengthening, stabilization, and balance restoration in the abdominal wall) along with anti-inflammatory medications, deep massage, heat or ice, and prolonged rest followed by gradual return to activity.[7] However, nonsurgical treatment has not been found to be overly successful.[7] In patients whose pain continues after 6 to 8 weeks of nonsurgical management, surgical repair of the weak posterior inguinal wall with conventional or laparoscopic techniques may be performed. Surgical treatment is successful in 80% to 97% of cases. When adductor abnormalities are not effectively treated preoperatively, an adductor tenotomy may be performed to treat pelvic muscle imbalance because of a contracted or overdeveloped adductor muscle. Following surgical treatment, most athletes return to sports participation 2 to 6 weeks after laparoscopic repair and within 1 to 6 months after open repair.[7]

Stress Fractures of the Pelvis and Femoral Neck

A stress fracture of the femoral neck is a rare but severe injury that often is the result of muscle fatigue or repetitive overload, which can lead to delayed union, non-

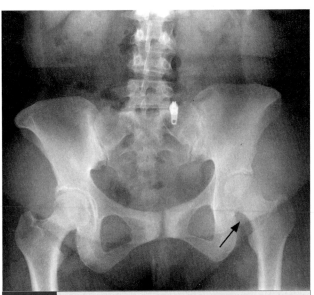

Figure 1 Stress fracture of the left femoral neck was not identifiable on the patient's plain radiographs (arrow points to area of stress fracture).

union, or osteonecrosis of the femoral head.[9] Stress fractures of the pelvis may occur in the sacrum or pelvic rami, particularly at the ischium and inferior pubic ramus junction, and are characterized by worsening pain with activity.[3] Stress fractures of the pelvis or femoral neck often occur in long-distance runners, professional athletes, military personnel, and ballet dancers.[9] Patients with stress fractures of the pelvis may present with localized pain that is relieved with rest, whereas patients with stress fractures of the femoral neck may describe a more ill-defined pain.[9] Stress fractures of the femoral neck often are associated with painful internal rotation of the hip and an inability to hop on the affected limb. In stress fractures of the pelvis, the patient may feel pain with palpation over the pubic ramus, as well as with one leg standing or jumping.[3] Plain radiographs (**Figure 1**) may be useful, but a negative result in a symptomatic patient may require an MRI or a bone scan to determine the presence of an occult stress fracture of the pelvis or femoral neck[10] (**Figure 2**).

Most stress fractures of the pelvis and femur can be treated nonsurgically with rest and subsequent activity modification.[3,10] It is also important that contributory factors to the onset of the stress fracture be addressed, including training errors such as continually increasing the training regimen to exceed the rate of bone repair. In addition, special attention should be placed on proper nutrition and hormonal deficiencies, particularly in female athletes, who are at risk of amenorrhea and resulting bone loss. Patients in whom dietary-based osteopenia is an associated factor will need restoration of proper nutrition to aid in a quicker return to activity. Rehabilitation for stress fractures to the femoral neck and pelvis involves a stepwise process of gradual return

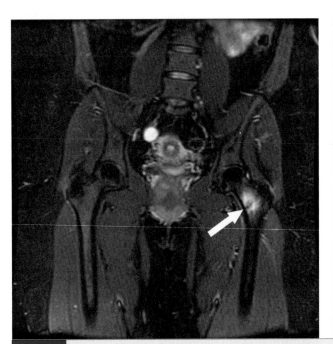
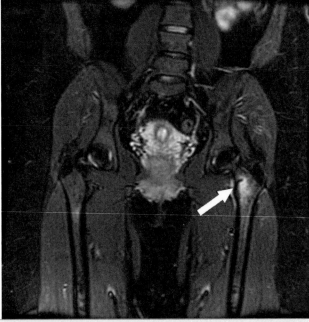

Figure 2 **A** and **B,** MRIs of the patient in Figure 1, showing a stress fracture of the left femoral neck (arrow).

to activity.[3,10] Stress fractures may require surgical management with open reduction and internal fixation, particularly in patients with a stress fracture in the superior portion (tension side) of the femoral neck. In these instances, surgical fixation is important in avoiding possible complications such as complete fractures, displacement, and subsequent osteonecrosis.[3]

Osteitis Pubis

Osteitis pubis is a painful inflammatory condition that may be caused by infection.[11] The condition is rare and involves the pubic bone, symphysis, and surrounding structures.[12] Noninfectious osteitis pubis is believed to be the result of repetitive microtrauma from the pull of the rectus abdominis muscle and is most common in athletes participating in running, hockey, soccer, and tennis.[11,13] The condition causes sharp or aching anterior pelvic pain over the symphysis pubis, in the lower abdominal muscle or in the perineum, and can radiate along the adductor region of the thigh. The pain is especially aggravated by walking or arising from a seated position. In addition, the patient may present with a waddling gait and hip stiffness.[11]

To determine if pain is the result of osteitis pubis, a lateral compression test should be performed by applying force at the iliac wing with the patient in the lateral decubitus position. This maneuver applies stress to the ipsilateral crossed extremity while the contralateral iliac wing is used to stabilize the pelvis.[11] Although the radiographic characteristics specific to osteitis pubis are difficult to define, plain radiographs and CT scans may show joint space narrowing, subchondral irregularity, sclerosis, and subchondral cysts. In addition, MRI scans show joint space alterations, articular surface irregularity, para-articular marrow edema, and extrusions of the symphyseal disk.[11] Occasionally, osteitis is caused by instability that can be identified with radiographs of the pelvis (one-legged stork views).[1]

Osteitis pubis is initially treated nonsurgically with rest, anti-inflammatory medications including oral and injected steroids, antibiotics (for the infectious form), and physical therapy.[11] The rehabilitation program should include correction of mechanical abnormalities that may have contributed to the onset of the condition.[13] When nonsurgical treatment is unsuccessful, surgery is indicated. Types of surgical intervention include curetting the joint, arthrodesis of the pubis symphysis in instances of instability, wedge resection, and complete resection of the joint. Curettage of the joint is considered the least aggressive surgical option but is associated with an increased risk of infection. Wedge resection of the symphysis pubis is less aggressive than complete resection, which is associated with posterior pelvic instability and pain. Wedge resection takes advantage of the strong reinforcing ligamentous structures anteriorly and inferiorly.[11]

Adductor Strain

Adductor strain includes any of the three adductors (adductor longus, adductor brevis, or adductor magnus) and has been suggested as the main cause of groin pain, responsible for approximately 62% of chronic groin pain in athletes.[14] Adductor strains often occur in athletes involved in kicking sports or activities that require quick starts and rapid changes of direction with pivoting, such as ice hockey and tennis.[14,15] Patients often have aching groin or medial thigh pain, aggravated by resisted adduction of the lower extremity. The patient may also have tenderness to palpation and focal swelling along the adductor muscle.[14] To test for an adductor strain, the patient should be assessed for pain on palpation of the involved muscle and with resisted adduction.[4] Plain radiographs can be used to exclude other conditions, including fractures and avulsions. In acute strains, MRI may be used to show increased muscle signaling from hemorrhaging, which is highly correlated with patient symptoms. In chronic cases, MRI also can be used to show traction periostitis or stress fracture and tenoperiosteal granulation tissue.[4]

Nonsurgical management includes rest, ice, and compression initially, to reduce associated hemorrhaging and edema.[14] Once the patient is no longer experiencing pain, rehabilitation, including range-of-motion exercises followed by muscle strengthening to prevent future injury can be initiated. The patient can resume activity when both range of motion and muscle strength are fully restored. The use of anti-inflammatory medication remains controversial, with reports of initial improvement followed by adverse effects on long-term function.[14] A tenotomy may be indicated for chronic strains that do not respond to 6 months or more of conservative treatment and when all other possible conditions have been ruled out. It should be noted that only 63% of athletes are able to return to their previous level of sports participation following a tenotomy. Additionally, in rare instances when the tendinous insertion has been completely torn from the bone, surgical repair may be indicated.[4]

Hip Pointer

A hip pointer is a contusion to the iliac crest, often the result of a direct blow.[1] This condition most often occurs in football players, resulting from a direct hit to the iliac crest; however, it can be the result of a fall during any activity.[1] The patient may have severe pain on movement, especially with coughing, deep breathing, sneezing, or running. The condition may cause severe disability, with localized tenderness over the iliac crest and potential swelling or ecchymosis.[16]

The patient should be assessed for tenderness in the area of the iliac crest, as well as ecchymosis and muscle spasms.[2] MRI may be used to show ill-defined areas of diffuse edema within the muscle.[1] Initial treatment

2: Hip

should attempt to minimize swelling and bleeding with the application of ice and compression.[2] The hip should then be rested, and crutches should be used to ambulate. A gradual physical therapy program should include exercises to strengthen and stretch adjacent muscles before return to activity.[1] Also, repeated injury should be avoided by protecting the area with appropriate padding.[2]

Coxa Saltans/Internal and External Snapping Hip Syndrome

Snapping hip syndrome or coxa saltans is characterized by an audible and sometimes palpable snapping, popping, or clicking of the hip that is not always associated with pain.[17,18] Snapping hip syndrome is often the result of overuse or overtraining in such activities as running and ballet or caused by internal and external rotation in activities such as martial arts, gymnastics, soccer, and football. There are three main types: intra-articular, internal, and external.[17,18]

Intra-articular conditions can be difficult to differentiate from internal conditions because both are similar in presentation.[6] Intra-articular conditions are caused by loose bodies, synovial osteochondromatosis, acetabular labral tears, osteochondral fractures, and transient subluxation of the femoral head.[19] Patients with intra-articular snapping hip present with reports of clicking or catching.[18] MRI has been a useful assessment tool because it shows abnormalities of the iliopsoas tendon, anterior capsule, bursa, and musculature of the iliopsoas mechanism that correlate with the location of symptoms. Also, plain films or CT scans can be used if snapping is the result of fractured bodies, bony and cartilaginous changes, or for delineating bone changes, including prominent iliopectineal eminence.[19]

Internal snapping hip is caused by the iliopsoas tendon slipping over either the femoral head or the iliopectineal eminence when the hip is extended from the flexed position, causing a snap at the anterior part of the groin.[20] Iliopsoas tendinitis is the inflammation associated with internal snapping hip syndrome, which can present in concert with iliopsoas bursitis, a condition with identical clinical characteritistics.[20] Patients report snapping, repetitive clicking, or sometimes clunking in the groin area that is often reproducible and palpable with hip flexion and extension.[16] The patient is considered symptomatic when there is associated pain, often at the musculotendinous junction during resisted hip flexion or hyperextension.[6,17] Dynamic testing of range of motion to reproduce snapping, such as flexion, abduction, and external rotation to extension, adduction, and internal rotation is useful in evaluating patients for internal snapping hip.[18,19] In addition, with the patient supine and raising the heels off the table to approximately 15°, tenderness can be assessed by palpating the psoas muscle below the lateral inguinal ligament at the femoral triangle.[4] Dynamic ultrasound or fluoroscopy

during motion of the hip can effectively demonstrate an abnormal jerk of the iliopsoas tendon.[18]

Internal snapping is normally treated nonsurgically through activity modification, anti-inflammatory medications, rest, and a subsequent physical therapy program that initially involves exercises to stretch the hip flexors and rotators, followed by exercises to improve hip rotation strength.[18,20,21] In addition, it is critical that any contributory mechanical abnormalities also be treated to prevent future recurrence. Once patients are no longer symptomatic and strength is restored, they may return to sports participation. If the problem persists, corticosteroid injections have been shown to be effective.[4] If conservative treatment is unsuccessful, surgical options include open techniques to release or lengthen the iliopsoas muscle-tendon unit or endoscopic techniques to release the psoas tendon at the hip joint, the hip capsule, or inside the psoas bursa closer to the lesser trochanter at the tendon portion.[17] The endoscopic method involving iliopsoas tendon release at the lesser trochanter has reportedly been effective and comparable to standard open procedures at short-term follow-up.[17] A more proximal release through an arthroscopic capsular incision at the hip periphery allows the muscle portion to remain intact, resulting in less reduction in flexion strength (**Figure 3**). It also allows direct evaluation of the snapping portion of the tendon to determine if enough lengthening has been achieved to prevent the iliopsoas tendon from snapping.[17] Recent studies have shown that more than 50% of the cases of internal snapping hip treated arthroscopically are associated with intra-articular pathology, including labral tears.[6,17] Complications after open techniques have reportedly been as high as 50% and include recurrent snapping, persistent hip pain, weakness, and sensory nerve injuries from the incision.[6] Although endoscopic techniques reduce the risk of wound complications and allow direct examination for intra-articular conditions, they have associated complications, including recurring snapping and some loss of flexion strength immediately after surgery.[17]

External snapping hip syndrome is the most common form and is caused by slippage of the thickened portion of the iliotibial (IT) band over the posterior edge of the greater trochanter.[18,21] In flexion, the IT band slides anteriorly over the greater trochanter; when the thickened portion passes over the greater trochanter, it snaps to an anterior position. Extension then brings it back to the posterior position, repeating the snapping phenomenon. The greater trochanter bursa lies between the IT band and the greater trochanter over the tendinous insertion of the gluteus medius and the origin of vastus lateralis muscles and may become inflamed with reproducible snapping, causing pain.[18,21] Physical examination is important for both diagnosing external snapping hip syndrome and eliminating other causes of hip pain. Clinical assessment should include the Ober test, which is useful in evaluating IT band tightness.[19]

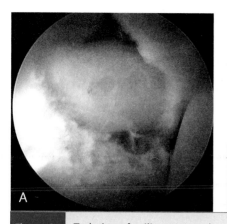
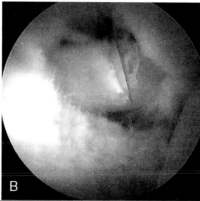
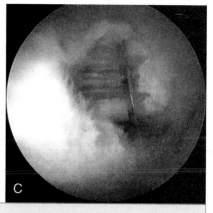

Figure 3 Technique for iliopsoas tendon release to treat internal snapping hip syndrome arthroscopically. **A,** Intact tendon. **B,** Partially cut tendon. **C,** Released tendon.

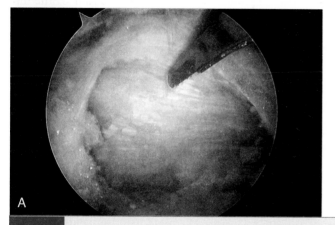
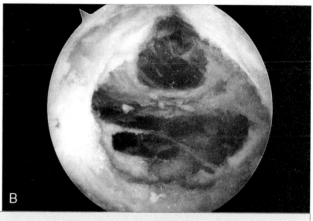

Figure 4 IT band lengthening to treat external snapping hip syndrome arthroscopically. **A,** Intact IT band. **B,** Lengthened IT band.

As with internal snapping hip, the external form should initially be treated nonsurgically, paying special attention to any mechanical abnormalities that may have led to the condition.[21] If nonsurgical treatment is unsuccessful, possible surgical options include open resection of the greater trochanter bursa combined with either Z-plasty lengthening of the proximal third of the IT band or open or endoscopic partial release of the IT band.[21] The endoscopic technique involves partial IT band release using a vertical cut, followed by a transverse cut at the middle of the vertical release by a beaver blade under arthroscopic visualization, to create a cross-shape in the IT band. The resulting four flaps are then resected, forming a diamond-shaped defect (**Figure 4**). Although endoscopic partial release has been criticized because of the need for endoscopic hardware and for increased surgical time, it is effective and minimally invasive.[21]

Piriformis Syndrome

Piriformis syndrome is a rare condition believed to be caused by anatomic abnormalities of both the pirifor-

mis muscle and the sciatic nerve, causing irritation of the sciatic nerve by the piriformis muscle.[22] Piriformis syndrome is composed of six characteristics: history of trauma to the sacroiliac and gluteal region; pain in the sacroiliac joint region, greater sciatic notch, and piriformis muscle, which extends down the leg and may cause difficulty walking; acute exacerbation of pain by stooping or lifting and moderately relieved by traction; palpable sausage-shaped mass over the piriformis muscle, which is tender to the touch; positive Lasègue sign (pain on voluntary hip flexion, adduction, and internal rotation); and possible gluteal atrophy.[22,23]

The patient should be evaluated in a standing position for pelvic tilt and then palpated for tenderness in the buttock from the medial edge of the greater sciatic foramen to the greater trochanter.[22] A spindle-shaped mass may occasionally be felt in the buttock. A helpful finding is pain with voluntary flexion, adduction, and internal rotation of the hip. Finally, the patient should be tested for pain on forced internal rotation of the extended thigh, as well as pain and weakness on resisted abduction of the hip when seated.[22] Electromyography can demonstrate myopathic and neuropathic changes, including a prolonged H reflex. CT scans can show

2: Hip

enlargement or abnormal uptake by the piriformis muscle, whereas MRI can be used to confirm an enlarged piriformis muscle.[22]

Initial treatment of piriformis syndrome includes physical therapy, along with anti-inflammatory medication, analgesics, and muscle relaxants. In addition, activity modification, massage, heat, and ultrasound treatment may be used to relieve pain.[24] Biomechanical abnormalities that impact posture, pelvic obliquities, and leg-length inequalities should be corrected. Physical therapy programs should initially involve stretching exercises, followed by hip abductor strengthening once pain has subsided. If physical therapy is ineffective, local anesthetic and/or steroid injections can be used.[22] Surgery may be indicated for patients unresponsive to nonsurgical treatment or in the presence of anatomic abnormality of the piriformis muscle; this structure may be thinned, divided, or excised.[22] Surgical treatment includes release of the piriformis muscle, which has been occasionally reported to cause compression of the sciatic nerve.[23]

Gluteus Medius Syndrome

Gluteus medius syndrome is normally caused by overuse and characterized as a cause of greater trochanteric pain syndrome. Gluteus medius injury can vary in severity and include peritendinitis, tendinosis, and partial or complete tears.[25] Gluteus medius syndrome occurs more commonly in women, particularly those who participate in running or step aerobics, although it can be the result of a direct blow to the gluteus medius.[26] Patients may have dull pain in the lateral hip and point tenderness adjacent to the greater trochanter, with additional weakness with hip abduction.[25] Frequently, there is pain with attempts to climb or descend stairs.

The patient should be tested for pain with resisted abduction, as well as with passive hip adduction and internal rotation.[27] Patients with more severe symptoms will have weakness and a positive Trendelenburg maneuver with one-legged stance. MRI and ultrasound have been useful for detecting soft-tissue edema, an early sign of gluteus medius syndrome.[25,26] Nonsurgical management includes activity modification, massage, ice, and stretching exercises, in addition to anesthetic or steroid injections to treat associated pain.[27] Surgery may be indicated for recalcitrant symptoms in patients with partial or full tears. If the gluteus medius tendon has a full- or partial-thickness tear, it can be repaired by excision of the degenerative tear tissue, curettage of the bone surface attachment, and then reattachment using bone anchors in combination with direct side-to-side repair of the tendon.[26]

Summary

The groin and pelvis make up a complex anatomic region that plays a critical role in various athletic activities and is traversed by forces greater than six to eight times body weight, even with light activity, making this region particularly prone to sports injuries. Because many groin and pelvis injuries have similar presentations and many patients have coexisting injuries, it is imperative that clinicians be knowledgeable of the differences between the conditions and the treatment options to provide the most effective treatment.

Annotated References

1. Nelson EN, Kassarjian A, Palmer WE: MR imaging of sports-related groin pain. *Mag Reson Imaging Clin N Am* 2005;13:727-742.

   The authors present a review of various conditions that may contribute to sports-related groin pain and the applicable imaging techniques for diagnosing specific conditions.

2. Anderson K, Strickland S, Warren R: Hip and groin injuries in athletes. *Am J Sports Med* 2001;29:521-533.

3. Morelli V, Espinoza L: Groin injuries and groin pain in athletes: Part 2. *Prim Care Clin Office Pract* 2005;32:185-200.

   The authors present part II of a two-part review of common injuries that can cause groin pain in athletes and include a discussion on the presentation of injury, diagnostic methods, and treatment options.

4. Morelli V, Weaver V: Groin injuries and groin pain in athletes: Part 1. *Prim Care Clin Office Pract* 2005;32:163-183.

   The authors present part I of a two-part review of common injuries that can cause groin pain in athletes and include a discussion on the presentation of injury, diagnostic methods, and treatment options.

5. Brittenden J, Robinson P: Imaging of pelvic injuries in athletes. *Br J Radiol* 2005;78:457-468.

   The authors review pelvic injuries in athletes and indicated imaging methods for the diagnosis and treatment of such injuries.

6. Flanum ME, Keene JS, Blankenbaker DG, Desmet AA: Arthroscopic treatment of the painful "internal" snapping hip: Results of a new endoscopic technique and imaging protocol. *Am J Sports Med* 2007;35:770-779.

   The authors present a cases series assessing an imaging protocol and a new endoscopic technique for the treatment of internal snapping hip syndrome. Level of evidence: IV.

7. Farber AJ, Wilckens JH: Sports hernia: Diagnosis and therapeutic approach. *J Am Acad Orthop Surg* 2007;15:507-514.

   The authors present a review of sports hernia, including a description of the condition and the diagnostic and therapeutic approaches used to treat the condition.

8. Ahumada LA, et al: Athletic pubalgia: Definition and surgical treatment. *Ann Plast Surg* 2005;55:393-396.

   The authors present a retrospective review to assess diagnostic approaches and the use of an open approach using mesh as a surgical treatment of athletic pubalgia. Level of evidence: IV.

9. Lee CH, Huang G, Chao KH, Jean JL, Wu SS: Surgical treatment of displaced stress fractures of the femoral neck in military recruits: A report of 42 cases. *Arch Orthop Trauma Surg* 2003;123:527-533.

   The authors present a prospective cohort to assess the efficacy of surgical treatment of stress fractures of the femoral neck in a military population at an average follow-up of 5.6 years. Level of evidence: II.

10. Miller C, Major N, Toth A: Pelvic stress injuries in the athlete: Management and prevention. *Sports Med* 2003;33:1003-1012.

    The authors present a review of stress fractures of the pelvis, including the mechanism of injury, diagnosis, treatment, and prevention.

11. Mehin R, Meek R, O'Brien P, Blachut P: Surgery for osteitis pubis. *Can J Surg* 2006;49:170-176.

    The authors present a retrospective review of four surgical treatment options for osteitis pubis, and a review of literature pertaining to osteitis pubis. Level of evidence: IV.

12. Paajanen H, Heikkinen J, Hermunen H, Airo I: Successful treatment of osteitis pubis by using totally extraperitoneal endoscopic technique. *Int J Sports Med* 2005;26:303-306.

    The authors present case reports of athletes with osteitis pubis and describe the outcome of surgical treatment using a totally extraperitoneal endoscopic technique. Level of evidence: IV.

13. McCarthy A, Vicenzino B: Treatment of osteitis pubis via the pelvic muscles. *Man Ther* 2003;8:257-260.

    The authors present a case report of osteitis pubis and describe an alternative approach for assessment, as well as rehabilitation methods for treating the condition. Level of evidence: IV.

14. Strauss EJ, Campbell K, Bosco JA: Analysis of the cross-sectional area of the adductor longus tendon: A descriptive anatomic study. *Am J Sports Med* 2007;35:996-999.

    The authors present a basic science study of the anatomic features of the adductor longus tendon and the relationship between the structure's anatomy and adductor strain.

15. Holmich P: Long-standing groin pain in sportspeople falls into three primary patterns, a "clinical entity" approach: A prospective study of 207 patients. *Br J Sports Med* 2007;41:247-252.

    The authors present a prospective, case-control study to test the reliability of clinical examination techniques in assessing pathology in the adductors, iliopsoas, and rec-

tus abdominis in a cohort of athletes. Level of evidence: IV.

16. Blazina ME: The "hip-pointer," a term to describe a specific kind of athletic injury. *Calif Med* 1967;106:450.

17. Ilizaliturri VM Jr, Villalobos FE, Chaidez PA, Valero FS, Aguilera JM: Internal snapping hip syndrome: Treatment by endoscopic release of the iliopsoas tendon. *Arthroscopy* 2005;21:1375-1380.

    The authors present a case series to assess the efficacy of treating internal snapping hip syndrome by endoscopic release of the iliopsoas tendon. Level of evidence: IV.

18. Wahl CJ, Warren RF, Adler RS, Hannafin JA, Hansen B: Internal coxa saltans (snapping hip) as a result of overtraining: A report of 3 cases in professional athletes with a review of causes and the role of ultrasound in early diagnosis and management. *Am J Sports Med* 2004;32:1302-1309.

    The authors present case reports of patients with internal snapping hip syndrome and the use of ultrasound for early diagnosis and management. Level of evidence: IV.

19. Winston P, Awan R, Cassidy JD, Bleakney RK: Clinical examination and ultrasound of self-reported snapping hip syndrome in elite ballet dancers. *Am J Sports Med* 2007;35:118-126.

    The authors present a cross-sectional study that involved a questionnaire completed by elite ballet dancers to establish the prevalence, associated factors, and mechanism of the snapping hip, as well as the efficacy of physical and ultrasound examination methods. Level of evidence: III.

20. Overdeck KH, Palmer WE: Imaging of hip and groin injuries in athletes. *Semin Musculoskelet Radiol* 2004;8:41-55.

    The authors present a review of common hip and groin injuries in athletes and the imaging techniques indicated for the various conditions discussed.

21. Ilizaliturri VM Jr, Martinez-Escalante F, Chaidez PA, Camacho-Galindo J: Endoscopic iliotibial band release for external snapping hip syndrome. *Arthroscopy* 2006;22:505-510.

    The authors present a prospective case series to assess the treatment of external snapping syndrome by endoscopic iliotibial band release. Level of evidence: IV.

22. Benzon HT, Katz J, Benzon HA, Iqbal MS: Piriformis syndrome: Anatomic considerations, a new injection technique, and a review of the literature. *Anesthesiology* 2003;98:1442-1448.

    The authors present a basic science study of the piriformis muscle's anatomic features and a new injection technique. In addition, a retrospective review assessing injection site and depth, as well as patient response, and a literature review are presented.

23. Windisch G, Braun EM, Anderhuber F: Piriformis muscle: Clinical anatomy and consideration of the piriformis syndrome. *Surg Radiol Anat* 2007;29:37-45.

    The authors present a basic science study of pertinent anatomic features of the piriformis muscle as well as a review of clinical presentation treatment options for piriformis syndrome.

24. Yoon SJ, Ho J, Kang HY, et al: Low-dose botulinum toxin type A for the treatment of refractory piriformis syndrome. *Pharmacotherapy* 2007;27:657-665.

    The authors present a prospective, nonrandomized trial testing the efficacy of low-dose botulism toxin type A for the treatment of refractory piriformis syndrome. Level of evidence: II.

25. Kong A, Van der Vliet A, Zadow S: MRI and US of gluteal tendinopathy in greater trochanteric pain syndrome. *Eur Radiol* 2007;17:1772-1783.

    The authors present a review of the efficacy of MRI and ultrasound in the diagnosis of gluteal tendinopathy and describe the anatomic features of the gluteus minimus and medius muscles.

26. Connell DA, Bass C, Sykes CJ, Young D, Edwards E: Sonographic evaluation of gluteus medius and minimus tendinopathy. *Eur Radiol* 2003;13:1339-1347.

    The authors present a case-control study that tested the efficacy of sonography in patients with gluteus medius and minimus tendinopathy by comparing symptomatic patients to asymptomatic control subjects. Level of evidence: III.

27. Hammer WI: The hip and thigh, in Hammer WI (ed): *Functional Soft Tissue Examination and Treatment by Manual Methods*, ed 3. Boston, MA, Jones and Bartlett Publishers, 2007, pp 286-287.

    The author reviews pertinent descriptions, diagnostic approaches, and treatment options for various hip and thigh conditions.

2: Hip

Chapter 8

Hip Joint Injuries

*Marc R. Safran, MD

Introduction

Hip pain in the athletic population is commonly diagnosed as a simple hip strain or pull. However, the management of hip injuries has evolved substantially with better understanding of the hip and its pathomechanics and advances in diagnostic modalities such as MRI and hip arthroscopy, with new techniques and flexible instrumentation. Hip pain can be caused by an injury to the joint itself or the soft tissue surrounding the joint or by referred pain. Hip injuries can be divided into intra-articular, extra-articular, or central pubic. Intra-articular sources of hip pain include labral tears, chondral damage, ligamentum teres tears, loose bodies, femoroacetabular impingement, hip displasia, and hip instability.

Disabling intra-articular hip pain in the athletic population is most often the result of a labral tear. However, labral tears may occur as an isolated phenomenon and often are the result of a bony abnormality, such as femoroacetabular impingement or dysplasia.

Evaluation of the Athlete With Hip Pain

The differential diagnosis of hip pain is quite broad in the athletic population. Without an appropriate work-up, hip pain in an athlete should not be simply diagnosed as muscle strain or soft-tissue contusion. A detailed history and physical examination help to narrow the differential diagnosis. Careful evaluation is critical to delineate the source of the pain. Soft-tissue pain can be caused by trochanteric bursitis, muscle tears, contusions, iliopsoas bursitis, snapping hip, and piriformis syndrome. Remote sites leading to referred pain can include the spine, the abdomen, the genitourinary system, and the knee. Pain from the hip joint itself can be caused by arthritis, stress fractures, synovial pathology, labral injuries, trauma, fractures, dislocation, chondral lesions, loose bodies, osteonecrosis, stiffness, and instability.

*Mark R. Safran, MD or the department with which he is affiliated has received research or institutional support from Smith & Nephew; holds stock or stock options in Cool Systems, Inc; and is a consultant for or an employee of Cool Systems, Inc.

Patient History

A careful history should include the qualitative nature of the discomfort (clicking, catching, stiffness, instability, decreased performance, weakness), the location of the discomfort, and the precipitating cause of symptoms (insidious or traumatic onset). It is important to determine if the symptoms are acute and began after an inciting event or have been ongoing. Pertinent findings include a history of trauma; instability; inciting or aggravating activities; mechanical symptoms; or weakness. The location of the pain, such as over the groin, thigh, or greater trochanter, may provide a clue to the diagnosis. Intra-articular pathology is frequently manifested as groin pain. Details about medical history, surgical history, social history, and medications provide pertinent information. Further, questions about sports participation are important because certain types of sports activities are associated with hip pathology, such as golf, running, ballet, and football.

Physical Examination

The physical examination should determine if the pain originates from intra-articular or extra-articular pathology and confirm that the pain is not referred from a remote source, such as the spine, genitourinary system, or abdomen. Most intra-articular pathologies can be aggravated by passive motion of the hip joint such as log-rolling, and placement of the hip in the impingement position (flexion, internal rotation, and adduction). Extra-articular conditions more typically will be aggravated by localized palpation or resisted muscular contraction.

For physical examination of the hip, the patient should undress to shorts or undergarments. During the first part of the examination, gait and posture are observed. The way a patient sits (slouched to reduce hip flexion, off to one side to unload a hip) may provide a clue about the source of hip pain. The way a patient arises from a chair may also provide important information, particularly whether the hands must be used to raise up, and whether hip flexion or standing on the affected leg is avoided. It is important to observe and evaluate for an antalgic or Trendelenburg gait; a positive Trendelenburg sign indicates hip abductor weakness.

During the next part of the examination, palpation over the site of pain can help determine whether the

2: Hip

pain is deep, muscular, or bursal related, or possibly caused by trochanteric bursitis, an anterior superior iliac spine avulsion fracture, or osteitis pubis.

After palpation and with the patient supine, both active and passive ranges of motion, including flexion, abduction, and internal and external rotation, should be tested. Strength should be tested and compared with that of the contralateral side.

Finally, hip-specific and provocative tests that should be performed include a resisted straight-leg raise, the Ober test (for hip abductor tightness), the Thomas test (for flexion contracture), the Patrick test (placing the leg in a figure-of-4 position while the patient is supine to assess for sacroiliac joint conditions and psoas pain or tightness from hip pathology), the labral stress test (extending, adducting, and internally rotating the hip while it is flexed, abducted, and externally rotated, as well as extending, abducting, and externally rotating

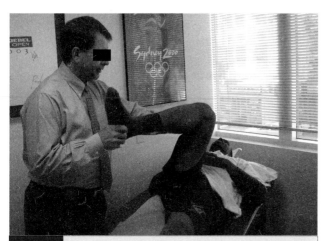

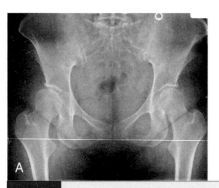

| Figure 1 | The impingement test of the hip is performed with the patient supine. The hip is flexed to 90°, then adducted, and finally internally rotated. A positive test is defined as pain with internal rotation in this position. |

the flexed, adducted, and internally rotated hip to assess for pain and/or clunk). The impingement test (passive flexion and gradual internal rotation of the adducted hip) will elicit groin pain (**Figure 1**) that corresponds to labral tears, and a positive impingement test may be seen with femoroacetabular impingement. Log rolling of the lower extremity can be performed to test for intra-articular hip pain. A positive McCarthy sign (with both hips fully flexed, the pain is reproduced by extending the affected hip first in external rotation, then in internal rotation) also corresponds to intra-articular pathology.

Radiographic Evaluation
Plain Radiographs
According to a 2004 study, 87% of patients with labral tears had evidence of osseous abnormalities detected on plain radiographs.[1] An AP pelvic and true (cross table) lateral (or Dunn lateral) radiographs of the hip may show evidence of abnormalities in bony contour and shape, such as malunited femoral neck fractures, osteonecrosis, developmental dysplasia, slipped capital femoral epiphysis, Legg-Calvé-Perthes disease, and femoroacetabular impingement (**Figure 2**). If underlying dysplasia is suspected, a false-profile view should be obtained.

The AP pelvic radiograph allows comparison between both proximal femora. The center edge angle, the acetabular version, the head-neck angle, and the femoral offset all can be measured. Radiographs should be evaluated for joint space narrowing, osteophytes, cysts, erosions, osseous lesions, and calcification. Specific signs such as the figure-of-8 sign or crossover sign indicate excess anterior bony rim and relative retroversion of the acetabular roof.[2] In addition, attention should be paid to the head-neck junction, and the anterolateral neck should be compared with that of the unaffected side to identify reactive bone changes and bone associated with femoroacetabular impingement (**Figure 2, A** and **B**).

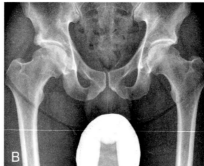
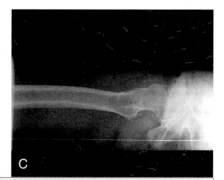

| Figure 2 | Bony variants associated with hip pain. **A,** Radiograph from a 32-year-old woman with right hip pain and evidence of hip dysplasia. **B,** AP radiograph of the pelvis of a 40-year-old man showing bony changes consistent with combined type femoroacetabular impingement. The femoral head-neck junction reveals reduced offset laterally; coxa profunda and a positive crossing sign are seen, findings that are consistent with relative retroversion of the upper acetabulum. **C,** Radiograph from the same patient with an obvious bump at the anterior femoral head-neck junction, seen with cam impingement. |

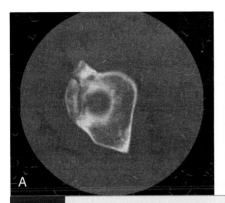 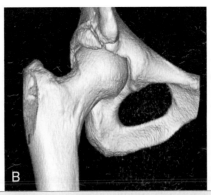 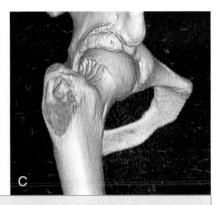

Figure 3 CT scans of the hip of a 36-year-old man who plays competitive football and has right hip pain and evidence of a superolateral acetabular stress fracture. **A,** Axial cut CT scan. **B** and **C,** Three-dimensional CT reconstructions showing mild cam femoroacetabular impingement and clearly demonstrating the fracture fragment.

Lateral radiographs may help determine loss of femoral head-neck offset in femoroacetabular impingement and evaluate dysplasia. Plain radiographs will show signs of trauma, including fractures, dislocations, and loose bodies.

Avulsion fractures from the anterosuperior iliac spine, the anteroinferior iliac spine, or the ischial tuberosity may all be seen on plain radiographs. Osteitis pubis has classic radiographic findings of cystic changes and sclerosis at one or both margins of the pubic symphysis.

Stress fractures can occur as a result of chronic loading and high stress to the femoral neck and may lead to serious complications, including complete and displaced fracture with possible resultant osteonecrosis of the femoral head. Fractures may be seen on plain radiographs; if not, a bone scan or MRI may confirm the presence of fractures. Other stress fractures, including those of the acetabular roof, ischium, sacrum, and pelvis, may occur about the hip.

To assess trauma about the hip, inlet and outlet views as well as Judet views may be helpful. Additional imaging studies may be warranted if intra-articular pathology or underlying bony impingement or dysplasia are suspected.

Bone Scans

Bone scans are more sensitive than plain radiographs for assessing bony injury and may be positive within 24 hours after injury. Bone scans allow a survey view of the entire pelvis and lower extremities and can be used to determine the presence of fractures, arthritis, neoplasms, and infections but have a low specificity for intra-articular abnormalities such as loose bodies, labral tears, and chondral defects.

Computed Tomography

CT can help delineate the osseous geometry of the hip. After hip dislocation, CT helps define fractures and loose bodies.[3] CT also can be used for preoperative planning for acetabular fractures. In patients with femoroacetabular impingement, CT (particularly three-dimensional CT) can show bony anatomy, including the acetabular version and bony prominence of the anterior femoral head-neck junction (**Figure 3**).

Magnetic Resonance Imaging

MRI helps differentiate soft tissue, myotendinous injuries, inflammation, synovitis, neoplasms, infections, and stress fractures. Magnetic resonance arthrography detects intra-articular pathology of the hip, such as labral tears, chondral injuries, and ligamentum teres. The sensitivity and accuracy of magnetic resonance arthrography for the diagnosis of a hip labral tear (**Figure 4**) may approach 100% and 95%, respectively.[4,5] At some institutions, high-contrast imaging has reportedly been achieved without intra-articular contrast agents. MRI has high specificity and sensitivity for labral lesions; chondral softening, chondral delamination, and small defects are less consistently detected by MRI.

Fluoroscopically-Guided Injections

Fluoroscopically-guided intra-articular injection of local anesthetic as an adjunct to clinical and radiographic examination has been the most highly sensitive indicator of an intra-articular abnormality, with a reliability of greater than 90%.[6] This finding has led to the use of intra-articular anesthetic along with gadolinium during magnetic resonance arthrography as an adjunctive diagnostic tool.

Specific Diagnoses of Intra-articular Sources of Hip Pain

The more common sources of intra-articular pain in athletes are labral tears and chondral lesions, which may be seen together in patients with femoroacetabular impingement and/or hip dysplasia, ligamentum teres tears, and loose bodies. Other sources of hip pain in athletes include hip dislocations, more subtle hip instability such as hip subluxation, and adhesive capsulitis.

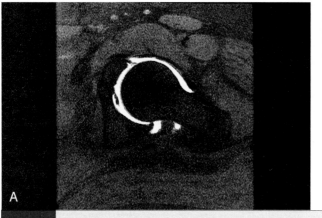
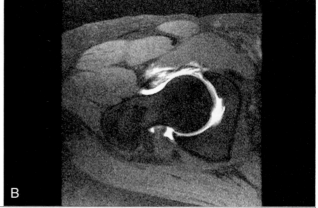

Figure 4 | Magnetic resonance arthrography of a labral tear. **A,** MRI of a 40-year-old woman with evidence of labral chondral separation. **B,** MRI of a 46-year-old woman with evidence of an intrasubstance labral tear.

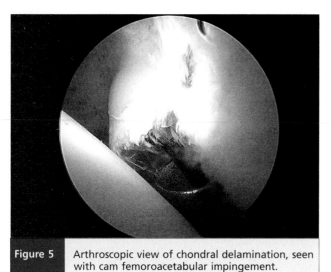

Figure 5 | Arthroscopic view of chondral delamination, seen with cam femoroacetabular impingement.

Femoroacetabular Impingement

Femoroacetabular impingement occurs when there is abnormal abutment between the femur and the acetabulum.[7] It has recently received increased attention as a structural entity associated with early arthritis of the hip.[8] Predisposing factors associated with femoroacetabular impingement include altered femoral neck morphology (which may be caused by slipped capital femoral epiphysis; anteverted femoral neck, femoral neck nonunion, developmental dysplasia of the hip, Legg-Calvé-Perthes disease, osteonecrosis, a pistol grip femoral neck, and coxa vara as well as acetabular morphologic variants such as a retroverted acetabulum and a deep acetabular socket (coxa profunda and protrusio). Impingement can occur as a result of femoral-sided impingement (cam impingement), acetabular rim impingement (pincer impingement), or, most commonly, a combination of both. Cam lesions on the femoral head-neck region lead to shear forces of the nonspherical portion of the femoral head against the acetabulum, resulting in a characteristic pattern of anterosuperior car-

tilage loss over the femoral head and corresponding dome, as well as labral tears.[9] Labral tears associated with cam impingement are more commonly labral-chondral separation lesions affecting the transition zone cartilage that leave the labral tissue in fairly good condition. The chondral damage tends to begin with softening, followed by debonding and delamination of the articular cartilage from the underlying acetabular bone (**Figure 5**). These chondral lesions are located in the anterosuperior region of the acetabulum and extend deeper into the acetabulum than chondral lesions because of pincer impingement.

Pincer type lesions result from repetitive contact stresses of a normal femoral neck against an abnormal anterior acetabular rim as a result of overcoverage. This situation results in degeneration, ossification, and tearing of the anterosuperior labrum, as well as the characteristic posteroinferior contrecoup pattern of cartilage loss over the femoral head and corresponding acetabulum.[9] In this setting, the acetabular labrum failure leads to degeneration and eventual ossification, which worsens the overcoverage. Overall, the pincer type lesion has chondral damage that is limited to near the rim but occurs more globally around the circumference of the acetabulum in comparison with the deep chondral injury associated with cam impingement.

Patients with femoroacetabular impingement commonly present with anterior groin pain, and deep hip pain that is worse with hip flexion and internal rotation. The typical patient is middle aged and is younger than the typical patient with degenerative joint disease. The typical patient with a cam lesion is a young adult male in his 20s, whereas the typical patient with a pincer lesion is an active middle-aged female in her 40s.[9] The pain and symptoms usually are related to activity. On physical examination, patients often exhibit decreased internal rotation and adduction with the hip flexed to 90°. The impingement test is positive, and there is pain with passive adduction and gradual internal rotation of the flexed hip (**Figure 1**).

Plain radiographs detect pistol grip deformity; flattening of the femoral head; synovial herniation pits; and prior deformity of the femoral head, neck, and acetabulum in young patients with hip pain. A positive figure-of-8 sign seen on an AP hip radiograph may suggest relative acetabular retroversion.[2,7] MRI can show anterosuperior labral tears and anterosuperior cartilage defects on the acetabulum. The α angle is an MRI measurement that indicates abnormal offset at the head-neck junction.[10] Normal α angles are less than 50°, with elevated values leading to increased cartilage and labral pathology consistent with the described mechanism of impingement.[10,11]

Nonsurgical treatment such as anti-inflammatory medications and activity modification may improve hip impingement symptoms, but because the pain is caused by a mechanical block, surgery is likely necessary. Unless the impingement is caused by an anteverted pelvis (seen with increased lumbar lordosis), physical therapy usually is not beneficial.[12] When patients have symptoms attributable to an intra-articular source (pain relieved with intra-articular anesthetic) and the bony anatomy of impingement, the treatment is usually surgical, either arthroscopic or open.

Hip Dysplasia

Hip dysplasia occurs when there is less acetabular bony coverage over the femoral head (**Figure 2, C**). Often, the acetabular labrum will be hypertrophied to compensate for the deficient bony coverage (**Figure 6**). Concomitant femoral head enlargement is occasionally present. Although deficient bony coverage of the roof is a common sequelae of congenital hip dislocation, many individuals will function well with a properly reduced hip joint. Some sports activities (such as ballet) select for individuals who have greater hip motion such as that seen in hip dysplasia, where there is reduced bony constraint. However, increased stresses on the labrum may result when there is increased anteroposterior mobility of the femoral head within the acetabulum. This abnormal mechanical stress leads to a labral degeneration or tearing, resulting in further motion within the joint and edge loading of the acetabulum, resulting in chondral damage and premature arthritis.[13] Further, lateral subluxation of the femoral head within the acetabulum caused by loss of bony constraint also can cause damage to the ligamentum teres. As a result, patients with hip dysplasia more commonly suffer from labral tears, chondral damage, and ligamentum teres hypertrophy, elongation, or tears.

The typical patient is a woman in her 30s or early 40s with hip pain that may worsen with physical activity. The patient often has groin pain or mechanical symptoms. Pain is reproduced with the impingement sign as well as by hyperextending the hip or placing the hip in the FABER (flexion-abduction external rotation) position; the leg is placed in a figure-of-4 position while the patient is supine. There often is increased range of motion of both hips, although the affected hip may have less motion, limited by pain. Plain radiographs

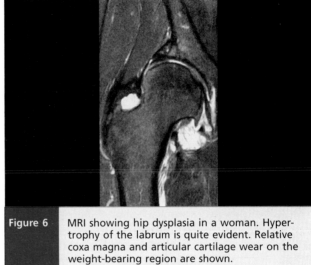

Figure 6 — MRI showing hip dysplasia in a woman. Hypertrophy of the labrum is quite evident. Relative coxa magna and articular cartilage wear on the weight-bearing region are shown.

will show the signs of dysplasia, including a reduced center-edge angle and retroversion; CT may help confirm this. Magnetic resonance arthrography can help identify the labral damage, although coexistent chondral damage, beginning at the acetabular rim, is often present but may not be seen on MRI.

Although arthroscopy may detect the damage to the labrum, ligamentum teres, and/or chondral flaps, treatment is focused on the bony deficiency, which is currently beyond the realm of arthroscopy. Return to sports participation, especially at the elite level, after surgery for dysplasia is not likely.

Hip Instability

Hip instability is much less common than that of the shoulder. The hip is subject to both traumatic and atraumatic instability. The hip relies less on soft-tissue stability because of the intrinsic stability provided by the bony architecture. Previous hip dislocations lead to capsular laxity of the hip and the possibility of recurrent hip instability. Traumatic hip instability is typically the result of a posteriorly directed force, such as landing on a bent knee or being tackled with the hip and knee flexed. The spectrum of injury ranges from subluxation to dislocation with or without concomitant injuries. Most athletic-related dislocations are posterior, and the classification is the same as with trauma, whether there is an associated fracture or not.

In addition to a standard radiographic workup, the evaluation should include an MRI that may demonstrate the characteristic triad of findings seen with hip dislocation: hemarthrosis, a posterior acetabular lip fracture or posterior labral tear, and an iliofemoral ligament disruption.[14] Anterior labral pathology is often present and may represent a traumatic avulsion of the labrum or indicate the presence of some underlying bony impingement. The presence of a significant hemarthrosis may warrant aspiration under fluoroscopy to decrease intracapsular pressure. MRI also is useful to detect osteonecrosis and helps determine which patients may return safely to sports activity.

Hip subluxations and dislocations have been described in athletes participating in a variety of sports activities, such as football, rugby, skiing, jogging, basketball, soccer, biking, and gymnastics. Most of these hip dislocations are pure dislocations and, because of the relatively low-energy mechanism, usually have no associated fractures or small acetabular rim fractures. Hip subluxation may be more subtle in its presentation and has been described with both contact injuries (such as a fall on a flexed knee) as well as noncontact injuries (such as occurs while running or during cutting and pivoting maneuvers).

Hip dislocations are treated with prompt reduction, with sedation or general anesthesia, to reduce the risk of osteonecrosis. After reduction, the hip is assessed for stability and smoothness of motion. Dislocations without fracture are inherently stable; in these hips, surgical stabilization is often not warranted. Postreduction radiographs are obtained to confirm concentric reduction and to look for intra-articular fragments and associated fractures. CT can be used to confirm the absence of intra-articular loose bodies and rule out fracture. Hip arthroscopy may play a role after dislocation and subluxation to treat femoral head pathology, loose bodies, chondral injuries, and associated labral pathology. The optimal timing of the procedure is debatable because of the concern of placing a hip in traction and capsular distention for hip arthroscopy in the acute phase of injury.

Controversy exists regarding management after reduction. Rest for up to 48 hours is often recommended, with a knee immobilizer or hip abduction pillow to prevent a position of possible redislocation, although active and passive range of motion can begin as soon as tolerated by the patient. Controversy also exists regarding weight bearing after dislocation, although protected weight bearing for 2 to 6 weeks is recommended after reduction of dislocation, with return to sports after approximately 3 months.

Atraumatic instability is a spectrum ranging from overuse injuries leading to microinstability to generalized ligamentous laxity. Overuse injuries are common in athletes who participate in sports involving repetitive hip rotation with axial loading (such as golf, figure skating, football, tennis, baseball, ballet, martial arts, and gymnastics). However, preoperative diagnosis of this condition is unclear and quite subjective. The labrum or iliofemoral ligament may be damaged from these repetitive forces, and increased tension in the joint capsule can lead to painful labral injury, capsular redundancy, and subsequent microinstability. The hip must rely more on the dynamic stabilizers for stability once the static stabilizers of the hip such as the iliofemoral ligament or labrum are injured. The spectrum of atraumatic instability also includes patients with hip pain secondary to more generalized ligamentous laxity, or, in the extreme form, patients with connective tissue disorders such as Ehlers-Danlos syndrome or Marfan syndrome. Physical findings include local or generalized ligamentous laxity and increased external rotation of the hip in extension, during the log roll or during flexion, such as with the FABER maneuver. Activity modification and physical therapy to improve the strength and proprioception of the hip joint is the initial treatment. If this treatment fails, capsular plication may be warranted.

Labral Tears

Injuries to the acetabular labrum are the most consistent pathologic findings identified during hip arthroscopy in athletes, although labral tears have been found in more than 90% of cadaver specimens with an average age of approximately 80 years.[15] Although labral tears may occur as an isolated condition, they are usually associated with traumatic injuries such as hip dislocation or subluxation, or with bony abnormalities such as hip dysplasia and femoroacetabular impingement.[1] Labral tears less commonly may be the result of some other etiology, including atraumatic microinstability or capsular laxity, psoas impingement, or symptomatic internal coxa saltans.

The labrum is a triangular fibrocartilaginous structure attached at its base to the rim of articular cartilage surrounding the perimeter of the acetabulum. The labrum is absent inferiorly where the transverse acetabular ligament completes the rim. The labrum provides some structural resistance to lateral and vertical motion of the femoral head within the acetabulum and has an important sealing function that limits fluid expression from the joint space to protect the cartilage layers of the hip. The labrum likely also provides some proprioceptive feedback.

Labral tears have been classified in different ways. Although these tears had been defined as radial flap tears (most common, 57%), radial fibrillated labrum tears (22%), longitudinal peripheral tears (16%), and abnormally mobile tears (5.4%),[16] they are now described more functionally as intrasubstance tears and tears at the labral-chondral junction. The vascularity of the labrum comes from the capsule and bony acetabulum.[17] Unfortunately, many tears occur in the articular nonvascular zone, making healing of some labral repairs unlikely. Labral tears are frequently seen in conjunction with acetabular chondral lesions. Tears more commonly occur anterosuperiorly because of the association between labral pathology and underlying bony abnormalities such as impingement and dysplasia. Both femoroacetabular impingement and dysplasia lead to injury to the anterosuperior labrum, albeit through different mechanisms. With impingement, the anterosuperior labrum is compressed between the femoral head-neck region and the acetabular rim. With dysplasia, the anterosuperior labrum is overloaded because of a loss of acetabular bony coverage and subsequent capsular and labral decompensation. In most patients with dysplasia, the labral tissue is hyperplastic in an attempt to create a soft-tissue substitute for the loss of bony acetabular coverage and is thus even more vulnerable to degenerative tearing.

The location of the labral pathology in hip instability may be different than the most common anterosuperior location seen in the setting of impingement and dysplasia. Traumatic hip instability, usually the result of a posteriorly directed force, may result in a posterior labral tear, although an anterior labral injury may also be present, indicating a traumatic avulsion of the labrum. Hip subluxation may occur from the same mechanism as a dislocation or be the result of a cutting or pivoting maneuver. Atraumatic instability is a spectrum ranging from overuse injuries leading to microinstability to generalized ligamentous laxity and repetitive forces that may result in labral injury.

The diagnosis of labral tears can be quite difficult because history, symptoms, and physical examination vary among patients; there is also a lack of familiarity with the diagnosis. Many patients have mechanical symptoms such as buckling, clicking, catching, or painful restricted range of motion. Some can have dull pain with activity that does not improve with rest or change in position. Common presenting symptoms include insidious onset of moderate to severe groin pain that may be aggravated with pivoting and walking or other activities. The patient may also notice the pain to be reproducible when the hip is brought into extension from flexion, such as when arising from a seated position or climbing stairs.

Pain with hyperflexion, internal rotation, and adduction (impingement position) is present in most patients. The pain and/or clunk may also be reproduced with the labral stress test and/or a resisted straight leg raise.

Patients who have had persistent pain for more than 4 weeks, in whom nonsurgical treatment has failed, and who have imaging findings consistent with a labral tear are candidates for hip arthroscopy. The goal of arthroscopic débridement of a torn labrum is to relieve the pain by eliminating the unstable flap. Although débridement of labral tears will lead to pain relief, labral tears can be repaired to maintain the chondroprotective function of the labrum. Because the healing capacity is likely related to the vascularity, the labrum has its greatest healing potential in the periphery, and because of the poor vascularity in its midsubstance, tears in this area are not considered viable for repair. Regardless of whether a torn labrum is repaired or removed, underlying bony pathology that is left untreated has a greater chance of failure.

Chondral Damage

Articular cartilage injuries in the hip have received considerably less attention than other joints, mostly because an accurate diagnosis is difficult without surgery and the inability to objectively assess treatment techniques. Nonarthritic cartilage injuries in the hip refer to focal chondral defects on either the femoral or acetabular side of the joint. Focal chondral defects on the femoral side are relatively uncommon; however, they

may result from axial loading or shear injury of the head within the acetabulum. Hip subluxation and dislocation may result in a shear injury to the cartilage surfaces of the femoral head. Recently, acute isolated surface injuries have been reported to occur from lateral impact loading across the hip joint.[18] The typical patient is a physically fit young adult male with little soft tissue and subcutaneous tissue surrounding the greater trochanter. The lateral impact injury occurs after a fall or blow to the greater trochanter that dissipates the force and energy through to the acetabulum and femoral head, leading to full-thickness articular cartilage loss caused by either shear or compressive forces on the medial aspect of the femoral head or chondronecrosis in the superomedial weight-bearing portion of the acetabulum, without osseous injury.

Cartilage injuries on the acetabular side are more common and typically present as localized cartilage delamination in the anterosuperior weight-bearing zone of the acetabular rim.[7,8] The most common underlying condition resulting in these types of cartilage defects is femoroacetabular impingement, which leads to damage of the transition zone cartilage with extension, over time, into the articular cartilage of the acetabulum caused by cam lesions entering the hip joint during flexion and rotation.[9]

When there is no associated bony lesion, such as with impingement, physical examination findings are nonspecific. These cartilage lesions may be treated with simple débridement of chondral flaps to a stable rim, abrasion chondroplasty, or microfracture.

Ligamentum Teres

The ligamentum teres is a triangular-shaped structure with a broad-based attachment to the posteroinferior portion of the cotyloid fossa of the acetabulum; its function is not fully known. It provides blood supply to the developing hip through a small artery to the fovea of the femoral head. There is no known mechanical function, although it has been suggested that this ligament plays a biomechanical role that contributes significantly to the stabilization of the hip.[19] Analysis of the material properties of this ligament has demonstrated similarities to other ligaments and confirms its ability to resist dislocation forces applied to the femoral head. It is tight in adduction, flexion, and external rotation. Disruption of the ligamentum teres can be associated with trauma and dislocation of the hip or may occur without dislocation.[19] Disruption of the ligamentum teres also may occur with degenerative arthritis.[19] Patients with ligamentum rupture as a result of trauma or dislocation will often experience instability and pain.

The incidence of ligamentum teres ruptures seen at arthroscopy is more common than would be expected, with an 8% incidence in one study.[20] Acute disruptions of the ligamentum teres are believed to occur as a result of exaggerated movements of adduction and external rotation, although hip abduction is often the injury mechanism described with patient history. Diagnosis of these injuries can be difficult, and a high index of suspicion with careful attention to the injury mechanism and the physical examination are critical for accurate evaluation.

Ligamentum teres injuries in high-impact sports such as football may lead to recurrent subluxation of the hip. The high incidence of degenerative arthritis associated with complete ligamentum teres ruptures has been attributed to the original injury; however, recurrent instability and subluxation episodes may cause repetitive injury to the femoral head and account for an increased incidence of osteonecrosis in these patients. Arthroscopy of persistently symptomatic lesions can clearly demonstrate ligamentum teres pathology, and athletes respond well to arthroscopic débridement of the disrupted and entrapped fibers.[21]

Loose Bodies

Loose bodies in the hip joint are the most clear indication for arthroscopy. Loose bodies are common after trauma, including hip dislocations, and may occur in the presence of dislodged osteophytes, foreign bodies, or synovial chondromatosis.

Patients with loose bodies may have mechanical symptoms such as locking, catching, or clicking; these bodies can be seen on AP pelvis radiographs, CT, MRI, or magnetic resonance arthrography. Nonossified loose bodies may be difficult to see on plain radiographs and are easier to see on CT or MRI scans. A high incidence of loose bodies is associated with traumatic hip dislocations, including loose bodies not seen on plain radiographs.[3] When persistent symptoms are present even in the absence of clear evidence of ossified loose bodies, arthroscopy is a way to confirm the diagnosis suggested by clinical examination as well as provide simultaneous treatment with minimal associated morbidity.

Summary

Sports-related hip pathology has gained increased recognition as a more complete understanding of the wide variety of intra- and extra-articular hip conditions has evolved. Currently the role of hip arthroscopy in the management of intra-articular injuries allows reproducible surgical treatment for athletes in whom nonsurgical treatment has failed. Appropriate indications for hip arthroscopy include management of central compartment pathology involving the labrum, chondral surfaces, ligamentum teres, capsular tissue, and centrally located loose bodies. Peripheral compartment arthroscopy is effective for the treatment of peripheral loose bodies, displaced labral flaps, and the treatment of both cam and rim impingement lesions associated with femoroacetabular impingement. Pathologic conditions of the iliopsoas tendon can be addressed via the central or peripheral compartment. The peritrochanteric space or lateral compartment of the hip can be accessed endoscopically for effective treatment of recalcitrant trochanteric bursitis, external snapping hip, and symptomatic abductor tendon tears.

Annotated References

1. Wenger DE, Kendell KR, Miner MR, Trousdale RT: Acetabular labral tears rarely occur in the absence of bony abnormalities. *Clin Orthop Relat Res* 2004;426: 145-150.

   The authors reviewed 31 consecutive patients with acetabular labral tears. Twenty-seven of the 31 patients (87%) had at least one abnormal finding, and 35% had more than one abnormality. Only 4 of the 31 patients (13%) had no identifiable structural abnormalities. Level of evidence: IV.

2. Jamali AA, Mladenov K, Meyer DC, et al: Anteroposterior pelvic radiographs to assess acetabular retroversion: High validity of the "cross-over-sign." *J Orthop Res* 2007;25:758-765.

   The authors studied the value of AP pelvis radiographs and the crossover sign in detecting relative acetabular retroversion. The sensitivity to detect acetabular anteversion of less than 4° was 96%, its specificity was 95%, and the positive predictive and negative predictive values were 90% and 98%, respectively.

3. Mullis BH, Dahners LE: Hip arthroscopy to remove loose bodies after traumatic dislocation. *J Orthop Trauma* 2006;20:22-26.

   In 36 patients with traumatic hip injuries, loose bodies were found with arthroscopy in 92%. Loose bodies were found in seven of nine patients in whom radiographs and CT scan found no loose bodies and a concentric reduction. Level of evidence: IV.

4. Chan YS, Lien LC, Hsu HL, et al: Evaluating hip labral tears using magnetic resonance arthrography: A prospective study comparing hip arthroscopy and magnetic resonance arthrography diagnosis. *Arthroscopy* 2005;21:1250.

   Using hip arthroscopy as the gold standard, these authors found the sensitivity and accuracy of magnetic resonance arthrography for the diagnosis of hip labral tear were 100% and 94%, respectively. Level of evidence: III.

5. Freedman BA, Potter BK, Dinauer PA, Giuliani JR, Kuklo TR, Murphy KP: Prognostic value of magnetic resonance arthrography for Czerny stage II and III acetabular labral tears. *Arthroscopy* 2006;22:742-747.

   Twenty-two of 23 tears (96%) were detected initially. On the basis of intraoperative findings, magnetic resonance arthrography yielded one false-positive result, one false-negative result, and one overstaging. On repeat interpretation, all 23 tears were identified. Level of evidence: IV.

6. Byrd JW, Jones KS: Diagnostic accuracy of clinical assessment, magnetic resonance imaging, magnetic resonance arthrography, and intra-articular injection in hip

arthroscopy patients. *Am J Sports Med* 2004;32:1668-1674.

Clinical assessment accurately determined the existence of intra-articular abnormality but was poor at defining its nature. Magnetic resonance arthrography was more sensitive than MRI at detecting lesions but had double false-positive results. The response to an intra-articular anesthetic was a 90% reliable indicator of intra-articular abnormality. Level of evidence: IV.

7. Parvizi J, Leunig M, Ganz R: Femoroacetabular impingement. *J Am Acad Orthop Surg* 2007;15:561-570.

The authors present a current review of femoroacetabular impingement.

8. Ganz R, Parvizi J, Beck M, Leunig M, Nötzli H, Siebenrock KA: Femoroacetabular impingement: A cause for osteoarthritis of the hip. *Clin Orthop Relat Res* 2003;417:112-120.

Femoroacetabular impingement was proposed as a mechanism for the development of early osteoarthritis for most nondysplastic hips. Level of evidence: IV.

9. Beck M, Kalhor M, Leunig M, Ganz R: Hip morphology influences the pattern of damage to the acetabular cartilage: Femoroacetabular impingement as a cause of early osteoarthritis of the hip. *J Bone Joint Surg Br* 2005;87:1012-1018.

Femoroacetabular impingement is divided into two mechanisms: cam impingement caused by a nonspherical head and pincer impingement caused by excessive acetabular cover. Cam impingement causes damage to the anterosuperior acetabular cartilage with labral-chondral separation, whereas pincer impingement results in narrow circumferential rim cartilage damage and the crushed labrum. Level of evidence: IV.

10. Nötzli HP, Wyss TF, Stoecklin CH, Schmid MR, Treiber K, Hodler J: The contour of the femoral head-neck junction as a predictor for the risk of anterior impingement. *J Bone Joint Surg Br* 2002;84:556-560.

11. Beaulé PE, Zaragoza E, Motamedi K, Copelan N, Dorey FJ: Three-dimensional computed tomography of the hip in the assessment of femoroacetabular impingement. *J Orthop Res* 2005;23:1286-1292.

The CT-derived α angle was greater for those with femoroacetabular impingement than for control subjects, and those femoroacetabular impingement patients with chondral lesions had higher α angles than femoroacetabular impingement patients without chondral lesions. Level of evidence: IV.

12. Jager M, Wild A, Westhoff B, Krauspe R: Femoroacetabular impingement caused by a femoral osseous head-neck bump deformity: Clinical, radiological, and experimental results. *J Orthop Sci* 2004;9:256-263.

The authors studied the surgical (47%; 8 patients—12 hips) and nonsurgical (53%; 9 patients—10 hips) approach for femoroacetabular impingement. There was a significant improvement in internal rotation and pain relief in patients who underwent surgical resection of the osseous bump. In contrast, no nonsurgically treated

patients improved. Level of evidence: IV.

13. Langlais F, Lambotte JC, Lannou R, et al: Hip pain from impingement and dysplasia in patients aged 20-50 years: Workup and role for reconstruction. *Joint Bone Spine* 2006;73:614-623.

The authors present a clinical, biomechanical, and treatment review of dysplasia and femoroacetabular impingement in young, active patients with long-term considerations in dysplasia.

14. Moorman CT III, Warren RF, Hershman EB, et al: Traumatic posterior hip subluxation in American football. *J Bone Joint Surg Am* 2003;85:1190-1196.

This article studies the injury mechanism, pathoanatomy, clinical and radiographic findings, and treatment of traumatic hip subluxation in an athletic population. The pathognomonic MRI findings include posterior acetabular lip fracture, iliofemoral ligament disruption, and hemarthrosis. Level of evidence: IV.

15. McCarthy JC, Noble PC, Schuck MR, Wright J, Lee J: The Otto E. Aufranc Award: The role of labral lesions to development of early degenerative hip disease. *Clin Orthop Relat Res* 2001;393:25-37.

16. Lage LA, Patel JV, Villar RN: The acetabular labral tear: An arthroscopic classification. *Arthroscopy* 1996;12:269-272.

17. Kelly BT, Shapiro GS, Digiovanni CW, Buly RL, Potter HG, Hannafin JA: Vascularity of the hip labrum: A cadaveric investigation. *Arthroscopy* 2005;21:3-11.

The authors studied labral vascularity with the modified Spalteholz technique. Overall, there was a relatively poor vascular supply to the labrum. Zone I (capsular contribution) had significantly more vascularity than zone II (articular side).

18. Byrd JW: Lateral impact injury: A source of occult hip pathology. *Clin Sports Med* 2001;20:801-815.

19. Rao J, Zhou YX, Villar RN: Injury to the ligamentum teres: Mechanism, findings, and results of treatment. *Clin Sports Med* 2001;20:791-799.

20. Gray AJ, Villar RN: The ligamentum teres of the hip: An arthroscopic classification of its pathology. *Arthroscopy* 1997;13:575-578.

21. Byrd JW, Jones KS: Traumatic rupture of the ligamentum teres as a source of hip pain. *Arthroscopy* 2004;20:385-391.

More than 50% of 41 patients studied had traumatic ruptures of the ligamentum teres. All had deep anterior groin pain. Nearly 50% experienced mechanical symptoms. The diagnosis of a ligamentum teres injury was made preoperatively in only two patients. Level of evidence: IV.

Chapter 9
Techniques for Arthroscopy of the Hip

*Bryan T. Kelly, MD

Introduction

Interest in hip arthroscopy has rapidly increased over the past 5 years, with a significant improvement in the understanding of various intra-articular and extra-articular disorders. Improvements in clinical examination skills and advances in radiographic imaging have led to more accurate assessment of different hip joint pathologies. Continued progress in instrumentation techniques has allowed easier access to the hip joint and periarticular compartments. Despite these advances, hip arthroscopy continues to be technically challenging, and a thorough understanding of hip anatomy and meticulous surgical technique are critical to safely perform the procedure. The basic steps for set up, portal placement, and surgical techniques within the central compartment, peripheral compartment, and peritrochanteric space (lateral compartment) need to be well understood before undertaking hip arthroscopy (Figure 1).

General Setup

Hip arthroscopy can be performed with the patient in either the supine or the lateral position. Patient positioning is based on surgeon preference. The most important factors are consistency of the setup and comfort level of the surgeon and the ancillary staff because most complications related to hip arthroscopy are associated with patient positioning and traction. Complications reportedly occur in 1% to 6% of patients. The most common complications reportedly involve neurapraxias of the lateral femoral cutaneous and pudendal nerves. The common goal of either a lateral or supine approach is distraction of the femoral head from the acetabulum to fully visualize the articular surfaces. A thorough understanding of the anatomic relationships around the hip joint, with special attention to neurovascular structures and tissue planes, is of paramount importance.

Specialized instruments—including flexible probes; extra-long cannulas; and extra-long shavers, burrs, drills; and loose body retrievers—all have improved accessibility to the joint and increased the versatility of procedures available to the surgeon (Figure 2). Careful initial placement of the cannulas and instruments will minimize the risk of iatrogenic cartilage injury to the femoral head or inadvertent injury to the labrum. Most of the intra-articular structures in the hip joint can be seen through the combined use of 30° and 70° arthroscopes as well as the interchange of portals.

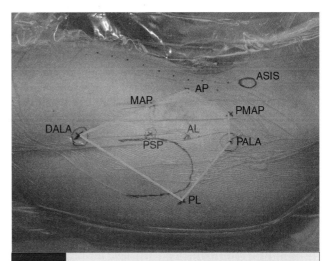

| Figure 1 | Standard and accessory portals for arthroscopic access to the hip joint. ASIS = anterosuperior iliac spine; AP = anterior portal; MAP = midanterior portal; AL = anterolateral (portal); PL = posterolateral (portal); PMAP = proximal midanterior portal; DALA = distal anterolateral accessory (portal); PSP = peritrochanteric space portal; PALA = proximal anterolateral accessory (portal). (*Reproduced with permission from Robertson WJ, Kelly BT: The safe zone for hip arthroscopy: A cadaveric assessment of central, peripheral, and lateral compartment portal placement. Arthroscopy 2008;24:1019-1026.*) |

Bryan T. Kelly, MD is a consultant for or an employee of Pivot Medical.

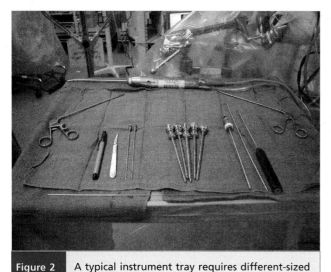

Figure 2 | A typical instrument tray requires different-sized cannulas and working instruments.

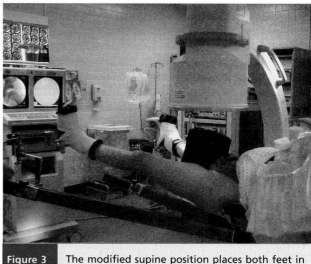

Figure 3 | The modified supine position places both feet in traction. The operative leg is positioned with approximately 20° of hip flexion and 15° of internal rotation through the foot, and neutral adduction.

Patient Positioning

Supine Position

The setup for the supine position is similar to that used for the fixation of hip fractures, using a fracture distraction table. The feet are well padded, and an extra-large perineal cushion is used to optimize distraction of the hip joint with the least amount of traction (Figure 3). Adequate traction under direct fluoroscopic visualization typically requires from 25 to 50 lb of force. The force necessary for distraction can be reduced by releasing the vacuum within the joint with arthrocentesis and injecting saline into the joint. The initial vector for traction runs parallel to the femoral neck rather than to the shaft of the femur and is applied with the hip in approximately 30° of abduction. The leg is kept in approximately 20° of flexion relative to the long axis of the body. Once the initial axial distraction is applied, the hip is brought into neutral adduction, which allows for a lateral distraction force to help displace the head from the socket. Adequate distraction is confirmed with fluoroscopic visualization of approximately 10 mm of joint space widening in the anteroposterior plane. Internal rotation of the hip is a final maneuver that decreases the tension on the anterior capsule and allows for easier instrument entry. Gentle traction is also applied to the contralateral limb to provide counterforce. Minor variations in the specific position of the hip joint with regard to flexion and extension, abduction and adduction, and internal and external rotation, have been described.[1]

Lateral Position

The main advantage of the lateral position is that fat drops away from the surgical site in this position (Figure 4). As with supine positioning, a fracture table is required to apply the necessary joint distraction. The principles of joint distraction are identical in both positions. Compared with the supine position, in which the

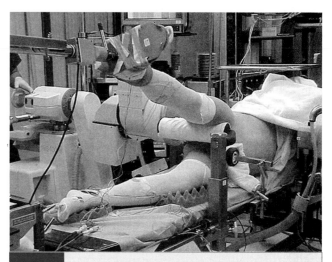

Figure 4 | The right leg of a patient is positioned in the foot piece of a traction device. The leg is positioned in slight flexion, abduction, and external rotation to relax the hip capsule. The perineal post is positioned upward against the medial side of the thigh so that it applies slight upward distraction and does not rest against the branch of the pudendal nerve that crosses over the ischium. (*Reproduced with permission from Glick JM: Hip arthroscopy by the lateral approach. Clin Sports Med 2001;20:733-747.*)

anterior portal is often used, the lateral position provides comfortable access to the hip joint via the anterolateral and posterolateral portals. Principles of portal placement and arthroscopic technique do not vary with position, and the choice of setup is based primarily on surgeon preference and training. Traction attachments are now available so that standard operating tables can be used in the surgery center setting.[2]

Portal Placement

Accurate portal placement is essential for optimal visualization and safe access to the hip joint. The standard portals that are used are the anterolateral peritrochanteric, the posterolateral peritrochanteric, and the anterior portals. Anatomic studies have demonstrated that the anterior portal has the greatest risk for nerve injury because of its close proximity to the lateral femoral cutaneous nerve. Other portals have been described and are useful for more advanced technical procedures.[3]

Anterolateral Portal

The anterolateral portal also has been described as the anterior peritrochanteric portal because it is referenced off the greater trochanter. This portal is placed approximately 1 to 2 cm superior and 1 to 2 cm anterior to the anterosuperior "corner" of the greater trochanter, depending on the patient's weight and size. The anterolateral portal should be established first and should be performed under fluoroscopic guidance. Initially, a spinal needle is placed in the appropriate position with the use of an image intensifier. The needle should be kept as close to the femoral head as possible, without hitting the cartilage surfaces. This placement will decrease the risk of injury to the labrum. Once placement of the needle in the joint is confirmed, the joint is distended with approximately 40 mL of saline solution. A good return of fluid confirms an intra-articular location of the needle. A guidewire is then placed through the spinal needle until it rests in the central foveal region within the acetabulum. A small diameter cannula and trochar set is passed over the guidewire, taking care not to bend or break the wire against the acetabulum. If this portal is placed too anterior or deep, the femoral neurovascular bundle is at risk for injury.

Anterior Portal

If used, the anterior portal is typically the second portal to be established and is obtained under direct visualization of the anterior triangle. The portal location was originally described in line with the anterolateral portal at the level of the anterosuperior iliac spine. Lateralization of this location by approximately 1 cm (modified anterior portal) appears to provide protection from the course of the lateral femoral cutaneous nerve and ensures avoidance of the femoral neurovascular structures. A spinal needle is directed 45° cephalad and 30° medially into the joint. Placement of the needle into the joint can be confirmed with an image intensifier, or may be directly visualized from the arthroscope in the anterolateral portal.

Posterolateral Portal

The posterolateral portal is also called the posterior peritrochanteric portal because it is also referenced off the greater trochanter. The entry site is 2 to 3 cm posterior to the tip of the greater trochanter at the same level as the anterolateral portal. Direct visualization of entry into the joint is possible with the scope in the anterolateral portal. The anterolateral and posterolateral portals should be established parallel to one another. The greatest risk with this portal is injury to the sciatic nerve, which lies approximately 3 cm away. Advancing the trocar with the femur in a neutral or slightly internally rotated position can protect the nerve, as this maneuver rotates the nerve away from the posterior margin of the greater trochanter.

Midanterior (Distal Lateral Accessory) Portal

The midanterior portal is placed midway between the anterior portal and the anterolateral portal, approximately 2 to 3 cm distally. The more distal location allows for an improved angle of entry into the central compartment, particularly in hips with significant acetabular retroversion. This portal is also useful for work within the peripheral compartment and peritrochanteric space.

Distal and Proximal Anterolateral Accessory Portals

Portal placement in line with the anterolateral portal in both distal and proximal directions allows for advanced arthroscopic procedures in the peripheral compartment and peritrochanteric space. The distal anterolateral accessory portal is placed 3 to 4 cm distal to the anterolateral portal and is particularly useful for femoral-sided decompressions for femoroacetabular impingement procedures. The proximal anterolateral accessory portal is placed 3 to 4 cm proximal to the anterolateral portal and is particularly useful for the treatment of peritrochanteric space disorders.

Studies of the proximity of neurovascular structures to the previously mentioned portals in cadavers confirm the safety of both the standard and accessory portals. Although the midanterior and anterior portals are in close proximity to a small terminal branch of the ascending lateral femoral cutaneous artery, the greatest risk in all of the portals discussed appears to come from the proximity of the anterior portal to the lateral femoral cutaneous nerve. Lateralization of this portal by 1 cm (modified anterior portal) seems to provide substantial benefits.

Central Compartment Pathology

The central compartment of the hip is the space between the femoral head and the acetabulum and can be seen arthroscopically only when the hip is placed in traction. Although the force of distraction should be minimized, typically a minimum of 10 mm of distraction is required to safely access the central compartment. Entry into the central compartment is performed by inserting a 70° arthroscope through the anterolateral portal using fluoroscopic assistance. The posterolateral peritrochanteric and anterior portals can then be obtained under direct visualization to avoid iatrogenic injury to the labrum or the cartilage surfaces. The midanterior portal is helpful in accessing the central compartment in patients with acetabular retroversion, pincer impingement, and profunda. Diagnostic arthroscopy within the central compartment should fully evaluate the entire labrum, the cartilaginous surfaces of the acetabulum and femoral head, the ligamentum teres, and the capsular structures. Loose bodies can be extracted from the central compartment and must be carefully looked for within the posterior recess as well as the central fovea.

Treatment of Labral Tears

Injuries to the acetabular labrum are the most consistent pathologic findings identified during hip arthroscopy in athletes. Treatment strategies for labral pathology include both labral débridement for irreparable tears and labral repair for healthy tissue with good healing potential. Vascularity studies have demonstrated that there is a good vascular supply to the labrum stemming from the capsular side; however, the articular portion of the labrum remains largely avascular.[4] With an increased understanding of the function of the labrum and its potential chondroprotective role, newer repair strategies have been described to improve the chance of labral preservation. It has become clear that the treatment of labral pathology in isolation, without treating underlying bony pathology has a greater chance of failure. Arthroscopic treatment of labral tears has been shown to have variable rates of effectiveness, with at least 67% and as high as 100% of patients satisfied with their outcomes.[5] Satisfied patients have been able to return to their preinjury level of athletic competition and have achieved good results on the Western Ontario and McMaster University Osteoarthritis Index (WOMAC) or Harris hip scores.

The most common location for labral injury in the athlete is in the anterosuperior zone and may be characterized as described in a 2001 study.[6] A type 1 tear is a detached labrum with displacement from the fibrocartilaginous labrum-cartilage junction, and a type 2 tear is an intrasubstance tear. Type 1 tears are probably more amenable to labral repair because of vascular penetration from the capsule. The presence of most labral tears in the anterosuperior location is related to the high correlation between labral pathology and underlying bony abnormalities such as impingement and dysplasia in this area.

Once the labral tissue is débrided of all nonviable tissue, the remaining labral tissue should be probed to determine if there is sufficient volume and quality to warrant refixation. The acetabular rim can be directly visualized and should be prepared to a bleeding bone bed with a motorized burr. Labral tears in a more lateral position (the 12 o'clock position) are most easily addressed with a 70° scope in the anterior or midanterior port and the working portal in the anterolateral or posterolateral portal. More medial tears (the 2 to 3

o'clock position) are most easily addressed with a 70° scope in the anterolateral portal and the working portal in the anterior or midanterior portal. Fluoroscopy can be used to assist anchor placement at the edge of the acetabulum. Care must be taken not to penetrate the joint. Once the anchor is placed, the suture is passed through the labrum using either suture penetrators or shuttle sutures. Restoration of labral function and anatomy is probably best achieved if the suture is passed through the tissue in a vertical mattress fashion, so that the suture material does not deform the labrum and is not in direct contact with the weight-bearing acetabular cartilage. This method of suture passing mimics the technique used for open labral refixation.[7]

Rim Decompression

Anterior overcoverage secondary to a pincer lesion also can be treated arthroscopically. Rim decompression can be performed in either the central compartment or the peripheral compartment. Rim impingement caused by acetabular retroversion or pincer impingement leads to a characteristic crushing of the labrum against the femoral neck and is usually associated with a flattened, degenerative, or cystic labrum. In isolated rim impingement, the acetabular cartilage is typically spared with primary injury to the labrum. This pattern of labral injury most likely corresponds to the type 2 intrasubstance injury pattern previously described.[6] If the tissue is viable, preservation of the labral tissue with labral refixation is optimal so that the suction seal effect of the labrum can be reestablished. In these instances, the rim decompression must be performed with careful protection of the labrum.

The margins of the pincer lesion are initially defined by probing with a flexible instrument. Fluoroscopy can be used during this portion of the procedure to clearly visualize the relationship between the anterior and posterior walls of the acetabulum. Resection of the rim lesion often leads to destabilization or requires detachment of the labrum to fully visualize the pathology. Preservation of the labrum during the rim resection can be accomplished using two different techniques. In the first, the labrum is sharply dissected off the acetabular rim in the region of the rim impingement and held in a protected position while the bone is resected. Once an adequate rim resection is completed, the labrum is refixed to the rim using the previously described bone anchoring technique. In the second method, the capsule overlying the rim lesion is cut in a longitudinal fashion and is peeled back to fully expose the bony overhang using a radiofrequency tissue ablator without frank detachment of the labrum. The rim is then resected over the labrum until the transition zone is reached, and the labrum is subsequently refixed in regions that have been destabilized (**Figure 5**).

Microfracture

Although relatively uncommon, focal chondral defects on the femoral side may result from axial loading or shear injury of the head within the socket. Hip subluxation and dislocation often will result in a shear injury to the cartilage surfaces of the femoral head. These cartilage injuries may be treated with arthroscopic techniques to stabilize loose cartilage flaps and microfracture areas of exposed bone, particularly if the injury is not in a weight-bearing zone. If the injury is in the weight-bearing zone of the femoral head, cartilage transplant procedures that in most cases must be performed as open procedures should be considered. These cartilage lesions may be treated with simple débridement to stabilize cartilage flaps, abrasion chondroplasty, or microfracture. Currently, there are no studies that provide long-term data on the usefulness of any of these techniques.

Treatment of Ligamentum Teres Rupture

Patients with ligamentum teres rupture as a result of trauma or dislocation will often have instability and pain. Although some authors have reported a low incidence of ligamentum teres ruptures seen at arthroscopy, authors of a 2004 study found these lesions to be the third most common complication encountered by athletes undergoing hip arthroscopy.[8] Arthroscopy of persistently symptomatic lesions can clearly demonstrate ligamentum teres pathology, and athletes have responded well to arthroscopic débridement of the disrupted and entrapped fibers.

Management of Loose Bodies

Hip arthroscopy is ideally suited for the removal of loose bodies. Loose bodies may or may not be ossified and are readily identified by radiographic studies only when calcium is present. If they are not evident on plain films, CT scans are highly sensitive for visualization; intra-articular fragments may be obscured with MRI. Symptoms are often described as mechanical locking or catching. When persistent symptoms are present even in the absence of clear evidence of ossified loose bodies, arthroscopy is a method to confirm the diagnosis suggested by clinical examination as well as provide simultaneous treatment with minimal associated morbidity.

Loose bodies may occur as an isolated fragment, such as after dislocation or with osteochondritis dissecans, or as multiple bodies or clusters such as that seen in synovial chondromatosis. With multiple loose bodies, it is essential to fully explore the joint and be sure to remove all fragments. Multiple loose bodies associated with synovial chondromatosis often adhere to the synovium around the fovea and must be morcellized before removal by arthroscopy.

Peripheral Compartment

Access to the peripheral compartment and its anatomy has been well described.[9] There are a variety of ways to enter the peripheral compartment for visualization of the

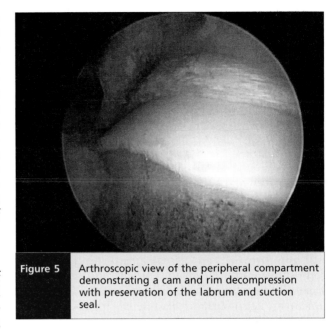

Figure 5	Arthroscopic view of the peripheral compartment demonstrating a cam and rim decompression with preservation of the labrum and suction seal.

anterior aspect of the femoral head-neck junction. Arthroscopy of the peripheral compartment is performed with the hip out of traction. The hip is typically flexed between 30° and 45°. Direct entry into the peripheral compartment can be achieved from the central compartment with the arthroscope in the anterior portal. As traction is released, the camera is swept anteromedially around the femoral head. The scope is then located in an anteromedial position within the peripheral compartment. Alternatively, entry can be achieved using the Seldinger technique over a guidewire with fluoroscopic assistance. With this technique the camera portal can be directed in the optimal location for treating the relevant peripheral compartment pathology that most often is a cam impingement lesion. If a capsulotomy is performed in the central compartment, the scope can be brought directly into the peripheral compartment with the camera in the anterolateral peritrochanteric portal with visualization through the capsulotomy.

Once in the peripheral compartment, standard arthroscopic evaluation should be performed with visualization of the medial synovial fold anteromedially, the zona orbicularis distally, the labrum proximally with evaluation of maintenance of the labral seal, and the lateral retinacular vessels in the superolateral location. The head-neck offset can be clearly seen in the peripheral compartment; with the assistance of fluoroscopic localization, the optimal position for cam decompression can be delineated. Complete evaluation of the peripheral compartment includes careful examination for loose bodies and displaced labral fragments. The posterior aspect of the peripheral compartment is hard to access arthroscopically because of tightening of the posterior capsule.

Femoroacetabular Impingement

The surgical goal of decompression of the femoral head-neck junction (cam decompression) is restoration of the normal head-neck junction offset and clearance of the femoral head within the acetabulum with full flexion and rotation. There are numerous techniques for achieving this goal; however, adequate visualization of the cam lesion within the peripheral compartment is essential, and fluoroscopic assistance can be helpful. With visualization of the cam lesion (typically through the anterolateral portal) a 5.5-mm burr is introduced through a second portal. The boundaries of the cam impingement lesion are marked, and then sequential removal of the cam lesion is performed to re-create a spherical femoral head. At the completion of the bone resection, all bone debris is removed from the peripheral compartment, and dynamic arthroscopy is performed to confirm the absence of any residual impingement. A resection of less than 30% of the head-neck junction is recommended because the load-bearing capacity of the femoral neck is preserved.[10,11]

Good results have been reported in the literature for patients treated arthroscopically for labral tears and associated femoroacetabular impingement, with as many as 93% of patients able to return to sports and 78% able to remain active at 1.5 years after surgery. Although some studies suggest that patients with associated chondral lesions fare worse than patients with isolated labral tears, larger series have been unable to detect a correlation between chondral injury and clinical outcomes.[12,13] Although the current volume and quality of outcomes literature is insufficient to conclude superior short-term outcomes when both the labral tear and underlying impingement are surgically treated compared with treatment of the labral tear alone, reports on revision hip arthroscopy have demonstrated that the highest failure rates are associated with patients who have residual untreated bony impingement pathology.[14,15]

Iliopsoas Tendon

Labral tears typically occur anterosuperiorly in association with femoroacetabular impingement or dysplasia. Less commonly, labral pathology may occur in an atypical direct anterior location in the absence of bony abnormalities. This direct anterior injury may be related to compression of the anterior capsule-labral complex by the psoas tendon as it crosses the anterior acetabular rim and results in a unique constellation of intra-articular findings reproducibly demonstrated at the time of arthroscopy. Arthroscopic findings are most notable for the intimate relationship between the labral pathology (inflamed labrum or frank tear with mucoid degeneration) and the iliopsoas tendon, which lies directly anterior to the labral abnormality and sometimes is adherent or scarred to the anterior capsule. Torn labra can either be débrided or reattached to the acetab-

ular rim depending on the pattern of the tear. Labral débridement or repair combined with lengthening of the iliopsoas has led to subjective improvement in symptoms and may be a logical treatment option for these patients.

Peritrochanteric Space

The peritrochanteric space or lateral compartment of the hip can be easily entered after routine evaluation and treatment of central and peripheral compartment disorders. Peritrochanteric space endoscopy can be performed in either the lateral or supine position. The first portal established is the anterior or midanterior portal. This portal is placed directly over the most prominent and lateral aspect of the greater trochanter and enters the space from an anterior to posterior direction. The cannula is then swept back and forth between the iliotibial band overlying the trochanteric bursa and the greater trochanter and is freely mobile in this space. Proper placement ensures that the cannula will not violate the gluteus medius or vastus lateralis musculature. Additional portals proximal and distal to the midanterior portal but in line with the anterolateral peritrochanteric portal provide complete access to the space (proximal and distal anterolateral accessory portals). These portals can be established under direct visualization using the Seldinger technique.[16]

Complete evaluation of the peritrochanteric space begins with identification of the gluteus maximus inserting onto the femur at the level of the linea aspera just below the vastus lateralis. This reproducible landmark provides good orientation within the space. It is typically unnecessary to work distal to the gluteus maximus tendon, and exploration posterior to the tendon should be avoided because the sciatic nerve lies within 2 to 4 cm. The camera light source is then directed to the lateral aspect of the femur where the longitudinal fibers of the vastus lateralis can be clearly seen and followed proximally to the vastus ridge. Proximal to this the insertion, the muscle belly of the gluteus medius is clearly defined. The gluteus minimus inserts more anteriorly and is mostly covered by the muscle fibers of the gluteus medius. Finally, with the camera pointed proximally and laterally, the iliotibial band is clearly identified. Care is taken to see the posterior fibers of the iliotibial band and its intimate relationship to the trochanter. The posterior third of the iliotibial band is typically the portion of the band implicated in external snapping.

A complete understanding of the insertional anatomy of the abductors on the facets of the trochanter aids in accurate arthroscopic assessment. Four separate facets can be identified on the greater trochanter. The anterior facet is the primary insertion site for the gluteus minimus. The gluteus medius has two distinct insertion sites. There is one robust insertion on the superoposterior facet and a second more broad-based insertion on the middle facet. The posterior facet of the trochanter has no distinct tendon insertion, but it is the primary location for the most prominent trochanteric bursae.

Trochanteric Bursectomy

In patients with recalcitrant trochanteric bursitis, débridement of the trochanteric bursa alone with a shaver can provide soft-tissue decompression and relieve symptoms. With the scope still in the midanterior portal and the shaver in the distal peritrochanteric space portal, a thorough trochanteric bursectomy is performed over the distal portion of the space. Distended bursal tissue and fibrinous bands are cleared off of the gluteus maximus tendinous insertion initially. The bursectomy is performed from distal to proximal. Care is taken to remove all visible thickened bursa.

Repair of the Gluteus Medius and Gluteus Minimus

The gluteus medius and minimus tendons can be examined in a manner similar to the subacromial space of the rotator cuff in the shoulder. The most common location for gluteus medius tears is along the middle facet. There may be extension of the tear toward fibers of the gluteus minimus insertion on the anterior facet. They are often high-grade partial thickness tears starting on the undersurface of the tendon. A thorough evaluation is required to identify the site of the tear. When a repairable tear is identified, the edges are débrided, and the attachment site of the tendon at the greater trochanter is prepared with a full-radius shaver in a manner similar to preparation of the rotator cuff footprint. Suture anchors are placed into the footprint of the abductor in a standard fashion. Fluoroscopy is helpful in directing the anchors in the appropriate direction. Once the anchors are placed, the sutures are retrieved and passed sequentially through the edges of the gluteus medius tendon with a suture passing device and tied under arthroscopic visualization with an arthroscopic knot pusher.

Iliotibial Band Release

If snapping of the iliotibial band (coxa saltans externus) has been refractory to nonsurgical treatment, a release can be performed along the posterolateral portion of the greater trochanter, beginning at the vastus tubercle insertion extending to the tip of the greater trochanter in a z-type or t-type release. Variations of this technique may be performed based on instrumented palpation of the fibers under the greatest amount of tension. The release can be performed either from within the peritrochanteric space with direct visualization of the trochanter and iliotibial band (inside-out), or from outside-in, where an elliptical section of the iliotibial band is excised directly over the prominent trochanter.

Studies have reported on successful outcomes after endoscopic trochanteric bursectomy and iliotibial band release.[17,18] Good and excellent results also have been reported after both open and arthroscopic abductor repairs in patients with persistent, symptomatic abductor tears that have failed conservative management.

Summary

Sports-related hip pathology has gained increased recognition as a more complete understanding of the wide variety of intra-articular and extra-articular hip conditions has evolved. Currently, the role of hip arthroscopy in the management of intra-articular injuries allows for reproducible surgical treatment of athletes in whom nonsurgical treatment has failed. Appropriate indications for hip arthroscopy include management of central compartment pathology involving the labrum, chondral surfaces, ligamentum teres, capsular tissue, and centrally located loose bodies. Peripheral compartment arthroscopy is effective for the treatment of peripheral loose bodies, displaced labral flaps, and both cam and rim impingement lesions associated with femoroacetabular impingement. Pathologic conditions of the iliopsoas tendon can be treated via the central or peripheral compartment. The peritrochanteric space or lateral compartment of the hip can be accessed endoscopically for effective treatment of recalcitrant trochanteric bursitis, external snapping hip, and symptomatic abductor tendon tears. A thorough understanding of both open and arthroscopic hip anatomy, as well as careful attention to technical considerations surrounding each of the described surgical interventions, are critical for successful outcomes in this rapidly evolving field.

Annotated References

1. Byrd JW: Hip arthroscopy: The supine position. *Instr Course Lect* 2003;52:721-730.

   This article details the merits and techniques of hip arthroscopy done with the patient in the supine position.

2. Glick JM: Hip arthroscopy using the lateral approach. *Instr Course Lect* 1988;37:223-231.

3. Robertson WJ, Kelly BT: The safe zone for hip arthroscopy: A cadaveric assessment of central, peripheral, and lateral compartment portal placement. *Arthroscopy* 2008;24:1019-1026.

   This article discusses knowledge and techniques of necessary portals for safe and accurate access into the central, peripheral, and peritrochanteric compartments of the hip.

4. Kelly BT, Shapiro GS, Digiovanni CW, Buly RL, Potter HG, Hannafin JA: Vascularity of the hip labrum: A cadaveric investigation. *Arthroscopy* 2005;21:3-11.

   This article discusses a cadaver investigation of the vascularity of the hip labrum, and treatment strategies when labral tears occur in a vascular zone.

2: Hip

5. Robertson WJ, Kadrmas WR, Kelly BT: Arthroscopic management of labral tears in the hip: A systematic review of the literature. *Clin Orthop Relat Res* 2007;455: 88-92.

    This article is a systematic review of outcomes studies analyzing the efficacy of hip arthroscopy on the management of labral tears in the hip.

6. Seldes RM, Tan V, Hunt J, Katz M, Winiasky R, Fitzgerald RA Jr: Anatomy, histologic features, and vascularity of the adult acetabular labrum. *Clin Orthop Relat Res* 2001;382:232-240.

    This article discusses the causal relationship between labral pathology and bony abnormalities of the hip.

7. Kelly BT, Weiland DE, Schenker ML, Philippon MJ: Arthroscopic labral repair in the hip: Surgical technique and review of the literature. *Arthroscopy* 2005;21: 1496-1504.

    This article reviews the technique of labral repair in the hip with a review of the relevant literature.

8. Byrd JW, Jones KS: Traumatic rupture of the ligamentum teres as a source of hip pain. *Arthroscopy* 2004;20: 385-391.

    Clinical characteristics of ligamentum teres and outcomes after arthroscopic treatment are presented.

9. Dienst M, Godde S, Seil R, Hammer D, Kohn D: Hip arthroscopy without traction: In vivo anatomy of the peripheral hip joint cavity. *Arthroscopy* 2001;17: 924-931.

10. Guanche CA, Bare AA: Arthroscopic treatment of femoroacetabular impingement. *Arthroscopy* 2006;22: 95-106.

    This article discusses the benefits of arthroscopic treatment of hip impingement caused by an abnormal head-neck offset.

11. Sussmann PS, Ranawat AS, Lipman J, Lorich DG, Padgett DE, Kelly BT: Arthroscopic versus open osteoplasty of the head-neck junction: A cadaveric investigation. *Arthroscopy* 2007;23:1257-1264.

    This article is a cadaveric investigation looking at the precision and accuracy of open and arthroscopic osteoplasty for femoroacetabular impingement.

12. Ilizaliturri VM Jr, Orozco-Rodriguez L, Acosta-Rodriguez E, Camacho-Galindo J: Arthroscopic treatment of cam type FAI: Preliminary report at 2 years minimum follow-up. *J Arthroplasty* 2008;23:226-236.

    This article discusses outcomes in patients treated with arthroscopy for hip impingement.

13. Bedi A, Chen N, Robertson W, Kelly BT: The management of labral tears and FAI of the hip in the young active patient. *Arthroscopy: J Arthrosc Relat Surg* 2008; 24:1135-1145.

    This article discusses the quality of literature assessing outcomes after surgical treatment of labral tears and hip impingement.

14. Heyworth BE, Shindle MK, Voos JE, Rudzki JR, Kelly BT: Radiologic and intraoperative findings in revision hip arthroscopy. *Arthroscopy* 2007;23:1295-1302.

    This article details radiologic and intraoperative findings on patients with persistent hip pain after hip arthroscopy. Possible causes include unaddressed hip impingement lesions and tight psoas tendons.

15. Philippon MJ, Schenker ML, Briggs KK, Kuppersmith DA, Maxwell RB, Stubbs AJ: Revision hip arthroscopy. *Am J Sports Med* 2007;35:1918-1921.

    This article describes reasons for revision hip arthroscopy, and persistent impingement as a common cause for revision surgery.

16. Voos JE, Rudzki JR, Shindle MK, Martin H, Kelly BT: Arthroscopic anatomy and surgical techniques for peritrochanteric space disorders in the hip. *Arthroscopy* 2007;23:1246.

    This article discusses the pathologies encountered with the peritrochanteric space of the hip (lateral compartment) and reviews different techniques for addressing these conditions.

17. Ilizaliturri VM Jr, Martinez-Escalante FA, Chaidez PA, Camacho-Galindo J: Endoscopic iliotibial band release for external snapping hip syndrome. *Arthroscopy* 2006; 22:505-510.

    This article discusses the surgical approach to treatment of external snapping hip and its outcome.

18. Baker CL Jr, Massie RV, Hurt WG, Savory CG: Arthroscopic bursectomy for recalcitrant trochanteric bursitis. *Arthroscopy* 2007;23:827-832.

    This article discusses the surgical management of trochanteric bursitis and its outcome.

2: Hip

Section 3

Knee and Leg

SECTION EDITOR:

DARREN L. JOHNSON, MD

Chapter 10

Muscle Injuries

Scott Mair, MD   M. Brennan Royalty, MD

Introduction

Muscle injuries are a common report of patients presenting to orthopaedic offices. Many of these injuries are associated with concomitant joint injuries, but isolated muscle injuries, usually strains and contusions, contribute to significant morbidity in active populations. Muscle injuries can be classified as either indirect or direct. Indirect muscle injuries occur when tensile forces act on a muscle, causing individual muscle fibers to be disrupted. Indirect muscle strains represent approximately 90% of all sports-related muscle injuries.[1] Direct injuries occur as a result of a direct blow to the muscle tissue and cause muscle contusions. These compressive force contusions are the most common direct muscle injuries. Muscle lacerations are the second type of direct injury. Lacerations are more commonly associated with motor vehicle injuries or assault.

Muscle Strains

Skeletal muscle consists of contractile muscle cells and a supportive scaffold. Individual muscle cells, or myofibers, are cordlike in shape, with varying lengths and diameters. Each myofiber terminates in a connective tissue band known as the myotendinous junction (MTJ). The MTJ represents a transition from muscle tissue to tendon tissue and is the point of application for the muscle unit (concentric or eccentric) force. Myofibers are grouped into functional units to translate individual contractions into one cohesive effort. The endomysium is a basement membrane connective tissue that surrounds each individual myofiber. Groups of myofibers are joined and surrounded by the perimysium. The entire muscle is further surrounded by a thick connective tissue known as the epimysium.[2]

Muscle strains most often occur in muscles undergoing eccentric contraction, those with bony insertions that cross two joints, and in muscles with a predominance of fast-twitch fibers. Commonly injured muscles include the hamstrings, the rectus femoris, the biceps brachii, and the gastrocnemius.[3] The injury location is predominantly at either the proximal or distal MTJ, but injuries at central tendons also occur. Muscle strains are diagnosed clinically as mild (grade 1), partial muscle tears (grade 2), and complete muscle tears (grade 3).

The response to muscle strain injuries has been extensively studied. Following injury, muscle tissue undergoes three stages of repair. During the destruction phase, myofibers lose their integrity as muscle sarcoplasms are ruptured. Although the muscle cell is a single unit, damage does not extend along the entire length. Studies have identified a specific cytoskeletal component, called a contraction band, that effectively seals the point of injury both proximally and distally. Necrosis of the muscle unit does not extend outside this contraction band. Muscle-supplying blood vessels torn during the injury provide access for clotting factors, inflammatory cells, and signaling agents. Fibrin and fibronectin form an initial clot and hematoma in the injured muscle. Macrophages invade the injured area, eliminate necrotic debris, and initiate repair and regeneration.[2]

Following the initial destruction phase, the phases of repair and remodeling commence nearly simultaneously. Newly synthesized granulation tissue forms a framework for fibroblasts to attach and begin reparative protein synthesis. Additionally, the granulation tissue provides strength and elasticity to the injured area to prevent further injury. As modeling and remodeling continue, the initial scar shrinks, and the surrounding extracellular matrix matures. Approximately 10 days after injury, the scar is no longer the most vulnerable portion of the muscle unit.[4,5]

Within the basal lamina of the myofiber is a reservoir of undifferentiated cells or satellite cells that serve to facilitate muscle regeneration. Under the direction of a complex growth fiber cascade, satellite cells multiply, mature into myoblasts, and then coalesce with existing remnants of injured myofibers to form new myofibers. Continued remodeling results in revascularization, neural reinnervation, and conversion of collagen from type 3 to type 1 in the existing scar. Gradually, the scar becomes minimized as new MTJs form on each of its sides.[6]

Treatment of an acute muscle strain traditionally involves the PRICE protocol (protection, rest, ice, compression, and elevation). Research evidence is equivocal regarding the benefits of ice and compression in treating acute muscle injuries.[7] Data indicate that an initial brief period of immobilization does help the newly formed scar develop strength to withstand initial contraction requirements. Active mobilization is then initiated to help orient newly forming myofibers and

3: Knee and Leg

facilitate capillary ingrowth. As pain decreases and mobility improves, isometric, isotonic, and dynamic exercises are sequentially added.[1]

The use of nonsteroidal anti-inflammatory drugs (NSAIDs) in the treatment of muscle injury has been under considerable scrutiny over the past several years. Traditionally, these medicines have been used for analgesia and for controlling inflammation after muscle injury. Although the analgesic effects are not disputed, the benefits of limiting inflammation in the acute stage have been questioned because a cascade of inflammatory mediators is released after muscle injury that appear to be beneficial for the optimal healing of injured muscle. The benefits are mediated largely through the activities of cyclooxygenase (COX) enzymes and cytokines such as transforming growth factor-beta 1 (TGF-β1). To date, at least three isoforms of COX enzymes have been identified. COX-1 is a ubiquitous protein in various physiologic processes of homeostasis. COX-2 is an isoform of COX-1 activated by tissue damage and subsequent inflammation. COX-3, yet another variant of COX-1, is apparently driven by the central nervous system during febrile responses. The products of COX-regulated processes are prostaglandins. These prostaglandins regulate the synthesis of new muscle proteins, and the degradation of damaged muscle proteins. TGF-β1 also appears to be a seminal component in the inflammatory process following muscle injury. It has been shown to prevent differentiation of myogenic precursors, inhibit myoblast fusion, stimulate collagen production, and promote fibroblast proliferation.

Recent data have indicated that NSAIDs and selective COX inhibitors may not hasten muscle recovery but may actually impede healing.[8] Studies have shown that the administration of both selective and nonselective COX inhibitors can inhibit the activity of satellite cells, promote fibrosis, and slow the development of mature myofibrils within the damaged muscle tissue.[9] These effects can be observed even with treatment duration limited to less than 5 days. The effects of treatment do, however, appear to be transient. Research has indicated that in treated and untreated muscle tissue, muscle fibers are nearly identical at 28 days after injury.[9] Studies have also shown that inhibition of COX-2 following resistance exercise can prevent subsequent muscle hypertrophy because of its negative effects on protein synthesis.[10] Long-term administration of anti-inflammatory medicines appears to further lengthen the delay in healing. Thus, it appears anti-inflammatory treatment may only delay healing, not prevent it, and may prevent muscle hypertrophy associated with resistance training.

Recently, investigations have focused on whether the growth of atrophied muscle tissue following injury is affected by anti-inflammatory medicines.[8] The growth of atrophied muscle is distinct from that of injured muscle and requires the restoration of existing myofibers to their original size and strength. Although mild damage to the myofibers may occur, myofiber degeneration is rare. Healing of the atrophied muscle requires cessation of existing catabolism of proteins and initiation of an anabolic state. This process is in contrast to that found in injured muscle, in which new muscle fibers must be regenerated. Because the two processes may coincide after injury, uniquely characterizing the effects of anti-inflammatory treatment is critical. To date, limited studies indicate anti-inflammatory medicines adversely affect healing and restoration of atrophied muscle. The basis for the adverse effects of NSAIDs, however, has not been clearly identified.[8-11]

The dilemma in using anti-inflammatory medications in the acute setting comes when weighing short-term patient comfort against long-term healing and performance. Effective pain control with anti-inflammatory agents may quicken a patient's return to activity. If actual tissue healing is delayed, however, the patient is likely at greater risk for further injury and long-term debilitation.

Current research focusing on techniques to improve muscle healing after injury has investigated the utility of antifibrotic agents. Animal studies have been performed to assess the possible role of suramin, relaxin, and gamma interferon. All were shown to have the potential to decrease muscle fibrosis, with the possibility of enhanced muscle regeneration and improved functional recovery.[12,13]

Muscle Contusions

Muscle contusions are second to muscle strains as the largest contributor to morbidity among athletes. These injuries are observed in contact sports such as American football, rugby, and soccer. Complications of muscle contusions can include myositis ossificans (mo) and compartment syndrome.

Muscle contusions are caused by blunt impact to the muscle belly and compression of the muscle tissue against underlying bone. Upon impact, the muscle microstructure is damaged, with myofibril rupture and sarcolemma distortion. Subsequently, edema and infiltration by polymorphonuclear neutrophils occur, similar to that observed in muscle strain injuries. Within 4 days, the number of inflammatory cells is significantly reduced, and phagocytosis of necrotic debris is nearly complete. Myoblastic proliferation begins at this point, as new myofibrils seek to repair the defect in the muscle microstructure. Normal muscle fibers are typically observed by 3 weeks.

Diagnosis of muscle contusions is clinical, with patient history paramount. Pain, swelling, and limits on contiguous joint motion are observed. Radiographs are negative in the acute stage. In quadriceps contusions, the injuries have classically been categorized based on the ability to flex the knee to 90° (mild), 45° to 90° (moderate), and less than 45° (severe). Prognosis following injury is dependent on severity, with the time to return to full activity ranging from a few days to several weeks.

The treatment of muscle contusions is conservative and follows the PRICE protocol. Original treatment protocols were developed using studies of West Point cadets and emphasized rest with joint motion restoration a primary goal. Subsequent studies indicated that early limited immobilization in flexion, followed by pain-free range-of-motion exercises, was more effective. Immobilization periods are 24 hours for mild and 48 hours for severe injuries. Patients are progressed to functional rehabilitation when motion returns to normal. Return to full activities is allowed when full, pain-free range of motion is achieved with normal strength. Protective padding and compression wraps are often used to protect the affected tissue following return to activity. These are reasonable approaches because studies have shown that compressed and contracted muscle tissue is able to absorb more force than in a relaxed state.[14,15]

Since the original landmark human studies, advances in the understanding of muscle contusion injuries have predominantly been achieved through animal models. Animal studies have supported the concept of limited immobilization by showing that tensile strength is improved and scar tissue is lessened by immobilization only in the acute phase (24 to 48 hours).[1] Longer periods of immobilization increase muscle atrophy and prevent maturation of the local scar tissue. Research also shows that subsequent to the initial injury, failure of the muscle to recurrent load occurs at the original injury site, as opposed to MTJ tears seen in primary muscle strains.[2] Animal studies typically have not supported the benefits of therapeutic ultrasound after muscle contusions.

The use of pharmaceutical intervention after muscle contusion injury remains controversial. Animal studies indicate NSAIDs and corticosteroids are somewhat effective in improving recovery during the first 7 days after injury. The improvement is attributed to a decreased inflammatory response and a reduced loss of muscle protein catabolism. These effects are transient, however, and are countered by declines in force generation at 4 weeks postinjury.[14]

Myositis Ossificans

MO is the abnormal formation of bone within muscle tissue. In the literature, it is often synonymous with heterotopic ossification and ectopic calcification. It is primarily a posttraumatic condition, although in approximately 40% of cases no trauma can be recalled. MO is also seen in patients with burn and spinal cord injuries. It predominates in the large muscles of the anterior thigh and the upper arm, with the quadriceps and brachialis most commonly affected, but it can occur in any muscle. Incidence data vary, with ranges

from 9% to 20% quoted for MO postquadriceps contusions.

The pathology of MO remains poorly understood. Following trauma, MO typically develops as either a broad, flat thickening of the periosteum in the vicinity of the trauma or as a stalk emanating from the bone. In these instances, it appears hematoma development within the periosteum, and subsequent rupture of the hematoma into adjacent muscles, leads to bone formation and symptoms. The release of osteocytes from the injured bone serves as the precursor for abnormal ossification within the muscle tissue.

MO lesions also develop after trauma in which underlying adjacent bone is not damaged. The origin of osteocytes within these muscles has been studied, and data indicate these are undifferentiated muscle cells lying dormant within muscle before injury.[16] The signal for their differentiation into osteocytes may be related to decreased oxygen tension within the tissue. A recent study investigating the basis for the development of heterotopic ossification in muscle tissue concluded impaired osteoblastic differentiation results in the phenomena.[14,17]

Patients with MO after quadriceps injury most often have prolonged pain and stiffness. Flexion at the knee is limited to 120° or less, and a palpable mass may be noted on examination. Risk factors for development include poor anterior thigh flexibility, occurrence of injury during American football, and previous MO. Aggressive postinjury stretching is also cited as a contributing factor to MO occurrence.[2,3,18]

Treatment of MO initially consists of conservative measures. Rest, ice, compression, and NSAIDs are used in the acute setting, and gentle range-of-motion exercises are begun as pain allows. The West Point flexion protocol has been developed to specifically assist in the treatment of MO. Patients are advanced through physical therapy as pain allows, with ultimate goals of full range of motion and strength. Surgical excision is recommended if continued pain or limits on range of motion occur. Surgery is not performed until the lesion has matured and ceased to grow. Radiographic studies are used to determine the best time for surgical excision.[18-22]

The use of NSAIDs to prevent MO has been studied primarily in patients undergoing total hip replacement. NSAIDs are thought to prevent MO development by reducing the levels of inflammatory prostaglandins in damaged muscle tissue. COX-1 and COX-2 reduction has been the means to reduce prostaglandins, primarily prostaglandin E_2.[23] Data have shown that indomethacin is an appropriate choice in this setting, with diclofenac and naproxen as appropriate alternatives.[24,25] A recent randomized controlled trial using animal models indicated trauma-induced heterotopic ossification may be controlled via the COX-2 mechanism alone, and selective COX-2 inhibitors may be more beneficial in certain patients.[26]

Bisphosphonates have been used in an attempt to

3: Knee and Leg

prevent MO after acute trauma.[25] Bisphosphonates disrupt the metabolism and physiologic activity of osteoclasts. They effectively prevent formation of hydroxyapatite crystals within the developing bone matrix.[27] Although typically used in the prevention of osteoporosis, their activity in the prevention of MO has been theoretically supported. Recent studies using various bisphosphonates have yielded contradictory results.[23,25] It appears these treatments can be beneficial; however, the specific drug and duration of treatment remains to be determined. A recent Cochrane Database Review stated insufficient data were available to make a recommendation for the use of bisphosphonates for the prevention of MO.[24,28]

Diagnosis of MO is based on clinical findings, but imaging may help characterize newly discovered lesions without a history of trauma or aid in identifying stable lesions amenable to surgical excision. Conventional radiographs are typically negative immediately after injury. Within 2 weeks, the first evidence of a soft-tissue mass often can be observed. By 4 weeks, mineralization allows opacity to be appreciated with a predominantly peripheral concentration. By 8 weeks, a well-demarcated opacity is observed. Over the ensuing 5 months, the mass may enlarge. By 6 months, the mass should stabilize.

CT also can be used to characterize MO lesions. Within 2 weeks, a noncalcified mass can be seen. By 6 weeks, a calcified rim is observed with a central area of decreased attenuation. CT is often helpful in delineating the mass in areas of complex bony anatomy, such as the pelvis, when surgical excision is being planned.

Bone scintigraphy is sensitive in detecting MO because of the deposition of calcium salts within the damaged muscle tissue. Uptake is observed in vascular and blood pool images. Bone scans can be used to identify stable lesions. Serial scans showing decreased uptake indicate maturation. Two scans showing normal uptake indicate a mature, stable lesion.

MRI is a sensitive study to identify and characterize lesions in the acute state, before active calcification occurs. Short tau inversion recovery (STIR) images usually exhibit a "lacy" appearance, in which edema surrounds a central area of hyperintensity. At 6 to 8 weeks, osteoid is apparent peripherally. Physiologic bone is observed as the lesion matures.

Muscle Lacerations

Muscle lacerations are common in high-energy collisions, primarily motor vehicle accidents, assaults, and combat. Muscle lacerations damage tissue in a manner similar to a severe muscle strain resulting in rupture. These injuries typically require surgical intervention. Data continue to support the incorporation of epimysium during primary repair for improved outcomes. Although novel data regarding muscle lacerations are limited, a recent animal study did provide guidance on the prevention of fibrosis following injury and repair.[17] According to the study, muscle regeneration is improved and fibrosis is limited when stretching is initiated on the 14th day after laceration.

Markers of Muscle Injury

The diagnosis of muscle injury is primarily clinical, relying on history and physical examination. With most injuries, these methods are sufficient to identify and treat the patient. In a minority of cases, however, these tools provide only limited data. In athletes, for example, muscle soreness, fatigue, and recovery are inherent in the training process. Repeated bouts of training facilitate adaptations of muscle growth and metabolism, which benefit the athlete. Although physiologic and exercise studies have improved training methods in general, athletes with prolonged soreness and decreased performance are difficult to assess. Because of this, recent studies have attempted to identify reliable biochemical and radiographic markers of muscle injury.[29,30]

The use of biochemical markers to identify acute or chronic muscle damage has been challenging. Early theories advocated the use of creatine kinase and lactate dehydrogenase as markers of skeletal muscle damage. These markers are intracellular proteins, whose presence in the blood is believed to indicate cell membrane damage. Subsequent studies, however, revealed these enzymes to be nonspecific for skeletal muscle.[31] Further, the concentrations of these enzymes were shown to be higher in noninjured active populations than in noninjured sedentary populations. Recently, studies in humans have shown promise for the use of α-actin as a biochemical marker of acute muscle injury. Data indicate that in injuries to quadriceps, biceps femoris, and lumbar muscles, α-actin effectively discriminates between injured and noninjured muscle tissue. Additional studies are needed to determine if α-actin can be used to identify subclinical muscle damage, stratify muscle injury severity, or provide a means to monitor muscle healing during rehabilitation.[30,31]

Radiographic markers of muscle injury have predominantly involved MRI. Because of its sensitivity in assessing muscular soft-tissue injury, MRI can be used to localize damaged tissue, identify focal scarring from chronic injuries, and follow muscle healing in rehabilitation (Figure 1). Muscle damage typically leads to edema. The edema is exhibited as an increase in water content via T2 lengthening and signal hyperintensity. T2 fast spin-echo with fat suppression, and STIR imaging most often provides the best visualization of muscle injuries.

Research continues to focus on using MRI to predict convalescence following muscle injury. A recent study of Australian football players used MRI to specifically identify the extent of quadriceps injury. The study

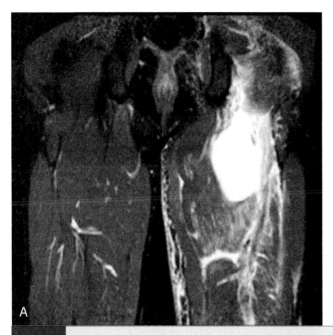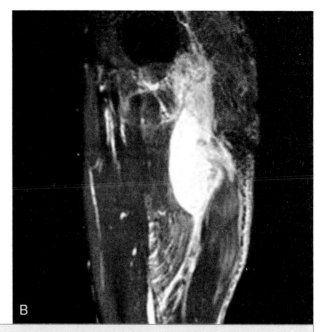

Figure 1 MRI studies showing a biceps femoris muscle tear. **A,** Coronal view. **B,** Sagittal view.

showed injuries to the quadriceps central tendon, and injuries to the middle portion of the quadriceps required a significantly longer rehabilitation time.[32] Research of the hamstring muscle complex has shown conflicting data regarding the use of MRI findings and prognosis.[33,34] Flexibility stretching exercises induce hamstring muscle complex injuries that seem to show no correlation of MRI findings and return to activity. Injuries during sprinting or kicking seem to correlate well with rehabilitation periods when comparing MRI findings of affected cross-sectional area, total volume, and length. One study indicated that length of injury alone can be predictive of recurrent hamstring injuries. Another MRI study of hamstring muscle strains found that proximity to the ischial tuberosity was associated with a longer time period to return to preinjury level of performance in sprinters.[34]

Summary

Muscle injuries can range from mild contusions to debilitating ruptures. Although these injuries can commonly be treated adequately using conservative measures, an increasing demand for optimizing recovery places additional emphasis on prompt diagnosis and novel therapeutic techniques. Comprehensive research continues to reveal the complex interplay of immune modulators and signaling proteins following muscle injury. Imaging studies are becoming more useful in injury identification and developing prognoses. Each of these areas will help advance knowledge regarding muscle injury and facilitate expeditious recovery.

Annotated References

1. Jarvinen MJ, Lehto MU: The effect of early mobilization and immobilization on the healing process following muscle injuries. *Sports Med* 1993;15:78-89.

2. Jarvinen TA, Jarvinen TL, Kaariainen M, Kalimo H, Jarvinen M: Muscle injuries: Biology and treatment. *Am J Sports Med* 2005;33:745-764.

    The authors review muscle injury mechanisms and pathology from cellular to macroscopic levels.

3. Armfield DR, Kim DH, Towers JD, Bradley JP, Robertson DD: Sports-related muscle injury in the lower extremity. *Clin Sports Med* 2006;25:803-842.

    The authors review presentation, evaluation, imaging findings, and treatment of muscle injuries in the lower extremity.

4. Hurme T, Kalimo H, Lehto M, Jarvinen M: Healing of skeletal muscle injury: An ultrastructural and immunohistochemical study. *Med Sci Sports Exerc* 1991;23:801-810.

5. Kaariainen M, Kaariainen J, Jarvinen TL, Sievanen H, Kalimo H, Jarvinen M: Correlation between biomechanical and structural changes during the regeneration of skeletal muscle after laceration injury. *J Orthop Res* 1998;16:197-206.

6. Hurme T, Kalimo H: Activation of myogenic precursor cells after muscle injury. *Med Sci Sports Exerc* 1992;24:197-205.

3: Knee and Leg

7. Bleakley C, McDonough S, MacAuley D: The use of ice in the treatment of acute soft-tissue injury: A systematic review of randomized controlled trials. *Am J Sports Med* 2004;32:251-261.

   The authors present a review of studies on the use of ice after muscle injury. It is concluded that little evidence exists that objectively suggests that ice has any effect on postinjury healing.

8. Bondesen BA, Mills ST, Pavlath GK: The COX-2 pathway regulates growth of atrophied muscle via multiple mechanisms. *Am J Physiol Cell Physiol* 2006;290: C1651-C1659.

   The authors present an animal study in which COX-2 null satellite cells exhibit less pronounced activation and proliferation than their wild-type counterparts. The authors suggest that the COX-2 path regulates muscle growth during recovery from atrophy and injury.

9. Shen W, Li Y, Tang Y, Cummins J, Huard J: NS-398, a cyclooxygenase-2-specific inhibitor, delays skeletal muscle healing by decreasing regeneration and promoting fibrosis. *Am J Pathol* 2005;167:1105-1117.

   An animal study on the effects of NSAIDs on muscle healing is presented. Results indicate that NSAIDs may adversely affect muscle healing because of their interaction with macrophages and neutrophils.

10. Weinheimer EM, Jemiolo B, Carroll CC, et al: Resistance exercise and cyclooxygenase (COX) expression in human skeletal muscle: Implications for COX-inhibiting drugs and protein synthesis. *Am J Physiol Regul Integr Comp Physiol* 2007;292:R2241-R2248.

    A case series investigating expression of COX variants following exercise in humans is presented. Results show that COX-1 and COX-2 are involved in postexercise metabolism, but COX-3 is not.

11. Smith CA, Stauber F, Waters C, Alway SE, Stauber WT: Transforming growth factor beta and myostatin signaling in skeletal muscle. *J Appl Physiol* 2007;102: 755-761.

    Results from an animal study indicate that TGF-β precursor levels are elevated after injury, but protein levels remain unchanged.

12. Ferry ST, Dahners LE, Afshari HM, Weinhold PS: The effects of common anti-inflammatory drugs on the healing rat patellar tendon. *Am J Sports Med* 2007;35: 1326-1333.

    The authors present the results of animal studies in which they demonstrate decreased failure loads at bone-tendon junctions following 14-day administration of various anti-inflammatory drugs.

13. Chan YS, Li Y, Foster W, Fu FH, Huard J: The use of suramin, an antifibrotic agent, to improve muscle recovery after strain injury. *Am J Sports Med* 2005;33:43-51.

    Animal study data indicate that the use of an antifibrotic agent after muscle injury can limit obstructive fibrosis and reduce healing time.

14. Beiner JM, Jokl P: Muscle contusion injury and myositis ossificans traumatica. *Clin Orthop Relat Res* 2002;403: S110-S119.

15. Crisco JJ, Hentl KD, Jackson WO, Goehner K, Jokl P: Maximal contraction lessens impact response in a muscle contusion model. *J Biomech* 1996;29:1291-1296.

16. King JB: Post-traumatic ectopic calcification in the muscles of athletes: A review. *Br J Sports Med* 1998;32: 287-290.

17. Hwang JH, Ra YJ, Lee KM, Lee JY, Ghil SH: Therapeutic effect of passive mobilization exercise on improvement of muscle regeneration and prevention of fibrosis after laceration injury of rat. *Arch Phys Med Rehabil* 2006;87:20-26.

    The authors discuss muscle fibrosis after laceration injury and the adjunctive use of decorin, an antifibrotic agent in healing.

18. Aronen JG, Garrick JG, Chronister RD, McDevitt ER: Quadriceps contusions: Clinical results of immediate immobilization in 120 degrees of knee flexion. *Clin J Sports Med* 2006;16:383-387.

    In this prospective case study, the authors conclude that early knee flexion after quadriceps contusion reduces time to return to play.

19. Ryan J: Quadriceps contusions. *Am J Sports Med* 1973; 55:299-304.

20. Jackson DW, Feagin JA: Quadriceps contusions in young athletes: Relation of severity of injury to treatment and prognosis. *J Bone Joint Surg Am* 1973;55: 96-105.

21. Parikh J, Hyare H, Saifuddin A: The imaging features of post-traumatic myositis ossificans, with emphasis on MRI. *Clin Radiol* 2002;57:1058-1066.

22. Miller AE, Davis BA, Beckley OA: Bilateral and recurrent myositis ossificans in an athlete: A case report and review of treatment options. *Arch Phys Med Rehabil* 2006;87:286-290.

    A case report on MO and a discussion of treatment approaches are presented.

23. Shafer DM, Bay C, Caruso DM, Foster KN: The use eidronate disodium in the prevention of heterotopic ossification in burn patients. *Burns* 2008;34:355-360.

    The authors present a retrospective analysis of eidronate disodium effects on burn patients, with the conclusion that using drug increased MO in the study population.

24. Fransen M, Neal B: Non-steroidal anti-inflammatory drugs for preventing heterotopic bone formation after hip arthroplasty. *Cochrane Database Syst Rev* 2004; 3:CD001160.

    The results of a systematic review regarding various NSAIDs following hip surgery are presented.

25. Schuetz P, Mueller B, Christ-Crain M, Dick W, Haas H: Amino-bisphosphonates in heterotopic ossification: First experience in five consecutive cases. *Spinal Cord* 2005;43:604-610.

A case study of pamidronate infusion in patients with spinal cord injury and a history of heterotopic ossification is presented. The authors detail success with pamidronate use but suggest that more data are needed to identify treatment method and length.

26. Rapuano BE, Boursiquot R, Tomin E, et al: The effects of COX-1 and COX-2 inhibitors on prostaglandin synthesis and the formation of heterotopic bone in a rat model. *Arch Orthop Trauma Surg* 2008;128:333-344.

The authors present an animal-based prospective case study of COX inhibitor involvement in heterotopic ossification, concluding that COX-2 is the sole COX inhibitor involved in traumatic heterotopic ossification.

27. Licata AA: Discovery, clinical development, and therapeutic uses of bisphosphonates. *Ann Pharmacother* 2005;39:668-677.

The author reviews the mechanism of action and therapeutic benefits of bisphosphonates on various bone pathologies.

28. Haran M, Bhuta T, Lee B: Pharmacologic interventions for treating acute heterotopic ossification. *Cochrane Database Syst Rev* 2004;18:CD003321.

The authors discuss a symptomatic review of treatment studies for heterotopic ossification.

29. Sorichter S, Mair J, Koller A, et al: Skeletal troponin I as a marker of exercise-induced muscle damage. *J Appl Physiol* 1997;83:1076-1082.

30. Martinez-Amat A, Boulaiz H, Prados J, et al: Release of alpha-actin into serum after skeletal muscle damage. *Br J Sports Med* 2005;39:830-834.

The authors describe α-actin levels after acute nonathletic injuries and conclude that the marker may be ideal for identifying muscle damage.

31. Martinez-Amat A, Marchal Corrales JA, Rodriguez Serrano F, et al: Role of alpha-actin in muscle damage of injured athletes in comparison with traditional markers. *Br J Sports Med* 2007;41:442-446.

The authors describe a prospective trial of athletic and nonathletic participants in which they conclude that α-actin is a more sensitive marker for muscle damage than troponin I or T, and lactate dehydrogenase in athletic injuries.

32. Cross TM, Gibbs N, Houang MT, Cameron M: Acute quadriceps muscle strains: Magnetic resonance imaging features and prognosis. *Am J Sports Med* 2004;32: 710-719.

The authors describe typical MRI findings of quadriceps strain and conclude that central tendon injury is associated with longer periods of healing and return to play.

33. Askling C, Saartok T, Thorstensson A: Type of acute hamstring strain affects flexibility, strength, and time to return to pre-injury level. *Br J Sports Med* 2006;40: 40-44.

The authors present a case series discussing hamstring injuries associated with slow-speed stretching in dancers and high-speed running injuries in sprinters. It was concluded that sprinters recover more quickly, though their associated injuries appear more debilitating initially.

34. Askling CM, Tengvar M, Saartok T, Thorstensson A: Acute first-time hamstring strains during high-speed running: A longitudinal study including clinical and magnetic resonance imaging findings. *Am J Sports Med* 2007;35:197-206.

The authors present a case series correlating injury severity with physical examination findings and MRI. It was concluded that proximal free tendon involvement and proximity to ischial tuberosity correspond to extended rehabilitation time and delayed return to play.

3: Knee and Leg

Chapter 11
Patellofemoral Joint Injuries

L. Daniel Latt, MD, PhD   Kian Raiszadeh, MD   Donald C. Fithian, MD

Structure and Function

The patellofemoral joint (PFJ) is a unique articulation with a complex architecture. Its motion is mainly composed of sliding rather than rolling, which differs from the motion of most other joints in the body. This motion places unique challenges on the articular cartilage. The most common disorders of the PFJ are believed to occur secondary to alterations in the mechanics of the joint, leading to cartilage overload or gross instability.

The tracking of the patella within the trochlear groove (TG) is ordinarily described by translation and tilt, both of which change with the knee flexion angle. As the knee begins to flex, the patella becomes engaged in the TG, which causes the patella to translate medially. At 20° of knee flexion, this translation is approximately 4 mm. With progressive flexion, the patella follows the TG laterally, leading to a laterally translated position of approximately 7 mm at 90° of flexion. While it is translating laterally, it also tilts medially in a progressive linear fashion and reaches approximately 7° at 90° of flexion. Deep in flexion, it is even more medially tilted with the odd (far medial) facet articulating with the medial trochlea. The patella flexes with the knee at a rate of approximagely 0.7° per degree of knee flexion.[1]

Maltracking may be caused by muscle weakness, soft-tissue deficiencies, abnormal joint geometry, or limb malalignment. Early in flexion, the medial retinaculum (specifically the medial patellofemoral ligament [MPFL]) provides much of the restraint to lateral displacement of the patella. Its contribution to patellar restraint decreases with flexion from 50% at 0° of flexion to 30% at 20°, as the patella begins to engage the femoral trochlea. The lowest force required to laterally displace the patella occurs at 30° of flexion. At this flexion angle, the vastus medialis obliquus is the most effective constraint, providing approximately 30% of the restraining force. With further flexion, the patella engages the TG, and trochlear geometry becomes the primary constraint to mediolateral patellar motion. In cadaver studies in which the trochlea has been modified (flattened) to simulate a dysplastic trochlea, the constraint of the patella is reduced by 70%.[2]

Overall limb malalignment can cause or exacerbate patellofemoral disorders. The lines of action of the quadriceps and the patellar tendon are not collinear;

the angular difference between the two is the Q angle. Because of this angle, the force generated by the quadriceps both extends the knee and pulls the patella laterally. The relative magnitude of this laterally directed force is proportional to the Q angle. External rotation of the tibia, internal rotation of the femur, and increasing knee valgus all cause an increase in the Q angle and an increase in the laterally directed force within the PFJ[3] (Figure 1).

Another form of malalignment, which is poorly recognized in the United States but has been studied elsewhere, is the abnormal vertical position of the patella or patella alta. In this condition, the patella enters the TG later in flexion. This leads to altered patellar

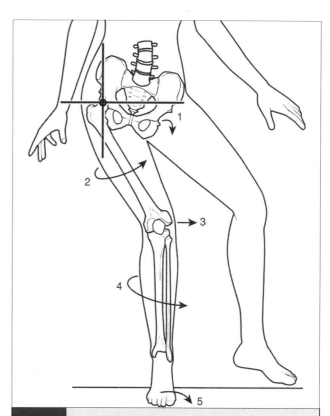

Figure 1   Diagrammatic representation of the various potential contributions of limb malalignment and malrotation to increased Q angle: (1) hip adduction, (2) femoral internal rotation, (3) genu valgum, (4) tibial internal rotation, and (5) pes planus.

3: Knee and Leg

tracking, decreased patellofemoral stability, and higher contact pressures at all flexion angles.[4]

History

A thorough patient history is essential for the successful treatment of patellofemoral disorders. The patient's specific reported symptoms should guide the work-up and dictate possible treatments. Patients most often report pain. Specific details of this pain, such as its chronicity, frequency, timing, character, inciting events, and mechanical symptoms are crucial to understanding the disorder. For example, a patient with daily aching pain has a very different disorder than a patient with occasion sharp pain associated with giving way. The relationship between knee flexion angle and symptoms is useful in helping to localize the pathology. Pain and catching in early flexion indicate an articular lesion at the inferior patella or proximal trochlea, whereas pain throughout the range of motion indicates a more diffuse or perhaps extra-articular process. The symptom of instability or giving way must be carefully scrutinized because a painful knee that occasionally gives way is quite different from a knee that becomes episodically painful secondary to pathologic laxity. As the clinician develops an understanding of the symptoms, one or more hypotheses can be developed, which then can be tested during the physical examination and with subsequent imaging studies. If objective evidence is not found, the patient should be treated nonsurgically.

Physical Examination

Because of the complex and delicate interactions between the knee extensor system and lower limb function, clinical evaluation of patellofemoral disorders can be challenging. After other disorders have been ruled out, specific testing for disorders of the PFJ can be performed. The patient should first be evaluated standing, walking, and stepping up and down from a small step. On standing examination, overall limb alignment should be noted. Hindfoot valgus also should be noted because valgus alignment can lead to tibial malrotation and consequent patellar malalignment. Determination of the Q angle is unreliable. An apparently increased Q angle should be used only as an indication to perform axial imaging to measure the offset between the tibial tuberosity and the TG.

During the seated or supine examination, patellar crepitus should be noted. Patellar grind and pain with resisted extension point to the retropatellar space as the source of pain. Careful palpation of both the medial and lateral retinaculum is helpful to localize tenderness. Studies have shown that 90% of patients with patellofemoral pain syndrome (PFPS) had pain in some portion of the lateral retinaculum.[5] The patella should be displaced to the side being examined so that during palpation of the fibers they are brought away from under-

lying structures to avoid confusion concerning the site of tenderness. The J sign is a useful but nonspecific sign of patellofemoral pathology; it is positive when the patella does not seat immediately as the knee is flexed. Many factors, such as trochlear dysplasia, patella alta, and medial retinacular laxity can contribute to the J sign. The flexibility of the iliotibial band should be evaluated using the Ober test. A tight iliotibial band may contribute to producing PFPS through its retinacular connection to the patella.

Patellar mobility is best assessed both at 0° and at 30° of flexion. The medial retinacular restraint, or the so-called checkrein, is easier to recognize at 0° because in this position the trochlea does not constrain the patella, making it easier to feel an endpoint as the patella is laterally displaced. The contribution of trochlear geometry is evaluated at 30° of knee flexion; at this angle the patella should be seated in the TG. Normal translation should be symmetric in each direction and not exceed 7 to 10 mm with a 5-lb load. Alternatively, the medial and lateral displacements can be quantified relative to the width of the patella, usually expressed in terms of quadrants (one quadrant equals one quarter of the width of the patella). If patients are apprehensive as the patella is moved, an examination under anesthesia can be helpful to confirm pathologic laxity before proceeding with surgical stabilization. Stabilization is never indicated unless excess laxity has been documented.

Imaging

Imaging begins with plain radiographic views of the knee, including AP, lateral, and axial views. Of these, the lateral view yields the most useful information. The presence of trochlear dysplasia is evaluated with the crossing sign. The crossing sign is positive when the floor of the TG crosses anterior to the projection of the condyles (**Figure 2**).

In a classic study comparing patients with objective patellar instability with a control group, the crossing sign was observed in 95% of patients with objective patellar instability; the mean trochlear prominence was 3.1 mm.[6] In the control group, crossing of the base of the groove with the lateral trochlear ridge was never seen; the mean trochlear prominence was 0.1 mm. The lateral radiograph should be performed with the PFJ in approximately 30° of knee flexion to ensure that the patellar tendon is under tension because measures of patellar height assume that the tendon is at its full length. Patellar height is best assessed using the Blackburne-Peel or the Caton-Deschamps ratio because they are more reproducible than other indices that have been described. The Caton-Deschamps ratio is the distance from the inferior patellar articular margin to the tibial plateau divided by the length of the patellar articular surface (**Figure 3**).

Tomographic imaging may be indicated if the physical examination or the lateral radiographs suggest an abnormality. If there is evidence of trochlear dysplasia

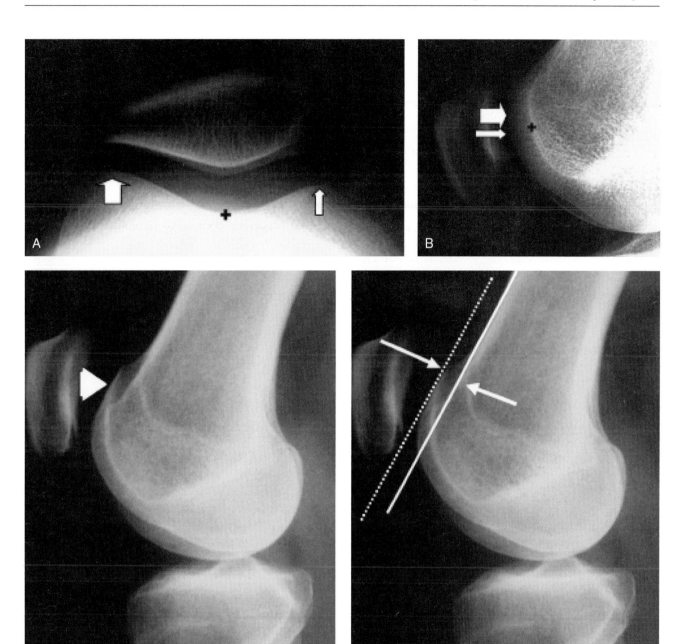

Figure 2 Radiographic criteria for trochlear dysplasia. Axial view **(A)** and lateral view **(B)** of a normal PFJ showing the radiographic lines that are used to determine the crossing sign. The floor of the trochlea (+) appears as a sclerotic, curved white line. Note that the curves representing the trochlear ridges (*arrows*) do not cross the curve of the trochlear floor. Accurate interpretation of the lateral view requires that the posterior condyles be aligned. **C,** Lateral radiograph showing the crossing sign, a simple qualitative criterion for trochlear dysplasia. The arrowhead indicates the point where the curve of the trochlear floor crosses the anterior contour of the lateral femoral condyle. By definition, the trochlea is flat at this level. This sign is of fundamental importance in the diagnosis. **D,** Lateral radiograph showing the quantification of trochlear prominence as the distance between the most anterior point of the trochlear floor (*dashed line*) and a line drawn along the distal 10 cm of the anterior femoral cortex (*solid line*). The prominence (bump) is a quantitative measure that is particularly useful in assessing trochlear dysplasia. The greater the trochlear prominence, the greater the dysplasia. (*Reproduced with permission from Fithian DC, Neyret P: Patellar instability: The Lyon experience.* Tech Knee Surg 2007;6:1-12.

(crossing sign or prominence) on the lateral radiograph, axial tomographic imaging (CT or MRI) is used to determine tibial tubercle (TT) to TG distance (TT-TG offset), which is a measure of the lateralizing force that is applied to the patella by the tibia via the patellar ten-don during quadriceps contraction (**Figure 4**). MRI is also particularly helpful in identifying patterns of wear or overload of the patellofemoral articulation. This can be useful in planning surgery in patients with patella alta and with trochlear dysplasia.

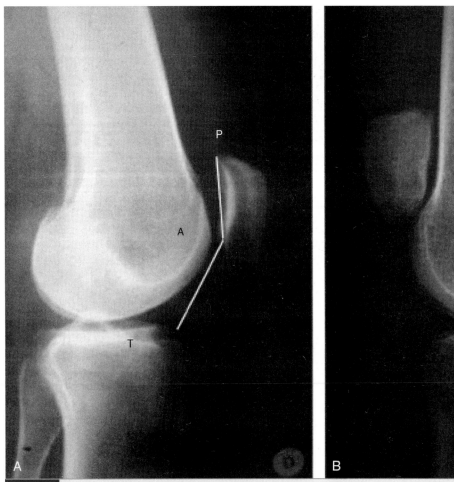
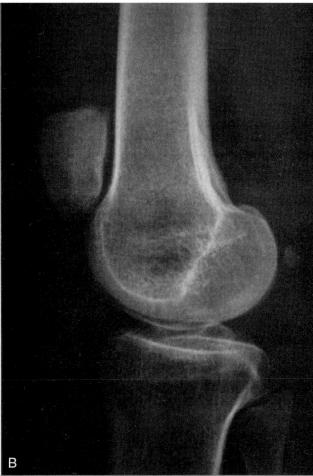

Figure 3 **A,** The height of the patella (A) is surprisingly difficult to measure reliably. The Caton-Deschamps ratio equals the distance between the lower edge of the patellar joint surface to the upper edge of the tibial plateau (AT) divided by the length of the patellar articular surface (AP). A ratio greater than 1.2 signifies patella alta. **B,** Radiograph showing severe patella alta.

A high Q angle or an increased TT-TG offset represents only one dimension of malalignment. The patella and femur relate to one another in three dimensions; thus, alignment could be measured in six degrees of freedom (rotation and displacement with respect to any of the three axes) with the potential for malalignment in any of these. Focusing solely on the medial-lateral alignment can lead to a dogmatic approach, with medialization of the tibial tuberosity as the mainstay of treatment. A recent study showed that patella alta by itself is associated with high contact stress near full knee extension, lateral shift, and increased tilt of the patella.[4] Patella alta represents the most frequently identified form of malalignment that is ignored in the treatment of patellofemoral disorders.

Malalignment is believed to cause symptoms by uneven distribution of forces that may result in overload of a particular region of the patellofemoral articulation. Evidence of significant overload can usually be documented on imaging studies that demonstrate physiologic stress, such as single photon emission computed tomography, MRI, or technetium bone scanning. Bone scanning is an excellent study to localize a presumed area of overload because it shows increased metabolic activity (**Figure 5**). If surgical correction is being considered, objective evidence should be sought using these modalities. In addition to confirming the hypothesis that local articular overload is the cause of the pain, this approach can help the surgeon develop a rationale for offloading the stressed area.

Patellofemoral Pain Syndrome

Diagnosis

PFPS is frequently diagnosed but poorly understood. This disorder occurs most commonly in adolescent and young adult females. The syndrome is defined by a symptom complex consisting of diffuse peripatellar or retropatellar pain that is exacerbated by specific daily activities such as squatting, stair climbing, kneeling, or prolonged sitting. Typical patients with PFPS have no

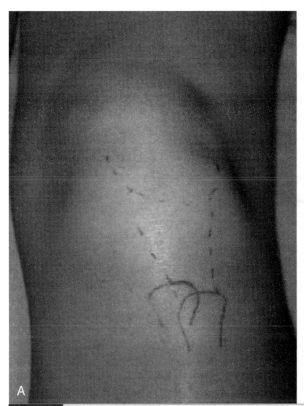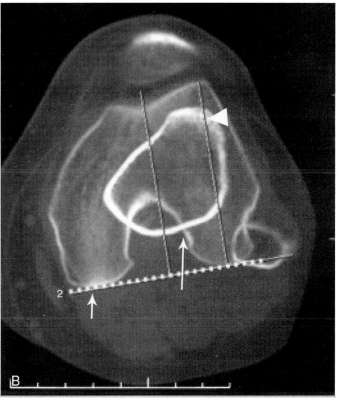

Figure 4	Measuring TT-TG offset. **A,** The lateral offset of the TT is suspected clinically, but the analysis is qualitative. **B,** A CT scan (or an MRI scan) allows a reliable and reproducible measurement. Two axial cuts (slices) are superimposed: one through the apex of the TT and the other through the femur at the level where the notch posteriorly resembles a curved Roman arch (*long arrow*). The TT-TG offset (*arrowhead*) is the distance between the most anterior point of the TT and the apex of the TG, along a line parallel to the posterior condylar line (*short arrow*).

history of antecedent trauma, ligament insufficiency, or instability. In these patients, the diagnosis is confirmed with physical examination findings of pain with resisted extension, pain with patellar compression underload (grind), and pain with palpation of the undersurface of the patella.

Etiology

The etiology of PFPS is a subject of significant controversy. Numerous factors have been proposed, including limb malalignment, muscle weakness, patellar maltracking, and chondral lesions.

Many studies have attempted to link PFPS to alterations in lower extremity kinematics, such as genu valgum, femoral internal rotation, tibial external rotation, or pes planus.[3,5,7-11] Theoretically, these malalignments increase the Q angle, which can lead to increased contact pressure between the lateral facet of the patella and the lateral trochlea, which may play a role in causing PFPS.[3] However, despite numerous investigations, gait analysis has not demonstrated any differences in the hindfoot or tibial kinematics between patients with and those without PFPS.[7,8] Gait studies have shown that the femur is slightly more internally rotated and the frontal plane moments are slightly higher in patients with PFPS.[8,9]

Weakness of the hip abductors can lead to dynamic valgus during gait. One study showed that young women with PFPS have hip abductors that are 26% weaker and hip external rotators that are 36% weaker than age-matched female controls who were pain free.[10]

Subtle patellar maltracking also may be associated with PFPS. One study reported that a TT-TG distance greater than 25 mm and a lateral patellofemoral angle of less than 8° (as measured on MRI) were predictive of anterior knee pain with a specificity of 95% and a sensitivity of 64%.[12]

Another potential source of PFPS is chondral lesions of either the patella or the trochlea. Many investigations have attempted to establish this link. Some have found an association with large or full-thickness lesions, but most have failed to demonstrate any association.[11] The difficulty in establishing this link is that asymptomatic lesions of the PFJ are exceedingly common. Thus, it may be more worthwhile to determine why some patients compensate well for their chondral lesions, whereas others do not.

Many factors have been investigated as potential causes of PFPS, and some of these have been found to be weakly associated with the condition; however, the true cause of PFPS remains elusive.

3: Knee and Leg

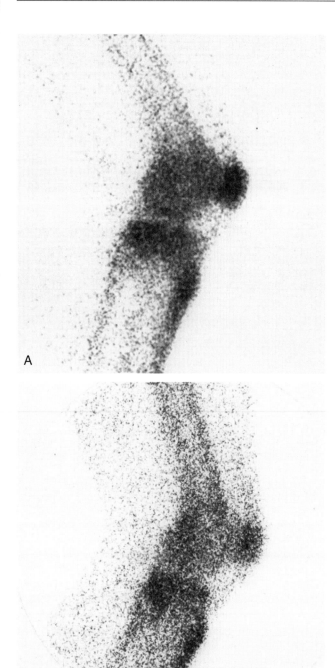

Figure 5 **A,** A technetium bone scan of a 28-year-old man with anterior knee pain shows a diffusely positive bone scan. **B,** A repeat technetium bone scan of the same patient 4 months later, after resolution of symptoms with conservative treatment. (*Reproduced with permission from Dye SF: The pathophysiology of patellofemoral pain. Clin Orthop Relat Res 2005;436:100-110.*)

Treatment

The appropriate treatment of patients with PFPS is controversial. Many types of treatment have been studied, but the evidence supporting the efficacy of most is weak.[13] The various treatments can be grouped into pharmacotherapy, bracing or taping, strengthening exercises, and surgery.

Pharmacotherapy for the treatment of patients with PFPS has been the subject of numerous articles. A Cochrane review reported some evidence that nonsteroidal anti-inflammatory drugs provide short-term pain relief but found no effect for steroids or glycosaminoglycans.[14]

The effectiveness of bracing or taping and potential mechanisms by which these treatments exert their effects have been the subject of intense interest. It has been shown that taping is effective at reducing pain, but it does not produce medial displacement of the patella and thus must act through some other mechanism.[15] A recent study showed that bracing, like taping, is effective in controlling pain.[16] It was shown that bracing does not reduce contact stress but instead acts by increasing the contact area and thus shifting some of the load onto the healthier medial cartilage. Another study showed that the patella tracking brace is useful in treating and preventing PFPS in previously pain-free individuals.[17] Despite numerous studies, a systematic review reported that there was insufficient evidence to draw conclusions about the effectiveness of this form of treatment.[18]

Exercise therapy is used frequently in the treatment of PFPS. A recent Cochrane review found that there is some evidence for its effectiveness.[19] Open (straight leg raise, leg extensions) and closed kinematic chain (leg press, step-ups) exercises are equally effective.[20]

Surgical treatment is indicated only in a small subset of patients with PFPS—those who have persistent pain despite a reasonable trial (at least 6 months) of nonsurgical therapy and have evidence of a discrete lesion that can be specifically treated with surgery. The two patterns that respond best to surgical treatment are lateral overload secondary to a tight lateral retinaculum, which can be treated with lateral release, and distal overload secondary to patella alta, which can be treated with distalization. The region of overload on the patella can be determined on bone scans, single photon emission computed tomograms, or MRIs. Suspected lateral retinacular tightness should be confirmed on CT scans taken at progressive degrees of flexion (5°, 20°, and 40°) showing lateral tilting and a taut lateral retinaculum (**Figure 6**). Lateral tilting and a slack retinaculum seen on CT scans suggest that lateral wear is the cause of the tilting. Unless the work-up reveals a taut lateral retinaculum, lateral release should not be expected to relieve symptoms. Similarly, patella alta should be confirmed with CT or MRI. An algorithmic approach is useful in helping to determine the optimal treatment for patellofemoral pain refractory to conservative care (**Figure 7**).

Patellofemoral Instability

Primary Dislocation

Nonsurgical treatment is recommended for the management of first-time traumatic patellar dislocations except when complicated by an osteochondral fracture

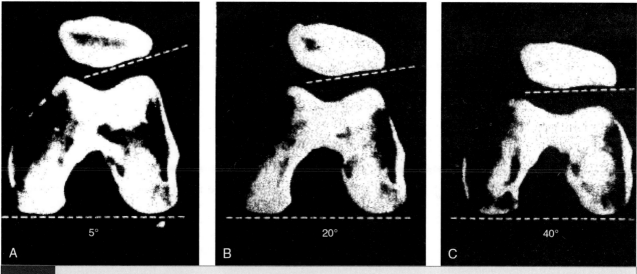

Figure 6 CT images from a patient with progressive patellar tilting beginning at 5° **(A)**, 20° **(B)**, and 40° **(C)** of flexion. The lateral patellofemoral angle is seen to decrease with increasing flexion, indicating a tight lateral retinaculum.

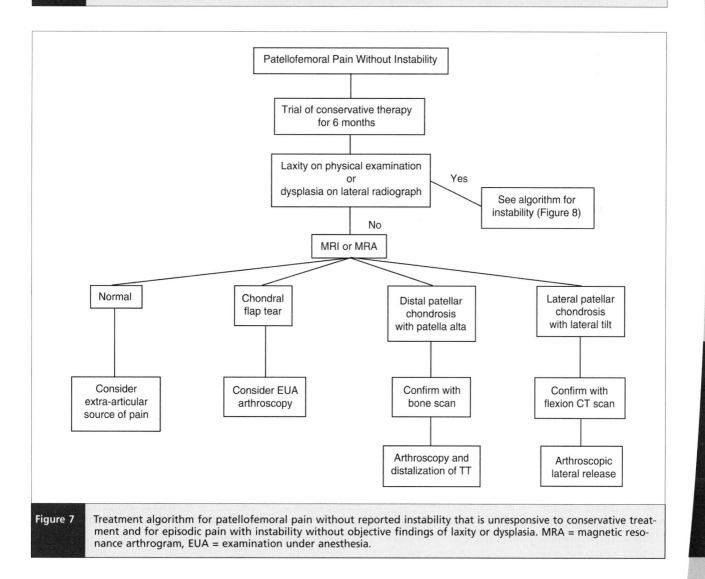

Figure 7 Treatment algorithm for patellofemoral pain without reported instability that is unresponsive to conservative treatment and for episodic pain with instability without objective findings of laxity or dysplasia. MRA = magnetic resonance arthrogram, EUA = examination under anesthesia.

3: Knee and Leg

with a loose body or complete disruption of the medial retinaculum (including the MPFL, the vastus medialis obliquus, and the adductor mechanism) with free communication between the joint and the subcutaneous space.[21] Complex dislocation should be suspected when there is a tense effusion or when a joint aspiration yields gross blood. MRI should then be used to confirm this suspicion.

Redislocation occurs infrequently after primary dislocation, with 17% of those with a primary dislocation having a second event in the next 2 to 5 years.[22] This is not the case after a second subluxation or dislocation; 50% of patients will have a third dislocation over the same time period (2 to 5 years). Interestingly, MRI evidence of MPFL injury does not correlate with the risk of subsequent redislocation among first-time dislocators. Patients with a retinacular injury, as demonstrated on MRI, are only 50% as likely to have subsequent patellar instability as those who do not have a retinacular injury. This may result from the association between predisposing factors (trochlear dysplasia and malalignment) and recurrent patellar instability and is consistent with the view that traumatic dislocations carry less risk of subsequent instability than nontraumatic dislocations. Another potential factor in redislocation is the method of nonsurgical treatment. One study reported that patients immobilized for 6 weeks had lower recurrence rates than those who wore braces and for whom full motion was allowed.[23]

Surgical treatment is infrequently needed after an initial dislocation, even in the setting of an osteochondral fracture. In a review of 1,765 first-time traumatic dislocations, the average rate of osteochondral fracture was 24.3%.[21] The fracture fragment most often originates from the medial facet of the patella and is best seen on the Merchant view. However, the bone fragments are usually in layer two, are extracapsular, and thus do not require excision. Surgical treatment is indicated for intra-articular fractures (fat fluid level on MRI) of either the patella or lateral femoral condyle. The decision of whether to fix or excise the fragment is often difficult and should be based on the size of the fragment, the degree of comminution, and the chance of obtaining adequate fixation with either 1.5-mm bioabsorbable implants or 4-mm cannulated screws.

Recurrent Instability

Patients with at least one prior episode of patellar dislocation have a 50% risk of redislocation over the subsequent 2 to 5 years.[24] Patellar instability is associated with four major factors: trochlear dysplasia, patellar height, lateral offset, and medial retinacular restraint. Although trochlear dysplasia is probably the most significant factor in terms of patellar constraint, it is rarely addressed in the treatment algorithm. Correction of trochlear dysplasia is not attempted except in rare revision cases because it is technically difficult and is usually not necessary for a successful outcome if other factors are corrected.

The treatment of patellar instability consists of quantifying and then attempting to correct the three remaining factors. Patella alta with a Caton-Deschamps ratio greater than 1.2 is corrected to between 0.8 and 1.0 by distal transfer of the TT. In planning the distal transfer based on radiographs, the surgeon should be careful to account for image magnification to avoid excessive distal transfer. Similarly, TT-TG distance greater than or equal to 20 mm is corrected to between 10 and 15 mm by medialization of the TT. The TT-TG distance should never be reduced to less than 10 mm.

Although more challenging to quantify, the competency of the medial soft-tissue tethers must be determined. MPFL reconstruction is used to treat episodic, lateral patellar instability caused by excessive laxity of medial retinacular patellar stabilizers because the MPFL is ideally oriented to resist lateral displacement of the patella. In the absence of trochlear dysplasia or patella alta, medial retinacular repair or reefing may be sufficient to stabilize the patella. However, when either patella alta or trochlear dysplasia is present and uncorrected by surgery, the demands on the native medial retinacular tissues will be greater. MPFL reconstruction rather than repair should be considered as a way to augment preexisting retinacular restraints. MPFL laxity should be documented by physical examination before proceeding with the reconstruction. If the patient is too apprehensive to allow an adequate examination, an examination under anesthesia should be done to confirm the diagnosis at the time of the procedure. An examination under anesthesia and arthroscopy routinely precede the reconstruction to objectively document laxity (without guarding or apprehension) and to stage cartilage lesions that may affect outcomes. If the median ridge of the patella can be displaced past the lateralmost aspect of the trochlea during arthroscopy, the diagnosis of medial retinacular insufficiency is confirmed.

Treatment of recurrent patellar instability remains controversial. TT osteotomy has been used frequently but long-term results have been mixed.[25] There are few studies in the literature comparing the efficacy of TT osteotomy with soft-tissue surgery. Basic science studies have demonstrated that soft-tissue reconstructions are sufficient to reestablish patellar constraint.

Isolated MPFL reconstruction without TT osteotomy has not been shown to lead to an increase in patellofemoral contact forces. In a cadaver study of specimens with normal trochlear anatomy with an experimentally created lateralized patella (TT-TG = 24 to 26 mm), overload of the medial femoral trochlea was not noted after MPFL reconstruction.[26] This study suggests that correction of malalignment may not be necessary if medial soft-tissue tethers are reestablished. Of particular interest is a recent study of isolated MPFL reconstruction in patients with trochlear dysplasia.[27] Eighty-eight percent of patients had Dejour type I, II, or III trochlear dysplasia. MPFL reconstruction alone provided satisfactory pain relief and stability in the presence of trochlear dysplasia. This study supports

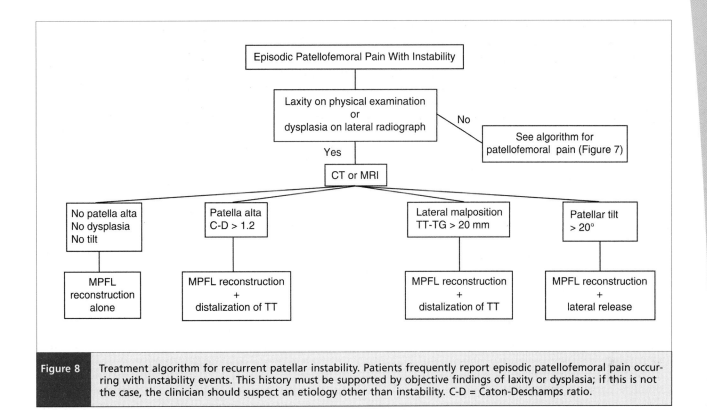

Figure 8 Treatment algorithm for recurrent patellar instability. Patients frequently report episodic patellofemoral pain occurring with instability events. This history must be supported by objective findings of laxity or dysplasia; if this is not the case, the clinician should suspect an etiology other than instability. C-D = Caton-Deschamps ratio.

the use of MPFL reconstruction in patients with deficient bony constraints.

It appears that stabilization of the patella should always include a repair or reconstruction of the MPFL to restore passive patellar restraint. MPFL reconstruction may be a more durable technique than medial retinacular repair for preventing recurrent patellar instability. It is indicated for any patient with at least two documented patellar dislocations and a physical examination indicating excessive lateral patellar mobility. The goal of MPFL reconstruction is to restore passive stability to the patella so that the patella may freely glide laterally up to 9 mm, with further displacement restricted by the reconstructed ligamentous tether (in other words, a checkrein on patellar motion has been restored). Patella alta, patellar tilt, and lateral offset are secondary factors that can contribute to patellar instability and, if present, should be treated at the time of surgery.[28] A treatment algorithm may be used as an aid in deciding which factors require surgical treatment (Figure 8).

Patellofemoral Cartilage Lesions and Osteoarthritis

Osteoarthritis

Osteoarthritis (OA) of the PFJ is a common condition. In patients age 60 years or older, its reported prevalence (based on joint-space narrowing to less than 3 mm on radiographs) is 33% in men and 36% in women. This condition exists in isolation (without tibiofemoral OA) in 15% of men and 14% of women.[29] Cartilage loss occurs more rapidly in women, those with a higher body mass index, and those with high pain scores.[30]

The symptoms of patellofemoral OA are distinct from those of tibiofemoral OA. Patients with patellofemoral OA report aching retropatellar pain that is worse with knee flexion under load, such as during stair climbing or squatting. The condition is usually characterized by tenderness with palpation of the affected facet of the patella. A complete examination also should include an assessment of lower extremity alignment, gait, and quadriceps strength.[31,32]

Patellofemoral OA often develops in the setting of PFJ derangements; specifically, a history of instability or PFPS, abnormal patellar tilt, and valgus limb malalignment are associated with OA of the PFJ.[33-35] Valgus malalignment is associated with the progression of lateral patellofemoral OA, whereas varus malalignment is associated with the progression of medial patellofemoral OA.[36]

There is significant debate concerning which radiographic views should be included in the work-up of patellofemoral OA. Some physicians obtain both lateral and axial views; others believe that a lateral view alone is sufficient. One recent study showed that the lateral view is less sensitive than the axial view in detecting OA.[29] However, another study compared two views with arthroscopy and found no difference between the sensitivity or specificity of the two views.[37] The same study also found that patellofemoral crepitus is a more reliable sign of patellofemoral OA. A third study found that the decrease in joint space over time, as measured on lateral radiographs, was better correlated with the change in cartilage thickness seen on MRI scans than on axial radiographs.[38] It appears the axial view provides no additional information about the presence of patellofemoral OA.

Effective nonsurgical treatments for patellofemoral OA include regular light exercise (150 minutes per week), weight loss, medializing patellar taping, varus-producing braces, and physical therapy for quadriceps strengthening.[31] Surgical treatment options include lateral release, osteophyte removal, partial or complete patellectomy, patellofemoral arthroplasty, and total knee arthroplasty.[32] Unloading of diseased cartilage can sometimes be accomplished through soft-tissue release or TT transfer (anterior displacement with or without medialization).[39] Cadaver studies have shown that anteromedialization reduces the mean total contact pressure while shifting contact pressures proximally and medially.[40,41] This can be useful if the lesion is small and distal but is less effective if the lesion is more extensive. Preoperative MRI or staging arthroscopy can be useful to ascertain the extent and location of cartilage loss. Complete patellectomy profoundly alters knee function by weakening the quadriceps/patellar tendon, reducing peak extensor torque, and increasing tibiofemoral loads. The patella should never be sacrificed, except perhaps in cases of severe trauma.[32]

In patients with disabling OA limited to the PFJ with full-thickness cartilage loss on both articulating surfaces, arthroplasty may be considered. In patients older than 60 years, total knee arthroplasty generally is preferred for durability and simplicity.[42] In younger patients, patellofemoral unicompartmental arthroplasty may be considered if the surgeon is experienced and comfortable with the technique. Most failures of patellofemoral unicompartmental arthroplasty have been attributed to uncorrected malalignment or progression of OA in the tibiofemoral compartments. Recent studies suggest that technical errors, such as overstuffing and malrotation, may lead to inferior outcomes.[43,44] Even when performed by an experienced surgeon, patellofemoral unicompartmental arthroplasty provides less reliable outcomes than total knee arthroplasty. The patient's disability should justify the risk of patellofemoral unicompartmental arthroplasty, and the patient should be informed that functional outcomes (pain, swelling, and activity level) may be disappointing even if the surgery is done well.[42]

Focal Lesions of Cartilage

Focal lesions of the cartilage of the PFJ often arise from trauma but also may occur in the setting of chronic derangements, such as instability or overload. Symptomatic focal chondral defects are difficult to treat nonsurgically. Surgical strategies can be classified into débridement (chondroplasty), unloading and/or realignment, and cartilage restoration.

As is the situation in patients with OA, unloading the diseased cartilage can be accomplished through soft-tissue release or TT transfer. Lateral release is indicated for patients with a tight lateral retinaculum resulting in lateral tilting of the patella and mild lateral facet chondrosis. It is contraindicated in patients with excessive laxity or a history of patellar instability. Anteromedial TT transfer is successful in treating patients with chondral lesions located on the distal or lateral portions of the patella; however, medial, central, diffuse, and proximal lesions do not improve and may actually be made worse with anteromedialization.[45]

There are many cartilage restoration procedures, including microfracture, mosaicplasty (osteochondral autograft transplantation), autologous chondrocyte implantation, and osteochondral shell allografts. There are only a few studies that have focused on the use of these techniques in the PFJ. Microfracture does not provide durable results for either patellar or trochlear lesions regardless of the patient's age.[46] In contrast, autologous chondrocyte implantation has shown some promising early results for lesions of the trochlea.[47] Early results with autologous chondrocyte implantation of the patella also have been promising and are improved with the performance of a concomitant realignment procedure.[48] Osteochondral autograft transplantation has shown good results in the trochlea but very poor results in the patella.[49] Fresh osteochondral allografts have been used in the PFJ; however, the technique involves replacement of the entire surface of the patella, trochlea, or both and is better suited to treating more diffuse chondral lesions.[50]

Despite the lack of conclusive evidence for the efficacy of using any of the cartilage restoration procedures in the PFJ, some general principles have emerged and are useful in making treatment decisions. First, any cartilage restoration procedure performed on the PFJ will tend to have worse results than the same procedure performed on a similar lesion in the tibiofemoral joint because of differences in the mechanical environment to which the repaired tissue will be subjected. Second, before embarking on any cartilage restoration procedure, the lesion must be fully characterized. Several questions should be answered. (1) Is the cartilage affected on only one side of the joint (monopolar) or are kissing (bipolar) lesions present? (2) Is the lesion well shouldered (surrounded by healthy cartilage) or is the surrounding cartilage also diseased? (3) Is there an associated trochlear dysplasia, maltracking, or alta? These malalignments provide an opportunity to unload or bypass the lesion.

Summary

The PFJ is a biomechanically complex articulation. The most common disorders—pain, instability, and OA—are usually associated with mechanical derangements. Most patients will respond to nonsurgical therapies, and these should be the first line of treatment. For those in whom nonsurgical treatment is unsuccessful, a thorough patient history and physical examination are needed. The choice of surgical treatment should be based on the patient's reported symptoms, which must correlate with the objective evidence obtained from the physical examination and imaging studies. Using this approach, the surgeon can be successful in treating these challenging disorders.

Annotated References

1. Amis AA, Senavongse W, Bull AM: Patellofemoral kinematics during knee flexion-extension: An in vitro study. *J Orthop Res* 2006;24:2201-2211.

   In a cadaver study of patellofemoral tracking during loading of the quadriceps, the authors found that the patella translates 4 mm medial from 0° to 20°, then translates 7 mm lateral from 20° to 90°. Tilt is progressive in a linear fashion to 7° at 90° of knee flexion. Patellar flexion is 0.7 times knee flexion.

2. Senavongse W, Amis AA: The effects of articular, retinacular, or muscular deficiencies on patellofemoral joint stability. *J Bone Joint Surg Br* 2005;87:577-582.

   The authors report on a cadaver study of the roles of muscle, soft tissue, and bone in patellar restraint and quantify the relative contributions of the lateral femoral condyle, the vastus medialis obliquus, and the medial retinaculum at various flexion angles. The trochlea dominated as the primary constraint to patellar displacement. The medial retinaculum was the second most important constraint. Vastus medialis obliquus contributed to a minor degree up to 20° of flexion but not at higher flexion angles.

3. Powers CM: The influence of altered lower-extremity kinematics on patellofemoral joint dysfunction: A theoretical perspective. *J Orthop Sports Phys Ther* 2003;33:639-646.

   An excellent review of how alteration in lower extremity alignment affects PFJ forces is presented. Increasing tibial external rotation, femoral internal rotation, and genu valgum lead to increases in the Q angle and a subsequent increase in lateral patellofemoral pressure. These lower extremity malalignments occur dynamically during gait, landing, or stair stepping. They are likely the result of proximal weakness or poor neuromuscular control. These findings suggest that treatments used to manage patellofemoral disorders should focus on the hip rather than the knee.

4. Ward SR, Terk MR, Powers CM: Patella alta: Association with patellofemoral alignment and changes in contact area during weight-bearing. *J Bone Joint Surg Am* 2007;89:1749-1755.

   With the quadriceps contracted, patients with patella alta (Insall-Salvati ratio > 1.2) had, on average, 19% less contact area than control patients without patella alta over the range of 0° to 60° of flexion. Patients with patella alta also had 20% more lateral patellar displacement and 39% more lateral patellar tilt than subjects with a normal patellar position at 0° of flexion. The association between patella alta and malalignment was seen only with the knee in full extension; however, decreased contact area leading to increased joint reactive forces were measured in all knee flexion angles from 0° to 60°. The authors considered patella alta to represent a form of malalignment because of its affect on patellofemoral weight-bearing surface area.

5. Fulkerson JP: The etiology of patellofemoral pain in young, active patients: A prospective study. *Clin Orthop Relat Res* 1983;179:129-133.

6. Morphologic factors in patellar instability: Clinical, radiologic, and tomographic data. *Journe'Es Du Genou* 1987;6:25-35.

7. Levinger P, Gilleard W: Tibia and rearfoot motion and ground reaction forces in subjects with patellofemoral pain syndrome during walking. *Gait Posture* 2007;25:2-8.

   Three-dimensional hindfoot and tibial rotation and ground reaction forces were examined in 13 patients with PFPS and compared with 14 age-matched controls. The authors reported no difference in hindfoot kinematic angles but found differences in timing, with peak eversion occurring later and peak dorsiflexion occurring earlier in the gait cycle for PFPS patients. In the kinetics analysis, they found a decreased peak medial ground reaction force in PFPS (0.04 compared with 0.06 times body weight). It was concluded that a delay in eversion (and more rapid dorsiflexion) helps patients with PFPS to attenuate shock.

8. Powers CM, Chen PY, Reischl SF, Perry J: Comparison of foot pronation and lower extremity rotation in persons with and without patellofemoral pain. *Foot Ankle Int* 2002;23:634-640.

9. Stefanyshyn DJ, Stergiou P, Lun VM, Meeuwisse WH, Worobets JT: Knee angular impulse as a predictor of patellofemoral pain in runners. *Am J Sports Med* 2006;34:1844-1851.

   This biomechanical study compared 20 runners with PFPS to 20 who were asymptomatic; it also evaluated a group of 140 runners in an epidemiologic study. Frontal plane moments about the knee during the stance phase of running were examined. They found that runners with PFPS have significantly higher knee abduction impulses than asymptomatic runners, and runners in whom PFPS develops have higher knee abduction impulses than comparable uninjured runners. It was concluded that increased frontal plane impulses lead to increased joint contact stress.

10. Ireland ML, Willson JD, Ballantyne BT, Davis IM: Hip strength in females with and without patellofemoral pain. *J Orthop Sports Phys Ther* 2003;33:671-676.

   A dynamometer was used to compare hip abduction and internal rotation strength in young women with PFPS and an age-matched control group. The authors found that the PFPS group was 26% weaker in abduction and 36% weaker in external rotation. They concluded that a valgus and internally rotated femur may

3: Knee and Leg

cause the patella to track laterally and thus increase PFJ contact pressure. A role for proximal strengthening in the rehabilitation of patients with PFPS was postulated.

11. Kettunen JA, Visuri T, Harilainen A, Sandelin J, Kujala UM: Primary cartilage lesions and outcome among subjects with patellofemoral pain syndrome. *Knee Surg Sports Traumatol Arthrosc* 2005;13:131-134.

   Two groups of patients with PFPS were examined (one retrospectively and the other prospectively) to determine an association between the severity of chondral lesions and PFPS symptoms. Lesions with an area greater than 5 cm² or Outerbridge grade 4 were considered severe. The Kujala score and pain on the visual analogue scale were evaluated after the performance of 10 squats. In both groups, patients with severe lesions had more symptoms and limitations than patients without lesions or those with small lesions—a different finding from other studies evaluating PFJ cartilage lesions and PFPS.

12. Wittstein JR, Bartlett EC, Easterbrook J, Byrd JC: Magnetic resonance imaging evaluation of patellofemoral malalignment. *Arthroscopy* 2006;22:643-649.

   This clinical case control study used MRI to compare the patellar height, tilt, and lateral offset in 14 patients (10 female and 4 male) with anterior knee pain with 20 patients (14 male and 6 female) with other internal derangements of the knee. The authors found that the knees of the patients with anterior knee pain had significantly greater lateralization, tilt, and alta. The changes in these measurements may be associated with anterior knee pain. The conclusions are limited by the small sample size and the lack of gender matching between the patients in the two groups.

13. Bizzini M, Childs JD, Piva SR, Delitto A: Systematic review of the quality of randomized controlled trials for patellofemoral pain syndrome. *J Orthop Sports Phys Ther* 2003;33:4-20.

   A systematic review of randomized trials for various methods of conservative treatment of patellofemoral pain is presented. The authors report that acupuncture, quadriceps strengthening, resistive bracing, soft foot orthotics, and the combination of exercise with patellar taping and biofeedback for treating patients with excessive pronation are all useful; however, the quality of the studies reviewed was generally poor.

14. Heintjes E, Berger MY, Bierma-Zeinstra SM, et al: Pharmacotherapy for patellofemoral pain syndrome. *Cochrane Database Syst Rev* 2004;3:CD003470.

   The authors present a Cochrane database review of evidence for pharmacotherapy in treating patellofemoral pain. There is limited evidence that nonsteroidal anti-inflammatory drugs provide short-term pain relief. No effect was found for steroids or glycosaminoglycans.

15. Pfeiffer RP, DeBeliso M, Shea KG, et al: Kinematic MRI assessment of McConnell taping before and after exercise. *Am J Sports Med* 2004;32:621-628.

   The authors present the results of a kinematic study of healthy young women using MRI to assess whether McConnell taping is effective in medially displacing the patella before and after exercise. They found that taping creates medial displacement before exercising (1 to 1.6 mm), but the effect is lost after exercising. It was concluded that taping produces pain relief by some other mechanism.

16. Powers CM, Ward SR, Chen YJ, Chan LD, Terk MR: Effect of bracing on patellofemoral joint stress while ascending and descending stairs. *Clin J Sport Med* 2004;14:206-214.

   An experimental study was performed to determine whether bracing leads to decreased patellofemoral stress during provocative exercise (stair climbing). Fifteen patients with patellofemoral pain were evaluated with MRI at 0°, 20°, 40°, and 60° flexion with a 25% weight-bearing load to assess patellofemoral contact with and without a brace. Patients then performed a stairclimbing task (with and without the brace) with force plate and kinematic analysis of the pelvis, the thigh, the leg, and the foot while ascending and descending stairs. The authors reported that although bracing increased the contact area, the calculated PFJ reaction force increased, keeping the stress basically unchanged. Despite this finding, there was a 50% decrease in pain. It was concluded that bracing shifts the load onto the healthier medial cartilage, permitting higher forces and more work. The authors' use of static measurements of the contact area and their modeling of reaction forces using a nonlinear model should be validated by further studies.

17. Van Tiggelen D, Witvrouw E, Roget P, et al : Effect of bracing on the prevention of anterior knee pain: A prospective randomized study. *Knee Surg Sports Traumatol Arthrosc* 2004;12:434-439.

   A prospective randomized control trial was undertaken to determine whether a dynamic patellofemoral brace is effective in preventing acute knee pain in healthy men in military basic training. Recruits were randomized to a bilateral brace in comparison with a control group with no brace. The authors reported that acute knee pain developed in 18.5% of recruits in the brace group and 37% of those in the control group. The authors concluded that patellofemoral bracing is effective in preventing PFPS, but they were uncertain of the mechanism and could not exclude the placebo effect.

18. D'hondt NE, Struijs PA, Kerkhoffs GM, et al: Orthotic devices for treating patellofemoral pain syndrome. *Cochrane Database Syst Rev* 2002;2:CD002267.

19. Heintjes E, Berger MY, Bierma-Zeinstra SM, et al: Exercise therapy for patellofemoral pain syndrome. *Cochrane Database Syst Rev* 2003;4:CD003472.

   A Cochrane database review of clinical trials of exercise therapy for treating patellofemoral pain is presented. The authors found weak evidence for exercise in treating patellofemoral pain (based on one strong study and one study that was problematic because of the control group). They found strong evidence that open- and closed-chain exercises were equally effective.

20. Witvrouw E, Danneels L, Van Tiggelen D, Willems TM, Cambier D: Open versus closed kinetic chain exercises in patellofemoral pain: A 5-year prospective randomized study. *Am J Sports Med* 2004;32:1122-1130.

    The authors present the results of a prospective study of open- versus closed-chain exercise programs for PFPS. Twenty-four patients were randomized into a 5-week open-chain exercise program and 25 into a closed-chain program, followed by a home exercise program. Follow-up at 5 weeks, 3 months, and 5 years assessed subjective pain, functional tasks, and muscle strength measurements. The authors found poor compliance with the home exercise program, good subjective and overall functional results, and no significant differences between the groups at 5-year follow-up.

21. Stefancin JJ, Parker RD: First-time traumatic patellar dislocation: A systematic review. *Clin Orthop Relat Res* 2007;455:93-101.

    Seventy studies were systematically reviewed to determine when patients with first-time traumatic dislocations should receive initial surgical treatment. The authors concluded that first-time traumatic dislocation should be treated nonsurgically except in the presence of an osteochondral fracture, substantial disruption of the medial patellar stabilizers, a laterally subluxated patella with normal alignment of the contralateral knee, a second dislocation, or in patients not improving with appropriate rehabilitation.

22. Fithian DC, Paxton EW, Stone ML, et al: Epidemiology and natural history of acute patellar dislocation. *Am J Sports Med* 2004;32:1114-1121.

    In this prospective cohort study of acute patellar dislocations, 189 patients were followed for a period of 2 to 5 years. Patients presenting with a prior history of instability were more likely to be female and were older than patients with first-time dislocations. Fewer first-time dislocators (17%) had episodes of instability during follow-up than patients with a previous history of instability (49%). After adjustment for demographics, patients with a prior history of instability had a seven times higher risk for subsequent instability episodes during the follow-up period than patients with first-time dislocations (adjusted odds ratio = 6.6, P < 0.001). The authors concluded that patellar dislocators who present with a history of patellofemoral instability are more likely to be female, older, and have a greater risk of subsequent patellar instability episodes than patients with first-time patellar dislocations. Risk of recurrent patellar instability episodes in either knee is much higher in this group than in first-time dislocators.

23. Mäenpää H, Lehto MU: Patellar dislocation: The long-term results of nonoperative management in 100 patients. *Am J Sports Med* 1997;25:213-217.

24. Fithian DC, Neyret P: Patellar instability: The Lyon experience. *Tech Knee Surg* 2007;6:112-123.

    An algorithm for work-up and management of a patient with patellar instability is presented. Treatment decisions are based on objective evidence of trochlear dysplasia obtained from a strict lateral radiograph taken at 30° of knee flexion. If the crossing sign is present, CT images are obtained to evaluate the three principal factors in objective patellar instability. Correction of each factor is planned according to the measurements taken from the CT images. TT-TG distance greater than 20 mm is corrected to between 10 and 15 mm by medialization of the TT. Patella alta is corrected to between 0.8 and 1.0 by distal transfer of the TT. A patellar tilt greater than 20° is corrected by lateral release or vastus medialis oblique advancement.

25. Carney JR, Mologne TS, Muldoon M, Cox JS: Long-term evaluation of the Roux-Elmslie-Trillat procedure for patellar instability: A 26-year follow-up. *Am J Sports Med* 2005;33:1220-1223.

    A case series evaluating recurrent instability and functional outcome in patients treated with the Roux-Elmslie-Trillat procedure at a mean follow-up of 26 years was compared with the prevalence reported at the mean follow-up of 3 years. Recurrent subluxation or dislocation occurred in only 7% of patients; despite this, functional scores decreased from 73% good-to-excellent results at 3 years to 54% at 26 years.

26. Bicos J, Carofino B, Andersen M, et al: Patellofemoral forces after medial patellofemoral ligament reconstruction: A biomechanical analysis. *J Knee Surg* 2006;19: 317-326.

    A cadaver study of MPFL reconstruction in knees with normal trochlear anatomy but a distal malalignment showed that MPFL reconstruction restored the position and tilt of the patella to the intact-state values. The load on the medial femoral trochlea was not increased relative to the intact state in either the lateralized or the MPFL reconstructed states.

27. Steiner TM, Torga-Spak R, Teitge RA: Medial patellofemoral ligament reconstruction in patients with lateral patellar instability and trochlear dysplasia. *Am J Sports Med* 2006;34:1254-1261.

    In this case study of 34 patients with chronic patellar instability and trochlear dysplasia treated with MPFL reconstruction, patients were evaluated preoperatively and postoperatively with Kujala, Lysholm, and Tegner scores. The authors found that MPFL reconstruction prevents recurrent dislocation and provides excellent long-term pain relief and functional outcomes.

28. Servien E, Verdonk PC, Neyret P: Tibial tuberosity transfer for episodic patellar dislocation. *Sports Med Arthrosc* 2007;15:61-67.

    A review of surgical treatments for episodic patellar dislocation is presented. A treatment algorithm is proposed based on anatomic factors—trochlear dysplasia, patella alta, patellar tilt, and an excessive TT-TG distance. The roles of TT transfer, MPFL reconstruction, and trochleoplasty are discussed.

29. Davies AP, Vince AS, Shepstone L, Donell ST, Glasgow MM: The radiologic prevalence of patellofemoral osteoarthritis. *Clin Orthop Relat Res* 2002;402: 206-212.

3: Knee and Leg

30. Cicuttini F, Wluka A, Wang Y, Stuckey S: The determinants of change in patella cartilage volume in osteoarthritic knees. *J Rheumatol* 2002;29:2615-2619.

31. Hinman RS, Crossley KM: Patellofemoral joint osteoarthritis: An important subgroup of knee osteoarthritis. *Rheumatology (Oxford)* 2007;46:1057-1062.

The presentation, diagnosis, and treatment of OA of the PFJ are presented as well as a good summary of the biomechanics of the PFJ. A history of dislocation, subluxation, abnormal tilt, and valgus malalignment are all associated with OA of the PFJ. Symptoms include retropatellar pain that is worse with flexion, tenderness to palpation of a facet, malalignment, abnormal gait, and poor quadriceps strength. Treatment consists of patellar taping or bracing and possibly physical therapy.

32. Donell ST, Glasgow MM: Isolated patellofemoral osteoarthritis. *Knee* 2007;14:169-176.

The authors present a review of OA of the PFJ, including anatomy, alignment, clinical presentation, work-up, and treatments (lateral release, patellectomy, osteotomy, patellofemoral arthroplasty, and total knee arthroplasty). It was concluded that weight loss and quadriceps strengthening are effective in most patients; however, no good evidence was found.

33. Utting MR, Davies G, Newman JH: Is anterior knee pain a predisposing factor to patellofemoral osteoarthritis? *Knee* 2005;12:362-365.

The authors try to determine if adolescent anterior knee pain is related to the development of OA of the PFJ. One hundred fifty patients treated with patellofemoral arthroplasty and 150 treated with medial unicompartmental arthroplasty were surveyed about the existence of anterior knee pain, injury, and instability as children. The authors report that patients with OA of the PFJ more frequently recalled having had anterior knee pain (22% compared with 6%) and instability symptoms (14% compared with 1%) as children. They concluded that adolescent PFPS or instability may not be benign.

34. Cahue S, Dunlop D, Hayes K, et al: Varus-valgus alignment in the progression of patellofemoral osteoarthritis. *Arthritis Rheum* 2004;50:2184-2190.

A clinical study that examined the relationship between limb alignment and progression of medial or lateral patellofemoral OA is presented. The authors examined 397 knees over an 18-month period and found that 30% of those studied had progression of lateral patellofemoral OA; if valgus alignment was present, the odds ratio for progression was 1.64. In contrast, 15% of knees studied had progression of medial patellofemoral OA; those with a varus alignment had an odds ratio of 1.85. It was concluded that valgus alignment is associated with the progression of lateral patellofemoral OA and varus alignment with the progression of medial patellofemoral OA.

35. Christoforakis JJ, Strachan RK: Internal derangements of the knee associated with patellofemoral joint degeneration. *Knee Surg Sports Traumatol Arthrosc* 2005;13:581-584.

In this study, 854 patients who were treated with knee arthroscopy were found to have chondral lesions of the PFJ. Isolated patellofemoral degeneration occurred in a higher proportion of patients with maltracking (64.7%) than those with normal tracking (18%). An increased incidence of OA of the PFJ also was found in knees with plica versus those without (24.7% compared with 15.5%, respectively). Ligamentous and meniscal injuries were negatively associated with isolated OA of the PFJ.

36. Harilainen A, Lindroos M, Sandelin J, Tallroth K, Kujala UM: Patellofemoral relationships and cartilage breakdown. *Knee Surg Sports Traumatol Arthrosc* 2005;13:142-144.

The authors present the results of a clinical study comparing the location of chondral lesions found at arthroscopy to radiographic measurements of patellar height and lateral position in two groups of patients (24 patients with PFPS and 21 with meniscal tears). The authors found that patella alta was associated with central patellar lesions, and lateral patellar position was associated with both lateral patellar and lateral trochlear lesions in both groups. In the PFPS group, the patella was more likely to be laterally positioned. There were no differences between groups with respect to patellar height or tilt.

37. Bhattacharya R, Kumar V, Safawi E, Finn P, Hui AC: The knee skyline radiograph: Its usefulness in the diagnosis of patello-femoral osteoarthritis. *Int Orthop* 2007;31:247-252.

The authors present the results of a study comparing patellofemoral crepitus as a clinical sign and skyline and lateral radiographs in diagnosing OA of the PFJ in 77 patients reporting knee pain. The lateral and skyline radiographs were found to have a sensitivity of 82% and 79%, respectively, and a specificity of 65% and 80%, respectively; this was not statistically significant. Crepitus was found to be 89% sensitive and 82% specific. It was concluded that the skyline radiograph adds no additional information; of the three indicators, crepitus best correlates with the operative appearance of the cartilage.

38. Cicuttini FM, Wluka AE, Hankin J, Stuckey S: Comparison of patella cartilage volume and radiography in the assessment of longitudinal joint change at the patellofemoral joint. *J Rheumatol* 2004;31:1369-1372.

The results of a study comparing measurements of longitudinal changes at the PFJ on lateral and skyline radiographs to MRI measurements in a 2-year follow-up study of 102 patients with OA of the PFJ are presented. Joint space measured on lateral radiographs better correlated with the MRI assessment of cartilage loss than measurements from skyline radiographs.

39. Fulkerson JP: Alternatives to patellofemoral arthroplasty. *Clin Orthop Relat Res* 2005;436:76-80.

A review of nonarthroplasty treatment options for isolated OA of the PFJ is presented. After failed conservative treatment and the failure of basic procedures such as débridement, release, and realignment, the surgical options are TT transfer, patellectomy, cartilage resurfacing, and arthroplasty. Straight anteriorization leads to skin necrosis, nonunion, and the risk of compartment syndrome. Anteromedialization is useful in patients with lateral facet arthrosis because it shifts pressure onto the medial facet and unloads the joint. It is not useful in treating proximal patellar lesions because it tends to shift the load proximally. Patellectomy leads to chronic weakness and trochlear wear and should be used only as a last resort when the patella is severely degenerated and the trochlea is intact. Autologous chondrocyte implantation has not been well studied in the PFJ. Cartilage transplantation combined with anteromedialization is a good alternative, but there are no studies to demonstrate its long-term success.

40. Ramappa AJ, Apreleva M, Harrold FR, Fitzgibbons G, Wilson DR, Gill TJ: The effects of medialization and anteromedialization of the tibial tubercle on patellofemoral mechanics and kinematics. *Am J Sports Med* 2006; 34:749-756.

The authors of a controlled laboratory study of TT osteotomies on 10 human cadaver knees found that straight medialization and anteromedialization are equivalent in correcting patellar mechanics and kinematics.

41. Ballester J, Muñoz MC, Vazquez J, Torres J: Biomechanical effects of different surgical procedures on the extensor mechanism of the patellofemoral joint. *Clin Orthop Relat Res* 1995;320:168-175.

42. Saleh KJ, Arendt EA, Eldridge J, et al: Symposium: Operative treatment of patellofemoral arthritis. *J Bone Joint Surg Am* 2005;87:659-671.

Reviews of treatment options for isolated OA of the PFJ, including osteotomy, patellofemoral arthroplasty, and total knee arthroplasty, are presented.

43. Nicol SG, Loveridge JM, Weale AE, Ackroyd CE, Newman JH: Arthritis progression after joint replacement. *Knee* 2006;13:290-295.

In this prospective study, 103 patients treated with PFJ replacement were evaluated to determine the frequency of conversion to total knee arthroplasty secondary to progression of symptomatic tibiofemoral OA. The authors reported that 14% of these patients were revised to total knee arthroplasty at a mean revision time of 55 months. Knees with trochlear dysplasia were less likely to need revision to total knee arthroplasty.

44. Leadbetter WB, Ragland PS, Mont MA: The appropriate use of patellofemoral arthroplasty: An analysis of reported indications, contraindications, and failures. *Clin Orthop Relat Res* 2005;436:91-99.

The authors present a systematic review of the indications, contraindications, and factors contributing to the failure of patellofemoral arthroplasty from 12 studies. Commonly cited contraindications are tibiofemoral arthritis, uncorrected patellofemoral or tibiofemoral malalignment, and inflammatory arthritis. The highest failure rates were reported in patients with progression of OA in other compartments or persistence of congenital or surgically uncorrected malalignment.

45. Pidoriano AJ, Weinstein RN, Buuck DA, Fulkerson JP: Correlation of patellar articular lesions with results from anteromedial tibial tubercle transfer. *Am J Sports Med* 1997;25:533-537.

46. Kreuz PC, Erggelet C, Steinwachs MR, et al: Is microfracture of chondral defects in the knee associated with different results in patients aged 40 years or younger? *Arthroscopy* 2006;22:1180-1186.

A case series of 85 patients with full thickness chondral lesions treated with microfracture is presented. Patients were divided into six groups based on patient age (older or younger than age 40 years) and lesion location (femoral condyles, tibia, and PFJ). Patients were evaluated preoperatively and 6, 18, and 36 months postoperatively with Cincinnati and International Cartilage Repair scores. Outcomes were best and did not deteriorate over time for young patients with defects on the femoral condyles or the tibia. The results were worse and deteriorated over time (regardless of patient age) for lesions located in the trochlea or on the patella.

47. Mandelbaum B, Browne JE, Fu F, et al: Treatment outcomes of autologous chondrocyte implantation for full-thickness articular cartilage defects of the trochlea. *Am J Sports Med* 2007;35:915-921.

A case study of 40 patients (with 2-year follow-up) who were treated with autologous chondrocyte implantation for full thickness cartilage lesions of the trochlea is presented. Lesion size averaged 4.5 cm². Improvements occurred in the Cincinnati score, and patients had decreased pain and swelling. The results did not decrease over time. Eleven of the 40 patients required subsequent procedures.

48. Henderson IJ, Lavigne P: Periosteal autologous chondrocyte implantation for patellar chondral defect in patients with normal and abnormal patellar tracking. *Knee* 2006;13:274-279.

A clinical study comparing clinical outcomes at 2-year follow-up for patients with patellar chondral lesions treated with autologous chondrocyte implantation compared with those treated with autologous chondrocyte implantation and extensor realignment found that patients with malalignment and thus concomitant extensor realignment had better outcomes. The authors concluded than an unloading osteotomy may be beneficial for patients with normal alignment.

49. Bentley G, Biant LC, Carrington RW, et al: A prospective, randomised comparison of autologous chondrocyte implantation versus mosaicplasty for osteochondral defects in the knee. *J Bone Joint Surg Br* 2003;85: 223-230.

A prospective randomized clinical trial of autologous chondrocyte implantation versus mosaicplasty for the treatment of chondral defects of the knee is presented. Clinical and arthroscopic follow-up at 1 year showed poor results for patients treated with mosaicplasty of the patella.

50. Torga Spak R, Teitge RA: Fresh osteochondral allografts for patellofemoral arthritis: Long-term follow-up. *Clin Orthop Relat Res* 2006;444:193-200.

3: Knee and Leg

A clinical study of bipolar osteochondral allografts for the treatment of patellofemoral OA in 14 knees in 11 women age 55 years or younger with more than 2-year follow-up are presented. Treatment failure was defined as conversion to total knee arthroplasty. The procedure was deemed to be successful in 8 of 14 knees. Two failures were caused by graft segmentation and collapse, 1 was caused by recurrent dislocation, and 3 were caused by progression of tibiofemoral OA. The authors reported good functional results; however, many revisions were necessary.

Chapter 12

Knee Ligament Injuries

David M. Junkin Jr, MD   *Darren L. Johnson, MD   Freddie H. Fu, MD   *Mark D. Miller, MD
Melissa Willenborg, MD   Gregory C. Fanelli, MD   Daniel C. Wascher, MD

Anterior Cruciate Ligament Injury

With approximately 400,000 anterior cruciate ligament (ACL) reconstructions annually in the United States, improved treatment of this severe knee injury is of great focus and interest. Despite conventional surgical reconstructive measures, both short- and long-term studies have shown an increased incidence and progression of osteoarthritis after so-called successful reconstruction.[1-4] Radiographic evidence of osteoarthritis has been reported in 79% to 90% of patients in as few as 7 years after reconstruction.[2,5] The rate of progression is dependent on multiple factors, including age and associated meniscal, osteochondral, or other ligamentous pathology.

Nonsurgical treatment, particularly in the young, active patient, has produced unsatisfactory results. The articular cartilage changes in contact areas in the ACL-deficient knee lead to an acceleration of chondral wear and increased incidence of meniscal tears, which contribute to the progression of osteoarthritis.[6] Functional bracing in the ACL-deficient patient, while possibly reducing the incidence of instability events, has not prevented the progression of degenerative changes in the knee.

Long-term evaluation of ACL graft integrity and anteroposterior stability is good to excellent according to several studies.[2,5] Kinematic studies and gait analysis studies have demonstrated near-normal flexion-extension moments in the ACL-reconstructed knee more than 1 year after surgical reconstruction.[7] However, other studies have investigated the tibiofemoral rotational moments about the knee during low- and high-demand activities in the ACL-reconstructed knee in hopes of identifying the causes of osteoarthritis.[7-9] All patients in these studies underwent surgical reconstruction with either a bone-patellar tendon-bone or hamstring autograft. Anterior translation was similar in the uninjured and reconstructed knees but normal internal-external tibial rotation was not restored, par-

ticularly during activities such as running, jumping, or pivoting.

As outcome measures and studies continue to demonstrate the short- and long-term development of osteoarthritis, in addition to the expansion of knowledge of normal joint biomechanics and anatomy, surgical techniques for ACL reconstruction will continue to evolve. A focus on a more anatomic reconstruction has emerged over the past few years, and its clinical significance currently is being defined. The degree of anatomic precision of surgical techniques is unknown. In acetabular fracture surgery, anatomic reduction within 2 mm of perfect is required for optimal outcome. With clinical outcome scores resulting in a normal International Knee Documentation Committee (IKDC) score of only 33% for contemporary single tunnel hamstring autograft reconstructions and 41% of bone-patellar tendon-bone autograft reconstructions, additional investigation of a more anatomic reconstruction is warranted.[2]

Diagnosis

The Lachman test is the most clinically sensitive examination for a complete ACL rupture, with a predictability equal to or greater than MRI. The pivot shift test, most easily done with the patient under anesthesia, confirms the absence of a competent functioning ligament and is the most specific physical examination finding that correlates with return to play of the level 1 athlete. Sagittal MRI remains the standard for noninvasive diagnostic modalities. Improved MRI technology has allowed improved visualization of the ACL and its individual anteromedial and posterolateral bundles.[10]

Associated injuries are common, particularly meniscal tears, osteochondral lesions, and collateral ligament injuries. Missed fibular collateral ligament and posterolateral corner injuries are increasingly recognized as a cause of failed ACL reconstruction because secondary instabilities greatly increase the stress on the replacement graft substitute with resultant late failure. Meniscal tears have a long-term impact on the injured knee with the associated progression of osteoarthritis. Injuries to the medial collateral ligament (MCL) are commonly associated with ACL tears, particularly in patients who participate in contact sports. Grade I injuries pose little concern because no valgus instability

*Darren L. Johnson, MD or the department with which he is affiliated has received research or institutional support from Smith & Nephew Endoscopy. Mark D. Miller, MD or the department with which he is affiliated has received royalties from WB Saunders/Elsevier.

3: Knee and Leg

Table 1

Consensus Statements: 2005 Hunt Valley II Meeting Prevention Programs

• There is good level II evidence that neuromuscular training including plyometrics, balance, and technique training, as well as a heightened awareness of injury biomechanics, reduces the risk of serious knee injuries in female athletes. What specific exercises or sequence of exercises or what intensity and duration of exercise are most important is still unknown.

• All reported prevention programs for ACL noncontact injuries center on alteration of neuromuscular risk factors, but each is unique. Some are sport specific; some are general; some are age specific; some are not. Most have been designed for and tested with female athletes.

• The underlying mechanism by which intervention programs are effective is not clearly understood; however, existing evidence points to changes in balance, strength, and neuromuscular coordination as possible contributors.

• Training may facilitate neuromuscular adaptations that provide increased joint stabilization and muscular preactivation and reactive patterns that may protect the athlete's ACL from increased loading.

(Data from Griffin LY, Albohm MJ, Arendt EA, et al: Understanding and preventing noncontact anterior cruciate ligament injuries: A review of the Hunt Valley II Meeting. January 2005. Am J Sports Med 2006;34:1512-1532.)

---

is present. Numerous studies support nonsurgical treatment of the MCL in associated grade II injuries because no increased incidence of instability can be observed in comparison with patients without an associated MCL injury.[11] Complete tears of the MCL have continued to impact ACL reconstruction results, with concerns about continued valgus instability. Surgical and nonsurgical treatment of grade III MCL ruptures with concurrent ACL reconstructions were compared in a prospective randomized study.[12] Both groups had good to excellent results with no residual valgus instability; however, the location of the MCL rupture was not reported. Another study showed that patients with ruptures of the superficial layer of the MCL isolated to the femoral attachment regained valgus stability with nonsurgical treatment, whereas those patients with superficial layer injuries extending distally to the joint line or a complete tibial avulsion required combined ACL/MCL reconstructive surgery to regain valgus stability.[13] The location of the MCL grade III injury must be considered before reconstruction of the ACL because the combined procedure may be necessary for restoring knee stability in these rare injuries.

Prevention

With the increasing number of noncontact ACL injuries, several prevention strategies have been evaluated for their efficacy. In female athletes, the risk of noncontact ACL injury is three to four times that of male athletes participating in the same sport.[14] There are no level I studies to show the benefit of prevention training among athletes to reduce noncontact ACL injuries. However, significant level II evidence shows that high-intensity plyometrics coupled with balance training and strengthening improves neuromuscular feedback, which appears to reduce ligamentous strain during pivoting and landing activities.[15,16] Plyometric training improves muscular and neurologic activity, resulting in the improved stretch-shortening cycle muscle activation and better body mechanics, thereby reducing ligamentous strain and potential injury. The successful cohort

studies also incorporated education regarding injury mechanics and awareness of dangerous positions placing increased strain on the ACL. Visual or verbal reinforcement during the training period was provided by supervising athletic trainers and was believed to contribute to the reduction of ACL injuries in trained compared with nontrained study groups.

For the training regimen to be effective, high-intensity plyometric exercises must be included, with a minimum of one session per week for 6 weeks. Balance training alone failed to show any reduction in ACL injuries. The cohorts lacking the plyometric exercises and reinforcement education reported no reduction in risk.[15,17]

This level II evidence supports the consensus statement of the 2005 Hunt Valley II Meeting regarding ACL injury prevention strategies[15] summarized in **Table 1**.

Anatomy

Two distinct functional bundles comprise the ACL: anteromedial and posterolateral. In extension, the bundles are oriented vertically and parallel to each other, whereas in 90° of knee flexion the bundles are oriented horizontally and crossed (**Figure 1**). In flexion the anteromedial bundle tightens but in extension and with internal or external tibial rotation the posterolateral bundle tightens.[18] It is important to understand the relationship of the two bundles to each other because the ACL usually is shown with the knee in extension; however, much of the surgery to reconstruct the ligament is done with the knee at or near 90° of flexion.

The femoral origin of the anteromedial bundle is anteroproximal in the intercondylar notch, near the over-the-top position, and inserts anteriorly and medially within the anterior intercondylar area of the tibia.[19] The posterolateral bundle originates more posteriorly and distally in the notch and inserts posteriorly and laterally within the anterior intercondylar area of the tibia.[19] The bony landmarks for the femoral origins of the individual bundles are bony ridges on the lateral femoral condyle.[20] A resident's ridge on the lateral femoral

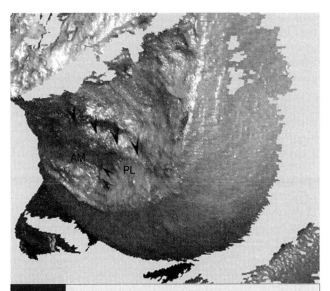

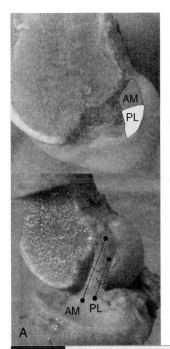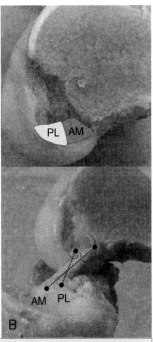

Figure 1 **A,** With the knee in extension, the anteromedial (AM) and posterolateral (PL) femoral insertions are oriented vertically and the bundles are parallel. **B,** With the knee in 90° of flexion, the anteromedial and posterolateral insertions are oriented horizontally and the bundles are crossed. (*Reproduced with permission from Chhabra A, Starman JS, Ferretti M, Vidal AF, Zantop T, Fu FH: Anatomic, radiographic, biomechanical, and kinematic evaluation of the anterior cruciate ligament and its two functional bundles. J Bone Joint Surg Am 2006;88:2-10.*)

Figure 2 A three-dimensional laser digitization of the lateral intercondylar notch of a human cadaver specimen in 90° of flexion. The large arrowheads point to the lateral intercondylar ridge, which marks the superior border of the ACL attachment with the knee in 90° of flexion. The small arrowheads point to the lateral bifurcate ridge, which separates the anteromedial (AM) and posterolateral (PL) bundle femoral attachments. (*Reproduced with permission from Fu FH, Jordan SS: The lateral intercondylar ridge: A key to anatomic anterior cruciate ligament reconstruction. J Bone Joint Surg Am 2007;89: 2103-2104.*)

condylar wall has previously been described. The ridge currently denotes the lateral intercondylar ridge and marks the most anterior and superior extent of the femoral origins.[20] A second ridge identified as the lateral bifurcate ridge, running nearly perpendicular to the lateral intercondylar ridge, separates the origins of the anteromedial and posterolateral bundles and is found in 30% of patients[21] (**Figure 2**).

Current single-bundle ACL reconstruction techniques mimic the function of the anteromedial bundle only and therefore may not treat rotational instability entirely in some patients. In vivo and cadaver studies have demonstrated continued rotational laxity after traditional single-bundle reconstruction. In vitro anatomic double-bundle reconstruction techniques, when compared with single-bundle reconstruction, have had much better restoration of rotational kinematics that more closely resembles the native ACL.[22]

Surgical Technique
The standard surgical technique of the single-bundle reconstruction has yielded excellent results with objective scores such as the KT-1000 arthrometer and the restoration of anteroposterior stability assessed with the

Lachman test. However, results of subjective scoring questionnaires have shown lower levels of satisfaction with normal IKDC scores lower than 50%. Long-term studies confirm the restoration of anteroposterior stability, but osteoarthritis eventually develops in most ACL-reconstructed knees. Many high-demand athletes are unable to return to preinjury level of competition after "successful" ACL reconstruction. An evaluation of National Football League wide receivers and running backs after ACL reconstruction showed only 80% of the athletes were able to return to play.[23] Of those returning to the National Football League, there was a documented 30% decrease in statistical performance as measured by parameters such as yards gained, games played, and number of touchdowns.

The traditional endoscopic single-bundle technique popularized in the early 1990s is done with the tibial bone tunnel placed posteriorly in the ACL native tibial footprint. This posteriorly placed tunnel is within the native insertion of the posterolateral bundle. The femoral tunnel is then drilled via the tibial tunnel at or near the 11 o'clock (right knee) or 1 o'clock (left knee) position, which is quite superior to the origin of the anteromedial bundle, often missing the native footprint. The resulting graft position (posterolateral on the tibia to anteromedial on the femur) is more vertically oriented than the native ACL. This vertical post adequately pre-

3: Knee and Leg

vents anterior translation of the tibia as measured by the Lachman test, anterior drawer test, and KT-1000 arthrometer; however, excessive tibial rotation as measured by the pivot shift test is often retained, particularly during high-demand activities such as running, cutting, and jumping.[7-9]

In vivo and cadaver studies have demonstrated the continued excessive tibial rotation following this traditional endoscopic reconstruction technique.[7-9] It is believed that this lack of rotatory stability may lead to unsatisfactory clinical results, particularly in high-demand athletes. This opens the debate as to the usefulness of objective measures such as the KT-1000 arthrometer, which only measures anteroposterior laxity, for determining the success of the reconstruction. This continued pathologic tibial rotation that alters articular cartilage contact stress may be one of the contributing factors for the development of osteoarthritis.[24,25]

These findings have led to the focus of the anatomic insertions of the ACL both on the femur and tibia. The transtibial drilling technique for the femoral tunnel does not afford easy access to the lateral wall of the femoral intercondylar notch and may result in nonanatomic placement of the graft. A nonanatomic reconstructed ligament may not function similarly to the native ACL. The "standard endoscopic technique" may reconstruct the ACL in a nonanatomic location.

Tunnel Placement

Placement of the femoral tunnel has long been a topic of debate. Using the clock face as a reference, the graft has traditionally been placed at the 1 o'clock or 11 o'clock position. This is easily accomplished with the transtibial technique; however, many now advocate using the anteromedial or far accessory anteromedial portal for placement of the anatomic femoral tunnel.[26] This allows for lower positioning of the femoral tunnel at either the 2 o'clock or 10 o'clock positions, independent of the tibial tunnel, and thereby affords an enhanced mechanical advantage for restoring normal tibial rotation kinematics. Furthermore, the lower lateral position places the tunnel in a more anatomic position consistent with the native ACL femoral footprint. Studies on femoral tunnel position have shown the lower, more lateral positioning of the tunnel does not appreciably change the anteroposterior translation.[27] However, this new graft position results in improved functional scores with less rotational laxity.[28-30] This more lateral, lower positioning of the femoral tunnel via the anteromedial portal allows the added advantage of placing the interference screw for femoral fixation through this anteromedial portal. In doing so the screw is placed in a position parallel to the tunnel, which is easier to accomplish with less risk of a divergent screw placement or graft laceration.

Anatomic Double-Bundle Reconstruction

Long-term results of the anatomic reconstruction are needed to determine any additional benefit to the traditional single-bundle technique. This more anatomic technique is well described in the literature with some surgeons adopting the technique in all cases. Short-term results are encouraging. No significant difference in short-term subjective scores has been identified; however, level I and II evidence has shown improved objective results such as the KT-1000 measurements and pivot shift findings.[22,30-32] Anatomic reconstruction has shown kinematics more similar to the native knee. Improved rotational stability has been objectively documented with the double-bundle anatomic reconstruction, with a negative pivot shift test in up to 97% of patients.[31] Currently there is no accepted standard regarding tunnel placement for the double-bundle reconstructions because different surgical techniques exist within the literature. With additional investigative studies such standardization may be developed; however, the unique ACL anatomic variability among the population must be kept in mind. Anatomic studies have described arthroscopic and radiographic landmarks to aid in identifying the anatomic footprint insertions of the ACL both on the lateral femoral wall and on the tibial plateau to assist in surgery.[19,33,34]

Partial ACL tears, which are of unknown frequency and are far less common than complete tears, can be treated with an anatomic approach. In such instances, examination under anesthesia or arthroscopic evaluation may identify a single-bundle tear, sparing the second bundle from injury. Knowledge of the anatomic double-bundle technique can enable the surgeon to augment the uninjured bundle by reconstruction of the single injured bundle, restoring either the anteroposterior or rotatory stability.

Revision Surgery

Revision surgery for a failed reconstruction occurs an estimated 5% to 20% annually in the United States, with the most common cause attributed to technical failure (tunnel placement) of the primary reconstruction.[35] Results vary following revision reconstruction; approximately 60% of patients return to athletic activity but with a decrease in the level of performance.[35]

ACL revision reconstruction poses technical difficulties ranging from hardware removal to tunnel expansion and osteolysis with poor bone quality. The question of bone grafting in a single-stage compared with a two-stage procedure is largely unanswered and is specific to the surgeon or patient. The degree of osteolysis and positioning of the previous tunnels will dictate the correct approach. In the event of a revision reconstruction of a failed endoscopic reconstruction, anatomic placement of the femoral tunnel via an accessory far anteromedial portal may result in a tunnel that does not communicate with the previously placed tunnel, alleviating the concerns of stable fixation while simultaneously allowing for bone grafting of the old tunnel without staging the procedure.

Augmentation of the previously placed graft may be an alternative in certain patients. Many traditional endoscopic single-bundle reconstructions with failed results may have an intact and partially functioning graft on arthroscopic inspection. The single bundle placed within the femur in the high position of either 11 o'clock or 1 o'clock can be retained if there is anteroposterior stability and augmentation with a graft placed in the lower lateral position on the femoral wall to provide rotational stability.[26] Results of such an augmentation procedure are relatively unknown, but early case reports supporting such approaches have yielded favorable outcomes.[26] Augmenting procedures should be approached with caution. The previous graft must be intact and provide stability to the knee in either the anteroposterior or rotational direction. The augmentation can then be customized to fit the patient's need to restore stability whether the anteromedial or posterolateral bundle is replaced.

Graft Selection

No single graft selection clearly stands out as superior. There are numerous studies comparing hamstring and bone-patellar tendon-bone autografts and evaluating autografts and allografts. There is consensus that the graft choice must be individualized to the patient, taking into account the patient's age and desired level of activity after surgery. No level I study comparing autograft to allograft currently exists in the literature, nor would such a study be possible because of the confounding factors in graft selection, most importantly the patient's decision. Meta-analyses comparing hamstring autografts and bone-patellar tendon-bone autografts concluded that there was no significant difference in functional outcome scores or stability between the groups; however, the patellar tendon group experienced a greater incidence of anterior knee discomfort following reconstruction and greater incidence of osteoarthritis.[36,37]

No functional differences in outcome scores among the different grafts, whether autograft or allograft, have been demonstrated.[38-40] However, the allograft group experienced less pain during the first year after reconstruction.[40] A meta-analysis recently demonstrated that abnormal stability, represented by a failed graft, was two to three times higher for allografts than for autografts.[14] This increased incidence of graft failure or resultant instability has been attributed to the possible immune response to the allograft tissue, alterations in the tissue caused by tissue processing or preparation, secondary sterilization, storage, and the age of the donor. According to a 2007 study, the catastrophic failure rate was 33% within 1 year after reconstruction with irradiated (2.0 to 2.5 mRad) Achilles allograft compared with a 2.4% failure rate with nonirradiated Achilles allografts.[41] These findings led the authors of the study to abandon the use of irradiated allograft tissue. Another study evaluated the use of anterior tibialis allografts in primary endoscopic ACL reconstruction.[42] The reoperation/failure rate was 24% in patients older than 25 years and 55% in patients younger than 25

years. All soft-tissue allografts in patients younger than 25 years who want to return to ACL-dependent sports should be used with caution. No studies have been done comparing outcome of different allograft tissues; bone-patellar tendon-bone compared with Achilles tendon; or bone compared with all soft-tissue allografts. The potential advantages and disadvantages of each individual graft substitute, whether autograft or allograft, must be recognized. The graft choice must be tailored to the age and activity level of the patient and not the surgeon.

Posterior Cruciate Ligament Injuries

Posterior cruciate ligament (PCL) injuries are challenging to treat. Unlike for ACL injuries, advances in research and surgical techniques for PCL injuries have been slow. The PCL is the primary stabilizer to posterior translation of the tibia. It is also a secondary stabilizer in varus, valgus, and rotatory stability. PCL injuries may represent up to 30% of all knee ligament injuries.

Anatomy and Biomechanics

The PCL is composed of a larger anterolateral bundle and the smaller posteromedial bundle. The anterolateral bundle is tight in flexion, lax in extension, and has twice the cross-sectional area of the posteromedial bundle. It also has 140% the strength of the posteromedial bundle.[43] The posteromedial bundle has the reciprocal pattern of tightness. The average intra-articular length and width of the PCL is 38 mm and 13 mm, respectively.[44] The PCL is intra-articular but extra-synovial, with reflected synovium covering all but the posterior aspect of the ligament. The PCL functions as the primary stabilizer of posterior tibial translation on the femur and is a secondary stabilizer of external rotation. Sectioning of the PCL results in increased posterior translation of the tibia that is most pronounced at 90° of flexion and most subtle in full extension. Valgus, varus, and rotatory instability are much less pronounced from an isolated PCL in comparison with multiple ligamentous injuries.[45] The PCL works synergistically with the posterolateral corner structures for knee stability. Reconstruction of a PCL injury while neglecting a posterolateral corner injury would lead to residual instability.

The meniscofemoral ligaments form a Y-shaped sling around the PCL. The anterior meniscofemoral ligament is known as the ligament of Humphry and the posterior ligament is known as the ligament of Wrisberg. These ligaments, which may be the same volume as the anterolateral bundle of the PCL, arise from the posterior horn of the lateral meniscus and insert on the femur with the PCL. These ligaments have a stiffness and ultimate load higher than that of the posteromedial bundle.[44] Their role in knee stability and kinematics has not yet been established.

Epidemiology

The incidence of PCL injuries varies by study from 5% to 37% of ligamentous knee injuries. The mechanisms of injury to the PCL are commonly a dashboard type injury with a direct blow to the anterior tibia or hyperflexion. The hyperflexion mechanism injures the anterolateral bundle preferentially. Hyperextension injuries are more likely to result in ACL and PCL injuries and affect the posteromedial bundle initially. Studies have shown that 50% of patients treated without surgery are able to return to preinjury level of athletic activity.[46] Combined ligament injuries and grade 3 injuries have poorer outcomes with nonsurgical treatment, and surgical reconstruction is recommended. A PCL-deficient knee has increased forces directed through the patellofemoral and medial compartment of the knee. Increased degenerative changes have been observed radiographically in the compartments of PCL-deficient knees.

Evaluation

Evaluation of an injured knee includes obtaining a detailed history regarding the direction of the applied force, keeping in mind dashboard type injuries are more likely to cause multiligament injuries. Physical examination should include evaluation for possible multiple ligament injury, meniscus pathology, and neurovascular status. Radiographs and MRI scans should be used as an adjunct and not a substitute for a thorough physical examination.

Physical Examination

Physical examination should be performed systematically by observing for deformity or swelling, palpating the joint, evaluating range of motion, and then testing for instability and other injuries. The most obvious finding is the posterior sag sign. Patients with acute injuries may have anterior tibial trauma and popliteal ecchymosis. With chronic injuries, patients may have tenderness to palpation of the patellofemoral and medial compartments because of degenerative changes. The posterior drawer test is used to classify the severity of the injury based on tibial translation in comparison with the femoral condyles. A grade 1 injury has less than 5 mm of displacement and the tibia is anterior to the femoral condyles. A grade 2 injury has 5 to 10 mm of displacement and the tibia is flush with the condyles. A grade 3 injury has more than 10 mm of displacement and the tibia is posterior to the condyles. The quadriceps active test will show correction of the posterior displacement of the tibia. The dial test must be performed at 30° and 90° to evaluate for the possibility of an associated posterolateral corner injury. If a posterolateral corner injury is present, the laxity will be most pronounced at 30°. Examination under anesthesia should remain part of the evaluation in the operating room before reconstruction is performed. Evaluation of peroneal and posterior tibial nerve function and distal pedal pulses is required to assess neurovascular function.

Radiographic Evaluation

Plain radiographs including AP, lateral, sunrise, and oblique views should be obtained to evaluate for signs of dislocation or subluxation of the joint. A possible avulsion of the PCL also can be seen. With posterolateral corner injuries, an avulsion of the fibular head, avulsion of the Gerdy tubercle, or medial tibial plateau fractures may be seen. In chronic injuries, degenerative changes of the patellofemoral and medial compartments may be seen. Telos stress radiography (Telos GmbH, Marburg, Germany) is a useful tool for quantifying the amount of laxity compared with the unaffected knee. A recent study showed that more than 12 mm of difference from side to side is indicative of a concurrent posterolateral corner injury.[47]

MRI is used to evaluate the possibility of posterolateral corner and other associated ligamentous injuries. It may also reveal meniscal or other intra-articular pathology and can determine whether one or both of the bundles are disrupted. In patients with chronic injuries, a bone scan may evaluate for increased uptake in the patellofemoral and/or medial compartments, indicative of degenerative changes.

Treatment

Treatment depends on the severity of the injury and time from injury to presentation. Isolated grade 1 or 2 injuries can be treated nonsurgically. Grade 3 or multiligament injuries are best treated surgically.

Nonsurgical Treatment

In patients with grade 1 and 2 isolated PCL injuries, an extension brace is worn, weight bearing is protected, and quadriceps strengthening is emphasized. Most patients are able to return to sports activity in 2 to 4 weeks after injury. Patients with grade 3 injuries who are treated nonsurgically are at risk of degenerative changes of the patellofemoral and medial compartments.

Surgical Repair and Reconstruction

Trends over the past few years have been focused on more aggressive treatment of PCL injuries, especially in the athletic population. The best method of reconstruction is controversial. There is still a paucity of long-term studies comparing techniques and their outcomes. An acute avulsion of the PCL can be repaired primarily. Most often the PCL is avulsed from the femoral condyle and can be treated with a posterior approach. Large fragments can be treated with screw fixation and smaller fragments can be repaired with suture through drill holes. Follow-up studies show consistently good results.

Tibial Inlay Technique

This technique is believed to re-create the anatomy of the PCL more accurately than the transtibial technique; abrasion of the anterior edge of the graft, or the killer angle effect, that can cause graft failure is avoided. A posterior approach to the knee theoretically places the neurovascular structures at greater risk of injury. This approach may not be an option if there is a large amount of soft tissue or vascular injury. The bone block shows faster graft incorporation than the soft tissue used in the transtibial technique. The most recent technique has been the arthroscopic transtibial technique that uses a reverse reamer through the tibia to create the bone block. The inlay is secured using suture fixation and a button. This method can be used to create a single- or double-bundle construct.[48,49] Long-term studies to evaluate the efficacy of this technique currently are lacking.

Transtibial Technique

This approach involves an ACL-type approach with a transtibial tunnel oriented anterior to posterior. The neurovascular structures are at risk of injury while the tunnel is drilled. The location of the structures is 4 mm posterior to the posterior horn of the lateral meniscus. The tunnel should be drilled using arthroscopic and fluoroscopic visualization. The posterior cortex can be hand-reamed for better control. The killer angle effect is possible and can be lessened by placing the tibial tunnel in the maximally vertical and the intra-articular opening in the more distal of the tibial upslope reproducing the insertion of the anterolateral bundle.[50] Studies have shown that hamstring and quadriceps-patellar bone autograft have similar outcomes when laxity and radiographic stability are assessed.[51,52] Double-bundle constructs are superior to single-bundle reconstructions. Single-bundle constructs should re-create the anterolateral bundle anatomy. Comparison studies of transtibial and tibial inlay reconstructions have shown no significant difference in laxity or short-term outcomes.[53,54]

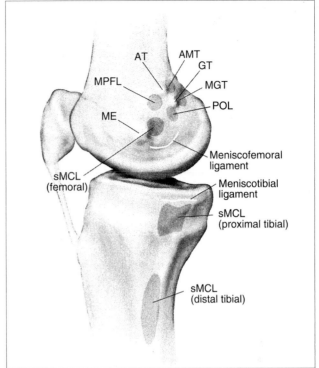

Figure 3 Illustration of the femoral osseous landmarks and attachment sites of the main medial knee structures. AT = adductor tubercle, GT = gastrocnemius tubercle, ME = medial epicondyle, AMT = adductor magnus tendon, MGT = medial gastrocnemius tendon, sMCL = superficial medial collateral ligament, MPFL = medial patellofemoral ligament, and POL = posterior oblique ligament. (*Reproduced with permission from LaPrade RF, Engebretsen AH, Ly TV, Johansen S, Wentorf FA, Engebretsen L: The anatomy of the medial part of the knee. J Bone Joint Surg Am 2007;89:2000-2010.*)

Multiple/Collateral Knee Ligament Injuries

The knee with multiple ligament injuries is challenging to treat. Traditionally, these injuries were identified by clinical or radiographic evidence of a complete tibiofemoral dislocation. It is now well recognized that the knee is reduced in 50% of these injuries.[55-57] The incidence of neurovascular injury is just as high in these "reduced" knee dislocations as in those knees that are acutely dislocated at presentation. Whenever a clinician encounters a grossly unstable injured knee with clinical and imaging evidence of multiple ligament injuries, the knee must be treated as a knee dislocation.

The goal of treatment of the knee with multiple ligament injuries is to prevent additional injury to the extremity and restore normal anatomy and function as best as possible. Immediate recognition and prompt treatment of arterial injuries is necessary to minimize the risk of amputation. In addition to the surgical treatment of the cruciate ligaments, the surgeon must be familiar with nonsurgical treatment and repair and re-

construction techniques for the collateral ligaments. Failure to restore stability to the collateral ligaments will jeopardize the results of cruciate ligament reconstructions in the multiply injured knee.

Anatomy and Biomechanics

It is conceptually useful to view the knee as containing four distinct ligament complexes: the ACL, PCL, medial structure, and posterolateral complex.

The primary structures providing stability to the medial aspect of the knee are the superficial and deep MCL, and the posteromedial capsule including the posterior oblique ligament. Their attachment sites are consistent and well defined[58,59] (**Figure 3**). The superficial MCL is the primary restraint to valgus and external rotation loads throughout flexion. The deep MCL functions as a secondary restraint to valgus loads and provides some restraint to external rotation beyond 30° of flexion. The posteromedial capsule resists 32% of the valgus load at full extension but its contribution to valgus stability drops quickly with knee flexion.[60] The

3: Knee and Leg

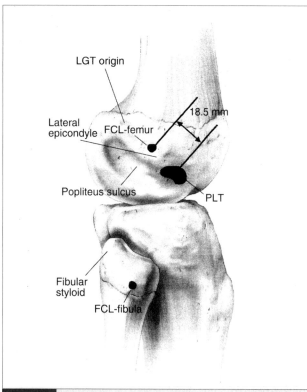

Figure 4   The attachment sites of the fibular collateral ligament (FCL) on the femur and fibula and the popliteus tendon (PLT) in the popliteus sulcus of the femur (lateral view, right knee). In addition, the average distance between the femoral attachment sites is noted. LGT lateral gastrocnemius tendon. (*Reproduced with permission from LaPrade RF, Ly TV, Wentorf FA, Engebretsen L: The posterolateral attachments of the knee. Am J Sports Med 2003;31:854-860.*)

posteromedial capsule does not play a significant role in controlling external rotation.

The primary components of the posterolateral complex are the fibular collateral ligament, the popliteofibular ligament, and the popliteus tendon. The attachment sites of these structures have been well described recently[61] (**Figure 4**). The fibular collateral ligament is the primary restraint to varus loads at all flexion angles.[62,63] There is a reciprocal relationship in response to external rotation loads with the fibular collateral ligament seeing high forces at lower flexion angles (less than 60°) and the popliteofibular ligament and popliteus tendon seeing higher forces at 60° and 90° of flexion. Although several studies have shown the ability of posterolateral reconstructions to restore static stability to the posterolateral corner deficient knee, more detailed studies have shown an inability of combined PCL/posterolateral corner reconstructions to completely reproduce normal knee biomechanics.[64-68] Although posterolateral corner reconstructions lessen the forces seen on a PCL reconstruction, they tend to overconstrain varus rotation and have higher forces than the native ligaments.

Initial Assessment

The initial assessment of a knee with multiple ligament injuries should focus on the neurovascular status of the limb. Serial physical examination identifies all clinically significant vascular injuries.[69,70] An ankle-brachial index with a threshold of less than 0.90 has a positive predictive value of 100% for the presence of a vascular injury requiring surgical intervention.[71] Arteriography is indicated in patients with (1) any decrease in pedal pulses, lower extremity color or temperature; (2) an expanding hematoma about the knee; (3) a history of an abnormal physical examination before presentation in the emergency department; or (4) an ankle-brachial index less than 0.90. If a vascular injury is confirmed, urgent revascularization is required to prevent amputation. Initial documentation of nerve injuries is important because the prognosis for complete recovery is poor.[72]

Evaluation of the knee ligaments is done with a combination of physical examination and imaging studies.[55-57] Radiographs will identify major periarticular fractures and bony avulsions. MRI will accurately assess the location of ligament injuries and helps with planning surgical treatment; however, MRI does not determine ligament function in partial injuries. Ligament stress testing under anesthesia provides the best information about the functional competence of partially torn ligaments. After physical examination and imaging studies, the knee injury should be classified based on extent of ligamentous injury. This classification system facilitates planning surgical treatment.

Nonsurgical Treatment

Although most multiple ligament knee injuries benefit from surgical repair or reconstruction, there are instances when an initial nonsurgical approach is required. Examples include knees requiring revascularization, open knee dislocations, and patients with multiple trauma who require a prolonged stay in intensive care. After initial reduction and ensuring adequate limb perfusion, the physician should immobilize the limb in 30° of flexion. This can be accomplished with a splint or locked brace, or with a spanning external fixator. Whatever the method of immobilization, serial radiographs should be obtained to ensure maintenance of reduction. Mobilization of the knee should occur by 6 weeks to prevent arthrofibrosis. Fixator removal under anesthesia and a gentle closed manipulation can be done. Healing of partial ligament injuries and some complete MCL tears is possible with temporary immobilization. After motion has been restored, elective ligament reconstructions can be performed when the patient's overall condition allows.

Surgical Treatment

The decision to perform arthroscopic instead of open reconstruction in a complex knee injury depends on the timing of the surgery, as well as the nature of the injury itself. In patients with an open knee dislocation, irrigation, débridement, and repair of repairable lesions may be indicated in the first few weeks.[55] If a reconstruction or repair is done in the first few weeks, the capsular tissue may be torn, and open techniques may have to be used to avoid extravasation of fluid into compartments to prevent compartment syndrome. Bony avulsions of ligaments are generally best treated using open techniques early after injury.

Under ideal circumstances, preferred treatment of knee dislocations consists of arthroscopic ACL and PCL reconstruction, and open repair or reconstruction of the posterolateral and/or the medial complexes.

Surgical timing in the knee with acute multiple ligament injuries (dislocated knee) depends on the extremity vascular status, collateral ligament injury severity, degree of instability, open or closed injury, skin condition, meniscus and articular surface injuries, bony avulsions, severe capsular injuries, other orthopaedic injuries, and systemic injuries. Delaying surgical reconstruction for approximately 2 to 3 weeks has resulted in a decreased incidence of arthrofibrosis in some series.[73-75]

Some ACL/PCL/MCL injuries can be treated with a brace on the MCL followed by arthroscopic combined ACL/PCL reconstruction in 4 to 6 weeks after healing of the MCL. Other injuries require repair or reconstruction of the medial structures and must be assessed on an individual basis. Diffuse MCL injury or a Stener type MCL injury revealed by MRI are best treated surgically.

Combined ACL/PCL/posterolateral injuries should be treated surgically as early as is safely possible. ACL/PCL/posterolateral repair and reconstruction performed from 2 to 3 weeks after injury allows healing of capsular tissues to permit an arthroscopic approach, and still permits primary repair of injured posterolateral structures in addition to posterolateral reconstruction.

Open multiple-ligament knee injuries and dislocations may require staged procedures. The collateral or capsular structures are repaired and/or reconstructed after thorough irrigation and débridement, and the combined ACL/PCL reconstruction is done later, after the wound has healed. When reconstruction is delayed, care must be taken to maintain tibiofemoral joint reduction by splinting or external fixation.

Chronic multiple-ligament-injured knees may have progressive functional instability, posttraumatic arthrosis, and gait abnormalities. Gait analysis demonstrating varus or valgus thrust indicates the need for realignment osteotomy before performing knee ligament reconstructive surgical procedures. Meniscal transplantation and osteochondral grafting also may be necessary in these complex cases.

The ideal graft material is readily available, has low donor-site morbidity, is strong, is easy to pass, and achieves secure fixation. Available options are autograft and allograft sources. Several studies have demonstrated successful results using both allograft and au-

tograft tissue in the treatment of the multiple-ligament-injured knee.[73,74,76-81] Many authors advocate using allograft tissue to minimize further trauma to the knee.

The principles of reconstruction in the multiple-ligament-injured knee are to identify and treat all pathology, perform accurate tunnel placement, identify anatomic graft insertion sites, use strong graft material, secure graft fixation, and initiate a deliberate postoperative rehabilitation program. The PCL reconstruction can be performed as an arthroscopic transtibial tunnel technique, or by using the tibial inlay technique.

An accessory extracapsular extra-articular posteromedial safety incision is used during transtibial tunnel PCL reconstruction to protect the neurovascular structures and to confirm the accuracy of tibial tunnel placement.[55] The notchplasty is performed first and consists of ACL and PCL stump débridement, bone removal, and contouring of the medial wall of the lateral femoral condyle and the intercondylar roof. The curved over-the-top PCL instruments are used to sequentially lyse adhesions in the posterior aspect of the knee and elevate the capsule from the posterior tibial ridge.

The PCL is reconstructed first, followed by the ACL, the lateral side, and the medial side. A tensioning boot has been used for tensioning the ACL and PCL reconstructions with good results, but manual tensioning also is acceptable.[74,77,78] Fixation is achieved on the PCL femoral side using a resorbable interference screw and back-up fixation with a polyethylene knee ligament fixation button, or other secure method of fixation. Tension is placed on the PCL graft distally either manually or with a tensioning boot, and the knee is taken through full range of motion cycles to allow pretensioning and settling of the graft. The knee is placed in 70° to 90° of flexion, the normal tibial step-off is restored, and fixation is achieved on the tibial side of the PCL graft with a screw, spiked ligament washer, and an interference screw or other secure fixation method. The knee is maintained at 70° to 90° of flexion, and final fixation of the ACL graft is achieved. Lateral posterolateral and medial posteromedial reconstructions are performed as indicated (**Figure 5**).

Postoperative rehabilitation proceeds in a deliberate fashion that includes periods of immobilization; no weight bearing; progressive range of motion; progressive weight bearing; and strength and proprioceptive skills training. Return to sports and heavy labor may occur after 6 to 9 months when sufficient strength, proprioceptive skills, and range of motion have returned.[55,78] Many patients take much longer than 9 months to return to full activity, whereas others never return to their preinjury level of function.

Potential complications in the treatment of the multiple-ligament-injured knee include failure to recognize and treat vascular injuries (both arterial and venous), iatrogenic neurovascular injury at the time of reconstruction, iatrogenic tibial plateau fractures at the time of reconstruction, failure to recognize and treat all components of the instability, postoperative medial

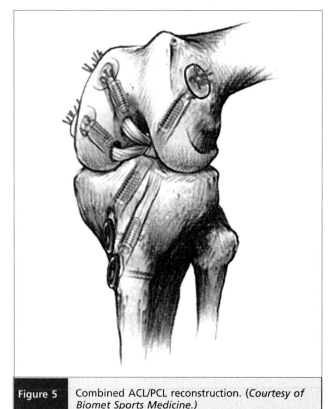

| Figure 5 | Combined ACL/PCL reconstruction. (*Courtesy of Biomet Sports Medicine.*) |

done for type I and type II injury patterns. The MCL is reconstructed for type III injury patterns and in cases of chronic MCL laxity. Most MCL reconstructions describe routing a soft-tissue graft between the attachment points of the superficial MCL, sometimes accompanied by a posteromedial capsule reefing.[82,86] Limited clinical data suggest that functional valgus stability is restored in most patients (**Figure 6**). Complications of MCL surgery include recurrent valgus laxity, stiffness, and saphenous nerve injury.

Lateral and Posterolateral Ligament Injuries of the Knee

Diagnosis

Lateral collateral ligament and posterolateral corner injuries have been historically difficult to diagnose. These injuries usually occur in combination with cruciate ligament tears that can divert the physician's attention. These patients often have acute pain about the posterolateral aspect of the knee. Patients with chronic pain may have no symptoms or functional instability.[87]

Several physical examination tests specific for injury to the posterolateral corner have been described. The external rotation recurvatum, posterolateral drawer, reverse pivot shift, and dial tests all have been used in the diagnosis of these injuries.[88]

Plain radiographs are usually normal; however, the presence of distinct abnormalities is suggestive of posterolateral corner injuries. The arcuate sign, a small avulsion fracture of the fibular styloid, is said to be pathognomonic for posterolateral corner injuries. Segond fractures and medial Segond fractures also have been seen in conjunction with PCL injuries.[89]

MRI is the primary study used to assess soft tissues in patients with a knee injury. Inconsistency in the anatomy of the PCL combined with the varying obliquity of the ligamentous structures can limit the utility of MRI, underscoring the need for a meticulous physical examination.[90]

Treatment of Acute Injury

Surgical treatment options for the acutely injured lateral collateral ligament or posterolateral corner are varied. Acute injuries without pathologic laxity can be treated nonsurgically with rehabilitation and careful observation. In patients with pathologic motion, surgical treatment is the mainstay. The goal of surgery should be to stabilize the knee by treating all injured structures. Surgery can involve primary repair of all injured ligaments, posterolateral capsular advancement, and/or augmentation of the lateral and posterolateral structures. Many surgical techniques have been described. Concomitant injuries to the ACL/PCL, menisci, articular cartilage, medial knee ligament, and tibial plateau, for example, should be identified.[91-93]

femoral condyle osteonecrosis, knee motion loss, skin and wound healing difficulty, infection, postoperative anterior knee pain, stiffness, and residual laxity.

Medial Side Injuries

The diagnosis of MCL injuries is accomplished with a combination of valgus stress testing and MRI.[82] An increase in valgus laxity greater than 1.0 cm without an end point indicates a grade III MCL injury. Involvement of the posterior oblique ligament is common in grade III MCL tears.[83] MRI will help localize the area of superficial MCL injury. Grade III MCL injuries have been divided into type I injuries located at the femoral attachment; type II are at the tibial insertion; and type III injuries occur where there is increased signal throughout the length of the superficial MCL. Nonsurgical treatment of type III injuries has been unsuccessful.[84]

Partial MCL injuries heal well with nonsurgical treatment. Even isolated grade III MCL injuries generally heal well with bracing and rehabilitation. Combined ACL/MCL injuries can be treated with early (in less than 21 days) reconstruction of the ACL only; results are equal to ACL reconstruction with MCL repair.[85] With initial management of the multiple-ligament-injured knee, there is a wide spectrum of healing of MCL injuries. When early surgery is performed, MCL and posteromedial capsule repair are

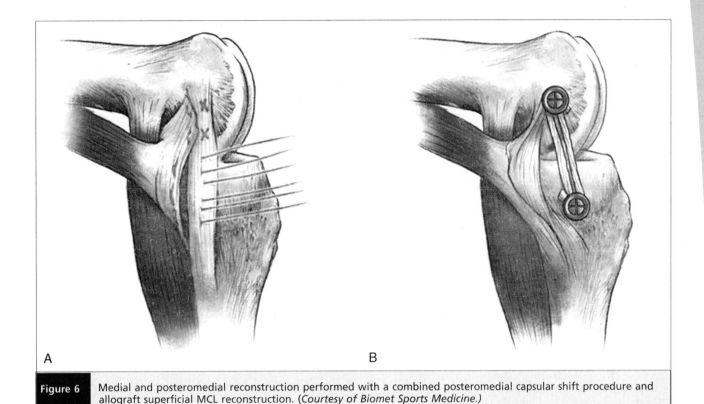

Figure 6 Medial and posteromedial reconstruction performed with a combined posteromedial capsular shift procedure and allograft superficial MCL reconstruction. *(Courtesy of Biomet Sports Medicine.)*

Treatment of Chronic Injury

If left untreated, significant injuries to the posterolateral corner may lead to posterolateral rotatory instability. Some have defined chronic posterolateral corner injuries to include those more than 3 weeks old, because after this period the quality of the tissues makes primary repair difficult. Numerous surgical options to reconstruct the posterolateral structures have been described. Local rotation of a strip of iliotibial band on a distally based pedicle has been used to reconstruct the popliteus while a central slip of the biceps tendon augments and reconstructs the popliteofibular ligament. Arcuate complex and capsular advancement procedures have been used to reapproximate anatomy and reduce capsular volume. Numerous autograft and allograft reconstructions have been described in the treatment of chronic posterolateral rotatory instability[94-96] (**Figure 7**). In the setting of a varus mechanical axis, undue stress will be placed on lateral and posterolateral reconstructions, leading to early failure. High tibial osteotomy before or at the time of the formal ligament reconstruction can improve results.[96]

Complications of PCL Injuries

Reported complications of PCL injuries include persistent or recurrent laxity, stiffness, infection, and pain. The risk of recurrent laxity can be minimized by treating all injured structures while ensuring neutral mechanical alignment. Particular attention must be paid to anatomic graft placement. A standardized and closely monitored rehabilitation protocol should be instituted

to maximize strength and range of motion while limiting risk to the repaired or reconstructed tissues.[97]

Summary

Advances in ACL reconstruction surgical techniques are continually evolving. With the long-term outcomes of good to excellent results averaging 65%, there is much room for improvement. The understanding of the importance of rotational stability and function of the native ACL has led to advances in tunnel placement and the evolution of the anatomic double-bundle reconstruction. Early results of these changes are encouraging as improved rotational stability and knee kinematics have been observed.

As the understanding of the anatomy and function of the ACL improves so too will surgical techniques and improvements in short- and long-term outcomes. However, easily reproducible objective measures are needed to evaluate outcomes in the clinical environment. The pivot shift test, though highly sensitive in the anesthetized patient, has poor reproducibility in the office setting. An easy-to-use standardized tool that measures the restoration of normal kinematics after knee ligament surgery must be developed. Until this is done the comparison of outcomes of different ACL surgical techniques will continue to be difficult.

With an increasing number of ACL injuries annually, especially in the female athlete, additional investigation in prevention strategies is warranted. Plyometric train-

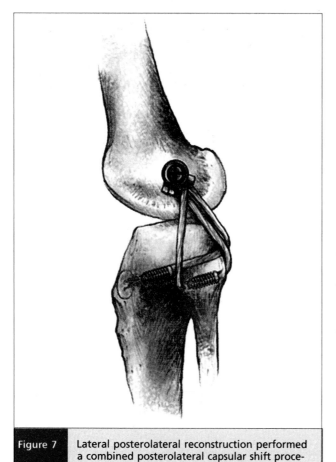

| Figure 7 | Lateral posterolateral reconstruction performed a combined posterolateral capsular shift procedure, figure-of-8 allograft through the fibular head, and allograft through the proximal tibia. (*Courtesy of Biomet Sports Medicine.*) |

ing and continued reinforcement of proper body mechanics by supervising athletic trainers or physical therapists are demonstrating effectiveness in reducing the incidence of injury.

Graft selection is left to the discretion of the surgeon and patient. Long-term comparisons of grafts have not identified any single graft option as superior in all patients. A thorough discussion of the risks and benefits of each graft must occur between the patient and the treating surgeon to allow proper graft selection.

Just as anatomic reduction of fractures supersedes the method of fixation in fracture surgery, re-creation of the native anatomy and function of the ACL should surpass graft choice or the method of fixation. It remains unclear which patients may benefit from anatomic double-bundle reconstruction rather than a single-bundle reconstruction with properly placed femoral and tibial tunnels.

In the future, the specific procedure may be individualized to the patient's unique anatomy, injury pattern, and degree of laxity, as no two patients or knee laxity patterns are exactly the same. A patient with a medial meniscus tear and a grade IV pivot shift may require an ACL reconstruction technique different from that per-

formed for a patient with intact secondary restraints and a grade I pivot shift. More research and long-term studies are required in this area.

More is being learned about the anatomy and biomechanics of the PCL for effective treatment. Based on this knowledge, reconstruction techniques continue to improve. The surgical treatment of PCL injuries remains an area of great controversy where further research is needed. The knee with multiple injured ligaments represents a tremendous treatment challenge for the orthopaedic surgeon. Thorough knowledge of collateral ligament anatomy and biomechanics is critical for understanding and treating these injuries. A thorough initial evaluation and a logical stepwise approach to surgical treatment can yield improved outcomes in most patients.

Acknowledgments

Drs. Fanelli and Wascher would like to thank Daniel Tomaszewski, MD; Mark McKenna, MD; and John Beck, MD for their help in the preparation of the chapter.

Annotated References

1. Lohmander LS, Englund PM, Dahl LL, Roos EM: The long-term consequence of anterior cruciate ligament and meniscus injuries: Osteoarthritis. *Am J Sports Med* 2007;35:1756-1769.

   The authors reviewed the long-term radiographic and functional outcomes 10 to 20 years after ACL reconstruction. Radiographic changes and functional impairment associated with osteoarthritis developed in approximately 50% of patients. The proposed pathogenic causes are presented in this review. Level of evidence: III.

2. Biau DJ, Tournoux C, Katsahian S, Schranz P, Nizard R: ACL reconstruction: A meta-analysis of functional scores. *Clin Orthop Relat Res* 2007;458:180-187.

   This meta-analysis comparing patellar with hamstring grafts after ACL reconstruction demonstrated no difference in final overall IKDC score or in the number of patients returning to full activity. At final follow-up, 41% of patients receiving a patellar graft and 33% of patients receiving a hamstring graft reported a normal IKDC score. Level of evidence: I.

3. Salmon LJ, Russell VJ, Refshauge K, et al: Long-term outcome of endoscopic anterior cruciate ligament reconstruction with patellar tendon autograft: Minimum 13-year review. *Am J Sports Med* 2006;34:721-732.

   The authors presented a case series of 67 patients who had undergone reconstruction with a patellar tendon autograft with a minimum of 13 years of follow-up. Seventy-nine percent of patients had radiographic degenerative changes, which commonly were associated with meniscectomy at the time of reconstruction, loss of extension postoperatively, and greater laxity measured by the Lachman test. Level of evidence: IV.

4. Laxdal G, Kartus J, Ejerhed L, et al: Outcome and risk factors after anterior cruciate ligament reconstruction: A follow-up study of 948 patients. *Arthroscopy* 2005; 21:958-964.

This retrospective case series of 948 patients following reconstruction using patellar tendon autograft reviewed outcomes at a median of 32 months postoperatively. Inferior results correlated with a longer period between the index injury and reconstruction and concomitant joint damage diagnosed at surgery. Level of evidence: IV.

5. Fithian DC, Paxton EW, Stone ML, et al: Prospective trial of a treatment algorithm for the management of the anterior cruciate ligament-injured knee. *Am J Sports Med* 2005;33:335-346.

This prospective nonrandomized clinical trial demonstrated ACL reconstruction within 3 months from the time of injury reduces the risk of worsening knee laxity, symptomatic instability, and meniscus tear. However, reconstruction did not prevent the appearance of late degenerative changes on radiographs. Level of evidence: II.

6. Tandogan RN, Taser O, Kayaalp A, et al: Analysis of meniscal and chondral lesions accompanying anterior cruciate ligament tears: Relationship with age, time from injury, and level of sport. *Knee Surg Sports Traumatol Arthrosc* 2004;12:262-270.

This multicenter study reviewed the associated risk of meniscal and chondral injuries in conjunction with an ACL injury. Analysis demonstrated that the time from injury and age are important predictors of meniscal tears and chondral lesions; however, time from injury was the better predictor of medial meniscal tears.

7. Stergiou N, Ristanis S, Moraiti C, Georgoulis AD: Tibial rotation in anterior cruciate ligament (ACL)-deficient and ACL-reconstructed knees: A theoretical proposition for the development of osteoarthritis. *Sports Med* 2007; 37:601-613.

The authors present a review of in vivo gait analyses of normal, ACL-deficient, and ACL-reconstructed knees. They proposed that the altered tibiofemoral rotations of the ACL-deficient and ACL-reconstructed knees are mechanisms for the development of osteoarthritis.

8. Ristanis S, Stergiou N, Patras K, et al: Excessive tibial rotation during high-demand activities is not restored by anterior cruciate ligament reconstruction. *Arthroscopy* 2005;21:1323-1329.

This case series of kinematic data compared in vivo knee rotational of ACL-deficient, ACL-reconstructed, and ACL-intact knees during jumping, landing, and pivoting activities. Significant differences were found between the ACL-reconstructed group and the healthy control group, and between the ACL-deficient group and the healthy control group.

9. Tashman S, Collon D, Anderson K, Kolowich P, Anderst W: Abnormal rotational knee motion during running after anterior cruciate ligament reconstruction. *Am J Sports Med* 2004;32:975-983.

Abnormal tibial rotation in ACL-reconstructed knees was demonstrated when compared with a patient's un-injured knee in this prospective study of knee kinematics. The reconstructed knees exhibited increased tibial external rotation while the patient ran on a treadmill.

10. Steckel H, Vadala G, Davis D, Musahl V, Fu FH: 3-T MR imaging of partial ACL tears: A cadaver study. *Knee Surg Sports Traumatol Arthrosc* 2007;15:1066-1071.

This cadaver study showed a high predictability to recognize partial ACL transections on oblique sagittal and oblique coronal planes using three-Tesla MRI technology.

11. Hara K, Niga S, Ikeda H, Cho S, Muneta T: Isolated anterior cruciate ligament reconstruction in patients with chronic anterior cruciate ligament insufficiency combined with grade II valgus laxity. *Am J Sports Med* 2008;36:333-339.

This cohort study showed no clinically significant valgus laxity in patients with an associated grade II MCL injury compared with a patient group consisting of an isolated ACL tear. All patients regained valgus stability with nonsurgical treatment of the MCL and ACL reconstruction. Level of evidence: II.

12. Halinen J, Lindahl J, Hirvensalo E, Santavirta S: Operative and nonoperative treatments of medial collateral ligament rupture with early anterior cruciate ligament reconstruction: A prospective randomized study. *Am J Sports Med* 2006;34:1134-1140.

Patients with a combined grade III MCL injury and ACL tear were prospectively randomized into surgical and nonsurgical treatment groups of the MCL injury. No statistical difference in regard to subjective function was determined between the two groups.

13. Nakamura N, Horibe S, Toritsuka Y, et al: Acute grade III medial collateral ligament injury of the knee associated with anterior cruciate ligament tear: The usefulness of magnetic resonance imaging in determining a treatment regimen. *Am J Sports Med* 2003;31:261-267.

In this prospective cohort, patients identified by MRI with tears of the superficial MCL distal to the joint line continued to have valgus instability after nonsurgical treatment of the MCL. Surgical treatment of such MCL tears had more favorable outcomes.

14. Prodromos CC, Han Y, Rogowski J, Joyce B, Shi K: A meta-analysis of the incidence of anterior cruciate ligament tears as a function of gender, sport, and a knee injury-reduction regimen. *Arthroscopy* 2007;23:1320-1325.

This meta-analysis concluded a threefold greater incidence of ACL injury among female athletes in soccer and basketball. Female athletes who participate in both soccer and basketball have an ACL injury rate of approximately 5%.

15. Griffin LY, Albohm MJ, Arendt EA, et al: Understanding and preventing noncontact anterior cruciate ligament injuries: A review of the Hunt Valley II Meeting. January 2005. *Am J Sports Med* 2006;34:1512-1532.

This article discusses the current knowledge of risk factors associated with noncontact ACL injuries, ACL in-

3: Knee and Leg

jury biomechanics, and existing ACL prevention programs.

16. Myer GD, Ford KR, McLean SG, Hewett TE: The effects of plyometric versus dynamic stabilization and balance training on lower extremity biomechanics. *Am J Sports Med* 2006;34:445-455.

    In a controlled laboratory study, plyometric training and dynamic stabilization exercises improved the landing and jumping mechanics with a decrease in valgus moments exhibited by the lower extremities, both in double- and single-leg maneuvers.

17. Pfeiffer RP, Shea KG, Roberts D, Grandstrand S, Bond L: Lack of effect of a knee ligament injury prevention program on the incidence of noncontact anterior cruciate ligament injury. *J Bone Joint Surg Am* 2006;88: 1769-1774.

    No reduction in the incidence of noncontact ACL injuries was recorded in the prevention group in comparison with the control group in this study. Plyometric-based training was provided twice weekly in-season for the athletes. Level of evidence: II.

18. Chhabra A, Starman JS, Ferretti M, et al: Anatomic, radiographic, biomechanical, and kinematic evaluation of the anterior cruciate ligament and its two functional bundles. *J Bone Joint Surg Am* 2006;88:2-10.

    This cadaver study describes the detailed anatomy of the ACL and biomechanical function of the individual bundles.

19. Luites JW, Wymenga AB, Blankevoort L, Kooloos JG: Description of the attachment geometry of the antero-medial and posterolateral bundles of the ACL from arthroscopic perspective for anatomical tunnel placement. *Knee Surg Sports Traumatol Arthrosc* 2007;15:1422-1431.

    This anatomic study provides a geometric description of the center of the attachment sites of the two individual ACL bundles relative to arthroscopically visible landmarks.

20. Farrow LD, Chen MR, Cooperman DR, Victoroff BN, Goodfellow DB: Morphology of the femoral intercondylar notch. *J Bone Joint Surg Am* 2007;89:2150-2155.

    The authors characterize the osseous anatomy of the femoral intercondylar notch with specific attention to the morphology of the ridge on the lateral wall of the intercondylar notch and the posterolateral rim of the intercondylar notch.

21. Fu FH, Jordan SS: The lateral intercondylar ridge: A key to anatomic anterior cruciate ligament reconstruction. *J Bone Joint Surg Am* 2007;89:2103-2104.

    The authors present an editorial response to further describe the intercondylar femoral ridge and identification and characterization of the lateral bifurcate ridge.

22. Yagi M, Kuroda R, Nagamune K, Yoshiya S, Kurosaka M: Double-bundle ACL reconstruction can improve rotational stability. *Clin Orthop Relat Res* 2007;454:100-107.

    This randomized study analyzed rotational stability in patients who had double-bundle ACL reconstruction compared with patients who received a single-bundle reconstruction. The double-bundle group demonstrated greater rotational instability as determined by the pivot shift test. Level of evidence: II.

23. Carey JL, Huffman R, Parekh SG, Sennett BJ: Outcomes of anterior cruciate ligament injuries to running backs and wide receivers in the National Football League. *Am J Sports Med* 2006;34:1911-1917.

    ACL injury and reconstruction data from the National Football League were collected over a 5-year period for running backs and wide receivers. Approximately 80% of players returned to professional sports but with an average one third reduction in performance.

24. Logan MC, Williams A, Lavelle J, Gedroyc W, Freeman M: Tibiofemoral kinematics following successful anterior cruciate ligament reconstruction using dynamic multiple resonance imaging. *Am J Sports Med* 2004;32: 984-992.

    Anteroposterior tibiofemoral motion was assessed using open-access MRI in this case series of 10 patients with an isolated ACL reconstruction in one knee and a normal contralateral knee. The authors concluded successful ACL reconstruction reduces sagittal laxity to within normal limits but does not restore normal tibiofemoral kinematics.

25. Logan M, Dunstan E, Robinson J, et al: Tibiofemoral kinematics of the anterior cruciate ligament (ACL)-deficient weightbearing, living knee employing vertical access open "interventional" multiple resonance imaging. *Am J Sports Med* 2004;32:720-726.

    Anteroposterior tibiofemoral motion was assessed using open-access MRI in this case series of 10 patients with an isolated ACL rupture in one knee and a normal contralateral knee. The authors concluded rupture of the ACL changes tibiofemoral kinematics producing anterior subluxation of the lateral tibial plateau without changing the medial tibiofemoral relationship.

26. Brophy RH, Selby RM, Altchek DW. Anterior cruciate ligament revision: Double-bundle augmentation of primary vertical graft. *Arthroscopy* 2006;22:683.e1-e5.

    The authors describe a surgical technique whereby augmenting the primary vertically placed graft with a more anatomically placed graft to restore rotation stability.

27. Jepsen CF, Lundberg-Jenson AK, Faunoe P: Does the position of the femoral tunnel affect the laxity or clinical outcome of the anterior cruciate ligament-reconstructed knee? A clinical, prospective, randomized, double-blind study. *Arthroscopy* 2007;23:1326-1333.

    This study demonstrates different femoral tunnel positions for ACL reconstruction do not impact sagittal laxity but improve rotational stability with a femoral tunnel placed at the 2 o'clock (low) position instead of a 1 o'clock (high) position. Level of evidence: I.

28. Musahl V, Plakseychuk A, Van Scyoc A, et al: Varying femoral tunnels between the anatomical footprint and

isometric positions: Effect on kinematics of the anterior cruciate ligament-reconstructed knee. *Am J Sports Med* 2005;33:712-718.

ACL reconstructions performed in cadaver knees with the femoral tunnel placed in either the anatomic footprint or a position for best graft isometry were compared. Although neither tunnel placement restored normal knee kinematics, the tunnel within the anatomic footprint more closely resembled that of the intact knee.

29. Yamamoto Y, Hsu WH, Woo SL, et al: Knee stability and graft function after anterior cruciate ligament reconstruction: A comparison of a lateral and an anatomical femoral tunnel placement. *Am J Sports Med* 2004; 32:1825-1832.

ACL reconstructions performed in cadaver knees with a single laterally placed femoral tunnel compared with an anatomic reconstruction were subjected to various forces and compared to ACL-intact knees and ACL-deficient knees. Greater rotatory stability was obtained with the anatomic reconstruction.

30. Muneta T, Koga H, Mochizuki T, et al: A prospective randomized study of 4-strand semitendinosus tendon anterior cruciate ligament reconstruction comparing single-bundle and double-bundle techniques. *Arthroscopy* 2007;23:618-628.

A randomized clinical study comparing double-bundle and single-bundle ACL reconstructions with four-strand semitendinosus tendon presents evidence of superior anterior and rotational stability of double-bundle reconstructions. However, the study failed to show any subjective difference between the two groups. Level of evidence: I.

31. Siebold R, Dehler C, Ellert T: Prospective randomized comparison of double-bundle versus single-bundle anterior cruciate ligament reconstruction. *Arthroscopy* 2008;24:137-145.

This randomized clinical trial demonstrated superior anterior and rotational stability with double-bundle ACL reconstruction when compared with single-bundle reconstruction. Subjective scoring among the two groups showed no difference.

32. Streich NA, Friedrich K, Gotterbarm T, Schmitt H: Reconstruction of the ACL with a semitendinosus tendon graft: A prospective randomized single blinded comparison of double-bundle versus single-bundle technique in male athletes. *Knee Surg Sports Traumatol Arthrosc* 2008;16:232-238.

This prospective comparison of double- versus single-bundle reconstructions showed no significant clinical or subjective differences after 2 years in high-demand male athletes. A single-bundle reconstruction with a more horizontally placed femoral tunnel showed equal clinical and subjective results.

33. Edwards A, Bull AM, Amis AA: The attachments of the anteromedial and posterolateral fibre bundles of the anterior cruciate ligament: Part 2. Femoral attachment. *Knee Surg Sports Traumatol Arthrosc* 2008;16:29-36.

The authors performed a cadaveric study describing the locations of the femoral attachments of the antero-medial and posterolateral bundles of the ACL. The attachment sites were measured and described in terms of the clock positions parallel to the femoral long axis and parallel to the roof of the intercondylar notch.

34. Edwards A, Bull AM, Amis AA: The attachments of the anteromedial and posterolateral fibre bundles of the anterior cruciate ligament: Part 1. Tibial attachment. *Knee Surg Sports Traumatol Arthrosc* 2007;15:1414-1421.

The authors performed a cadaveric study describing the locations of the tibial attachments of the anteromedial and posterolateral bundles of the ACL.

35. Battaglia MJ III, Cordasco FA, Hannafin JA, et al: Results of revision anterior cruciate ligament surgery. *Am J Sports Med* 2007;35:2057-2066.

The authors present a case series of 95 patients who underwent revision ACL reconstruction. Approximately 60% of patients returned to sports but with a decrease in performance. The degree of radiographic arthritis was proportional to the duration of instability symptoms after primary failure.

36. Goldblatt JP, Fitzsimmons SE, Balk E, Richmond JC: Reconstruction of the anterior cruciate ligament: Meta-analysis of patellar tendon versus hamstring tendon autograft. *Arthroscopy* 2005;21:791-803.

This meta-analysis shows the incidence of instability is not significantly different between the patellar tendon and hamstring grafts. Patellar tendon grafts were more likely to result in normal objective measurements with less significant flexion loss. Hamstring grafts had a reduced incidence of patellofemoral crepitance, kneeling pain, and extension loss. Level of evidence: I.

37. Sajovic M, Vengust V, Komadina R, Tavcar R, Skaza K: A prospective, randomized comparison of semitendinosus and gracilis tendon versus patellar tendon autografts for anterior cruciate ligament reconstruction: Five-year follow-up. *Am J Sports Med* 2006;34:1933-1940.

At the 5-year follow-up, both hamstring and patellar tendon autografts provided good subjective outcomes and objective stability in this study. More than 80% of patients were able to return to their preinjury level of activity. Level of evidence: I.

38. Poehling GG, Curl WW, Lee CA, et al: Analysis of outcomes of anterior cruciate ligament repair with 5-year follow-up: Allograft versus autograft. *Arthroscopy* 2005;21:774-785.

This prospective cohort study demonstrated similar objective and subjective outcomes at 5 years for allografts and autografts. However, allograft patients reported less pain, better function within the first year, and fewer activity limitations throughout the follow-up period. Level of evidence: II.

39. Barrett G, Stokes D, White M: Anterior cruciate ligament reconstruction in patients older than 40 years: Allograft versus autograft patellar tendon. *Am J Sports Med* 2005;33:1505-1512.

The authors present a cohort of patients older than 40 years comparing allograft and autograft patellar tendon. They concluded that neither graft was superior but the allograft group had a quicker return to activities despite greater laxity compared with the autograft group.

40. Kustos T, Bálint L, Than P, Bárdos T: Comparative study of autograft or allograft in primary anterior cruciate ligament reconstruction. *Int Orthop* 2004;28:290-293.

   No statistical difference in objective and subjective comparison of allografts and autografts were reported in this patient group. The revision rates between the groups were equivalent.

41. Rappé M, Horodyski MB, Meister K, Indelicato PA: Nonirradiated versus irradiated Achilles allograft: In vivo failure comparison. *Am J Sports Med* 2007;35:1653-1658.

   The failure rate during the first 6 months following ACL reconstruction of irradiated Achilles allografts was 33% compared with 2.4% for the nonirradiated Achilles allografts. Level of evidence: III.

42. Singhal MC, Gardiner JR, Johnson DL: Failure of primary anterior cruciate ligament surgery using anterior tibialis allograft. *Arthroscopy* 2007;23:469-475.

   The use of anterior tibialis allografts in ACL reconstructions was evaluated. The revision/failure rate was 24% in patients older than 25 years and 55% in patients younger than 25 years.

43. Harner CD, Xerogeanes JW, Livesay GA, et al: The human posterior cruciate ligament complex: An interdisciplinary study. Ligament morphology and biomechanical evaluation. *Am J Sports Med* 1995;23:736-745.

44. Van Dommelen BA, Fowler PJ: Anatomy of the posterior cruciate ligament: A review. *Am J Sports Med* 1989;17:24-29.

45. Miller MD, Harner CD: The anatomic and surgical considerations for posterior cruciate ligament reconstruction. *Instr Course Lect* 1995;44:431-440.

46. Shelbourne KD, Davis TJ, Patel DV: The natural history of acute, isolated, nonoperatively treated posterior cruciate ligament injuries: A prospective study. *Am J Sports Med* 1999;27:276-283.

47. Sekiya JK, Whiddon DR, Zehms CT, Miller MD: Clinically relevant assessment of posterior cruciate ligament and posterolateral corner injuries: Part I. Evaluation of isolated and combined deficiency. *J Bone Joint Surg Am* 2008;90:1621-1627.

   In this cadaveric study, stress radiographs were taken sequentially with intact knees, PCL-deficient knees, and PCL and posterolateral corner-deficient knees. Posterior displacement was measured demonstrating approximately 10 mm of displacement with PCL deficiency and 20 mm of displacement with combined PCL and posterolateral corner-deficient knees. PCL deficiency resulted in minimal rotational instability. Combined PCL and posterolateral corner deficiency resulted in significant rotational instability.

48. Jordan SS, Campbell RB, Sekiya JK: Posterior cruciate ligament reconstruction using a new arthroscopic tibial inlay double-bundle technique. *Sports Med Arthrosc* 2007;15:176-183.

   The authors present a review of a new arthroscopic tibial inlay double-bundle technique and short-term outcomes.

49. Campbell RB, Jordan SS, Sekiya JK: Arthroscopic tibial inlay for posterior cruciate ligament reconstruction. *Arthroscopy* 2007;23:1356.

   The authors discuss arthroscopic tibial inlay for PCL reconstruction.

50. Noyes FR, Barber-Westin SD: Treatment of complex injuries involving the posterior cruciate and posterolateral ligaments of the knee. *Am J Knee Surg* 1996;9:200-214.

51. Cooper DE, Stewart D: Posterior cruciate ligament reconstruction using single-bundle patella tendon graft with tibial inlay fixation: 2- to 10-year follow-up. *Am J Sports Med* 2004;32:346-360.

   The authors prospectively studied patellar tendon grafts in PCL reconstruction with improvement in posterior drawer test and Telos radiographs, and no difference between allograft and autograft.

52. Chan YS, Yang SC, Chang CH, et al: Arthroscopic reconstruction of the posterior cruciate ligament with use of a quadruple hamstring tendon graft with 3- to 5-year follow-up. *Arthroscopy* 2006;22:762-770.

   The authors studied outcomes of hamstring graft reconstructions using Lysholm and Tegner scores, as well as flexor and extensor strength ratios, and found improvement in all these areas postoperatively.

53. Margheritini F, Mauro CS, Rihn JA, et al: Biomechanical comparison of tibial inlay versus transtibial techniques for posterior cruciate ligament reconstruction: Analysis of knee kinematics and graft in situ forces. *Am J Sports Med* 2004;32:587-593.

   Cadaver knees were used to evaluate the kinematics of the different reconstructions, and both reconstructions restored posterior tibial translation of the knee without significant difference between the groups.

54. Seon JK, Song EK: Reconstruction of isolated posterior cruciate ligament injuries: A clinical comparison of the transtibial and tibial inlay techniques. *Arthroscopy* 2006;22:27-32.

   A retrospective case series studying the differences in posterior drawer, Lysholm scores, radiologic stability of the knee, and Tegner activity test found no significant difference between the two groups.

55. Fanelli GC, Orcutt DR, Edson CJ: The multiple-ligament injured knee: Evaluation, treatment, and results. *Arthroscopy* 2005;21:471-487.

The authors present a thorough overview of their approach to evaluation and treatment of knee dislocations in this current concepts review.

56. Rihn JA, Groff YJ, Harner CD, Cha PS: The acutely dislocated knee: Evaluation and management. *J Am Acad Orthop Surg* 2004;12:334-346.

    A thorough review of the literature on evaluation and management of knee dislocations is presented.

57. Robertson A, Nutton RW, Keating JF: Dislocation of the knee. *J Bone Joint Surg Br* 2006;88:706-711.

    This review paper focuses on the initial evaluation and management of the dislocated knee.

58. LaPrade RF, Engebretson AH, Ly TV, Johansen S, Wentorf FA, Engebretsen L: The anatomy of the medial part of the knee. *J Bone Joint Surg Am* 2007;89:2000-2010.

    The authors present a detailed anatomic description of the attachment points of the major components of the medial side of the knee.

59. Robinson JR, Sanchez-Ballester J, Bull AM, Thomas Rde W, Amis AA: The posteromedial corner revisited: An anatomical description of the passive restraining structures of the medial aspect of the human knee. *J Bone Joint Surg Br* 2004;86:674-681.

    Anatomic dissections were performed in which oblique fibers were identified in the posteromedial capsule, but the authors could not identify a discrete posterior oblique ligament.

60. Robinson JR, Bull AM, Thomas RR, Amis AA: The role of medial collateral ligament and posteromedial capsule in controlling knee laxity. *Am J Sports Med* 2006;34: 1815-1823.

    The authors present a sequential cutting study evaluating contributions and functions of the deep and superficial MCL and the posteromedial capsule.

61. LaPrade RF, Ly TV, Wentorf FA, Engebretsen L: The posterolateral attachments of the knee: A qualitative and quantitative morphologic analysis of the fibular collateral ligament, popliteus tendon, popliteofibular ligament, and lateral gastrocnemius tendon. *Am J Sports Med* 2003;31:854-860.

    A detailed anatomic description of the attachment points of the major components of the posterolateral aspect of the knee is presented.

62. LaPrade RF, Bollom TS, Wentorf FA, Wills NJ, Meister K: Mechanical properties of the posterolateral structures of the knee. *Am J Sports Med* 2005;33:1386-1391.

    In this laboratory study, the posterolateral components were loaded to failure. Ultimate tensile loads were fibular collateral ligament 295 N, popliteofibular ligament 298 N, and popliteus tendon 700 N. Stiffness values were 33.5 N/m, 28.6 N/m, and 83.7 N/m, respectively.

63. LaPrade RF, Tso A, Wentorf FA: Force measurement on the fibular collateral ligament, popliteofibular ligament,

and popliteus tendon to applied loads. *Am J Sports Med* 2004;32:1695-1701.

    In this laboratory study, forces were measured using buckle transducers on the posterolateral components. For external rotation, the fibular collateral ligament had higher loads at lower flexion angles and the popliteus complex was noted to have higher loads at higher flexion angles.

64. LaPrade RF, Johansen S, Wentorf FA, Engebretsen L, Esterberg JL, Tso A: An analysis of an anatomical posterolateral knee reconstruction: An in vitro biomechanical study and development of a surgical technique. *Am J Sports Med* 2004;32:1405-1414.

    A technique for reconstructing the major components of the posterolateral corner with allograft is described, and cadaver mechanical testing demonstrates restoration of static stability.

65. Nau T, Chevalier Y, Hagemeister N, Deguise JA, Duval N: Comparison of 2 surgical techniques of posterolateral corner reconstruction of the knee. *Am J Sports Med* 2005;33:1838-1845.

    Reconstruction of all major posterolateral corner components is compared with a figure-of-8 reconstruction of the fibular collateral ligament and popliteofibular ligament in a laboratory study. Both reconstructions were able to restore static laxity to the posterolateral sectioned knee.

66. Markolf KL, Graves BR, Sigward SM, Jackson SR, McAllister DR: Effects of posterolateral reconstructions on external tibial rotation and forces in a posterior cruciate ligament graft. *J Bone Joint Surg Am* 2007;89: 2351-2358.

    In a laboratory study, posterolateral reconstructions lessened forces on a PCL graft. An isolated fibular collateral ligament graft could not decrease PCL graft forces to normal. Popliteofibular ligament and popliteus tendon grafts were able to decrease PCL forces to normal but at the expense of overconstraining external rotation.

67. Coobs BR, LaPrade RF, Griffith CJ, Nelson BJ: Biomechanical analysis of an isolated fibular (lateral) collateral ligament reconstruction using an autogenous semitendinosus graft. *Am J Sports Med* 2007;35:1521-1527.

    A surgical technique and laboratory study are described in which an isolated fibular collateral ligament reconstruction was able to restore static stability to a knee with isolated fibular collateral ligament sectioning.

68. Markolf KL, Graves BR, Sigward SM, Jackson SR, McAllister DR: How well do anatomical reconstructions of the posterolateral corner restore varus stability to the posterior cruciate ligament-reconstructed knee? *Am J Sports Med* 2007;35:1117-1122.

    Three different posterolateral reconstructions in a cadaver study were shown to overconstrain varus rotation if tensioned at 30 N at 30° flexion.

69. Stannard JP, Sheils TM, Lopez-Ben RR, McGwin G Jr, Robinson JT, Volgas DA: Vascular injuries in knee dis-

3: Knee and Leg

locations: The role of physical examination in determining the need for arteriography. *J Bone Joint Surg Am* 2004;86:910-915.

In a prospective study, the ability of serial physical examinations to predict the need for arteriography was assessed in a large group of patients with knee dislocations. Nine of ten patients with an abnormal physical examination had significant arterial injuries on arteriography. None of the patients (124 knees) with normal serial examinations developed significant acute arterial problems.

70. Klineberg EO, Crites BM, Flinn WR, Archibald JD, Moorman CT III: The role of arteriography in assessing popliteal artery injury in knee dislocations. *J Trauma* 2004;56:786-790.

In a retrospective analysis of 55 patients (57 knees) with knee dislocation, none had a normal physical examination and those with an ankle-brachial index greater than 0.8 had a significant popliteal artery injury.

71. Mills WJ, Barei DP, McNair P: The value of the ankle-brachial index for diagnosing arterial injury after knee dislocation: A prospective study. *J Trauma* 2004;56:1261-1265.

In a prospective study of 38 patients with a knee dislocation, an ankle-brachial index less than 0.9 was used as a criterion for performing arteriography. An ankle-brachial index less than 0.9 has a 100% positive predictive value and ankle-brachial index greater than 0.9 had a 100% negative value for the presence of a significant arterial injury.

72. Niall DM, Nutton RW, Keating FF: Palsy of the common peroneal nerve after traumatic dislocation of the knee. *J Bone Joint Surg Br* 2005;87:664-667.

Fifty-five patients with a knee dislocation were retrospectively reviewed. The incidence of peroneal nerve injury was 25%. Of those with peroneal nerve injury, 21% had full recovery, 29% had partial recovery, and 50% had no useful recovery of motor function. Patients with the nerve in continuity and less than 7 cm of nerve involvement had the best prognosis.

73. Fanelli GC, Giannotti BF, Edson CJ: Arthroscopically assisted combined anterior and posterior cruciate ligament reconstruction. *Arthroscopy* 1996;12:5-14.

74. Fanelli GC, Edson CJ: Arthroscopically assisted combined ACL-PCL reconstruction: 2 to 10 year follow-up. *Arthroscopy* 2002;18:703-714.

75. Blevins FT, Salgado J, Wascher DC, Koster F: Septic arthritis following arthroscopic meniscus repair: A cluster of three cases. *Arthroscopy* 1999;15:35-40.

76. Fanelli GC, Giannotti BF, Edson CJ: Arthroscopically assisted posterior cruciate ligament/posterior lateral complex reconstruction. *Arthroscopy* 1996;12:521-530.

77. Fanelli GC, Edson CJ: Combined posterior cruciate ligament–posterolateral reconstruction with Achilles tendon allograft and biceps femoris tendon tenodesis: 2-10 year follow-up. *Arthroscopy* 2004;20:339-345.

The authors present a case series on PCL-based multiple ligament reconstruction using allograft Achilles tendon and the arthroscopic transtibial PCL reconstruction surgical technique. Excellent results were demonstrated using stress radiography, KT 1000 arthrometer, and physical examination. Level of evidence: IV.

78. Fanelli GC, Edson CJ, Orcutt DR, Harris JD, Zijerdi D: Treatment of combined anterior cruciate-posterior cruciate ligament-medial-lateral side knee injuries. *J Knee Surg* 2005;18:240-248.

The authors describe the evaluation and treatment of the multiple-ligament-injured knee.

79. Cooper DE, Stewart D: Posterior cruciate ligament reconstruction using single bundle patellar tendon graft with tibial inlay fixation: 2 to 10 year follow-up. *Am J Sports Med* 2004;32:346-360.

The authors present a case series on PCL reconstruction in the multiple-ligament-injured knee using the tibial inlay surgical technique. Level of evidence: IV.

80. Wascher DC, Becker JR, Dexter JG, Blevins FT: Reconstruction of the anterior and posterior cruciate ligaments after knee dislocation: Results using fresh-frozen nonirradiated allografts. *Am J Sports Med* 1999;27:189-196.

81. Garofalo R, Jolles BM, Moretti B, Siegrist O: Double bundle transtibial posterior cruciate ligament reconstruction with a tendon-patellar bone-semitendinosus tendon autograft: Clinical results with a minimum 2 years' follow-up. *Arthroscopy* 2006;22:1331-1338.

The authors describe double-bundle PCL reconstruction in this case series.

82. Azar FM: Evaluation and treatment of chronic medial collateral ligament injuries of the knee. *Sports Med Arthrosc* 2006;14:84-90.

The diagnosis and surgical treatment options available for MCL reconstruction are outlined.

83. Sims WF, Jacobson KE: The posteromedial corner of the knee: Medial-sided injury patterns revisited. *Am J Sports Med* 2004;32:337-345.

Ninety-three patients with surgically treated medial side injuries are retrospectively reviewed. In these knees, there was injury to 99% of the posterior oblique ligaments, 70% of the semimembranosus capsular attachments, and 33% of the tibial collateral ligaments. Thirty percent of patients had complete peripheral detachment of the meniscus.

84. Nakamura N, Horibe S, Toritsuka Y, Mitsuoka T, Yoshikawa H, Shino K: Acute grade III medial collateral ligament injury of the knee associated with anterior cruciate ligament tear: The usefulness of magnetic resonance imaging in determining a treatment regimen. *Am J Sports Med* 2003;31:261-267.

Seventeen patients with ACL/MCL injury were assessed in a retrospective cohort study. MRI evidence of diffuse injury of the length of the superficial MCL predicted persistent valgus laxity after nonsurgical treatment that required MCL reconstruction.

3: Knee and Leg

85. Halinen J, Lindahl J, Hirvensalo E, Santavirta S: Operative and nonoperative treatments of medial collateral ligament rupture with early anterior cruciate ligament reconstruction: A prospective randomized study. *Am J Sports Med* 2006;34:1134-1140.

Forty-seven patients were randomized to surgical or nonsurgical treatment of MCL injuries. Patients received early ACL reconstruction (after less than 3 weeks) and MCL repair or bracing. The groups had similar laxity measurements and outcome scores. Level of evidence: I.

86. Yoshiya S, Kuroda R, Mizuno K, Yamamoto T, Kurosaka M: Medial collateral ligament reconstruction using autogenous hamstring tendons: Technique and results in initial cases. *Am J Sports Med* 2005;33:1380-1385.

In a retrospective analysis of 24 patients with acute and chronic MCL injuries (12 ACL/MCL, 7 PCL/MCL, 3 ACL/PCL/MCL, and 2 isolated MCL), the MCL was reconstructed using autogenous hamstring graft. The technique is described in detail. At 2-year follow-up, results showed normal or nearly normal laxity and range-of-motion measurements in all patients.

87. Bahk MS, Cosgarea AJ: Physical examination and imaging of the lateral collateral ligament and posterolateral corner of the knee. *Sports Med Arthrosc* 2006;14:12-19.

The authors discuss the diagnosis of posterolateral corner injuries in regard to physical examination, radiographic signs, and MRI findings.

88. LaPrade RF, Wentorf F: Diagnosis and treatment of posterolateral knee injuries. *Clin Orthop Relat Res* 2002;402:110-121.

The authors review the anatomic structures, radiographic imaging, physical examination, surgical timing, and surgical techniques involved in treatment of posterolateral knee injuries.

89. Lee J, Papakonstantinou O, Brookenthal KR, Trudell D, Resnick DL: Arcuate sign of posterolateral knee injuries: Anatomic, radiographic, and MR imaging data related to patterns of injury. *Skeletal Radiol* 2003;32:619-627.

The authors present a cadaver study and retrospective review of patients and show that specific radiographic and MRI findings of the posterolateral corner may suggest injuries to specific structures inserting on the fibular head. Level of evidence: IV.

90. Theodorou DJ, Theodorou SJ, Fithian DC, Paxton L, Garelick DH, Resnick D: Posterolateral complex knee injuries: Magnetic resonance imaging with surgical correlation. *Acta Radiol* 2005;46:297-305.

MRI is well suited for demonstrating the presence and extent of injuries of the major structures of the posterolateral complex of the knee. Level of evidence: III.

91. Fanelli GC, Edson CJ, Orcutt DR, Harris JD, Zijerdi D: Treatment of combined anterior cruciate-posterior cruciate ligament-medial-lateral side knee injuries. *J Knee Surg* 2005;18:240-248.

An algorithm for an approach to ACL, PCL, and medial-sided knee injuries in regard to imaging, surgical approach, and overall treatment is discussed in this review article.

92. Fanelli GC, Orcutt DR, Edson CJ: The multiple-ligament injured knee: Evaluation, treatment, and results. *Arthroscopy* 2005;21:471-486.

A systematic approach and algorithm are presented for assessment, timing, and techniques of treatment and outcomes of multiple-ligament-injured knees.

93. Fanelli GC, Tomaszewski DJ: Allograft use in the treatment of the multiple ligament injured knee. *Sports Med Arthrosc* 2007;15:139-148.

The evaluation and treatment of a multiple-ligament-injured knee with assessment of allograft reconstruction is reviewed.

94. Flandry F, Sinco SM: Surgical treatment of chronic posterolateral rotatory instability of the knee using capsular procedures. *Sports Med Arthrosc* 2006;14:44-50.

The authors review how capsular redundancy and elimination with capsular shift-type reconstruction will decrease instability and increase durability of posterolateral reconstruction.

95. Chen FS, Rokito AS, Pitman MI: Acute and chronic posterolateral rotatory instability of the knee. *J Am Acad Orthop Surg* 2000;8:97-110.

The authors discuss the complex anatomy and biomechanics of the posterolateral corner of the knee. In addition, surgical techniques and long-term functional results of both repair and reconstruction are analyzed.

96. Phisitkul P, Wolf BR, Amendola A: Role of high tibial and distal femoral osteotomies in the treatment of lateral-posterolateral and medial instabilities of the knee. *Sports Med Arthrosc* 2006;14:96-104.

How varus or valgus alignment can affect success and longevity of ligamentous reconstruction in the knee is discussed.

97. Noyes FR, Barber-Westin SD, Albright JC: An analysis of the causes of failure in 57 consecutive posterolateral operative procedures. *Am J Sports Med* 2006;34:1419-1430.

The authors suggest greater emphasis during the index operation on anatomic graft reconstruction of one or more of the posterolateral structures as necessary, restoration of all ruptured cruciate ligaments, and correction of varus malalignment. Level of evidence, IV.

3: Knee and Leg

Chapter 13

Articular Cartilage Lesions/Osteoarthritis

Michael J. Angel, MD   *Nicholas A. Sgaglione, MD   Christian Lattermann, MD

Articular Cartilage Lesions

Recent trends indicate that a rise in physical activity among adult patients of all ages has led to an increase in symptomatic osteochondrol lesions that require treatment. In one study, cartilage damage was noted in approximately 63% of patients undergoing knee arthroscopy.[1] Similarly, chondral or osteochondral defects were found in 610 of 1,000 patients undergoing knee arthroscopy, most often in the medial femoral condyle.[2] Because of the reported frequency of this injury, the practicing orthopaedist should be comfortable with treatment.

Basic Science
Structure/Function
Articular cartilage is a complex viscoelastic structure that provides a smooth, low-friction surface that transmits variable loads across the joint while minimizing peak stress on the underlying subchondral bone. In the knee, these load-bearing characteristics are shared with the meniscus. The medial and lateral meniscus transmits 50% and 70% of the load, respectively. Thus, partial or complete injury to the meniscus dramatically transmits loads to the articular surface, rendering it more vulnerable to substantial injury and degeneration.

Response to Damages
The healing response in articular cartilage is poor, largely because of its limited vascular supply and capacity for chondrocyte division and migration. Superficial or partial-thickness cartilage injury will result in a cellular insult with decreased matrix production by the underlying chondrocytes with little healing. Full-thickness defects will respond in similar fashion. A defect that penetrates the subchondral plate, an osteochondral lesion, results in an influx of marrow contents including inflammatory cells, undifferentiated mesen-

chymal cells, cytokines, and growth factors.[3,4] This will result in a healing response that more closely mimics normal healing; however, the resultant repair typically resembles fibrocartilage instead of hyaline cartilage.

Natural History
The natural history of chondral injury is not completely understood. The process begins with the disruption of the integrity of articular cartilage, resulting in volume loss and leading to pathologic edge loading of the surrounding perimeter. The elevated contact pressures on the surrounding surfaces can result in joint degradation. Although the literature often does not make a distinction between partial-thickness and full-thickness chondral defects because of their similar healing response, a full-thickness defect is more likely to expand. An osteochondral defect will result in a healing response filling the defect with fibrocartilage, a substance biomechanically inferior to hyaline. Although fibrocartilaginous healing may be tolerated clinically in smaller defects, larger insults are more likely to lead to significant degeneration and osteoarthritis.

Clinical Evaluation and Presentation
History
Clinical evaluation begins with a precise history. A patient who recalls a single injury or series of injuries is likely to have incurred a focal chondral or osteochondral lesion, whereas a patient who may not recall an event is likely to have a degenerative chondral lesion. If the patient recalls an injury, details surrounding the injury may help in determining the extent of the lesion. With a history that is suspicious for injury to the ligaments (the classic "pop" associated with anterior cruciate ligament injury or reports of instability), an associated chondral lesion is likely present. In addition, mechanical symptoms such as locking or catching may be associated with a pathologic chondral or osteochondral defect.

Physical Examination
Inspection of the knee begins with an evaluation of gait and alignment of the limb. Antalgia and precise evaluation of varus/valgus alignment are key elements of the

*Nicholas A. Sgaglione, MD or the department with which he is affiliated holds stock or stock options in Arthrocare and is a consultant for or an employee of Smith & Nephew Endoscopy, ConMed Linvatec, Arthrocare, and Musculoskeletal Tissue Foundation.

3: Knee and Leg

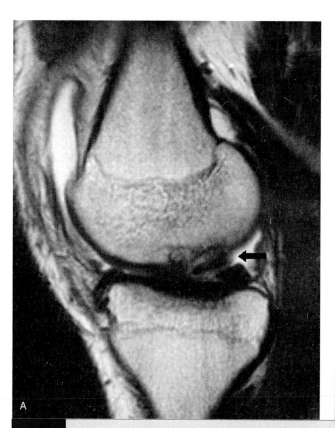
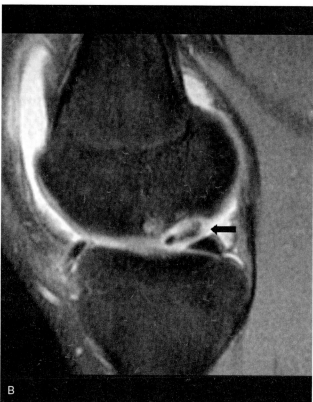

Figure 1 | T1- and T2-weighted sequence MRI images of osteochondral lesions of the knee showing "fluid tracking" indicative of an unstable lesion.

examination. Range of motion is tested, evaluating for mechanical symptoms such as locking, popping, or crepitus. The Wilson sign is performed with the knee flexed to 90° and the tibia internally rotated; gradual extension of the joint leads to pain at approximately 30° of flexion.[5] External rotation of the tibia at this point relieves the pain. The symptoms result from impingement of the tibial eminence on the chondral lesion on the medial femoral condyle. An effusion may also be detected. A thorough examination of the knee should assess for instability or pinpoint other associated injuries.

Radiologic Studies

Radiographic examination includes a standing AP, lateral, Merchant, and 45° flexion PA views. In addition to a focal osteochondral defect, the radiographs may show associated pathology such as osteophytes, joint space narrowing, fractures, or signs of ligamentous injury. The identification of associated degenerative joint disease is essential because it may affect decisions about surgical treatment options.

MRI can be used for evaluation of cartilage lesions and concomitant pathology or osteochondritis dissecans lesions. The presence of edema tracking around the cartilage defect is a significant radiographic sign that indicates the presence of an unstable cartilage lesion that may require surgical fixation (**Figure 1**). Al-

though there is no consensus on the best pulse sequence, fat-suppressed T2, proton density, and T2-weighted fast spin-echo sequences appear to result in improved sensitivity and specificity of cartilage lesions over standard sequences.

Bone scintigraphy may also be useful but has been supplanted in recent years by MRI. Bone scan has a significant advantage over MRI as a prognostic indicator because of its higher degree of osseous uptake, correlating with healing potential of an osteochondral lesion.

Arthroscopic Grading

The most accurate assessment of location, size, depth, shape, and stability of articular cartilage is obtained arthroscopically. The Outerbridge classification is a widely used classification system for grading chondral lesions. This classification of chondral wear was initially described as four grades: grade I, softening and swelling of the cartilage; grade 2, fragmentation and fissuring in an area half an inch or less in diameter; grade 3, same as grade 2, but involving greater than half an inch of cartilage; grade 4, erosion of cartilage down to bone.[6] This classification was later modified (**Table 1**). More recently, however, the International Cartilage Repair Society has proposed a universal grading system that offers a more precise description of chondral and osteochondral lesions, including size, depth, and location of injured cartilage[7] (**Figure 2**).

Nonsurgical Treatment

The initial management of articular cartilage lesions should consist of rest, analgesics to control pain, and anti-inflammatory medications. Although physical therapy is often used for strengthening and conditioning, it is often less effective in reducing symptoms. The use of steroid injections, hyaluronic acid, and glucosamine and chondroitin sulfate remains controversial. Although they may provide temporary pain relief, healing of cartilage is not likely. Although hyaluronic acid injections are used to treat early stages of degenerative arthritis, there are no current data to support its application with isolated focal articular cartilage lesions. Bracing can be used to treat an associated malalignment. Although an unloader brace may improve symptoms by decreasing the load incurred by the affected compartment, symptom relief is typically unsatisfactory in younger and more active patients.

Surgical Techniques

Débridement

Arthroscopic débridement and lavage is a temporizing first-line arthroscopic treatment of chondral lesions used in an attempt to reduce pain, inflammation, and mechanical symptoms caused by loose chondral fragments and inflammatory cytokines such as interleukin-1 and tumor necrosis factor-α.[8] Arthroscopic lavage alone has shown to provide short-term benefits in 50% to 70% of patients.[8-10] Although patients have improved results when arthroscopic lavage is combined with a formal chondroplasty, the studies to date have usually focused on patients with more degenerative conditions of the knee. Arthroscopic débridement remains a viable surgical alternative for a subset of patients with advanced degenerative conditions in the knee and for patients who cannot readily comply with the strict postoperative protocols required for cartilage restoration procedures. Chondroplasty is done using an arthroscopic shaver and meniscal biter, débriding loose chondral fragments while carefully preserving the intact surrounding cartilage.[11]

Fixation Techniques

Fixation of an osteochondral defect is a decision that depends on many characteristics of the lesion, including size, shape, and location along with the condition of the remaining fragment. Fixation is generally recommended for symptomatic, unstable fragments with adequate subchondral bone. MRI allows an accurate evaluation of the fragment and its stability in determining its suitability for fixation.

Osteochondral fixation begins with precise preparation. The nonviable or necrotic tissue underneath the fragment is débrided with a rasp, shaver, or curet. Depending on the condition of the underlying subchondral defect, bone graft may be used and obtained from Gerdy's tubercle or (less preferably) the intercondylar notch. The fragment must be reduced anatomically for effective fixation. Accessory portals are often needed to

Table 1	

Description of Outerbridge Classification

Grade	Description
0	Normal cartilage
I	Softening and swelling
II	Partial thickness defect, fissures less than 1.5 cm diameter
III	Fissures that reach subchondral bone, diameter greater than 1.5 cm
IV	Exposed subchondral bone

improve exposure, reduction, and fixation. After preparation and reduction, drilling or passage of a small Kirschner wire may help obtain subchondral bleeding and promote healing. Care must be taken during drilling and placement of the fixation devices to avoid open physis and penetration of and damage to normal articular cartilage.

Fixation may be achieved with both absorbable and nonabsorbable devices. Although nonabsorbable fixation devices provide optimal compression, they must be removed at a later date, requiring a second surgery. Successful healing has been achieved in 80% to 90% of patients with the use of headless metallic cannulated screws.[8] This device may be countersunk and provides excellent compression across the fracture site. Staple fixation, on the other hand, has had poor results, with 50% healing and 30% staple breakage.[8] The biosorbable devices, such as SmartNail (ConMed Linvatec, Largo, FL) or Biotrak resorbable screws (Acumed, Sports Medicine, Hillsboro, OR) are a lower profile and require smaller perforations in the articular surface; however, fixation and compression strength remain a concern for many surgeons. In addition, the rapid breakdown of the polymers has led to localized inflammatory reactions and joint irritation.

Marrow Stimulation Techniques

Marrow stimulation techniques include osteochondral drilling, abrasion arthroplasty, and microfracture. The goal of marrow stimulation is the delivery of progenitor cells from the marrow below the subchondral plate to the articular surfaces, which differentiate and form fibrocartilage tissue. Fibrocartilage consists primarily of type I collagen, whereas native hyaline cartilage consists of type II collagen, a biomechanically superior matrix. This is typically used as a first-line treatment of small, focal lesions with grade III or IV changes.

The technique involves débriding the damaged and unstable cartilage on the surface, removing the calcified cartilage below with a shaver or curet and creating a well-contained lesion to optimize clot adhesion.[12,13] The awls are then placed perpendicular to the surface, approximately 2 to 3 mm apart, and driven in with a mal-

ICRS Grade 0 - Normal   ICRS Grade 1 - Nearly Normal   ICRS Grade 2 - Abnormal

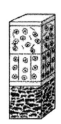
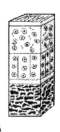
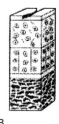
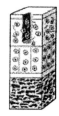

A   B

Superficial lesions. Soft indentation (A)   Lesions extending down to < 50 %
and/or superficial fissures and cracks (B)   of cartilage depth

ICRS Grade 3 - Severely Abnormal   ICRS Grade 4 - Severely Abnormal

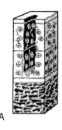
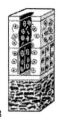
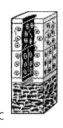
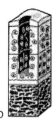
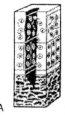
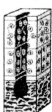

A   B   C   D   A   B

Cartilage defects extending down > 50% of cartilage depth (A) as
well as down to calcified layer (B) and down to but not through the
subchondral bone (C). Blisters are included in this Grade (D).

Figure 2   Classification system as described by the International Cartilage Repair Society. (*Reprinted with permission from the International Cartilage Repair Society, Switzerland.*)

let to a level of 2 to 4 mm (**Figure 3**). Fat droplets or blood typically are seen when the appropriate depth has been reached. Younger patients with smaller lesions have shown the potential for optimal outcomes. In carefully selected patients, microfracture is a cost-effective procedure that can provide symptomatic relief and improve function without making other restoration procedures infeasible.

Osteochondral Autograft Transplantation

This procedure involves the transfer of an osteochondral plug from a non–weight-bearing region to the symptomatic cartilage lesion. The typical harvest sites include the lateral or medial trochlea or the perimeter of the intercondylar notch[14] (**Figure 4**). The goal is to provide a structure that grossly and histologically matches the native tissue; the use of an autograft has a higher probability of healing to the surrounding recipient tissue. The preservation of chondrocyte viability, found in an autograft, is of paramount importance to the success of this surgery. Donor site availability and morbidity dictate the limitations of autologous transplantation. Focal, symptomatic grade IV lesions of the distal femoral condyle between 1 to 4 cm² represent the ideal lesion to treat using this technique; defects up to 2.5 cm² in size also can be treated. When lesions are of

significant size, multiple small osteochondral cylinders will be transferred to the recipient site (**Figure 5**). The lack of appropriate donor sites and lesions greater than 2 cm² are absolute contraindications to autologous transplantation.

The surgery is performed arthroscopically or arthroscopically assisted with an arthrotomy. A medial or lateral parapatellar miniarthrotomy is used to expose and assess the lesion. Assessment of the lesion determines the location, size, and shape of the defect. The lesion site is then prepared by drilling and shaping to provide a clean cylindrical recipient site with no loose fragments of cartilage or subchondral bone. Selection of the autograft site is based on tissue that will match the shape, contour, and size of the recipient site. Procurement of the autograft is then performed; several proprietary equipment systems have been developed to assist in this technique including MosaicPlasty (Smith & Nephew, Andover, MA), Osteochondral Autograft Transfer System (OATS, Arthrex, Naples, FL), and the COR Osteochondral Cartilage Repair System (DePuy Mitek, Westwood, MA).[14] The grafts are then placed in press-fit fashion into the recipient site. Each system has its own method of transferring the graft in a manner that retains the graft shape and limits significant impaction on the articular surface, a technique that sustains

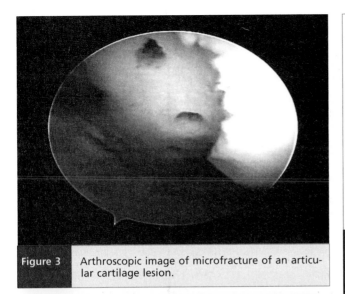

Figure 3 Arthroscopic image of microfracture of an articular cartilage lesion.

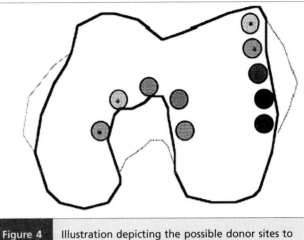

Figure 4 Illustration depicting the possible donor sites to be used for autologous chondrocyte transplantation. (*Reproduced with permission from Simonian PT, Sussman PS, Wickiewicz TL, Paletta GA, Warren RF: Contact pressures at osteochondral donor sites in the knee. Am J Sports Med 1998;26:491-494.*)

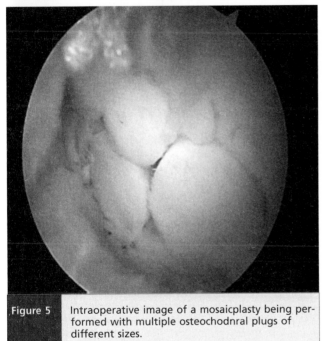

Figure 5 Intraoperative image of a mosaicplasty being performed with multiple osteochodnral plugs of different sizes.

chondrocyte viability. Graft height is positioned to sit flush with the native tissue. Grafts that are placed proud or countersunk lead to poor results.

TruFit Bone Graft Substitute Plugs (Smith and Nephew, Andover, MA) are porous polygraft material composed of a patented blend of polylactide-co-glycolide, calcium sulfate and polyglycolide fibers which may be used to backfill the bony defect at the harvest site. TruFit plugs are biomechanically stable scaffolds that allow ingrowth of new surface healing tissue and underlying subchondral bone, which may reduce donor site morbidity.

Osteochondral Allografts

Osteochondral allograft transplantation is a valuable treatment alternative for osteochondral lesions larger than 2.5 cm². The use of fresh or cold-stored allograft is preferred over fresh-frozen grafts because both cartilage cells and matrix are preserved. Significant decreases in chondrocyte viability are appreciated 14 to 21 days after storage in physiologic culture media; however, recent studies have shown that the chondrocyte cell appearance and biomechanical properties of the allograft persist even at 4 weeks.[15]

The procedure is performed in a manner similar to autologous transplantation, either arthroscopically or arthroscopically assisted with a miniarthrotomy. Using specialized proprietary instrumentation, a cylindrical dowel graft is obtained from the donor tissue that matches the defect at the lesion site (**Figure 6**). Ideally, the donor graft is of the same joint (that is, hemi-condyle for weightbearing surfaces of the knee); more important, the shape and contour of the allograft should match the native site. The graft is similarly placed in press-fit fashion with no need for further internal fixation.[16,17]

Osteochondral allograft transplantation may provide fully formed articular cartilage and bone without size limitation or concern for donor site morbidity. Several concerns include graft availability, chondrocyte viability at the time of implantation, disease transmission, and graft rejection. The advantage of using an autologous graft is its low cost, availability, and absence of disease transmission. Clinical outcomes have suggested that patients with unipolar, isolated lesions secondary to trauma can expect the greatest improvement in symptoms. Patients with ligament instability, tibiofemoral malalignment, or meniscal pathology have had limited clinical success with this procedure. Therefore, osteochondral allograft transplantation remains a viable treatment option in carefully selected patients with lesions larger than 2.5 cm.

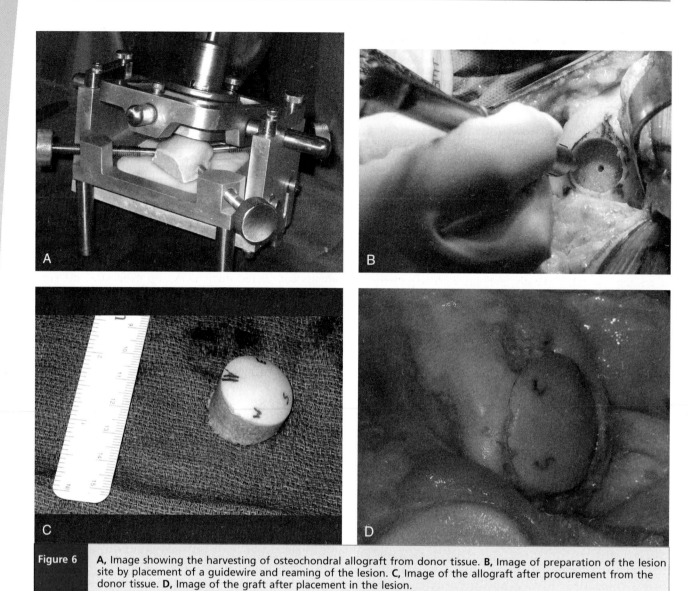

Figure 6 **A,** Image showing the harvesting of osteochondral allograft from donor tissue. **B,** Image of preparation of the lesion site by placement of a guidewire and reaming of the lesion. **C,** Image of the allograft after procurement from the donor tissue. **D,** Image of the graft after placement in the lesion.

Autologous Chondrocyte Implantation

Autologous chondrocyte implantation (ACI) is a cell-based procedure that attempts to repair the damaged chondral tissue by replacing it with viable autogenous chondrocytes. The first stage of the procedure involves arthroscopically obtaining a biopsy specimen of the articular cartilage to be implanted. This specimen typically is taken from the superomedial edge of the trochlea or the lateral side of the intercondylar notch and then sent for processing and cellular expansion. During the second stage of the procedure, the chondrocytes are reimplanted into the lesion underneath a periosteal patch approximately 6 to 8 weeks after the index harvest procedure. The chondrocytes can be preserved for up to 18 months, with cryopreservation limits up to 4 years.[18]

ACI can be used to treat lesions that are 2 to 10 cm². The ideal candidate has a focal, symptomatic, and unipolar defect with minimal subchondral bone loss. Marrow stimulation with an adequate amount of time for

recovery usually is unsuccessful in these patients. A bipolar kissing lesion is a relative contraindication to the ACI procedure. Ligamentous instability, malalignment, and meniscus pathology are not contraindications to the procedure as long as all of the pathology is treated during the index surgery.

Postoperative Management

The postoperative treatment of chondral lesions is fundamental to the success of the surgery. Each of these techniques requires a motivated and compliant patient who understands the significance of the treatment regimen.

The patient who undergoes a débridement and chondroplasty does not require a significant amount of restrictions. Full weight bearing is allowed immediately after surgery. Continuous passive motion (CPM) or physical therapy with active or active-assisted motion exercises begins early, and progression to low-impact strengthening protocols occurs after the swelling and pain subside, with a return to activities in 3 months or less.

In patients who undergo fixation of the lesion, weight bearing is restricted initially, with toe touch or partial weight bearing implemented with more stringent restrictions in larger lesions in the weight-bearing portions of the knee. Progression to full weight bearing is at approximately 8 to 12 weeks, with advancement in strengthening over the subsequent 3 months. Nonabsorbable fixation is removed in approximately 3 to 6 months, depending on relief of pain and swelling. After removal of the implants, partial weight bearing is instituted again for 6 weeks, with progression and return to activities in approximately 4 to 6 months.

The postoperative regimen for a marrow-stimulating procedure on the femoral condyle requires modification of weight bearing. Typically, patients with large lesions on the femoral condyle are restricted from bearing weight. Patients with lesions on the trochlea or patella typically may bear weight in full extension with limited flexion with the use of a flexion-stop brace. CPM immediately after surgery varies from 2 to 6 hours daily. Weight bearing is typically increased at approximately 6 to 8 weeks, with the goal of returning to full activities at approximately 6 months.

The postoperative regimen for osteochondral autograft or allograft transplants differs slightly. A hinged brace can be used immediately in patients with either transplant, and movement of the knee through an unrestricted range of motion either with or without a CPM machine is encouraged. Patients who undergo an osteochondral autograft transplant are restricted from bearing weight for 2 to 4 weeks, partial weight bearing is implemented for 4 to 6 weeks, and weight bearing is as tolerated at 6 to 8 weeks, whereas those with an osteochondral allograft are restricted from bearing weight for 2 to 3 months. Although not routinely obtained, serial cartilage-specific MRI studies can be used to assess graft healing and incorporation. Second-look arthroscopy can also be used to assess the quality of the graft and precise histomorphometry; however, this represents a second surgical procedure. Patients are allowed to return to sports only after careful clinical assessment and satisfactory progress, usually at 6 to 9 months.

Weight bearing after ACI is restricted for up to 8 to 12 weeks. CPM has been shown to improve the quality and quantity of defect fill and is instituted immediately. Strengthening exercises are initiated at approximately 6 to 8 weeks with increasing intensity over the next 3 to 6 months. Return to full athletic activities is typically achieved at 12 to 18 months after the chondrocyte implantation.

Results of Treatment

At this time, no consensus exists as to the most appropriate technique for each individual patient or lesion. Although the results to date show a significant amount of promise when each indicated technique is reported on, few controlled comparison studies exist (**Table 2**).

Although satisfactory results have been reported, others have found that the use of débridement or abrasion arthroplasty acts only as a temporizing measure with satisfaction typically deteriorating over time. In perhaps the most extensive study on abrasion arthroplasty, results of approximately 400 patients with an average age of 60 years were reported.[10] Sixty-six percent of these patients continued to have pain, and only 12% had complete relief of symptoms. In another study, there were 50% to 60% satisfactory results at 3- to 5-year follow-up after abrasion arthroplasty, with better results occurring in younger patients.[9]

In a 2003 study, the results of microfracture were reported in 72 patients age 45 years or younger with full-thickness chondral defects in a ligamentously stable knee.[19] At an average follow-up of 11.3 years, 80% of patients considered themselves improved after the surgery. Age was noted to be an independent variable because patients younger than 35 years reported better results. Significant improvements were found in the Lysholm and Tegner scores with good-to-excellent results in the Western Ontario and McMaster Universities (WOMAC) Osteoarthritis index. In another recent study, 48 full-thickness chondral defects of the knee were prospectively evaluated.[13] At an average follow-up of 41 months, 32 patients (67%) reported good or excellent subjective results, 12 (25%) had fair results, and only 4 (8%) reported poor function. In addition, MRI of 24 of these patients showed good repair tissue fill in 13 patients (54%), moderate fill in 7 (29%), and poor fill in 4 patients (17%). The fill grade also was noted to correlate with knee functional scores. Those knees with good tissue fill correlated with improved knee function, whereas poor fill was associated with poor subjective scores and decreasing function after 24 months.

The results of osteochondral autograft transplantation have been promising. Second-look biopsies were performed on 10 patients treated with osteochondral autografts at 2- to 12-month follow-up intervals.[14] Retention of the integrity of the grafts was demonstrated with living chondrocytes and osteocytes found histologically. Donor sites filled without grafting and were covered with fibrocartilagenous scar. No complications occurred in this group. In a 2003 study, 831 cases of mosaicplasty of the knee and ankle were reviewed over a 10-year period.[20] Good-to-excellent results were reported in 92% of patients with condyle lesions, 87% of those with tibial plateau lesions, and 94% of those with talar dome lesions. Long-term donor site morbidity occurred in only 3% of patients. In addition, 69 of 83 patients who were followed arthroscopically showed histologic evidence of survival of transplanted hyaline cartilage, congruent gliding surfaces, and fibrocartilage ingrowth at the donor sites. In a 2007 prospective study, 30 patients underwent arthroscopic mosaicplasty for the treatment of Outerbridge grade IV femoral condyle lesions less than 2.5 cm.[2,21] At 7 years, good-to-excellent results were seen in 76.7% of patients. MRI evaluation showed good integration of the

3: Knee and Leg

Table 2

Results of Treatment of Osteochondral Defects*

Year	Author	Study Design	Procedure	No. of Patients	Follow-up (months)	Results
2003	Hangody	Retrospective	OAT	831	120	Good-to-excellent results in 92% of pts treated for femoral lesions, 87% for tibial lesions, 79% for patella/trochlea lesions
2003	Peterson	Prospective	ACI	58	67	Good-to-excellent results in 91% of pts
2004	Steadman	Prospective	Microfracture	75	132	Eighty percent of patients consider themselves "improved." Lysholm increased from 59 preoperatively to 89 at follow-up
2005	Gudas	Prospective randomized	OAT vs microfracture	60	36	OAT had 96% good or excellent results compared to 52% with microfracture. Return to sport was 93% with OAT pts versus 52% of microfracture pts
2005	Mithoefer	Prospective	Microfracture	48	24	Good-to-excellent results in 67%, fair for 25% and poor for 8%
2005	Gross	Prospective	Fresh allograft	125	120	Femoral graft survivorship was 95% at 5 years, 85% at 10 years. Tibial graft survivorship was 95% at 5 years, 80% at 10 years, 65% at 15 years
2006	Barber	Retrospective	COR	14	24	Repeat arthroscopy showed good incorporation in all grafts (100%).
2007	Knutsen	Prospective randomized	ACI vs microfracture	80	60	No significant difference in overall satisfaction between both groups—77% satisfied
2007	Marcacci	Prospective	OAT	30	84	Good-to-excellent results in 76% of pts
2007	Williams	Prospective	Fresh allograft	19	48	MRI showed normal cartilage thickness preserved in 18 implanted grafts; trabecular incorporation of the allograft was complete or partial in 14 patients and positively correlated with Short Form-36 scores at the time of follow-up
2007	Miniaci	Prospective	OAT	20	18	MRI imaging showed healing of all grafts at 6 months. Pain scores reduced from 8.3/10 to 0.8/10 in 6 months and 0/10 at 1 year
2007	McCulloch	Prospective	Fresh allograft	25	35	Patients reported 84% satisfaction. Radiographically 88% of all grafts showed incorporation into host

*COR = chondral osseous autograft transplantation; OAT = osteochondral autograft transplantation; ACI = autologous chondrocyte implantation; pts = patients

graft into the host tissue in 60% of patients. Both lateral condyle lesions and younger patients were factors associated with better clinical outcomes.

The following results of osteochondral allograft transplantation have been encouraging. One study reported on 126 patients with traumatic chondral injuries to the knee.[16] The survivor rate was 85% at an average follow-up of 7.5 years. Two recent studies have demonstrated the effectiveness of using fresh allografts in treating osteochondral defects. In one study, 25 patients

had significant clinical improvement after osteochondral allograft transplantation with fresh allograft.[22] These patients were prospectively evaluated at an average follow-up of 35 months and patient satisfaction was reportedly 84%; 88% of grafts had radiographic evidence of incorporation into host bone. Similarly, another study prospectively evaluated 19 patients who underwent osteochondral allograft transplant with fresh stored allografts for large lesions (average size 6 cm^2).[23] At an average follow-up of 48 months, they

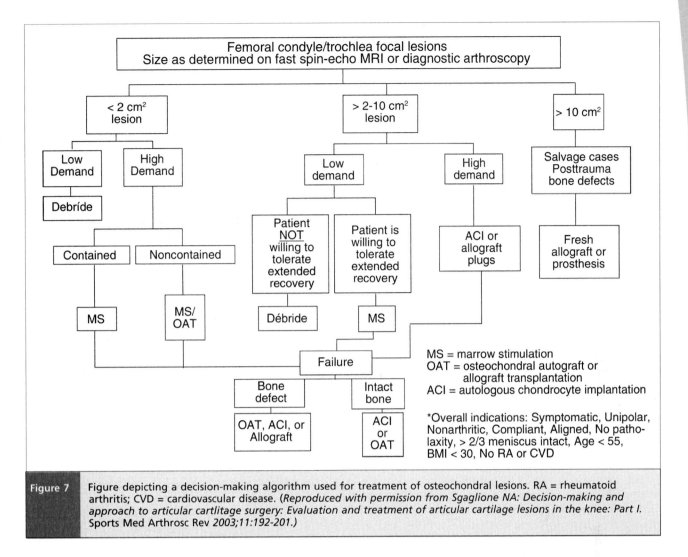

Figure 7 Figure depicting a decision-making algorithm used for treatment of osteochondral lesions. RA = rheumatoid arthritis; CVD = cardiovascular disease. (*Reproduced with permission from Sgaglione NA: Decision-making and approach to articular cartlitage surgery: Evaluation and treatment of articular cartilage lesions in the knee: Part I.* Sports Med Arthrosc Rev *2003;11:192-201.*)

demonstrated both clinical and radiographic improvement, with normal articular cartilage thickness preserved in all 18 of 19 grafts. As study results continue to show good graft incorporation, more surgeons will opt for the use of allografts.

Recent reports have compared treatment methods. Osteochondral autograft transplantation (OAT) and microfracture were compared in a prospective controlled study involving 60 athletes.[24] Autologous osteochondral transfer resulted in 96% of patients achieving good or excellent results compared with only 52% treated with microfracture. In addition, 93% of OAT patients returned to preinjury athletics at a mean of 6 months compared with 52% of microfracture patients. Another study prospectively compared osteochondral transplantation and autologous chondrocyte transplantation in 40 patients.[25] Although both treatments resulted in significant improvement of symptoms, histological analysis revealed defects treated with ACI to be filled primarily with fibrocartilage. Defects treated with autologous transfer retained their hyaline cartilage. The results of 80 patients randomized to undergo either ACI or microfracture with a 5-year follow-up period

were reported in a 2007 study.[26] Both groups had a 77% satisfaction rate, indicating no significant difference. In addition, both groups had similar histologic findings, failure rates, and progression of arthritic changes. Younger patients performed best and those with good histologic repairs had correlating clinical examinations.

Decision Making

Decision making regarding surgical options depends on patient goals, expectations, and compliance with rehabilitation as well as tolerance, expectation, and perception of methodology and prognosis. Surgeon preference will be shaped by experience and comorbidities. It is best to design a patient profile (including age, comorbidities, expectations, compliance, and so on) to assist in decision making. Although strict surgical indications can be used in some instances (**Figure 7**), careful consideration is required to select the best surgical treatment options.

Lesion size and patient's physical demands may be used to help determine the method of treatment (**Figure 7**). A low demand patient who has a lesion of relatively

3: Knee and Leg

insignificant size is best suited for débridement or lavage. The same lesion in a higher demand patient may best be suited for a marrow-stimulating procedure or OAT. The characteristics of the lesion as well as the patient profile may assist in deciding which to use. Lesions that are of larger size in the lower demand patient may best benefit from a reparative marrow-stimulating procedure if they are willing to comply with an extensive recovery regimen. The higher demand patient would undergo a restorative procedure (osteochondral autograft/allograft transplantation or ACI). The patient with a lesion greater than 10 cm^2, most often salvaged from primary failure or trauma, may require an allograft or prosthetic replacement.

One clinical entity that requires special mention is the young athlete (age 15 to 25 years) with a symptomatic osteochondritis dissecans lesion or osteochondral fracture. MRI is useful to evaluate the lesion for chondral stability, fragment size, and the presence of underlying bone and marrow involvement. If the lesion appears stable, juvenile patients may be managed nonsurgically with restricted weightbearing. With an unstable fragment that has maintained its position in the defect, internal fixation may be done.

Osteoarthritis

Basic Science
Histologic Changes
Structural changes caused by osteoarthritis can be seen macroscopically as changes in the consistency of cartilage (softening, fibrillation) or as complete loss of cartilage substance (erosions, ulcerations). These changes result from microscopic structural changes that relate to breakdown of the cartilage matrix, allowing fissures and cracks to occur through the cartilage matrix that reach and occasionally penetrate the subchondral bone. Deep lesions that involve the subchondral bone can stimulate a weak reparative response that leads to fibrocartilaginous scars. Histologically these changes are accompanied by an increase in chondrocyte death (apoptosis) as well as chondrocyte cloning and a duplication of the tide mark.[27]

Biochemical Changes
Cartilage matrix homeostasis is maintained through an intricate system that balances matrix production by the chondrocytes and matrix breakdown by degradative enzymes called metalloproteinases (MMPs). The breakdown of proteoglycans and collagen II mediated by MMPs is influenced directly by physiologic enzyme activators (cathepsin B and plasminogen activator/plasmin) and their inhibitors (tissue inhibitors of metalloproteinases, TIMPs). Proteoglycan breakdown seems to be mediated predominantly by stromelysin-1 (MMP-3) and aggrecanase-1 (encoded by the gene a disintegrin and metalloproteinase with thrombospondin motifs 4 [ADAMTS-4]), whereas collagen II is mainly degraded by collagenases 1 and 3 (MMP-1, MMP-13). It has been shown that in osteoarthritic cartilage there is an imbalance of this system, skewed toward matrix breakdown. Modifications of this imbalance may provide future treatment options.[28]

The direct cause of the onset of osteoarthritis is still unknown. It is likely that mechanical factors play a significant role in providing a trigger to start the process of matrix breakdown. Biomechanical studies have demonstrated that chondrocytes are directly affected by mechanical joint loading and may enter programmed cell death (apoptosis) if overloaded.[29,30] This effect seems to be most pronounced in the superficial zone of the articular cartilage. Certain loading conditions such as excessive cyclic loading may result in the overexpression of MMPs and thus could lead to the onset of osteoarthritis.[31]

Another recently reported factor in the development of early osteoarthritis may be related to boundary lubrication. Boundary lubrication is the ability to reduce friction between pressurized and opposed surfaces by a fluid independent of its viscosity. The lubricating effect of saline is usually used as a standard and is measured as a friction coefficient (μ) = 0. Normal synovial fluid has a significantly lower coefficient of friction than saline. After injury the coefficient of friction of synovial fluid increases significantly for several weeks and may therefore be a contributing factor to osteoarthritis. The protein closely associated with the ability to provide this low coefficient of friction is the soluble protein lubricin. Lubricin and its tissue-bound form, also known as superficial zone protein or SZP, are both a gene product of the PRG4 gene and can be broken down by elastases. The concentration of lubricin after injury or in patients with chronic effusions is significantly lower, whereas the concentration of elastase is higher. The breakdown of the lubricin-associated boundary lubrication could therefore play a significant role in the progression toward breakdown of the cartilage surfaces after injury.[32]

It remains unclear whether osteoarthritis is mediated through a primary inflammatory response originating in the cartilage matrix or the synovium. However, inflammatory cytokines such as IL-1β, TNF-α, and IL-6 play a key role in the initial disruption of cartilage homeostasis, shifting the balance toward an increased production of MMPs and subsequent matrix breakdown. These inflammatory cytokines can be secreted by synoviocytes, mononuclear cells in the synovial lining, and also chondrocytes. Although interleukin-1β (IL-1β) predominantly drives matrix degradation, tumor necrosis factor-α (TNF-α) maintains the inflammatory response. IL-6 leads to the increase of inflammatory cells in the synovial tissue. All of these proinflammatory cytokines therefore play a role in starting and maintaining an inflammatory reaction. This knowledge can be used clinically to monitor disease severity and to design therapeutic options aimed at selectively blocking these proinflammatory cytokines.

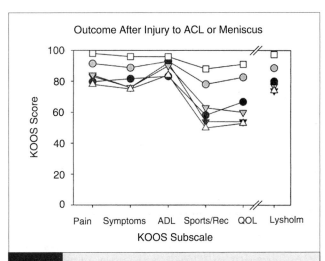

Outcome After Injury to ACL or Meniscus

Figure 8	The Knee Injury and Osteoarthritis Outcome Score subscale profiles for ACL and meniscus injury patients. Lysholm data for the same groups are given for comparison. Symbols: The gray circle represents 14-year follow-up of patients with traumatic meniscus tear; the black circle represents 14-year follow-up of patients with degenerative meniscus tear; the black triangle represents 12-year follow-up of patients with degenerative meniscus tear; the gray triangle represents 14-year follow-up of men with ACL rupture; the clear triangle represents 3-month follow-up of patients with partial meniscectomy; the square represents reference group with no knee injury and no knee osteoarthritis. ADL = activities of daily living; QOL = quality of life. (*Reproduced with permission from Lohmander LS, Englund PM, Dahl LL, Roos EM: The long-term consequence of anterior cruciate ligament and meniscus injuries: Osteoarthritis. Am J Sports Med 2007;35:1756-1769.*)	

Selective blockade of IL-1β with antagonist protein such as interleukin receptor antagonist protein has been used successfully in clinical trials. Current efforts focus on the use of highly sensitive C-reactive protein as a marker for the severity and progression of osteoarthritis. It has long been used as a marker for rheumatoid arthritis but may also correlate with disease activity in osteoarthritis.[33]

Epidemiology
Incidence/Prevalence of Osteoarthritis
Osteoarthritis is the most common inflammatory joint condition and is expected to have an increasing prevalence in middle-aged and elderly patients. Several longitudinal studies have attempted to identify the true incidence and prevalence of osteoarthritis in the general population. The Framingham study showed an incidence of clinically and radiographically symptomatic knee osteoarthritis of 1% per year in women and 0.7% in men.[34] A study based in Massachusetts evaluating blue-collar Caucasian individuals showed a 2:1 female-to-male ratio and a total incidence of 240 per 100.000 person-years.[34]

The prevalence of osteoarthritis depends on age group; there are subtle differences depending on the involved joint. Overall, however, there is a uniform trend in prevalence; although low (in women, 1% to 4%; in men, 1% to 6%), in individuals age 25 to 45 years the prevalence of osteoarthritis rises significantly to 53% to 55% in women and 22% to 33% in men older than 80 years.

One of the most important epidemiologic tasks is the identification of independent risk factors for the development of osteoarthritis. Both the Framingham and Chingford studies have shown that there is a clear relationship between body weight and osteoarthritis[34] Although higher body weight (upper body mass index [BMI] quintile) can lead to a higher risk of developing osteoarthritis, women who lose 2 BMI units over the previous 10-year period significantly reduce their odds of knee osteoarthritis (odds ratio, 0.46). Heavy manual labor is related to an increased risk of developing knee osteoarthritis, particularly if the labor involves knee bending and squatting of longer than 30 minutes per day. Previous injury frequently leads to osteoarthritis. Cross-sectional studies showed that previous injury is a stronger predictor than obesity. The strongest predictor is previous open meniscectomy, which has a prevalence of 48% compared with 7% in age-matched control subjects.[34] A subgroup of patients at risk for early development of osteoarthritis is those who had an anterior cruciate ligament (ACL) tear and underwent ACL reconstruction. At 12 years after ACL reconstruction, 75% of female athletes reported significant symptoms affecting their activities of daily living, and more than 40% had radiographic signs of osteoarthritis (**Figure 8**). These data are reproduced in men of the same age group and with the same treatment.[35]

Treatment
Health and Behavior Modifications
A basic first step in the treatment of osteoarthritis may include patient education about the disease so that the disease process and related limitations are understood. Although patient education is an often neglected aspect of the orthopaedic treatment protocol, the implementation of an arthritis self-management program can be effective for improving overall function and self-efficacy in patients with chronic osteoarthritis.[36]

Physical therapy is widely used to treat all stages of osteoarthritis. Although tightly controlled level I studies with validated outcome instruments are lacking, there is level I and II evidence for the efficacy of short courses of physical therapy (4 weeks) in patients with osteoarthritis. The maintenance of range of motion, gait corrections, and increase of flexibility have been beneficial, in addition to benefits derived from aerobic exercise.[37-39]

Bracing, particularly valgus bracing using an unloader brace to unload the medial compartment, is a treatment option in some patients with unicompartmental osteoarthritis. Bracing can lead to decreased

3: Knee and Leg

pain during activity and improve bipedal stance and swing of the involved leg during gait. The level of function in younger patients with unicompartmental osteoarthritis has increased with brace use.[40-42]

Drug Treatments

Various oral medications are available for the treatment of osteoarthritis, ranging from dietary supplements to nonsteroidal anti-inflammatory drugs (NSAIDs) and painkillers. Acetaminophen is often used as a first-line analgesic for mild pain related to osteoarthritis based on its overall cost, efficacy, and toxicity profile, and can be safely combined with various other drugs. Outcome studies have reported the efficacy of acetaminophen alone to be as efficient as that of NSAIDs.[43]

NSAIDs are recommended for moderate to severe arthritis pain related to arthritis. More than 17 clinical trials have assessed the efficacy of NSAIDs. It appears that NSAIDs have no disease-modifying effect overall but are effective for pain control in osteoarthritis. There is some evidence that NSAIDs may be as efficient in pain control when given at the lower, analgesic dose as when given in the higher anti-inflammatory dose. The major adverse effect of traditional nonselective NSAIDs is gastrointestinal toxicity, and the use of cyclooxygenase-2 (COX-2) inhibitors may be beneficial in these patients. Because of the cardiovascular risk associated with NSAIDs, they should be used as a secondary anti-inflammatory therapy. Their efficacy for the treatment of osteoarthritis is comparable to that of nonselective NSAIDs, with the added advantage of a once-a-day administration and higher gastrointestinal safety.[43]

The American Pain Society guidelines endorse the use of opiates for patients who do not respond to any other treatment of severe osteoarthritis-related pain. Treatment of osteoarthritis with opiates should be reserved for patients who are in severe pain and for whom surgical treatment is not recommended. Most patients with monoarthritic joint involvement should be counseled about joint arthroplasty therapy once the use of opiates becomes necessary.[42]

Glucosamine and chondroitin sulfate supplements may be useful in treating all stages of osteoarthritis but should be used early in the disease process because glucosamine and chondroitin sulfate possibly have a disease-modifying effect, although data have conflicting results. Several randomized clinical trials have been performed assessing the efficacy of these drugs. These drugs can be administered in combination with NSAIDs for added benefit. Glucosamine may be able to suppress IL-1β production in arthritic cartilage and may therefore have an anti-inflammatory effect. However, the latest recommendation from the National Institutes of Health based on the results of the Glucosamine/Chondroitin Intervention Trial (GAIT) is that glucosamine and chondroitin sulfate may have little to no effect above placebo. These substances may be of benefit in a small subset of patients with moderate to severe arthritis related pain.[44,45]

Injection-Based Treatments

Injection-based therapies that are currently available include corticosteroids and various forms of viscosupplementation. There is currently no clear guideline as to how many injections can or should be administered or if steroid injections should precede or follow viscosupplementation therapy.

Corticosteroid injection is indicated in patients with moderate to severe pain. The pain relief is usually transient and its duration can be unpredictable. Analysis of metadata suggests that the average length of pain relief is approximately 3 to 4 weeks. Corticosteroid injection can lead to severe adverse effects such as infection, crystal-induced synovitis, subcutaneous atrophy, and discoloration. Patient activity should be limited after an intra-articular steroid injection to avoid a postinjection flare. There are no clear data available about the total amount and frequency of steroid injections. Clinical opinion seems to suggest that a corticosteroid injection can be repeated every 3 to 4 months if necessary. Recently, there has been some concern about the use of local anesthetic depolarizing agents such as lidocaine or bupivacaine. The continuous infusion of these medications into the joint space have been implicated in the development of chondrolysis in the shoulder joint.[46] No such findings have been reported for the knee joint. In vitro and animal studies show that both lidocaine and bupivacaine cause dose-dependent chondrocyte death and decreased chonodrocyte metabolism.[47,48] However, there is no evidence to date that a single injection of cortisone diluted with lidocaine or bupivacaine has these effects in an arthritic joint.

Injection therapy with hyaluronan derivatives is called viscosupplementation. Viscosupplementation requires a series of injections[29-31] and is indicated in patients with moderate to severe disease. Viscosupplementation has been studied in multiple clinical trials and has been shown to be beneficial overall with regard to pain control. There is no evidence that viscosupplementation is a disease-modifying therapy. It can be used before or after therapy with steroid injections and can be combined with other nonsurgical and pharmacologic strategies. The proposed mechanism of action is thought to be better joint lubrication and the anti-inflammatory effect of hyaluronan on synoviocytes.[49]

Arthroscopic Treatment

Arthroscopy in patients with osteoarthritis has been a controversial topic. Although it is accepted that arthroscopy can provide short-term relief for patients with osteoarthritis, two randomized clinical trials indicate that arthroscopy does not provide long-term relief superior to nonsurgical treatment.[50,51] It is important to identify patients who have reproducible and site-specific mechanical symptoms, which may indicate an incarcerated meniscus tear, for example. Imaging is helpful for identifying possible loose body formation that can be treated successfully by arthroscopy. Patients in whom pain is the predominant symptom should be aware that they may experience short-term relief only.[50,51]

Summary

The treatment of articular cartilage lesions continues to be a difficult challenge for orthopaedic surgeons because there is no definitive treatment. Future treatments of articular cartilage lesions will depend on determining the most appropriate patient/lesion indications, identification of the best source of chondrocytes/osteochondral tissue, and development of bioactive factors that will enhance delivery as well as repair and restoration of chondral lesions. As more research is performed, the biomodular effects that cartilage experiences during damage and repair is revealed; this information will be invaluable in the future in directing treatment of cartilage lesions. Postinjury cartilage damage can lead to early osteoarthritis that can often be treated with some of the detailed articular cartilage repair and reconstruction procedures. Once global osteoarthritis is established, a careful treatment plan should include nonsurgical treatment using pain control and anti-inflammatory therapy to alleviate the patient's symptoms. Some disease-modifying agents that have recently been introduced are promising. It is important to understand that postinjury osteoarthritis is currently not preventable. Osteoarthritis is a continuum that can start early in life after a joint injury and may eventually lead to a total joint replacement. Physicians treating patients with osteoarthritis have to be prepared to present nonsurgical and surgical treatment options based on the course of the disease.

Annotated References

1. Curl WW, Krome J, Gordon ES, et al: Cartilage injuries: A review of 31,516 knee arthroscopies. *Arthroscopy* 1997;13:456-460.

2. Hjelle K, Solheim E, Strand T, Muri R, Brittberg M: Articular cartilage defects in 1,000 knee arthroscopies. *Arthroscopy* 2002;18:730-734.

3. Alford JW, Cole BJ: Cartilage restoration, Part 1: Basic science, histological perspective, patient evaluation, and treatment options. *Am J Sports Med* 2005;33:295-306.

   This article is a review and update of the presentation and basic science of articular cartilage lesions.

4. Marks PH, Donaldson ML: Inflammatory cytokine profiles associated with chondral damage in the anterior cruciate ligament–deficient knee. *Arthroscopy* 2005;21:1342-1347.

   Synovial fluid lavages were obtained from 31 patients with ACL-deficient knees. Four patients had lavages aspirated from their contralateral normal knee. These lavages were analyzed for interleukin (IL)-1α, IL-1β, IL-1ra, and tumor necrosis factor (TNF)-α. Concentrations of chondrodestructive IL-1β and TNF-α were significantly higher in patients with ACL ruptures than in the contralateral normal knees. The more severe the chondral damage, the higher the concentration of IL-1β and TNF-α.

5. Wilson JN: A diagnostic sign of osteochondritis dissecans of the knee. *J Bone Joint Surg Am* 1967;40:477-480.

6. Outerbridge RE: The etiology of chondromalacia patella. *J Bone Joint Surg Br* 1961;43-B:752-757.

7. Brittsberg M, Winalski CS: Evaluation of cartilage injuries and repair. *J Bone Joint Surg Am* 2003;85:58-69.

8. Alford JW, Cole BJ: Cartilage restoration, Part 2: Techniques, outcomes, and future directions. *Am J Sports Med* 2005;33:443-460.

   The authors present a review of current surgical techniques and results with a discussion of future techniques.

9. Friedman MJ, Berasi CC, Fox JM, et al: Preliminary results with abrasion arthroplasty in the osteoarthritic knee. *Clin Orthop Relat Res* 1984;182:200-205.

10. Johnson LL: Arthroscopic abrasion arthroplasty, in McGinty JB (ed): *Operative Arthroscopy.* New York, NY, Raven Press, 1991, pp 341-360.

11. Magnusson PB: Technique of debridement of the knee joint for arthritis. *Surg Clin North Am* 1946;26:249-266.

12. Rodrigo JJ, Steadman JR, Stilliman JF, Fulstone HA: Improvement of full-thickness chondral defect healing in the human knee after debridement and microfracture using continuous passive motion. *Am J Knee Surg* 1994;7:109-116.

13. Mithoefer K, Williams RJ III, Warren RF, et al: The microfracture technique for the treatment of articular cartilage lesions in the knee: A prospective cohort study. *J Bone Joint Surg Am* 2005;87:1911-1920.

   This article is a prospective study of the efficacy of the microfracture technique on articular cartilage lesions. Forty-eight patients with isolated full-thickness articular cartilage defects of the knee were evaluated with outcome studies performed at a minimum of 24 months. Knee function was rated good to excellent for 32 patients (67%), fair for 12 patients (25%), and poor for 4 patients (8%).

14. Barber FA, Chow JC: Arthroscopic chondral osseous autograft transplantation (COR procedure) for femoral defects. *Arthroscopy* 2006;22:10-16.

   This article is a retrospective review of a consecutive series of patients from two centers who were treated for full-thickness femoral articular cartilage lesions using a chondral osseous autograft transplantation technique. Full-thickness defects were greater than 1 cm and less than 2.5 cm in diameter and were followed for a minimum of 24 months. The average Lysholm score increased from 44 preoperatively to 84 at follow-up. Repeat arthroscopy in 14 patients showed good incorporation of the grafts in all cases. No radiographic examination showed arthritic changes.

15. Williams S, Amiel D, Ball S, et al: Prolonged storage effects on the articular cartilage of fresh human osteochondral allografts. *J Bone Joint Surg* 2003;85A:2111-2120.

16. Ghazavi MT, Pritzker KP, Davis AM, Gross AE: Fresh osteochondral allografts for post-traumatic defects of the knee. *J Bone Joint Surg Br* 1997;79:1008-1013.

17. Gross AE: Fresh osteochondral allografts for posttraumatic knee defects: Surgical techniques. *Oper Tech Orthop* 1997;7:334-337.

18. Brittberg M, Lindahl A, Nilsson A, et al: Treatment of deep cartilage defects in the knee with autologous chondrocyte transplantation. *N Engl J Med* 1994;331:889-895.

19. Steadman JR, Briggs KK, Rodrigo JJ, et al: Outcomes of microfracture for traumatic chondral defects of the knee: Average 11-year follow-up. *Arthroscopy* 2003;19:477-484.

This is a case series of 72 patients (75 knees) who underwent a microfracture for full thickness traumatic defects of the knee. Ninety-five percent were available for an average follow-up of 11 years. Significant improvement was recorded for clinical scores (Lysholm preoperative, 59; follow-up, 89; and Tegner preoperative, 3; follow-up, 6). At final follow-up, the SF-36 and WOMAC scores showed good to excellent results. At 7 years after surgery, 80% of the patients rated themselves as improved. Multivariate analysis revealed that age was a predictor of functional improvement.

20. Hangody L, Füles P: Autologous osteochondral mosaicplasty for the treatment of full-thickness defects of weight-bearing joints: Ten years of experimental and clinical experience. *J Bone Joint Surg Am* 2003;85-A:25-32.

This article describes the 10-year follow-up results of autologous osteochondral mosaicplasty in 831 patients. Good to excellent results were achieved in 92% of the patients treated with femoral condylar implantations, 87% of those treated with tibial resurfacing, 79% of those treated with patellar and/or trochlear mosaicplasties, and 94% of those treated with talar procedures. Sixty-nine of 83 patients who were followed arthroscopically had congruent gliding surfaces, histological evidence of the survival of the transplanted hyaline cartilage, and fibrocartilage filling of the donor sites.

21. Marcacci M, Kon E, Delcogliano M, et al: Arthroscopic autologous osteochondral grafting for cartilage defects of the knee: Prospective study results at a minimum

7-year follow-up. *Am J Sports Med* 2007;35:2014-2021.

This is a prospective study evaluating grade IV chondral lesions smaller than 2.5 cm^2 in 30 young patients treated with mosaicplasty. At 7-year follow-up, International Cartilage Repair Society scores showed 76.7% good and excellent results; however, there was a significant decrease in sport-related activities from the 2-year to 7-year results. MRI evaluation showed good integration of the graft in the host bone and complete maintenance of the grafted cartilage in more than 60% of patients.

22. McCulloch PC, Kang RW, Sobhy MH, Hayden JK, Cole BJ: Prospective evaluation of prolonged fresh osteochondral allograft transplantation of the femoral condyle: Minimum 2-year follow-up. *Am J Sports Med* 2007;35:411-420.

This is a prospective study evaluating the use of fresh osteochondral allograft transplantation in 25 patients (average age, 35 years) for the treatment of femoral condylar osteochondral defects. The average follow-up was 35 months. Improvements were seen for the Lysholm (39 to 67); International Knee Documentation Committee scores (29 to 58); the Knee Injury and Osteoarthritis Outcome Score (Pain, 43 to 73; Other Disease-Specific Symptoms, 46 to 64; Activities of Daily Living Function, 56 to 83; Sport and Recreation Function, 18 to 46; Knee-Related Quality of Life, 22 to 50); and the Short Form-12 physical component score (36 to 40). Patients reported 84% satisfaction (range, 25% to 100%) with their results. Twenty-two of the grafts (88%) had radiographic evidence of incorporation into host bone.

23. Williams RJ III, Ranawat AS, Potter HG, Carter T, Warren RF: Fresh stored allografts for the treatment of osteochondral defects of the knee. *J Bone Joint Surg Am* 2007;89:718-726.

The clinical outcome and graft morphology of patients who received fresh, hypothermically stored allograft tissue for the treatment of symptomatic chondral and osteochondral defects of the knee was assessed prospectively. Nineteen patients with symptomatic chondral and osteochondral lesions of the knee who were treated with fresh osteochondral allografts between 1999 and 2002 were prospectively followed. The mean lesion size was 6 cm^2. Follow-up at an average of 48 months showed improvement in the Activities of Daily Living Scale from 56 +/- 24 to 70 +/- 22. The mean Short Form-36 score increased from a baseline of 51 +/- 23 to 66 +/- 24. Cartilage-sensitive MRI demonstrated that normal articular cartilage thickness was preserved in 18 implanted grafts, and allograft cartilage signal properties were isointense relative to normal articular cartilage in 8 of the 18 grafts. Trabecular incorporation of the allograft was complete or partial in 14 patients and positively correlated with Short Form-36 scores at the time of follow-up.

24. Gudas R, Kalesinskas RJ, Kimtys V, et al: A prospective randomized clinical study of mosaic osteochondral autologous transplantation versus microfracture for the treatment of osteochondral defects in the knee joint in young athletes. *Arthroscopy* 2005;21:1066-1075.

Sixty young patients with an articular cartilage lesion of the knee who were randomized to undergo either an osteochondral autograft transplantation (OAT) or microfracture (MF) were assessed prospectively. At 12, 24, and 36 months after surgery, the Hospital for Special Surgery and International Cartilage Repair Society scores showed statistically significantly better results in the OAT group; 96% had excellent or good results compared with 52% for the MF procedure. MRI evaluation showed excellent or good results in 94% after OAT compared with 49% after MF. Twenty-six (93%) of OAT patients and 15 (52%) of MF patients returned to sports activities at the preinjury level at an average of 6.5 months (range, 4 to 8 months).

25. Horas U, Pelinkovic D, Herr G, Aigner T, Schnettler R: Autologous chondrocyte implantation and osteochondral cylinder transplantation in cartilage repair of the knee joint: A prospective, comparative trial. *J Bone Joint Surg Am* 2003;85-A:185-192.

The purpose of this study was to evaluate the clinical and histological outcomes of these two techniques. Forty patients were followed for 2 years after randomized treatment with either transplantation of an autologous osteochondral cylinder or implantation of autologous chondrocytes for articular cartilage lesions of the knee. The recovery after autologous chondrocyte implantation was histologically slower than after osteochondral transplantation at 6, 12, and 24 months. The clinical results were both good at 2-year follow-up. Histologically, the defects treated with autologous chondrocyte implantation were primarily filled with fibrocartilage, whereas the osteochondral cylinder transplants retained their hyaline character, although there was a persistent interface between the transplant and the surrounding original cartilage.

26. Knutsen G, Drogset JO, Engebretsen L, et al: A randomized trial comparing autologous chondrocyte implantation with microfracture: Findings at five years. *J Bone Joint Surg Am* 2007;89:2105-2112.

In a randomized prospective study, autologous chondrocyte implantation was compared with microfracture. Eighty patients who had a single chronic symptomatic cartilage defect on the femoral condyle in a stable knee without general osteoarthritis were included in the study. Forty patients were treated in each group. At 2 and 5 years, both groups had significant clinical improvement compared with the preoperative status. Both groups had nine failures and one third of the patients in both groups had radiographic evidence of early osteoarthritis at 5 years. As both groups obtained satisfactory results in 77% of patients, there was no significant difference in the clinical and radiographic results between the two treatment groups and no correlation between the histologic findings and the clinical outcome.

27. Pearle AD, Warren RF, Rodeo SA: Basic science of articular cartilage and osteoarthritis. *Clin Sports Med* 2005; 24:1-12.

This is a comprehensive overview of the current literature on the basic science of osteoarthritis.

28. Martel-Pelletier J: Pathophysiology of osteoarthritis. *Osteoarthritis Cartilage* 2004;12:S31-S33.

This is a comprehensive overview of the current literature on the basic science of osteoarthritis.

29. Chen CT, Bhargava M, Lin PM, Torzilli PA: Time, stress, and location dependent chondrocyte death and collagen damage in cyclically loaded articular cartilage. *J Orthop Res* 2003;21:888-898.

This is an experimental study on cartilage explant cultures examining the effect of different loading conditions on cell death and collagen damage throughout the different zones of articular cartilage. The study shows that low loading conditions do not lead to significant cell death, whereas high load conditions (5MPa) lead to significant cell death in the superficial zone. This study provides basic science evidence that alterations in loading conditions are clearly detrimental to articular cartilage and may play a role in the development of osteoarthritis.

30. Lucchinetti E, Adams CS, Horton WE Jr, Torzilli PA: Cartilage viability after repetitive loading: A preliminary report. *Osteoarthritis Cartilage* 2002;10:71-81.

31. Lin PM, Chen CT, Torzilli PA: Increased stromelysin-1 (MMP-3), proteoglycan degradation (3B3 and 7D4) and collagen damage in cyclically load-injured articular cartilage. *Osteoarthritis Cartilage* 2004;12:485-496.

This is a study investigating proteoglycan homeostasis in response to cyclic loading. The importance is the demonstration of adaptive biochemical changes because of loading conditions in the joint.

32. Elsaid KA, Jay GD, Warman ML, Rhee DK, Chichester CO: Association of articular cartilage degradation and loss of boundary-lubricating ability of synovial fluid following injury and inflammatory arthritis. *Arthritis Rheum* 2005;52:1632-1633.

This study investigated the changes in boundary lubrication caused by increased synovial fluid production and a decrease in viscosity as a result of the inflammatory response. This change affects the actual friction properties in the joint.

33. Wolfe F: The C-reactive protein but not erythrocyte sedimentation rate is associated with clinical severity in patients with osteoarthritis of the knee or hip. *J Rheumatol* 1997;24:1486-1488.

34. Sharma L, Kapoor D: Epidemiology of osteoarthritis, in Moskowitz RW, Altman RD, Buckwalter JA, Goldberg VM, Hochberg MC (eds): *Osteoarthritis: Diagnosis and Medical/Surgical Management*, ed 4. Philadelphia, PA, Lippincott Williams and Wilkins, 2007, pp 3-26.

This is a comprehensive book chapter providing an excellent overview of medical management of osteoarthritis.

35. Lohmander LS, Englund PM, Dahl LL, Roos EM: The long term consequence of anterior cruciate ligament and meniscus injuries: Osteoarthritis. *Am J Sports Med* 2007;35:1754-1769.

This is a meta-analysis of studies reporting on outcome of ACL surgery with respect to development of osteoarthritis and meniscectomy. It delineates carefully the progression of osteoarthritis after ACL surgery and meniscectomy as well as the rate of progression after different surgical procedures. It formulates an algorithm of development of osteoarthritis in these young patients.

36. Lorig K, Chastain RL, Ung E, Shoor S, Holman HR: Development and evaluation of a scale to measure perceived self-efficacy in people with arthritis. *Arthritis Rheum* 1989;32:37-44.

37. Deyle GD, Henderson NE, Matekel RL, Ryder MG, Garber MB, Allison SC: Effectiveness of manual physical therapy and exercise in osteoarthritis of the knee: A randomized controlled trial. *Ann Intern Med* 2000;132:173-181.

38. Petrella RJ: Is exercise effective treatment for osteoarthritis in the knee? *Br J Sports Med* 2000;34:326-331.

39. American Geriatrics Society Panel on Exercise and Osteoarthritis: Exercise prescription for older adults with osteoarthritis pain: Consensus practice recommendations: A supplement to the AGS Clinical Practice Guidelines on the management of chronic pain in older adults. *J Am Geriatr Soc* 2001;49:808-823.

40. Draper ER, Cable JM, Sanchez-Ballester J, Hunt N, Robinson JR, Strachan RK: Improvement in function after valgus bracing of the knee: An analysis of gait symmetry. *J Bone Joint Surg Br* 2000;82:1001-1005.

41. Ramsey DK, Briem K, Axe MJ, Snyder-Mackler L: A mechanical theory for the effectiveness of bracing for medial compartment osteoarthritis of the knee. *J Bone Joint Surg Am* 2007;89:2398-2407.

This is an experimental study of 16 subjects who were fitted with a medial unloader brace. Gait analysis was performed. Patients felt significantly less pain and were able to perform more activities of daily living with the use of the brace. The brace allowed them to function better during the day and it improved muscle co-contraction in the neutral position.

42. Lindenfeld TN, Hewett TE, Andriacchi TP: Joint loading with valgus bracing in patients with varus gonarthrosis. *Clin Orthop Relat Res* 1997;344:290-297.

43. Recommendations for the medical management of osteoarthritis of the hip and knee: 2000 update: American College of Rheumatology Subcommittee on Osteoarthritis Guidelines. *Arthritis Rheum* 2000;43:1905-1915.

44. National Center for Complimentary and Alternative Medicine: Glucosamine/Chondroitin Arthritis Intervention Trial (GAIT). *J Pain Palliat Care Pharmacother* 2008;22:39-43.

This is a large-scale study conducted by the National Institutes of Health to determine the efficacy of glucosamine/chondroitin sulfate compared with placebo. No significant effect of glucosamine/chondroitin sulfate could be found. One subgroup of patients with moderate to severe knee pain may see benefit from these drugs but the cohort was very small and requires verification.

45. Brief AA, Maurer SG, Di Cesare PE: Use of glucosamine and chondroitin sulfate in the management of osteoarthritis. *J Am Acad Orthop Surg* 2001;9:71-78.

46. Gomoll AH, Yanke AB, Kang RW, et al: Long-term effects of bupivacaine on cartilage in a rabbit shoulder model. *Am J Sports Med* 2008;37:72-77.

This study is a follow-up to an earlier short-term infusion study in rabbits. The authors show that the initial effects on proteoglycan production and chondrocyte viability after continuous bupivacaine infusion are reversible and lead to a prolonged reparative response. The authors point out that the continuous short-term infusion of bupivacaine alone is most likely not enough to inflict permanent chondral damage or cause chondrolysis in a rabbit model.

47. Gomoll AH, Kang RW, Williams JM, Bach BR, Cole BJ: Chondrolysis after continuous intra-articular bupivacaine infusion: An experimental model investigating chondrotoxicity in the rabbit shoulder. *Arthroscopy* 2006;22:813-819.

In this experimental study, continuous infusion of bupivacaine in the glenohumeral joint of rabbits was investigated. The articular cartilage was evaluated for proteoglycan production and content as well as dead/live staining. The study results showed that in an in vivo animal model the continuous infusion of bupivacaine leads to a significant reduction in chondrocyte metabolism and superficial cell death.

48. Chu CR, Izzo NJ, Coyle CH, Papas NE, Logar A: The in vitro effects of bupivacaine on articular chondrocytes. *J Bone Joint Surg Br* 2008;90:814-820.

This experimental study used bovine cartilage explant cultures of fresh articular cartilage. The cultures were exposed to different concentrations of bupivacaine and were evaluated for cellular viability and surface architecture. This study raised concerns about the effect of bupivacaine on the viability of chondrocytes.

49. Moreland LW: Intra-articular hyaluronan (hyaluronic acid) and hylans for the treatment of osteoarthritis: Mechanisms of action. *Arthritis Res Ther* 2003;5:54-67.

This is a review of the mechanism through which hyaluronan is thought to affect the knee arthritic joint. The author carefully delineates the different mechanisms of action.

50. Moseley JB, O'Malley K, Petersen NJ, et al: A controlled trial of arthroscopic surgery for osteoarthritis of the knee. *N Engl J Med* 2002;347:81-88.

This is a randomized controlled study using a placebo control group for the use of arthroscopic treatment in patients with osteoarthritis. One hundred eighty patients were studied in three groups receiving an arthroscopic lavage and débridement, arthroscopic lavage only, or a placebo surgery. The results did not suggest any significant difference between the three groups, indicating that arthroscopic treatment of osteoarthritis may not be superior to placebo.

51. Kirkley A, Birmingham TB, Litchfield RB, et al: A randomized trial of arthroscopic surgery for osteoarthritis of the knee. *N Engl J Med* 2008;359:1169-1170.

    This is the second reported randomized clinical trial comparing arthroscopy with nonsurgical treatment. The overall results of this study show that at 2-year follow-up there was no statistically significant difference between the groups. The authors caution surgeons to be specific in the diagnosis and identify other confounding factors such as instability related to unstable meniscus tears.

Chapter 14
Meniscal Injuries

Charles L. Cox, MD   *Kurt P. Spindler, MD

Basic Science

The menisci are crescent-shaped, fibrocartilaginous structures oriented between the articular cartilage of the tibial plateau and the femoral condyles (**Figure 1**). The intermeniscal ligament connects the medial and lateral menisci anteriorly, and the coronary ligaments anchor the periphery to the joint capsule. Posteriorly, meniscofemoral ligaments are variably present, attach the posterior aspect of the lateral meniscus to the medial femoral condyle, and insert anterior (ligament of Humphrey) or posterior (ligament of Wrisberg) to the posterior cruciate ligament. The lateral meniscus is more circular in shape than the medial meniscus and displays more mobility during knee range of motion, translating up to 11 mm in the anterior to posterior direction compared with 5 mm of normal translation in the medial meniscus.[1]

The menisci are biphasic, containing both a fluid and a solid phase; water comprises 65% to 75% of the meniscus. The solid phase of the menisci, comprising 60% to 70% of the dry weight, consists primarily of type I collagen with types II, III, V, and VI present in small amounts. The solid phase also includes polypeptides, known as proteoglycans, covalently bound to negatively charged polysaccharides, known as glycosaminoglycans. The associated charges allow water to bind, yielding a structure with one sixth to one tenth the permeability and half the elastic modulus of articular cartilage. This low compressive stiffness and low permeability allow the menisci to expand under compressive forces and increase the contact area between the articular surfaces of the knee joint.[2]

Branches of the medial and lateral genicular arteries (both superior and inferior) supply the peripheral 10% to 30% of the medial meniscus and the peripheral 10% to 25% of the lateral meniscus with a perimeniscal capillary plexus (**Figure 2**). The remainder of each meniscus receives its nutrition via diffusion and mechanical compression that occurs during normal joint motion. Neural elements are also unevenly distributed throughout the menisci, with concentrations greatest at the anterior and posterior horns, implying that the menisci possibly play a role in proprioception within the knee joint.

| Figure 1 | Section through a cadaver specimen displaying subchondral bone, articular cartilage, and wedge-shaped meniscus. (*Reproduced with permission from Warren RF, Arnoczky SP, Wickiewicz TL: Anatomy of the knee, in Nicholas JA, Hershman EB (eds): The Lower Extremity and Spine in Sports Medicine. St. Louis, MO, CV Mosby, 1986, pp 657-694.*) |

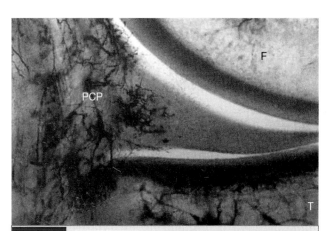

| Figure 2 | Sagittal section through the medial meniscus demonstrating penetrating blood vessels in the periphery. Note the avascular nature of the more central portions. F = femur; T = tibia; PCP = perimeniscal capillary plexus. (*Reproduced with permission from Arnoczky SP, Warren RF: Microvasculature of the human meniscus. Am J Sports Med 1982:10:90-95.*) |

*Kurt P. Spindler, MD or the department with which he is affiliated has received research or institutional support from NIH, DonJoy, Smith & Nephew, and Aircast.

3: Knee and Leg

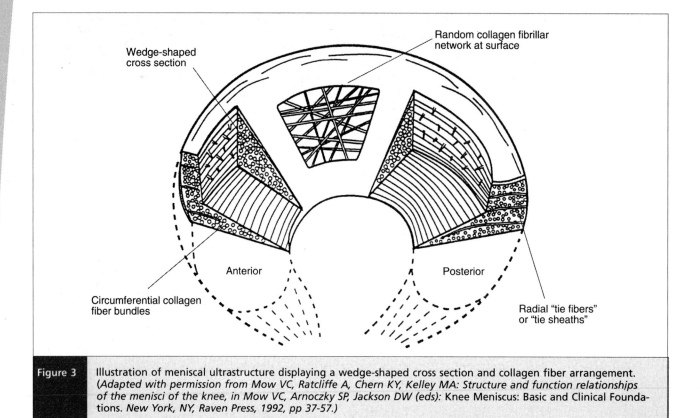

Figure 3 Illustration of meniscal ultrastructure displaying a wedge-shaped cross section and collagen fiber arrangement. (*Adapted with permission from Mow VC, Ratcliffe A, Chern KY, Kelley MA: Structure and function relationships of the menisci of the knee, in Mow VC, Arnoczky SP, Jackson DW (eds):* Knee Meniscus: Basic and Clinical Foundations. *New York, NY, Raven Press, 1992, pp 37-57.*)

Fibrochondrocytes, the cells that populate the meniscus, have characteristics of both fibroblasts and chondrocytes and are responsible for maintaining the extracellular matrix. The cells in the vascular periphery produce predominantly type I collagen, and the cells located more centrally in the avascular regions produce predominantly type II collagen. Cell contribution to intrinsic repair is also likely based on the location of the cell within the meniscus, as cells in the periphery respond better to growth factors than cells located centrally.[2]

The menisci consist of a collagen fiber ultrastructure that is wedge shaped in cross section. At the surface, the collagen fibers are randomly arranged. In the deep layers, the collagen fibers are oriented circumferentially and stabilized by periodic radial fibers (**Figure 3**). This ultrastructure allows the menisci to (1) dissipate hoop stresses that occur with axial loads upon the knee; (2) function in load transmission, distributing up to 50% of weight-bearing load in extension and up to 85% of weight-bearing load in 90° of knee flexion; (3) reduce stress on articular cartilage, functioning as shock absorbers and improving joint congruency; and (4) contribute to joint lubrication and nutrition. Studies have shown that total meniscectomy reduces joint surface contact area by 75% and increases peak local contact stresses by 235%; knees with intact menisci have 20% higher shock-absorbing capacity than those having undergone meniscectomy.[3] In the presence of an intact anterior cruciate ligament (ACL), the menisci play

no role in joint stability. However, in the setting of an ACL-deficient knee, the posterior horn of the medial meniscus acts as a secondary stabilizer to decrease anterior translation of the tibia relative to the femur. The lateral meniscus does not play a role in joint stabilization.[2,4]

Diagnosis

While obtaining the patient history, factors such as patient age, preinjury activity level, mechanism of injury, presence of mechanical symptoms such as locking or catching, and location and timing of pain should be carefully considered. Patients may report hearing or feeling a "pop" at the time of injury, and the examiner should inquire about the presence and timing of onset of effusion after injury. During physical examination, specific points relative to meniscal pathology include evaluation for the presence of an effusion, assessment of ACL status, and detection of joint line pain. According to a prospective study, a history of mechanical locking, joint line pain, and decreased ability to perform athletic activities is positively associated with meniscal pathology, whereas pain at rest is negatively correlated.[5]

Clinical pearls in evaluating the medial side of the knee include differentiating vertical versus horizontal orientation of pain. Vertically oriented pain (**Figure 4, *A***), associated with pain upon palpation of the medial femoral epicondyle and/or medial tibia extend-

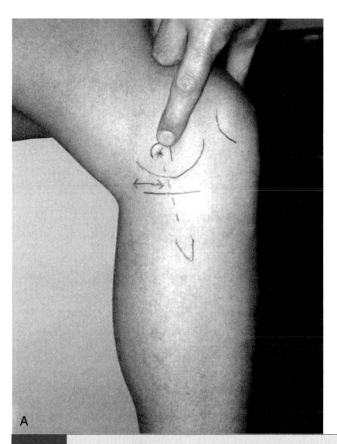
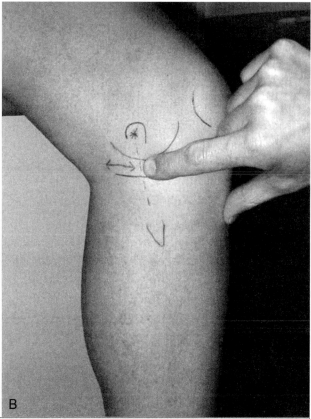

| Figure 4 | A, Photograph of the medial knee showing the vertical orientation of the medial collateral ligament coursing from the medial femoral epicondyle to the proximal medial tibia. B, Photograph of the medial knee showing the horizontal orientation of the joint line with the arrow representing the typical location of meniscal-type pain. Note that most pain from medial meniscus tears is oriented posterior to the medial collateral ligament. * = medial femoral epicondyle. |

ing up to 5 cm below the joint line, is more likely to be related to medial collateral ligament injury, whereas horizontally oriented pain (Figure 4, B), prominent with palpation of the joint line, is more likely to be meniscal in origin. Because most medial meniscal tears occur in the posterior horn, joint line tenderness is often greatest posterior to the midcoronal plane of the knee.

Clinical pearls in evaluating the lateral side of the knee again include a focus on superficial anatomy. By placing the leg into the figure-of-4 position, the lateral collateral ligament can be directly palpated originating on the lateral femoral epicondyle, crossing the joint line, and inserting onto the fibular head. Attention should again focus on the vertical orientation of this structure (Figure 5, A). The lateral meniscus differs from its medial counterpart in that tears occur in both the anterior and posterior horns, but joint line tenderness in the horizontal plane is again associated with tears (Figure 5, B).

Several tests have been described to assess for meniscal injury, and each attempts to re-create mechanical symptoms by trapping the torn meniscus under its associated condyle. During the McMurray test, the examiner internally and externally rotates the foot while taking the knee through varying degrees of flexion under an axial load. During the Apley test, the patient is positioned prone with the knee flexed to 90°, while the leg is internally and externally rotated under an axial load. During the Thessaly test, the patient is instructed to stand on the affected leg using one or two hands for balance followed by internal and external rotation of the leg and torso during varying degrees of knee flexion.

In a systematic review assessing the diagnosis of meniscal tears, joint line tenderness was associated with higher sensitivity but lower specificity; McMurray, Apley, and Thessaly tests at 5° were associated with higher specificity but lower sensitivity.[6] The physical examination tended to be less accurate in patients with associated ligamentous injuries or degenerative pathology, and accurate diagnosis was more likely in the hands of an experienced clinician when compared with an inexperienced examiner.[6] In the setting of acute ACL injuries and/or preexisting osteoarthritis, the presence or absence of joint line tenderness has been shown to be neither sensitive nor specific for the detection of meniscal pathology.[7]

Radiographic evaluation should begin with weightbearing films of bilateral knees, either standing AP

3: Knee and Leg

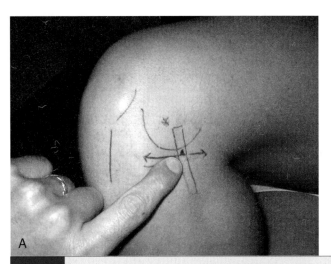
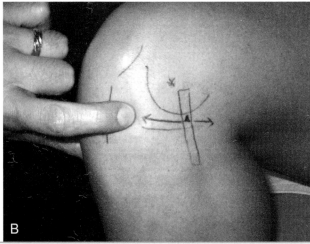

Figure 5 Photographs of the lateral knee demonstrating **(A)** the vertical orientation of the lateral collateral ligament and **(B)** the horizontal orientation of the joint line, with the arrow representing the typical location of meniscal-type pain. * = lateral femoral epicondyle; solid triangle = lateral collateral ligament.

Table 1

Diagnostic Performance of MRI in Evaluation of Lateral and Medial Meniscal Pathology

Diagnostic Performance of MRI	Accuracy (%)	Sensitivity (%)	Specificity (%)	Positive Predictive Value (%)	Negative Predictive Value (%)
Lateral meniscus	88.8	76	93.3	80.4	91.6
Medial meniscus	86.3	91.4	81.1	83.2	90.1

(Reproduced from Crawford R, Walley G, Bridgman S, Maffulli N: Magnetic resonance imaging versus arthroscopy in the diagnosis of knee pathology, concentrating on meniscal lesions and ACL tears: A systematic review. Br Med Bull 2007;84:5-23.)

films in extension or standing PA films in 45° of knee flexion. Merchant views of both patellae and a lateral view of the affected extremity also should be obtained. Radiographs should be examined for signs of osteoarthritis, with specific attention paid to the amount of joint space narrowing in comparison with the contralateral extremity. Additional radiographic evaluation options include ultrasonography, shown to be both sensitive and specific in the hands of a skilled operator, and MRI, which is the diagnostic procedure of choice. MRI has been evaluated as a diagnostic tool in two recent systematic reviews with the following findings: (1) MRI has a higher specificity than sensitivity and a higher negative than positive predictive value for identifying internal derangements in the knee, meaning that a negative MRI is likely to be a true negative result.[6,8] When assessing the false positive rate of MRI, findings consistent with an interpretation of meniscal tear were prevalent in 13% of asymptomatic individuals younger than 45 years and 36% of asymptomatic individuals older than 45 years.[9] (2) MRI has higher specificity for lateral meniscus tears and higher sensitivity for medial meniscus tears[8] (Table 1). (3) The accuracy of an experienced examiner in the diagnosis of meniscal tears approached that of MRI.[6] A negative MRI for the presence of a meniscal tear is a useful screening tool for avoiding unwarranted arthroscopy, and a positive MRI should not be used alone as an indication to proceed to the operating room because of the prevalence of false positives. Furthermore, the history and physical examination should correlate with MRI evidence of a tear. The optimal use of MRI clinically is for a diagnosis that remains in doubt after the history and physical examination.

Treatment

The treatment algorithm for meniscus tears begins with the classification of patients into one of two categories: young or middle aged. This classification is an attempt to categorize the presence or absence of arthritis because treatment outcome is inversely related to the amount of arthritis present in the knee joint. In the young patient population, attention should first focus on the evaluation of ACL integrity. In the context of chronic ACL deficiency, bucket-handle tears of the posterior horn of the medial meniscus are more likely caused by the reliance on the posterior horn as a sec-ondary stabilizer of anterior tibial translation relative to the femoral condyles. In the middle-aged patient population, degenerative meniscal pathology predomi-nates with varying degrees of preexisting osteoarthritis.

Treatment options include observation, excision, re-pair, or replacement. Treatment decisions should take into account tear stability, location, length, orientation, ligamentous stability, and the presence of articular car-tilage degeneration. Observation is a viable option in patients with partial, longitudinal tears less than 5 mm in length. This type of tear has a favorable prognosis with possibly good spontaneous healing potential in the setting of ACL reconstruction procedures. Unstable tears traversing the avascular zone, including radial, oblique, degenerative, complex, and flap tears, should be treated with partial excision.

The principles of arthroscopic partial meniscectomy include identifying mobile fragments with a probe and resecting to a stable base using mechanical and motor-ized instrumentation. The remaining meniscal tissue should then be sculpted to avoid sudden changes in contour, with care taken when possible to avoid com-plete rim section, which is the biomechanical equivalent of total meniscectomy resulting from complete disrup-tion of the circumferential fibers and resulting inability to dissipate hoop stress (**Figure 6**). In a frequently cited retrospective study, it was shown that osteoarthritic changes diagnosed via radiographic evaluation oc-curred in 38% of patients having undergone arthro-scopic partial medial meniscectomy and 24% of pa-tients having undergone arthroscopic partial lateral meniscectomy at an average 4-year follow-up.[10] Care should be taken when interpreting these results because 86% to 91% of the patients had good or excellent out-comes despite the radiographic presence of arthritis, and 33% of the patients who met the initial inclusion criteria were lost to follow-up.[10] Long-term results after partial meniscectomy have been shown to be inversely related to the amount of articular cartilage damage noted at the time of the index procedure.[11]

The goal of meniscal repair is to preserve function of the menisci in maintaining articular cartilage integrity. Unstable tears that occur in the periphery with a good vascular supply should be repaired. Longitudinal tears in the red-red zone are most amenable to repair. Tears traversing less vascularized areas have decreased heal-ing potential and are best treated with excision. The best prognosis for repairs occurs in conjunction with ligamentous surgery. Outcomes of repair are improved with concomitant ACL reconstruction, with healing rates ranging from 62% to 96%. Outcomes of meniscal repair in the setting of continued ACL deficiency are less favorable, ranging from 17% to 62%.[12]

Multiple techniques are available for meniscal repair. Preparation options include synovial abrasion, which induces peripheral bleeding in an attempt to promote migration of undifferentiated mesynchymal cells, and meniscal trephination, which attempts to create vascu-

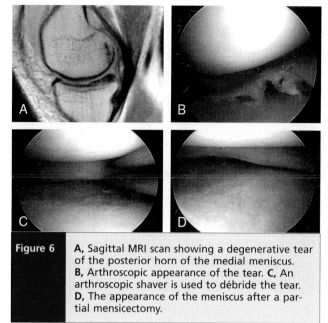

Figure 6 **A,** Sagittal MRI scan showing a degenerative tear of the posterior horn of the medial meniscus. **B,** Arthroscopic appearance of the tear. **C,** An arthroscopic shaver is used to débride the tear. **D,** The appearance of the meniscus after a par-tial mensicectomy.

lar channels through the induction of holes in the avas-cular portions of the meniscus. Attention should also be focused on proper reduction of meniscal segments. The choices for optimal repair include open, outside-in, inside-out, and all-inside techniques (**Figure 7**).

Open repair remains a viable option in surgical set-tings that necessitate an open approach to concomitant injuries. Tibial plateau fractures and multiligament knee injuries often allow easy exposure to the menis-cus, and suture anchors are helpful in meniscal stabili-zation. Retrospective studies of open repairs report 10- to 13-year survival rates ranging from 79% to 91%.[12]

Outside-in techniques involve passage of a spinal needle through the skin into the meniscus tear with ar-throscopic visualization. An arthroscopic knot is tied inside the joint, and multiple sutures are then tied to-gether outside the joint over the capsule, yielding com-pression at the site of the tear. Clinical success rates range from 74% to 98.6%, but biomechanical studies reveal that this type of construct is weak.[12]

Inside-out techniques remain the gold standard for meniscal repair, yielding reproducible, solid fixation without necessitating expensive implants. The disad-vantages include the required technical expertise and accessory incisions, which risk cutaneous nerve injuries. With this technique, sutures are placed from a cannula system inside the joint under direct arthroscopic visual-ization. Separate posteromedial or posterolateral inci-sions are made for suture retrieval and knot tying, us-ing retractors to protect cutaneous structures. With lateral meniscus repairs, the common peroneal nerve branches proximally 10% to 20% of the time, placing it at risk with joint line approaches. The incidence of common peroneal nerve injury approaches 3.4%, and thus inside-out techniques should be avoided for the lateral meniscus. Prospective studies report healing

3: Knee and Leg

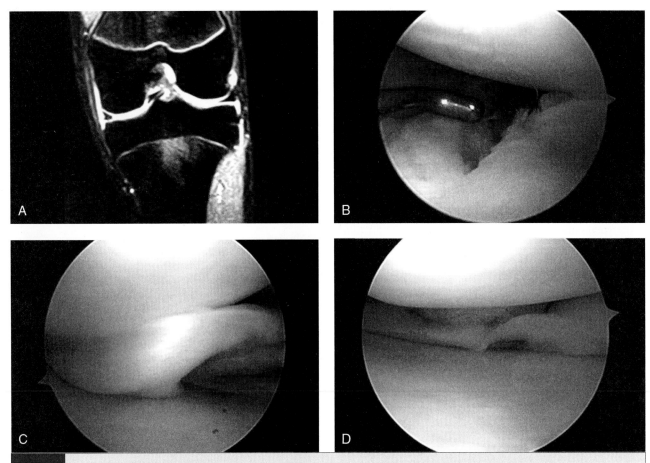

Figure 7 **A,** Coronal MRI scan showing a bucket-handle tear of the medial meniscus. Note the piece of meniscus displaced into the intercondylar notch. **B,** Probe demonstrating the excursion of the tear between the articular surfaces. **C,** Apex of the tear as seen medially. **D,** The appearance of the meniscus after all-inside repair with sutures.

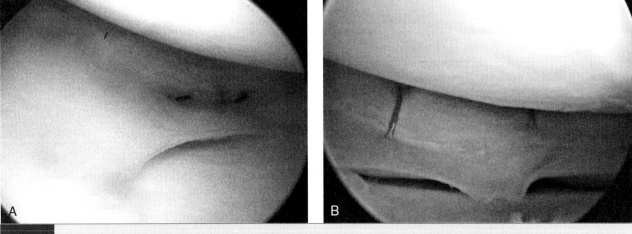

Figure 8 Arthroscopic photographs showing horizontal suture orientation (A) and vertical suture orientation (B) in meniscal repair.

rates ranging from 62% to 96% with the inside-out technique.[12]

Although the all-inside technique is relatively new and the least documented, it is probably the most common repair technique used, with repair devices including arrows, darts, screws, staples, and sutures (**Figure 8**). In a recent systematic review of outcomes associated with all-inside repair devices, no significant differences were found between the various repair devices, and failure rates did not increase with length of follow-up.

Only 13% of the identified studies were prospective in nature, and 75% of the studies defined failure as revision.[13]

Meniscus Allografts

Both medial and lateral meniscus allograft transplantation has been selectively performed for young to middle-aged patients with unicompartmental pain, limited degenerative change after total meniscectomy, and normal alignment and stability. However, a systematic review of 15 studies reporting results emphasized several important unknown factors, including the method of preoperative assessment and criteria for transplantation, the ideal method of graft preservation, graft sizing and the best method of fixation, and prospective outcomes data not confounded by concurrent procedures such as ACL reconstruction, high tibial osteotomy, and articular cartilage restoration.[14] Because most patients who have had meniscal allograft transplantation report pain and swelling during activities of daily living, the goal is relief of pain and not return to vigorous sports involving cutting and pivoting. Additional prospective studies are needed to clarify the return to high-impact sports and longevity of outcomes.

Recommendations from the systematic review are (1) use of a fresh-frozen allograft size-matched within 5% of normal, (2) implantation by a method that has rigid fixation of both horns (to preserve hoop stresses), and (3) multiple suture fixation of the peripheral rim to the capsule. Patients should expect to return only to light sports activity until further evidence is forthcoming, and they should be monitored for infection and immune reaction.

Summary

The menisci provide important biomechanical function for articular cartilage health. Current randomized controlled trials and prospective longitudinal cohorts will define at the highest level of evidence their role in patient outcomes, thus providing the clinically relevant goals for tissue engineers to improve repairs, develop functional scaffolds, and provide a living transplanted meniscus, all of which can improve a patient's outcome. These are exciting times as evidence-based medicine and tissue engineering work collaboratively to improve the relevant meniscus predictors of patient outcomes.

Annotated References

1. Thompson WO, Thaete FL, Fu FH, Dye SF: Tibial meniscal dynamics using three-dimensional reconstruction of magnetic resonance images. *Am J Sports Med* 1991;19:210-215.

2. Arnoczky SP, McDevitt CA: The meniscus: Structure, function, repair, and replacement, in Buckwalter JA, Einhorn TA, Simon SR (eds): *Orthopaedic Basic Science: Biology and Biomechanics of the Musculoskeletal System*, ed 2. Rosemont, IL, American Academy of Orthopaedic Surgeons, 2000, pp 531-545.

3. Baratz ME, Fu FH, Mengato R: Meniscal tears: The effect of meniscectomy and of repair on intraarticular contact areas and stress in the human knee: A preliminary report. *Am J Sports Med* 1986;14:270-275.

4. Greis PE, Bardana DD, Holmstrom MC, Burks RT: Meniscal injury: I. Basic science and evaluation. *J Am Acad Orthop Surg* 2002;10:168-176.

5. Abdon P, Lindstrand A, Thorngren KG: Statistical evaluation of the diagnostic criteria for meniscal tears. *Int Orthop* 1990;14:341-345.

6. Ryzewicz M, Peterson B, Siparsky PN, Bartz RL: The diagnosis of meniscus tears: The role of MRI and clinical examination. *Clin Orthop Relat Res* 2007;455:123-133.

   This systematic review evaluated 32 prospective cohort studies comparing MRI and clinical examination to arthroscopy in the diagnosis of meniscal pathology. The accuracy of an experienced examiner in diagnosing meniscal tears approached that of MRI, and the authors concluded that MRI is best used clinically when the diagnosis remains in doubt after history and physical examination. Level of evidence: II.

7. Shelbourne KD, Martini DJ, McCarroll JR, VanMeter CD: Correlation of joint line tenderness and meniscal lesions in patients with acute anterior cruciate ligament tears. *Am J Sports Med* 1995;23:166-169.

8. Crawford R, Walley G, Bridgman S, Maffulli N: Magnetic resonance imaging versus arthroscopy in the diagnosis of knee pathology, concentrating on meniscal lesions and ACL tears: A systematic review. *Br Med Bull* 2007;84:5-23.

   This systematic review scored the methodology of 59 articles comparing MRI and arthroscopy in the diagnosis of knee pathology, reporting on a total of 7,367 knee MRI scans and 5,416 arthroscopies. The authors concluded that MRI is the screening tool of choice for therapeutic arthroscopy with an accuracy of over 85% for meniscal tears, but the performance of MRI was different for diagnosing lateral versus medial meniscal pathology, with higher specificity for lateral meniscus tears and higher sensitivity for medial meniscus tears. Level of evidence: II.

9. Boden SD, Davis DO, Dina TS, et al: A prospective and blinded investigation of magnetic resonance imaging of the knee: Abnormal findings in asymptomatic subjects. *Clin Orthop Relat Res* 1992;282:177-185.

10. Rangger C, Klestil T, Gloetzer W, Kemmler G, Benedetto KP: Osteoarthritis after arthroscopic partial meniscectomy. *Am J Sports Med* 1995;23:240-244.

11. Schimmer RC, Brülhart KB, Duff C, Glinz W: Arthroscopic partial meniscectomy: A 12-year follow-up and two-step evaluation of the long-term course. *Arthroscopy* 1998;14:136-142.

12. McCarty EC, Marx RG, DeHaven KE: Meniscus repair: Considerations in treatment and update of clinical results. *Clin Orthop Relat Res* 2002;402:122-134.

13. Lozano J, Ma CB, Cannon WD: All-inside meniscus repair: A systematic review. *Clin Orthop Relat Res* 2007; 455:134-141.

    This systematic review evaluated 31 articles that studied all-inside meniscal repair devices. Clinical failure rates ranged from 0% to 43.5%, and no notable differences were seen between the devices studied with regard to failure rates. Definitive conclusions regarding outcomes could not be drawn because 77% of the studies were case series. Level of evidence: IV.

14. Matava MJ: Meniscal allograft transplantation: A systematic review. *Clin Orthop Relat Res* 2007;455: 142-157.

    This systematic review evaluated the clinical outcomes for meniscal allograft transplantation among 15 papers. The authors concluded that the ideal candidate is a ligamentously stable young to middle-aged adult with joint line pain, normal knee alignment, and minimal arthritis. The allograft should be matched to within 5% of the normal meniscus size and firmly implanted. Patients should be limited postoperatively to light sports pending further outcomes research. Level of evidence: IV.

Chapter 15

Overuse Injuries of the Lower Extremity

Robin Vereeke West, MD   James J. Irrgang , PhD, PT, ATC

Introduction

Overuse injuries of the lower extremity are extremely common and include a wide range of diagnoses, including iliotibial band syndrome, chronic exertional compartment syndrome, medial tibial stress syndrome, stress fractures, and tendinopathies. A brief overview of the most commonly encountered overuse injuries of the lower extremity is presented in **Table 1**. Several of these injuries are discussed in other chapters.

Iliotibial Band Syndrome

Iliotibial band (ITB) syndrome is caused by excessive friction between the ITB and the lateral femoral condyle. This syndrome typically affects long-distance runners and cyclists.

The ITB is a thick fascial extension of the tensor fascia lata and gluteus maximus muscles. It expands to join the lateral patellar retinaculum before crossing the lateral joint line to insert onto the Gerdy tubercle. It functions as a knee flexor and extensor, depending on the knee flexion angle. In knee extension, the ITB lies anterior to the lateral epicondyle. As the knee is flexed beyond 30°, the ITB passes over the bony prominence of the epicondyle to lie posterior to it. The impingement zone is at 30° of knee flexion.

Factors associated with ITB syndrome include training errors, anatomic factors, and footwear and surfaces. There is a high incidence of acute ITB syndrome development after a single, high-intensity training session or after an abrupt change in training routine. Malalignment arising from foot pronation or genu varum results in increased tension in the ITB over the epicondyle. Running on roads with excessive camber or hills can cause increase varus stress across the knee and increased ITB friction. ITB syndrome is more common in downhill long-distance runners than in sprinters because the knee is less flexed during downhill running. This decreased flexion angle results in greater impingement of the ITB at the epicondyle.[1]

Patients with ITB friction syndrome report pain over the lateral aspect of the knee during activity. The pain may limit activity and is usually initiated or exacerbated by running on banked surfaces, hills, or stairs, and may increase with increasing mileage. Repetitive flexion and extension during cycling may initiate the symptoms of ITB friction syndrome. Usually, the pain resolves with rest.

Examination findings include localized tenderness over the lateral epicondyle with the knee at 30° of flexion. The tenderness may be aggravated when the knee is brought into flexion with the patient either supine or standing. A single leg squat often reproduces the pain. Varus stress while rapidly extending the knee from 45° of flexion also may elicit pain. Swelling or localized crepitus may be present. Excessive iliotibial band tightness can be assessed with the Ober test.

Diagnostic testing can include a radiograph of the knee to detect associated pathology, such as medial compartment joint-space narrowing or patellar maltracking. An MRI also can be used to evaluate for any conditions that are associated with lateral-sided knee pain, including a lateral meniscal tear or cyst.

Treatment consists of activity modification and relative rest, stretching exercises, strengthening exercises for the hip, ice, nonsteroidal anti-inflammatory medications, and foot orthotics. The patient should be instructed to avoid activities that precipitate the pain, including activities that require repetitive flexion and extension of the knee. If running on a cambered road contributes to symptoms, the patient should be advised to run in the same direction on the opposite side of the road. The individual's activity level should be reduced to avoid the development of pain. If necessary to maintain conditioning, the athlete may supplement training with other forms of exercise that do not contribute to symptoms. Ice should be used after exercise and activity to control pain and swelling. Foot orthotics should be provided if abnormal pronation is believed to be a contributing factor to the patient's condition.

A detailed examination of all major muscle groups of the lower extremity to identify muscle tightness and weakness should include assessment of flexibility in the tensor fascia lata/ITB band complex using the Ober test as well as flexibility of the iliopsoas, rectus femoris, hamstrings, and gastrocnemius. The patient should be instructed to stretch tight muscles, performing three to five repetitions, each held for 30 seconds, twice daily.

Table 1

Common Overuse Injuries of the Lower Extremity

Disorder	Symptoms	Examination Findings	Diagnostic Testing	Treatment
Iliotibial Band Syndrome	Lateral-sided knee pain that increases with activity and improves with rest	Localized tenderness over epicondyle with knee at 30° flexion; pain aggravated with single-leg squat	Radiographs to assess prominent epicondyle, medial compartment degenerative joint disease; MRI to evaluate for associated patellar chondrosis, lateral meniscal tear	Activity modifications, stretching, strengthening, orthotics
Exertional Compartment Syndrome	Aching, cramping pain in leg that starts with exercise and improves with rest	Examination is usually normal but may have localized fullness or tenderness in compartment	Compartment pressure of 15 mm Hg or greater preexercise or 30 mm Hg or greater 1 minute after exercise	Avoid inciting activity or surgical intervention with fasciotomy or fasciectomy
Medial Tibial Stress Syndrome	Pain along posteromedial tibia that is exacerbated with activity	3- to 6-cm area of exquisite tenderness along the posterior medial distal third tibial border	Radiographs are normal, bone scan may show diffuse uptake and is nonspecific; MRI can differentiate fracture, stress reaction and periostitis	Activity modification, stretching, orthotics, strengthening
Tendinitis	Localized pain over tendon that worsens with activity	Tenderness, swelling over localized area and associated weakness		Activity modification, eccentric strengthening, nitroglycercin patches

The strength of the lower extremity muscles should be assessed, with particular emphasis on the strength of the gluteus medius and external rotators of the hip. Progressive resistance exercises should strengthen the weak muscles.[2]

Chronic Exertional Compartment Syndrome

Chronic exertional compartment syndrome (CECS) results from abnormally high intracompartmental pressure during and after exercise. The pathologic pressure develops secondary to increased intracellular and extracellular fluid accumulation with a noncompliant fascial compartment. Blood flow and oxygenation decrease as the compartment pressure increases. The metabolic demands of the muscle are not met, which results in pain. Dysesthesias from nerve compression may also develop.

The pathophysiology of CECS results from an increase in capillary surface area and pressure in the muscle during exercise. The diagnosis is based on patient history and compartment pressure findings. Typically, the patient will report reproducible pain during and immediately after exercise. The pain is described as aching or cramping and usually starts a few minutes into exercise and persists until after exercise has ceased. Rest usually decreases the intensity of the pain. Occasionally, numbness or tingling will be reported, which indicates neural compression in the involved compartment.

Examination findings are often normal. The patient may have localized tenderness in the involved compartment. Examination immediately after exercise may reveal localized tense and tender areas limited to the involved compartment. Associated periostitis is not uncommon and can result in tenderness over the posteromedial border of the tibia.

Radiographic evaluation may reveal associated findings such as a tibial stress fracture or stress reaction over the posteromedial border of the tibia. MRI is useful if the patient has associated findings on examination, such as tenderness over the posterior tibial border. MRI can be used to assess for an occult tibial stress fracture or reaction that is not seen on the radiograph. The clinical symptoms of CECS should be confirmed with a pressure transducer in the compartment before exercise and 1 minute and 5 minutes after exercise. When used correctly, the following compartment measurement methods show equal effectiveness: slit catheter, microtip pressure method, wick catheter, microcapillary infusion, and needle manometer. The pressure criteria for the diagnosis of CECS is a preexercise pressure of 15 mm Hg or greater, and/or a pressure 30 mm Hg or greater 1 minute after exercise, and/or a pressure 20 mm Hg or greater 5 minutes after exercise.[3]

Aside from activity modification or avoiding the inciting activity all together, nonsurgical treatment of

CECS has been unsuccessful. Surgical treatment of CECS is with fasciotomy of the involved compartment(s).[4] Numerous fasciotomy techniques have been described, including mini-incision, endoscopic, complete open, and fasciectomy, with reportedly high success rates, as long as a complete release of the involved compartment is performed. A fasciectomy may be useful in a failed fasciotomy.

Medial Tibial Stress Syndrome

Medial tibial stress syndrome (MTSS) is a complex of symptoms in athletes who experience exercise-induced pain along the distal posteromedial aspect of the tibia. Also known as shin splints, this condition usually involves inflammation of the fascial insertion of the soleus or a periostitis of the tibia beneath the posterior tibialis or flexor digitorum longus. This condition often coexists with deep posterior exertional compartment syndrome, tibial stress fractures, or other soft-tissue injuries.

The typical reports of MTSS include pain along the posteromedial border of the tibia at the junction of the middle and distal third. The pain is exacerbated by activity and relieved with rest. The pain may be dull or excruciating. Examination typically reveals a 3- to 6-cm area of exquisite tenderness along the posterior medial border of the distal third of the tibia. Range of motion and strength are typically normal, and vascular and neurologic signs are absent with MTSS.

A differentiation between the associated findings including stress fractures and compartment syndrome must be made. A well-defined area of localized bony tenderness and swelling may indicate a stress fracture, and vague, diffuse pain with associated neurologic symptoms may reveal an exertional compartment syndrome.

Radiographic studies are usually the most helpful in diagnosing the condition. Plain radiographs are normal. A bone scan may reveal diffuse, longitudinal tracer uptake in MTSS. More intense and localized uptake is seen in acute stress fractures. However, healing stress fractures may have a similar appearance as MTSS on the bone scan. MRI can be used to differentiate between a stress fracture, stress reaction, and periostitis. Compartment pressure testing can be done to rule out an exertional compartment syndrome.[5]

Rest is the basis for treatment of MTSS. Ice massage and anti-inflammatory medications are useful adjuncts to relative rest. The flexibility of the gastrocnemius and soleus muscles should be evaluated, making sure the subtalar joint is maintained in the neutral position. Gastrocnemius flexibility should be determined with the knee in full extension and should reveal at least 10° of ankle joint dorsiflexion without compensatory subtalar joint pronation. Soleus flexibility should be determined with the knee flexed. Stretching exercises for the gastrocnemius and soleus should be performed if examination reveals inadequate flexibility. Foot orthotics should be considered if abnormal pronation is believed to contribute to the individual's symptoms.[6] Eccentric function of the tibialis posterior is also important to control abnormal subtalar joint pronation, and thus strengthening exercises for the tibialis posterior should be considered for MTSS.

Summary

Most overuse injuries of the lower extremity can be managed with activity modifications, orthotics, stretching, strengthening, and functional training. Because of the multifaceted nature of most of these disorders, a thorough evaluation with clinical examination and diagnostic testing should be done.

Annotated References

1. Orchard JW, Fricker PA, Abud AT, Mason BR: Biomechanics of iliotibial band friction syndrome in runners. *Am J Sports Med* 1996;24:375-379.

2. Fredericson M, Weir A: Practical management of iliotibial band friction syndrome in runners. *Clin J Sports Med* 2006;16:261-268.

   This article outlines the practical management of ITB friction syndrome in the running athlete.

3. Pedowitz RA, Hargens AR, Mubarak SJ, Gershuni DH: Modified criteria for the objective diagnosis of chronic compartment syndrome of the leg. *Am J Sports Med* 1990;18:35-40.

4. Schepsis AA, Gill SS, Foster TA: Fasciotomy for exertional anterior compartment syndrome: Is lateral compartment release necessary? *Am J Sports Med* 1999;27:430-435.

5. Edwards PH, Wright ML, Hartman JF: A practical approach for the differential diagnosis of chronic leg pain in the athlete. *Am J Sports Med* 2005;33:1241-1249.

   An algorithmic approach is created to aid in the evaluation of patients with reports of lower leg pain and to assist in defining a diagnosis by providing recommended diagnostic studies for each condition.

6. Yates B, White S: The incidence and risk factors in the development of medial tibial stress syndrome among naval recruits. *Am J Sports Med* 2004;32:772-780.

   The authors identified a 35% incidence of MTSS in a group of naval recruits during a 10-week basic training period. MTSS was more likely to develop in female recruits than males (53% compared with 28%), and the biomechanical results indicated a more pronated foot type in the MTSS group than in the control group.

3: Knee and Leg

Chapter 16

Athletic Foot Disorders

*Mark Glazebrook, MSc, PhD, MD, FRCSC   Annunziato Amendola, MD

Hindfoot

Plantar Fasciitis/Heel Pain

The plantar fascia is a dense band of connective tissue that originates on the medial calcaneal tuberosity and inserts on the plantar plates of the metatarsophalangeal (MTP) joints and proximal phalangeals (**Figure 1**). The athletic population is particularly prone to injuring this structure because of repetitive overuse such as that experienced with long distance running and training regimens that involve excessive mileage. This repetitive trauma may result in forces that exceed the elastic limits of the collagen network of the plantar fascia. This may lead to damage at the molecular level and incite an inflammatory response that results in the clinical features of pain, swelling, and heat.

The pain is classically aggravated with activity and is worst on initial weight bearing when rising from bed in the morning or from a prolonged seated position. The pain is usually localized to the origin of the plantar fascia on the plantar medial aspect of the heel and also radiates along the plantar medial aspect. Tenderness is usually quite focal although sometimes diffuse; the tenderness is usually aggravated with stretching of the plantar arch and palpation.

Contributing factors have included a cavovarus foot and a triceps surae contracture. Common conditions in the differential diagnosis of plantar fasciitis include a calcaneal stress fracture and nerve entrapment. A complete listing of differential diagnoses is provided in **Table 1**.

A calcaneal stress fracture should be suspected if there is an acute exacerbation or a history of chronic pain. On examination, pain is present with compression of the heel and radiographs that show classic findings of a stress fracture. A bone scan or MRI often is indicated to rule out the injury.

Nerve entrapment also should be considered in the differential diagnosis. The clinical features include radiating, electriclike, stabbing pain with a Tinel sign that is pathognomonic. Most commonly implicated is the first branch of the lateral plantar nerve (Baxter nerve),

a mixed motor and sensory nerve to the abductor digiti quinti, with entrapment typically occurring between the abductor hallucis fascia and the quadratus planus muscle (**Figure 2**).

Treatment of Plantar Fasciitis
Nonsurgical methods, including activity modification, analgesics or nonsteroidal anti-inflammatory drugs

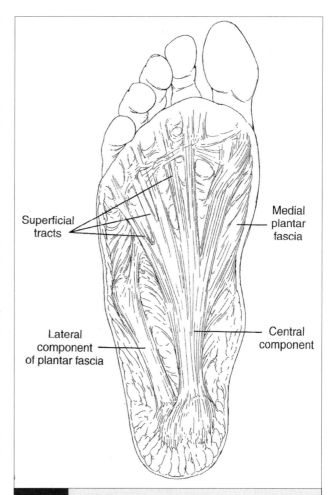

Figure 1   Anatomy of the plantar fascia. (*Reproduced from Anderson RB, James WC III, Lee S: Athletic foot disorders, in Garrick JG (ed): Orthopaedic Knowledge Update: Sports Medicine 3. Rosemont, IL, American Academy of Orthopaedic Surgeons, 2004, pp 249-262.*)

Mark Glazebrook, PhD, MD, FRCSC or the department with which he is affiliated has received research or institutional support from Arthrex and DePuy, holds stock or stock options in Stryker, Wright Medical Technologies, and Smith & Nephew, and is a consultant for or an employee of Conmed Linvatec.

Table 1

Differential Diagnosis for Plantar Fasciitis Heel Pain

Neurologic
Abductor digiti quinti nerve entrapment
Lumbar spine disorders
Problems with the medial calcaneal branch of the posterior tibial nerve
Neuropathies
Tarsal tunnel syndrome

Soft tissue
Achilles tendoniti
Fat pad atrophy
Heel contusion
Plantar fascia rupture
Posterior tibial tendinitis
Retrocalcaneal bursitis

Skeletal
Calcaneal epiphysitis (Sever disease)
Calcaneal stress fracture
Infections
Inflammatory arthropathies
Subtalar arthritis

Miscellaneous
Metabolic disorders
Osteomalacia
Paget disease
Sickle cell disease
Tumors (rare)
Vascular insufficiency

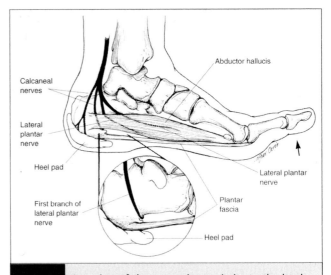

Figure 2	Location of the nerves in proximity to the heel. (*Reproduced from Anderson RB, James WC III, Lee S: Athletic foot disorders, in Garrick JG (ed): Orthopaedic Knowledge Update: Sports Medicine 3. Rosemont, IL, American Academy of Orthopaedic Surgeons, 2004, pp 249-262.*)

(NSAIDs), and physical therapy focusing on stretching of the plantar fascia and Achilles tendon complex are the mainstay of treatment.[1] Orthotic devices such as off-the-shelf or custom cushioned in-shoe orthoses to control heel motion and prevent splaying of the heel pad, or dorsiflexion night splints also are used. More invasive treatments include iontophoresis, steroid injections, and extracorporeal shock wave therapy (ESWT). Should these nonsurgical treatments fail, surgical treatment may be used.

There are limited studies examining the efficacy of oral NSAIDs. Twenty-nine patients were randomized to receive either placebo or NSAID as well as a conservative regimen that included heel-cord stretching, viscoelastic heel cups, and night splinting.[2] The results showed better pain relief with NSAIDs, providing some evidence that NSAIDs may increase pain relief and decrease disability in patients with plantar fasciitis when used with a conservative treatment regimen; however, current evidence is insufficient to allow definitive treatment recommendations.

A recent randomized controlled trial included 101 patients who had chronic proximal plantar fasciitis for at least 10 months.[3] Results showed that a program of stretching exercises specific to the plantar fascia with no weight bearing was superior to the standard program of weight-bearing Achilles tendon-stretching exercises for treating proximal plantar fasciitis. However, in another randomized controlled trial, 92 patients with plantar heel pain responded no better to a 2-week intervention period of prescribed calf muscle stretches and sham ultrasound compared with sham ultrasound alone.[4] In a third randomized controlled trial, 41 patients underwent stretching of the plantar fascia, calcaneal taping, sham taping, or no treatment.[5] The results of this study indicated that stretching was inferior to calcaneal taping. Another study provided limited data to support the use of night splints for the treatment of plantar fasciitis.[6]

Plantar fasciitis is often treated with foot orthoses; however, because studies of the effects of orthoses are limited, there is insufficient evidence to recommend or discourage their use. One study evaluated the short- and long-term effectiveness of foot orthoses in the treatment of plantar fasciitis.[7] One hundred thirty-five patients with plantar fasciitis were randomly allocated to receive a sham orthosis, a prefabricated orthosis, or a customized orthosis. The authors concluded that foot orthoses produced small, short-term benefits in function and possibly small reductions in pain, but there are no long-term beneficial effects in comparison with a sham device. The customized and prefabricated orthoses used in this trial showed similar effectiveness in the treatment of plantar fasciitis. These results were consistent with an earlier multicenter study that showed efficacy of a prefabricated shoe insert as part of the initial treatment of plantar fasciitis.[8]

Several studies provide evidence for and against the use of ESWT to treat chronic plantar fasciitis; other recent studies provide level II therapeutic evidence supporting the efficacy and safety for the use of ESWT.[9-16] One of these studies followed 2,293 patients randomized to receive high-energy electrohydraulic shock-wave treatments or placebo including subcutaneous anesthetic injections and nontransmitted shock waves by the same protocol.[15] The study concluded that treatment with electrohydraulic high-energy shock waves is a safe and effective noninvasive method of treating chronic plantar fasciitis, with effects lasting 1 year or longer. Another study compared the effectiveness of different energy densities of ESWT and concluded that the delivery of ESWT with a maximum tolerable energy density is a more effective treatment.[16] Other studies provide modest support for the use of corticosteroid injections for the treatment of plantar fasciitis.[6,17,18]

Surgical treatment of plantar fasciitis is reserved for chronic conditions when nonsurgical treatment has failed. A longitudinal plantar medial incision is made for removal of a 1-cm segment of the medial third of the plantar fascia to prevent arch collapse. Some surgeons also advocate removal of the calcaneal spur and release of the fascia surrounding the abductor hallucis muscle using this approach. Others advocate endoscopic plantar fascia release with the claim of a faster recovery time.[19] Most available evidence to support surgical treatment of plantar fasciitis is fair quality with no randomized controlled trials available; the efficacy of surgical treatment is based on level III and IV evidence.

Rupture of the Plantar Fascia

Rupture of the plantar fascia reportedly occurs after a sudden acceleration during athletic activities. Patients report a painful popping sensation of the medial arch. Existing evidence in the literature is insufficient to allow for definitive treatment recommendations. Nonsurgical treatment should include a short period of immobilization and no weight bearing (for 2 to 3 weeks) to allow resolution of pain and inflammation, followed by a gradual return to weight-bearing activity;[20] none of the 18 patients with a plantar fascia rupture who were treated with this regimen sustained reinjury, had postinjury sequelae, or needed surgery.

The possibility of medial arch collapse with this condition is cause for concern; however, this condition is not common. If arch collapse occurs, lateral column overload, which may cause stress fractures in the cuboid or lateral metatarsals, should be avoided. An orthotic for medial arch support may help prevent injury.

Posterior Ankle Impingement

Pain in the posterior aspect of the hindfoot may result from posterior ankle impingement, which causes pain localized to the posterior aspect of the ankle and is aggravated by forced plantar flexion. The most common pathologic diagnoses causing posterior ankle impingement are a symptomatic os trigonum and flexor hallucis longus tenosynovitis. Ankle osteochondritis, subtalar joint disease, and fracture are less common.

Os Trigonum Impingement

The os trigonum is an accessory bone located at the posterior aspect of the talus (**Figure 3**) that is present in 23.5% of the general population.[21] The os trigonum is often bilateral and may become symptomatic with or without an acute injury such as an ankle sprain, forced planter flexion, or repetitive overuse. Impingement is first suspected when deep posterior ankle pain is present that is aggravated with plantar flexion activities such as declined running, jumping, and dancing en pointe. Tenderness is localized anterior to the Achilles tendon and exacerbated with forced planter flexion and pronation of the foot. Often flexor hallucis longus irritation from the impingement, and therefore tenderness along the flexor hallucis longus tendon, is present. The presence of an os trigonum on lateral radiographs is not diagnostic unless translation or diastasis with dynamic imaging can be demonstrated. A bone scan or MRI may be helpful in diagnosis if positive at the os trigonum-talar junction. MRI can rule out soft-tissue pathology such as Achilles or other tendonopathies.

Some authors advocate a trial of nonsurgical treatment to include short periods of immobilization with steroid injection or oral NSAIDs.[22-24] If the os trigonum is mobile or symptoms persist despite 3 months of nonsurgical treatment, surgical excision through an open posterolateral, posteromedial, or posterior ankle arthroscopic approach may be warranted (**Figure 4**).

Flexor Hallucis Longus Tendinitis

Pain associated with flexor hallucis longus pathology can manifest anywhere along the length of the flexor hallucis longus from the posterior leg to the plantar foot and the hallux and may be associated with bony impingement or a mobile os trigonum. When the pain of posterior ankle impingement is more posteromedial, then flexor hallucis longus tendinitis is likely. The condition is more common in jumpers and en pointe dancers. Patients may also report clicking or locking with dorsiflexion and plantar flexion of the great toe. Nonsurgical treatment of flexor hallucis longus tendinitis with rest, NSAIDs, and physical therapy reportedly has been successful in 64% of patients studied.[24] Surgical treatment includes open surgical release of constricting structures and débridement or endoscopic flexor hallucis longus decompression.[25,26]

Midfoot

Lisfranc Fracture-Dislocation

The Lisfranc or tarsometatarsal joint is the articulation between the base of the five metatarsals distally and the

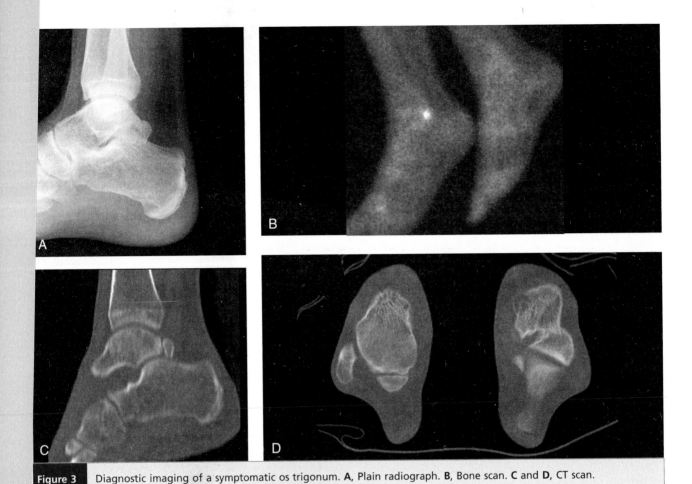

Figure 3 Diagnostic imaging of a symptomatic os trigonum. **A,** Plain radiograph. **B,** Bone scan. **C** and **D,** CT scan.

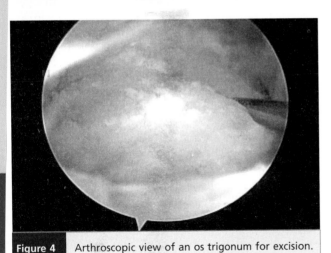

Figure 4 Arthroscopic view of an os trigonum for excision.

three cuneiforms and cuboid proximally. Stability of the tarsometatarsal joint is provided mainly by the bone and ligament anatomy, including a recessed base of the second metatarsal between the medial and lateral cuneiforms and a transverse geometry (resembling a Roman arch) for additional stability. Ligamentous supports to this joint include plantar, dorsal, and interosseous ligaments. The plantar ligaments are stronger than the dorsal ligaments, which may account for

dorsal dislocations. The intermetatarsal interosseous ligaments are the strongest of all the ligaments, with no intermetatarsal interosseous ligament between the second and first metatarsals, again making the joint more susceptible to disruption at this area. The Lisfranc ligament provides stability between the first and second metatarsal with its origin at the medial cuneiform and insertion at the base of the second metatarsal.

Mechanism of Injury and Classification

Injuries to the tarsometatarsal joint may be caused by indirect or direct forces. The indirect forces involve an axial loading mechanism or a twisting on a plantar-flexed foot. Examples include a fall from a height, an opponent falling on a plantar-flexed foot from behind, or a forefoot trapped in a strap or stirrup. Dislocation occurs at the weakest point, which is between the first and second metatarsal and in a dorsal direction. As the forces increase, the plantar aspect of the metatarsal base may fracture, possibly leading to progressive injury to the cuneiforms, cuboid, or metatarsals.

Direct injuries are less common and occur when a load is applied to the midfoot, resulting in less typical fracture patterns with a variable degree of bone and soft-tissue injuries. Direct injuries to the tarsometatarsal joint may also result in comminuted or compound

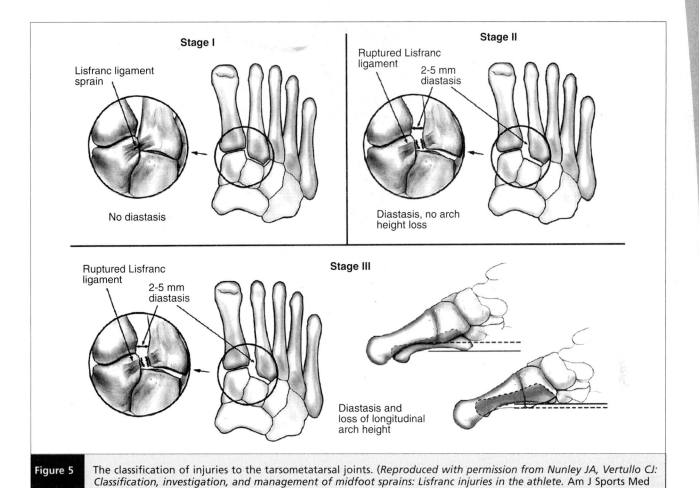

Figure 5 The classification of injuries to the tarsometatarsal joints. (*Reproduced with permission from Nunley JA, Vertullo CJ: Classification, investigation, and management of midfoot sprains: Lisfranc injuries in the athlete. Am J Sports Med 2002;30:817-878.*)

fractures that may be associated with compartment syndromes of the foot.

In athletes, there is a spectrum of injury from stable sprains (no radiographic displacement) to severe sprains with obvious widening between the base of the first and second metatarsal. A classification system helps the physician treating athletes with less severe injuries[27] (**Figure 5**). Patients with stage I injuries are unable to participate in sports because of pain in the Lisfranc joint and have nondisplaced weight-bearing radiographs with positive bone scan findings. Stage II patients have first to second metatarsal diastases of 1 to 5 mm but no evidence of loss of arch on weight-bearing radiographs. Stage III patients have first to second metatarsal diastases greater than 5 mm and evidence of loss of arch on weight-bearing radiographs.

History and Physical Examination
Although relatively uncommon, injuries to the tarsometatarsal joint often are misdiagnosed and thus require a high index of suspicion when there is a foot injury. Severe injuries with displacement are more obvious, but ligamentous injuries with minimal displacement are more likely to be missed.[28] Pain with weight bearing and swelling localized to the midfoot should be the first clue. Even with mild injuries, athletes will have difficulty pushing off. Physical examination will reveal swelling, ecchymosis, and localized tenderness to palpation or manipulation of the midfoot, particularily pronation-abduction or supination-adduction. Physical examination should also comprise neurovascular evaluation including dorsalis pedis pulse and deep peroneal nerve. Foot compartment syndromes should be ruled out or may need urgent treatment in severe Lisfranc fracture-dislocations.

Imaging
Diagnostic imaging of the foot with a suspected Lisfranc fracture-dislocation begins with AP, 30° oblique, and lateral views (**Figure 6**). These images are best obtained in the weight-bearing position or sometimes with stress to the Lisfranc joint to avoid missing a dislocation that has spontaneously reduced with soft-tissue disruption only. In some instances, weight-bearing radiographs may stabilize the Lisfranc joint, and widening or instability may not be apparent. In the normal foot, on any view, the first and second metatarsal should align with the medial, middle, and lateral cuneiform, respectively, and the fourth and fifth metatarsal bases should align with the cuboid. A consistent

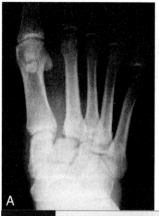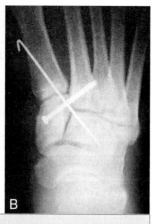

Figure 6 Preoperative **(A)** and postoperative **(B)** AP radiographs used to assess fracture-dislocation of the tarsometatarsal joints. *(Reproduced from Anderson RB, James WC III, Lee S: Athletic foot disorders, in Garrick JG (ed): Orthopaedic Knowledge Update: Sports Medicine 3. Rosemont, IL, American Academy of Orthopaedic Surgeons, 2004, pp 249-262.)*

relationship also should be present between the medial margin of the middle cuneiform and the medial aspect of the second metatarsal. On the oblique view, an unbroken line should exist between the medial base of the fourth and the medial margin of the cuboid. On the lateral view, an unbroken line should exist between the dorsum of the first and second metatarsals and the medial and middle cuneiforms. Flattening of the arch or a planus Meary angle is suggestive of a midfoot injury. Pathognomic signs of a Lisfranc fracture-dislocation include diastasis of the first and second metatarsal and a fleck sign (a small, bony avulsion fragment attached to the Lisfranc ligament seen in the space between the second metatarsal and the medial cuneiform). If a Lisfranc injury is suspected and plain radiographs are not diagnostic, a CT or MRI scan will be useful.[29,30] In mild injuries where routine radiographs are not diagnostic, stress views under anesthesia may be useful.

Treatment
The goal of treatment is to obtain and maintain anatomic reduction of the tarsometatarsal joint. In truly nondisplaced and stable Lisfranc sprains, use of a short leg cast with no weight bearing until tenderness resolves (approximately 6 weeks), followed by functional rehabilitation, is recommended. In the athlete, if there is concern about stability, stress radiographs may be helpful; if instability is demonstrated, fixation may prevent late collapse. In a displaced Lisfranc fracture-dislocation, an open reduction of all tarsometatarsal joints and internal fixation is recommended. Fixation devices should be positioned between the second metatarsal and the medial cuneiform and then through the metatarsals and their respective cuneiform or cuboid. In isolated sprains of the Lisfranc ligament (widening of the base of the first and second metatarsals) without

bony injury, percutaneous reduction and screw fixation may provide anatomic reduction and stable fixation.

There is no consensus on hardware removal; however, rather than an arthrodesis, hardware can be removed to allow motion at these joints. New internal fixation devices that use Endobuttons (Acufex microsurgical, Mansfield, MA) and suture material that provides resistance to tensile forces similar to those of metallic screws show early promise because they allow motion, and screw removal is no longer necessary. Most reports in the literature support open reduction and internal fixation of a Lisfranc fracture-dislocation.[31-33]

Forefoot

MTP Joint Injury/Turf Toe
The most common injury to the MTP joint involves the plantar plate (a thick, fibrous reinforcement of the plantar capsule firmly anchored to the plantar surface of the proximal phalanx and less firmly attached to the neck of the metatarsal). The classic description of a turf toe injury is an axial load applied to the hindfoot with the first MTP joint in a hyperextended position (**Figure 7**). This will cause a rupture of the plantar plate off the neck of the metatarsal or the proximal phalanx. However, in addition to hyperextension, varus and valgus injuries may occur. Factors associated with turf toe include artificial playing surfaces, sports requiring squatting and pushing off, and flexible shoe wear.

Diagnosis and Classification
Patients will usually have a history of an injury or multiple injuries to the great toe with resultant pain (worse with motion), ecchymosis, redness, and swelling around the MTP joint. Associated abnormal findings may include deformities such as hammering, subluxation, or hypermobility. Diagnostic imaging begins with standing AP and lateral radiographs of the MTP joint that often are normal but may reveal a tiny avulsion fracture of the plantar aspect of the proximal phalanx or the distal pole of the sesamoid. The position of the sesamoids on the AP and lateral radiographs may reveal proximal migration or increased distance between the base of the proximal phalanx and distal pole of the sesamoid that may increase with hyperextension of the MTP joint (**Figure 8**). Sesamoid views may also be useful to delineate a fracture of the sesamoids. MRI is the gold standard for assessing the extent of soft-tissue injury and associated osseous or cartilage injury.

Treatment
There is insufficient literature-based evidence to guide treatment recommendations, but some individual expert opinions exist.[34,35] Nonsurgical treatments include standard rest, ice, compression, and elevation in the acute setting. A classification system (**Table 2**) that grades the severity of the condition according to physi-

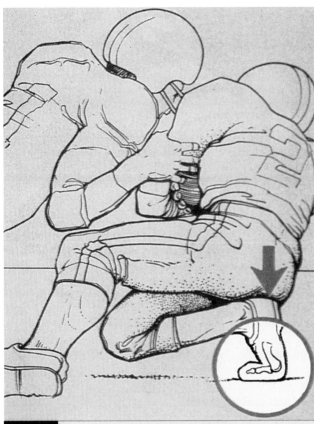

Figure 7 | Typical mechanism of injury (hyperdorsiflexion) to the first MTP joint that may cause turf toe. (Reproduced from Anderson RB, James WC III, Lee S: Athletic foot disorders, in Garrick JG (ed): Orthopaedic Knowledge Update: Sports Medicine 3. Rosemont, IL, American Academy of Orthopaedic Surgeons, 2004, pp 249-262.)

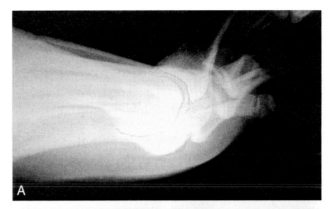

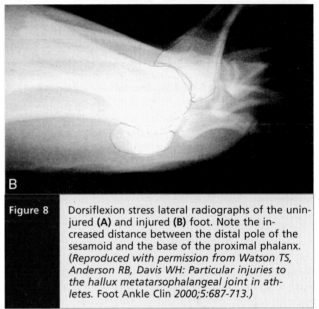

Figure 8 | Dorsiflexion stress lateral radiographs of the uninjured (A) and injured (B) foot. Note the increased distance between the distal pole of the sesamoid and the base of the proximal phalanx. (Reproduced with permission from Watson TS, Anderson RB, Davis WH: Particular injuries to the hallux metatarsophalangeal joint in athletes. Foot Ankle Clin 2000;5:687-713.)

cal findings is a useful guide for recommendations on treatment and activity restriction.[36,37] Grade 1 injuries may require shoe wear with a stiff insole and continuation in athletic events according to degree of pain. Grade 2 injuries may require rest in a cast boot or splint with restricted activities for 1 to 2 weeks, and grade 3 injuries may need protected weight bearing in a cast boot for up to 6 weeks.

Surgical treatment may be considered for large capsular avulsions, an unstable joint, diastasis of a bipartite or fractured sesamoid, retraction of sesamoids, or a loose body.

Sesamoid Disorder
The sesamoids of the great toe are particularly vulnerable to overuse disorders in the athlete. Pain can be caused by stress fractures, displaced fractures, sesamoiditis, arthrosis, osteochondritis, bipartite sesamoids, and osteomyelitis. Flexor hallucis brevis tendinitis and bursitis beneath the sesamoids may also occur in the athlete and may be confused with sesamoid injury. Diagnostic imaging using bone scan or MRI is recom-

mended to confirm the diagnosis and location of pathology.

Treatment recommendations include activity modification, immobilization, shoe wear modifications, orthoses, NSAIDs, and selective injections. When nonsurgical treatment fails, excision of the involved sesamoid is recommended. Excision of the sesamoid has been reported in several case series with satisfactory results, but residual pain can be problematic. As an alternative to hallux sesamoid excision, autogenous bone grafting was used in 21 patients in one study; successful bony union was achieved in all but 2 patients.[38]

Stress Fracture
A stress fracture is any fracture or microfracture that occurs as the result of repetitive loading to the bone rather than from a single traumatic event. A stress fracture can occur as the result of a marked increase in the load on a normal bone, such as an increase in a training regimen. Foot and ankle stress fractures are very common in athletes, and often the etiology is repetitive forces that outstrip the foot's ability to dissipate loads. However, stress fractures may occur from normal load-

Table 2

Clinical Classification System for Turf Toe Injury

Grade	Objective Findings	Activity Level	Treatment
1	Localized plantar or medial tenderness Minimal swelling No ecchymosis	Continued athletic participation	Symptomatic
2	More diffuse and intense tenderness Mild to moderate swelling Mild to moderate ecchymosis	Loss of playing time for 3 to 14 days	Walking boot and crutches, as needed
3	Severe and diffuse tenderness Marked swelling Moderate to severe ecchymosis Painful and limited range of motion	Loss of playing time for at least 4 to 6 weeks	Long-term immobilization in boot or cast versus surgical repair

(Reproduced with permission from Coughlin MJ, Mann RA (eds): Surgery of the Foot and Ankle, ed 7. St. Louis, MO, Mosby, 1999, vol 2, p 1186.)

ing patterns in bone that is abnormally weak or when the body's ability to repair and remodel microfractures is deficient because of chronic diseases such as metabolic bone disease, dietary deficiencies, or the female athletic triad (amenorrhea, disordered eating, and osteoporosis). Causative factors include poor training techniques, shoe wear or rigid playing surfaces, muscle imbalances, and foot and ankle malalignment.

Patient Evaluation

A high index of suspicion is always required with the insidious onset of foot pain. The history should include the location of pain and details about the training regimen, playing surface, and shoe wear of the athlete (especially recent changes). If a stress fracture is not diagnosed, later findings will include similar symptoms that are more intense and occur with less activity, or possibly during activities of daily living.

The physical examination should focus on the location of the pain because stress fractures in the athlete occur in common areas (such as the calcaneus, navicular, and metatarsals). Localized tenderness, swelling, and guarding are hallmark signs of stress fractures. Alignment of the lower extremity is important because malalignment can cause certain types of stress fractures. For example, a cavus foot promotes overload on the lateral border of the foot, possibly causing a fifth metatarsal stress fracture, whereas a planus foot may increase force in the midfoot, predisposing to metatarsal base fractures or navicular stress fractures.

Diagnostic imaging begins with plain radiographs that are often normal. Bone scans are very sensitive but not necessarily specific for diagnosing a stress fracture. MRI scans are both sensitive and specific for stress fractures in the foot and ankle. CT scans are usually better for assessment of healing of a stress fracture.

Treatment

Once the diagnosis of a stress fracture is made in the athlete, it is important to decide if it is a high-risk or low-risk fracture. For example, fractures of the navicular and base of the fifth metatarsal and fractures loaded in tension have a higher propensity for delayed union and a poor natural history and are therefore considered high risk. Thus, early surgical stabilization may be important, followed by a period of no weight bearing, to optimize the healing environment and prevent recurrent fracture. Calcaneal and second, third, and fourth metatarsals fractures can be considered low risk and early weight bearing can be allowed.

It is important to rule out or treat any pathologic process that may result in a deficiency in the body's ability to repair and remodel bone. Treatment may then be directed at unloading the bone by decreasing activity; this can be done aggressively in high-risk fractures with casting without bearing weight until pain is absent, or less aggressively in low-risk fractures by modifying activities that cause pain. A third option may include a cast boot that allows patients to unload the stress fracture of the foot when active and provide more convenience and comfort for activities that do not require weight bearing, such as sleeping.

Patients with high-risk stress fractures or evidence of nonunion (radiographs displaying fragmentation, sclerotic margins, or displacement) should be considered for surgery. Surgery may include fixation only in early fractures and/or open reduction with internal fixation after débridement and bone grafting of the fracture site in clear nonunions.

Distal Tibial Stress Fracture

Tibial stress fractures often occur in the proximal, middle, and distal third of the tibia. In contrast to midshaft diaphyseal fractures, which are high risk (anterior, tension side of the tibia), distal third fractures are low risk and are on the compressive side of the bone, are posteromedial, and generally heal with nonsurgical treatment. Fracture location may be related to specific etiologic factors. One study found that in 29 unilateral tibial stress fractures, 10 were anterior and 19 were posteromedial.[39] Nine of the 10 anterior mid-diaphyseal fractures occurred during pushoff or landing, and there was no difference in the posteromedial distal fracture group.

Distal third fractures may be a continuum of overuse in medial tibial stress syndrome periostitis. The typical longitudinal tenderness seen in medial tibial stress syndrome will become more focal and not subside with rest once the stress fracture occurs.

Medial malleollar stress fractures are uncommon but do occur from repetitive compressive loading. Treatment is similar to that of distal tibial stress fractures, and healing is expected with nonsurgical treatment. Tibia vara may predispose to medial overload, and in these situations treatment is necessary until healing occurs.

Clinical Evaluation

A tibial stress fracture should be suspected when an athlete reports leg pain and difficulty training or bearing weight that is not relieved with rest. The most important physical finding is localized tenderness over the fracture site, not diffuse longitudinal tenderness as with medial tibial stress syndrome. A thorough neurovascular examination should be done in any athlete with exercise-induced leg pain; however, this examination should be normal in an athlete with an isolated tibial stress fracture.

Imaging Studies

Plain radiographs can show evidence of bone response such as periosteal reaction, cortical thickening, or fracture lucency. When obvious findings are not present on plain radiographs, MRI is preferred.[36] A bone scan can also be helpful in diagnosis but is less specific because it does not necessarily differentiate medial tibial stress syndrome from a distal tibial stress fracture.

Treatment

The objectives of treatment are to decrease the repeated stress on the bone to allow it to rest and heal. Most distal tibial stress fractures can be healed with immobilization and varying degrees of rest.

In some cases, up to 8 weeks of cast immobilization may be necessary, but for many athletes relative rest and mobilization with a cast or brace may be all that is needed. In a study of soldiers, the use of a pneumatic brace did not improve healing time or function.[40] Although pulsed, low-intensity ultrasound has been suggested as an aid to healing tibial stress fractures,[37] in one prospective randomized double-blinded study of tibial stress fractures in military recruits, its use did not show any significant difference in time to healing in two similar groups.[41]

Navicular Stress Fracture

Navicular stress fractures are common in athletes who participate in sports involving repetitive loading, sud-

den acceleration, and deceleration (track and field, basketball, and football). Anatomic features that may predispose to stress fractures include a long second metatarsal or a short first metatarsal, anterior ankle impingement, or decreased ankle motion. The watershed area of the blood supply to the central portion of the navicular predisposes this area to stress fracture. Diagnosis can be difficult, but most patients will describe a history of vague pain in the ankle, the dorsum of the foot, or the medial aspect of the longitudinal arch that is worse with activity and improved with rest. Often there will be a history of an increase in the training pattern during the weeks or months prior to the onset of symptoms. Clinical findings mainly include tenderness and occasional swelling over the navicular.

Classification of navicular fractures include edema without cortical fracture, incomplete fracture, complete fracture (both dorsal and plantar cortex) and chronic nonunion (sclerosis).[42]

There are no randomized controlled trials that compare treatment protocols for navicular stress fractures, but level IV studies suggest that incomplete or nondisplaced complete navicular stress fractures should be treated in a short leg cast with no weight bearing until the tenderness over the navicular resolves (6 weeks or longer).[43] It would be prudent to confirm bony healing with CT before resuming athletic activity.

Surgical treatment of navicular stress fractures, including internal fixation with or without bone grafting, is recommended when nonsurgical treatment has failed or the fracture is displaced. Some authors suggest that high-performance athletes with partial or nondisplaced complete fractures may benefit from initial surgical intervention; however, the evidence to support or refute this claim is insufficient.

Second, Third, or Fourth Metatarsal Stress Fracture

Stress fractures are most common in the second metatarsal and occur in runners, hikers, and en pointe dancers who have experienced an increase in weight-bearing activities. These fractures are considered low risk and usually are located in the diaphyseal or metatarsal neck region, but also occur at the metatarsal base and sometimes extend intra-articularly in en pointe dancers.

Patients with metatarsal stress fractures usually have a history of pain in the forefoot and often an increase in symptoms after a change in training patterns. Physical examination reveals localized pain with palpation or metatarsal manipulation, and swelling may be present. Patients will avoid walking or walk with a limp. Toe walking is usually difficult or impossible because of the pain. Identification of early callus formation (after approximately 2 weeks) on AP or oblique radiographs of the foot is diagnostic. In patients with negative radiographs, a technetium Tc 99 bone scan may be diagnostic. Most metatarsal stress fractures can be effectively treated symptomatically with a short leg cast, cast boot, or possibly a stiff-soled shoe, with healing in 4 to 8 weeks.

Fifth Metatarsal Stress Fracture

Fractures of the fifth metatarsal are considered high risk and deserve separate discussion because of a unique subset of injury that occurs in the metaphyseal-diaphyseal junction (Jones fracture) that may not heal with nonsurgical treatment because of the watershed region, which has poor vascularity.

Several level III and IV studies support surgical and nonsurgical treatment of fifth metatarsal stress fractures. However level I or II studies providing evidence to recommend one over the other are limited. Thus it may be reasonable to suggest that noncompetitive athletes with these injuries should first be treated in a short leg cast with no weight bearing until signs of clinical and radiographic healing are present (6 weeks or longer).

Surgical treatment may be recommended[44] for those failing to respond to nonsurgical treatment or for competitive athletes who demand aggressive rehabilitation and return to play; these athletes should be made aware of nonsurgical treatment options and possible complications associated with surgery. Fixation of these fractures usually requires 4.0- to 7.0-mm half-threaded cancellous screws. Nonunions also may require bone grafting and possibly a bone stimulator. Refracture has been documented to occur in small numbers when return to sport occurs before radiographic healing.[45]

These fractures are caused by lateral foot overload, and treatment with an orthotic after healing should dissipate shock and prevent recurrence. Hindfoot varus or midfoot adductus may predispose to this type of stress fracture, and lateral forefoot orthotics are required. Osteotomy to correct deformity may be considered in patients with recurrent injury.

Calcaneal Stress Fracture

Calcaneal stress fractures are low risk because of their propensity to heal without complications. A delay in diagnosis is not uncommon because of a complex differential diagnosis including heel pain, atrophic heel pad, retrocalcaneal bursitis, Achilles insertional tendinosis, plantar fasciitis, and tarsal tunnel syndrome.

Patients with calacaneal stress fractures report heel pain that persists throughout the course of the day and is exacerbated by increased weight-bearing activities. Tenderness and swelling are usually medial and lateral on the calcaneus. Diagnostic imaging at 2 to 3 weeks may reveal sclerosis that interrupts normal trabecula on plain radiographs. A bone scan or MRI can confirm the diagnosis.

In adolescents, the term Sever disease refers to a phenomenon involving the calcaneal apophysis. In a recent study of children with a presumptive diagnosis of Sever's apophysitis and with continuing pain after nonsurgical treatment, MRI showed bone bruising within the trabecular bone of the metaphyseal region adjacent to the calcaneal apophysis.[46] Accordingly, the authors concluded that the disorder commonly referred to as Sever apophysitis may be a metaphyseal trabecular stress fracture, similar to the toddler's calcaneal stress fracture that has minimal or no involvement of the apophyseal ossification center, and thus should not be referred to as an apophysitis. Treatment recommendations include activity modification with early diagnosis or immobilization in a cast or cast boot until pain resolves (after 6 weeks). Long-term sequelae are rare.

Summary

Athletic foot disorders are a unique subset of orthopaedic foot and ankle pathologies requiring detailed management, ranging from acute injuries such as fractures or soft-tissue ruptures to chronic overuse injuries such as stress fractures and tendinopathies. The foot is one of the most frequent anatomic locations for injury, and a significant amount of time is lost from participation in athletic activities. Although the diagnosis and treatment of athletic foot disorders is similar to that of any other condition where a detailed history and physical examination are essential, in athletes certain areas of the history are more focused and the disorder is related to activity.

Annotated References

1. Neufeld SK, Cerrato R: Plantar fasciitis: Evaluation and treatment. *J Am Acad Orthop Surg* 2008;16:338-346.

   This article discusses characteristic features, differential diagnosis, and nonsurgical treatment of plantar fasciitis. Level of evidence: V.

2. Donley BG, Moore T, Sferra J, Gozdanovic J, Smith R: The efficacy of oral nonsteroidal anti-inflammatory medication (NSAID) in the treatment of plantar fasciitis: A randomized, prospective, placebo-controlled study. *Foot Ankle Int* 2007;28:20-23.

   Twenty-nine patients with plantar fasciitis were randomly assigned to a placebo group or a NSAID group and were treated with nonsurgical modalities including heel cord strengthening, night splints, and viscoelastic heel cups. Study results indicate that the use of an NSAID may increase pain relief and decrease disability in patients with plantar fasciitis when used in conjunction with nonsurgical treatment. Level of evidence: I.

3. Digiovanni BF, Nawoczenski DA, Malay DP, et al: Plantar fascia-specific stretching exercise improves outcomes in patients with chronic plantar fasciitis: A prospective clinical trial with two-year follow-up. *J Bone Joint Surg Am* 2006;88:1775-1781.

   Eighty-two patients with chronic proximal plantar fasciitis for more than 10 months were randomized to either a plantar fascia-stretching group or an Achilles tendon-stretching group. After 8 weeks, the plantar fascia-stretching group had better results than the Achilles tendon-stretching group. At 2-year follow-up, there was a marked decrease in pain and functional limitations and a high rate of satisfaction in the plantar fascia-stretching group. Level of evidence: II.

4. Radford JA, Landorf KB, Buchbinder R, Cook C: Effectiveness of calf muscle stretching for the short-term treatment of plantar heel pain: A randomised trial. *BMC Musculoskelet Disord* 2007;8:36.

    The authors studied the effectiveness of calf muscle stretching in 92 patients who were randomly assigned to either a group that received calf muscle stretching and sham ultrasound or sham ultrasound alone. Both treatment groups improved over the 2-week period of follow-up; however, there were no statistically significant differences in improvement between groups for any of the measured outcomes. Level of evidence: I.

5. Hyland MR, Webber-Gaffney A, Cohen L, Lichtman PT: Randomized controlled trial of calcaneal taping, sham taping, and plantar fascia stretching for the short-term management of plantar heel pain. *J Orthop Sports Phys Ther* 2006;36:364-371.

    The authors studied 41 patients who were treated with calcaneal taping, sham taping, plantar fascia stretching, and no treatment for plantar heel pain. Calcaneal taping was the most effective treatment.

6. Crawford F, Thomson C: Interventions for treating plantar heel pain. *Cochrane Database Syst Rev* 2003; 3:CD000416.

    The authors evaluated the effectiveness of various treatments for plantar heel pain. Level of evidence: I.

7. Landorf KB, Keenan AM, Herbert RD: Effectiveness of foot orthoses to treat plantar fasciitis: A randomized trial. *Arch Intern Med* 2006;166:1305-1310.

    The short- and long-term effectiveness of foot orthoses in the treatment of plantar fasciitis was evaluated in 135 patients. Although foot orthoses produce small short-term benefits in function and may also produce small reductions in pain for people with plantar fasciitis, there are no long-term beneficial effects compared with a sham device. Level of evidence: I.

8. Pfeffer G, Bacchetti P, Deland J, et al: Comparison of custom and prefabricated orthoses in the initial treatment of proximal plantar fasciitis. *Foot Ankle Int* 1999; 20:214-221.

9. Haake M, Buch M, Schoellner C, et al: Extracorporeal shock wave therapy for plantar fasciitis: Randomised controlled multicentre trial. *BMJ* 2003;327:75.

    The effectiveness of ESWT over placebo was studied in 272 patients with chronic proximal plantar fasciitis. After 12 weeks of treatment, the authors concluded that ESWT was ineffective. Level of evidence: I.

10. Kudo P, Dainty K, Clarfield M, et al: Randomized, placebo-controlled, double-blind clinical trial evaluating the treatment of plantar fasciitis with an extracoporeal shockwave therapy (ESWT) device: A North American confirmatory study. *J Orthop Res* 2006;24:115-123.

    The authors studied 114 adult subjects with plantar fas-

ciitis and determined that ESWT administered with the Dornier Epos Ultra is a safe and effective treatment for recalcitrant plantar fasciitis. Level of evidence: I.

11. Malay DS, Pressman MM, Assili A, et al: Extracorporeal shockwave therapy versus placebo for the treatment of chronic proximal plantar fasciitis: Results of a randomized, placebo-controlled, double-blinded, multicenter intervention trial. *J Foot Ankle Surg* 2006;45: 196-210.

    In a study of 172 patients with chronic proximal plantar fasciitis, it was determined that ESWT was efficacious and safe. Level of evidence: I.

12. Ogden JA, Alvarez RG, Levitt RL, Johnson JE, Marlow ME: Electrohydraulic high-energy shock-wave treatment for chronic plantar fasciitis. *J Bone Joint Surg Am* 2004;86-A:2216-2228.

    The authors performed a randomized, placebo-controlled, multiple blinded crossover study to assess the use of electrohydraulic high-energy shock waves in patients with chronic plantar fasciitis in whom nonsurgical treatment was unsuccessful. The treatment was found to be safe and effective, lasting up to and beyond 1 year. Level of evidence: I.

13. Rompe JD, Decking J, Schoellner C, Nafe B: Shock wave application for chronic plantar fasciitis in running athletes: A prospective, randomized, placebo-controlled trial. *Am J Sports Med* 2003;31:268-275.

    The authors studied 45 athletes with chronic plantar fasciitis who were divided into two treatment groups; half received three applications of low-energy shock waves and the other half received sham treatment. Low-energy shock wave therapy was successful, with a marked reduction in pain after 6 months. Level of evidence: I.

14. Speed CA, Nichols D, Wies J, et al: Extracorporeal shock wave therapy for plantar fasciitis: A double blind randomised controlled trial. *J Orthop Res* 2003;21:937-940.

    The authors studied the effects of moderate doses of shock wave therapy in two groups of patients with plantar fasciitis (active treatment and sham treatment). Both groups had significant improvement during the study, but there was no statistically significant difference in outcome measures over a 6-month period. Additional research is needed for evidence-based recommendations for the use of ESWT. Level of evidence: I.

15. Wang CJ, Wang FS, Yang KD, Weng LH, Ko JY: Long-term results of extracorporeal shockwave treatment for plantar fasciitis. *Am J Sports Med* 2006;34:592-596.

    One hundred forty-nine patients with plantar fasciitis were divided into two groups (ESWT treatment group and control group). Overall results were 69.1% excellent, 13.5% good, 6.2% fair, and 11.1% poor for the ESWT group. Level of evidence: I.

16. Chow IH, Cheing GL: Comparison of different energy densities of extracorporeal shock wave therapy (ESWT) for the management of chronic heel pain. *Clin Rehabil*

2007;21:131-141.

The authors determined that ESWT delivered with a maximum tolerable energy density was more effective in treating chronic heel pain and restoring functional activity than a fixed energy density. Level of evidence: I.

17. Porter MD, Shadbolt B: Intralesional corticosteroid injection versus extracorporeal shock wave therapy for plantar fasciopathy. *Clin J Sport Med* 2005;15:119-124.

The authors determined that corticosteroid injection was more effective than ESWT in treating plantar fasciopathy. Level of evidence: I.

18. Tsai WC, Hsu CC, Chen CP, et al: Plantar fasciitis treated with local steroid injection: Comparison between sonographic and palpation guidance. *J Clin Ultrasound* 2006;34:12-16.

The authors compared the effectiveness of sonographically-guided and palpation-guided steroid injection for the treatment of plantar fasciitis. Injection under sonographic guidance was associated with a lower recurrence of heel pain. Level of evidence: II.

19. Bazaz R, Ferkel RD: Results of endoscopic plantar fascia release. *Foot Ankle Int* 2007;28:549-556.

The authors determined that those patients who had more severe symptoms before endoscopic plantar fascia release and those with symptoms for 2 years or longer had worse results after treatment. Level of evidence: III.

20. Saxena A, Fullem B: Plantar fascia ruptures in athletes. *Am J Sports Med* 2004;32:662-665.

The authors evaluated 18 athletes with plantar fascia rupture who had received 2 to 3 weeks of nonsurgical treatment to determine feasibility for return to activity. All patients returned to activity after 2 to 26 weeks. Level of evidence: IV.

21. Cilli F, Akçaoğlu M: The incidence of accessory bones of the foot and their clinical significance. *Acta Orthop Traumatol Turc* 2005;39:243-246.

The authors evaluated AP and lateral foot radiographs of 464 male patients to determine the presence, incidence, and distribution of accessory bones. The three most common accessory bones were os perineum, os naviculare, and os trigonum.

22. Abramowitz Y, Wollstein R, Barzilay Y, et al: Outcome of resection of a symptomatic os trigonum. *J Bone Joint Surg Am* 2003;85-A:1051-1057.

Excision of an os trigonum that is symptomatic after 3 months of nonsurgical treatment was successful. Sural nerve injury is a main complication. Level of evidence: II.

23. Jerosch J, Fadel M: Endoscopic resection of a symptomatic os trigonum. *Knee Surg Sports Traumatol Arthrosc* 2006;14:1188-1193.

The technique and results of arthroscopic resection of symptomatic os trigonum via two posterior portals in 10 cases is described. Level of evidence: IV.

24. Willits K, Sonneveld H, Amendola A, et al: Outcome of posterior ankle arthroscopy for hindfoot impingement. *Arthroscopy* 2008;24:196-202.

The authors evaluated clinical outcomes of posterior ankle arthroscopy in patients with posterior ankle pain. Results suggest that this treatment is safe and effective. Level of evidence: IV.

25. Michelson J, Dunn L: Tenosynovitis of the flexor hallucis longus: A clinical study of the spectrum of presentation and treatment. *Foot Ankle Int* 2005;26:291-303.

The authors studied the presentation, physical examination findings, and treatment approach for flexor hallucis longus tendon pathology. Level of evidence: IV.

26. Keeling JJ, Guyton GP: Endoscopic flexor hallucis longus decompression: A cadaver study. *Foot Ankle Int* 2007;28:810-814.

The authors studied endoscopic flexor hallucis longus decompression in eight cadaver legs and determined that the procedure is technically demanding with significant risk to local neurovascular structures. Three of the eight flexor hallucis longus tendons were injured during the attempted release.

27. Nunley JA, Vertullo CJ: Classification, investigation, and management of midfoot sprains: Lisfranc injuries in the athlete. *Am J Sports Med* 2002;30:871-878.

28. Saab M: Lisfranc fracture-dislocation: An easily overlooked injury in the emergency department. *Eur J Emerg Med* 2005;12:143-146.

The authors studied Lisfranc fracture-dislocations, with an emphasis on diagnosis in the emergency department. Level of evidence: V.

29. Haapamaki V, Kiuru M, Koskinen S: Lisfranc fracture-dislocation in patients with multiple trauma: Diagnosis with multidetector computed tomography. *Foot Ankle Int* 2004;25:614-619.

The authors assessed the use of multidetector CT in the diagnosis of Lisfranc fracture-dislocation in 282 patients. This modality is recommended as a complementary examination for patients with high-energy injury or multiple trauma, or for patients in whom radiographic studies are equivocal. Level of evidence: V.

30. Lu J, Ebraheim NA, Skie M, Porshinsky B, Yeasting RA: Radiographic and computed tomographic evaluation of Lisfranc dislocation: A cadaver study. *Foot Ankle Int* 1997;18:351-355.

31. Myerson MS, Fisher RT, Burgess AR, Kenzora JE: Fracture dislocations of the tarsometatarsal joints: End results correlated with pathology and treatment. *Foot Ankle* 1986;6:225-242.

32. Calder JD, Whitehouse SL, Saxby TS: Results of isolated Lisfranc injuries and the effect of compensation claims. *J Bone Joint Surg Br* 2004;86:527-530.

The authors retrospectively studied 46 patients with Lisfranc injuries and determined that treatment results were often unsatisfactory. Level of evidence: IV.

33. Richter M, Thermann H, Huefner T, et al: Chopart joint fracture-dislocation: Initial open reduction provides better outcome than closed reduction. *Foot Ankle Int* 2004;25:340-348.

     The authors determined that an initial anatomic reduction improved results in patients with combined Chopart-Lisfranc joint fracture-dislocations. Level of evidence: IV.

34. Allen LR, Flemming D, Sanders TG: Turf toe: Ligamentous injury of the first metatarsophalangeal joint. *Mil Med* 2004;169:xix-xxiv.

     The authors reviewed the anatomy of the first MTP joint, mechanism of injury, and clinical presentation of turf toe. Level of evidence: IV.

35. Mullen JE, O'Malley MJ: Sprains: Residual instability of subtalar, Lisfranc joints, and turf toe. *Clin Sports Med* 2004;23:97-121.

     The authors reviewed the relevant anatomy, mechanism of injury, and diagnostic methods for foot sprains.

36. Gaeta M, Minutoli F, Scribano E, et al: CT and MR imaging findings in athletes with early tibial stress injuries: Comparison with bone scintigraphy findings and emphasis on cortical abnormalities. *Radiology* 2005;235: 553-561.

     The authors determined that MRI best assesses patients with possible tibial stress injuries.

37. Brand JC Jr, Brindle T, Nyland J, Caborn DN, Johnson DL: Does pulsed low intensity ultrasound allow early return to normal activities when treating stress fractures? A review of one tarsal navicular and eight tibial stress fractures. *Iowa Orthop J* 1999;19:26-30.

38. Anderson RB, McBryde AM Jr: Autogenous bone grafting of hallux sesamoid nonunions. *Foot Ankle Int* 1997; 18:293-296.

39. Ekenman I, Tsai-Felländer L, Westblad P, Turan I, Rolf C: A study of intrinsic factors in patients with stress fractures of the tibia. *Foot Ankle Int* 1996;17:477-482.

40. Rome K, Handoll HH, Ashford R: Interventions for preventing and treating stress fractures and stress reactions of bone of the lower limbs in young adults. *Cochrane Database Syst Rev* 2005;2:CD000450.

     The authors determined that shock-absorbing inserts in footware are likely to reduce the incidence of stress fractures in military personnel. Pneumatic bracing may help rehabilitation after tibial stress fracture, but additional evidence is needed. Level of evidence: I.

41. Rue JP, Armstrong DW III, Frassica FJ, Deafenbaugh M, Wilckens JH: The effect of pulsed ultrasound in the treatment of tibial stress fractures. *Orthopedics* 2004;27:1192-1195.

     The authors studied whether pulsed ultrasound was effective in reducing healing time of tibial stress fractures. Results indicated that there was no significant reduction in healing time. Level of evidence: I.

42. Saxena A, Fullem B, Hannaford D: Results of treatment of 22 navicular stress fractures and a new proposed radiographic classification system. *J Foot Ankle Surg* 2000;39:96-103.

43. Gehrmann RM, Renard RL: Current concepts review: Stress fractures of the foot. *Foot Ankle Int* 2006;27: 750-757.

     Diagnosis and treatment of stress fractures of the foot are reviewed. Level of evidence: V.

44. Mologne TS, Lundeen JM, Clapper MF, O'Brien TJ: Early screw fixation versus casting in the treatment of acute Jones fractures. *Am J Sports Med* 2005;33:970-975.

     The authors determined that cast treatment is associated with a high incidence of failure than early screw fixation in patients with acute Jones fractures; early screw fixation leads to faster return to sports participation.

45. Mironov SP, Bogutskaia EV, Lomtatidze E: Stress fractures of the metatarsal bone in sportsmen (Jones' fracture). *Ortop Traumatol Protez* 1989;11:21-24.

46. Ogden JA, Ganey TM, Hill JD, Jaakkola JI: Sever's injury: A stress fracture of the immature calcaneal metaphysis. *J Pediatr Orthop* 2004;24:488-492.

     The authors discuss the diagnosis and etiology of Sever injury. Level of evidence: I.

3: Knee and Leg

Chapter 17

Athletic Ankle Injuries

Marty E. Reed, MD   Jonathan B. Feibel, MD   Brian G. Donley, MD   Eric Giza, MD

Introduction

Epidemiology

Although ankle injuries are frequently treated nonsurgically, an understanding of the pathoanatomy involved is important to allow the sports medicine physician to guide appropriate nonsurgical treatment as well as recognize when surgery is the best solution. Ankle sprains are very common, but these injuries are not benign. According to the literature, from 32% to 76% of these injuries are followed by residual pain, instability, or swelling.[1,2]

Lateral Ankle Sprains

Anatomy

Lateral ankle stability is conferred by both static and dynamic restraints. The dynamic restraints include the peroneus longus and brevis. The static restraints include both bony architecture as well as the lateral ligamentous structures.

The bony architecture of the talus, with its trapezoidal shape, confers significant stability in full dorsiflexion. In this position, the flared anterior portion of the talus is locked into the mortise, which provides bony resistance to lateral displacement and inversion. This is in contrast to ankle plantar flexion, when the narrowest portion of the talus is in the mortise and requires more reliance on the lateral ligamentous structures.

The lateral ligamentous complex of the ankle joint comprises the anterior talofibular ligament (ATFL), the calcaneofibular ligament (CFL), and the posterior talofibular ligament (PTFL) (Figure 1). The ATFL, the primary restraint to inversion in plantar flexion and the weakest of the lateral ligaments, resists anterolateral translation of the talus in the mortise. When the ankle is in neutral or dorsiflexed position, the CFL is the primary restraint to inversion. The CFL is extra-articular and spans both the tibiotalar and subtalar joints, thereby restraining subtalar inversion. The PTFL, the strongest of the collateral ligaments, connects the posterolateral tubercle of the talus to the posterior aspect of the lateral malleolus.[3]

Mechanism and Grading of Injury

Because of the narrow diameter of the talus posteriorly, ankle instability occurs in plantar flexion and inversion. Failure occurs in the anterolateral joint capsule first, followed by rupture of the ATFL and the CFL as the arc of injury progresses laterally. The ATFL is injured in 85% of lateral ankle sprains; the CFL is injured in 20% to 40%. Injury to the PTFL is rare.

When evaluating amateur soccer players, it was found that more than 80% of ankle sprains are contact injuries. These injuries also tend to occur in the beginning of the season and toward the end of the first half or the end of the game.[4]

Grade I lateral ankle injuries involve stretching of the ATFL, with mild tenderness, no evidence of mechanical instability, and ability to bear weight with minimal discomfort. Grade II injuries are complete tears of the ATFL, usually accompanied by a partial injury of the CFL. Grade III injuries are complete ruptures of the ATFL and CFL. Patients have severe tenderness and pain, and weight bearing is difficult.

Nonsurgical Treatment

Many meta-analyses have evaluated the optimal treatment of acute lateral ankle sprains.[5,6] Although studies have shown good and excellent results after 1 year for surgically repaired grade III lateral ankle ligament sprains, it has been shown that functional treatment offers the same good and excellent outcomes with a faster return to full range of motion, work, and physical activity, without the inherent risks and cost associated with surgery.[7]

Current opinion, practice patterns, and the literature support functional, nonsurgical management as the preferred method of treatment for all lateral ankle sprains. The question remains as to the optimal nonsurgical management of various grades of ankle sprains. Recently, a randomized controlled study was done to assess which type of external support was most effective when instituting early, controlled motion in the treatment of first-time lateral ankle sprains.[7] A combination of elastic wrap with an Air-Stirrup brace (Aircast, Inc, Summit, NJ) was significantly faster at returning patients with grade I or II ankle sprains to preinjury function compared with an elastic wrap alone, an Air-Stirrup brace alone, or a walking cast used for 10 days. Patients with grade III sprains in this study showed no

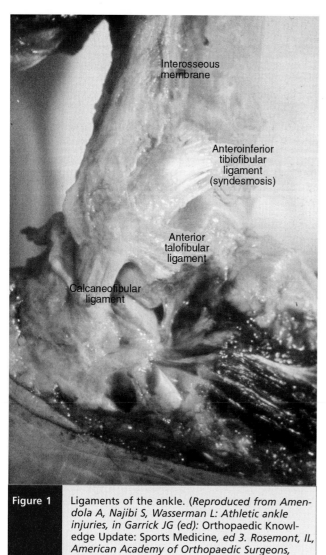

Figure 1 Ligaments of the ankle. (*Reproduced from Amendola A, Najibi S, Wasserman L: Athletic ankle injuries, in Garrick JG (ed): Orthopaedic Knowledge Update: Sports Medicine, ed 3. Rosemont, IL, American Academy of Orthopaedic Surgeons, 2004, pp 233-248.*)

Labels in figure: Interosseous membrane; Anteroinferior tibiofibular ligament (syndesmosis); Anterior talofibular ligament; Calcaneofibular ligament

difference in the time to return to normal function between an Air-Stirrup brace and a walking cast for 10 days. This is in contrast to previous studies, which have shown benefits with functional bracing over immobilization even for grade III lateral ankle sprains; however, the important distinction is the 10 days of immobilization in this group versus 4 to 5 weeks in other studies.[7]

Surgical Treatment

Lateral ligament rupture of the ankle has few indications for surgical repair. Even avulsion fractures of the distal fibula have been shown to heal readily without late instability when compared with purely ligamentous injuries.[8] Although there has historically been some controversy regarding grade III lateral ankle sprains as to whether they heal better with primary repair, there has been no recent literature that has shown definitively that surgical treatment is superior to nonsurgical treatment of grade III injuries.

Prevention

Several studies in the recent literature have examined the efficacy and cost of taping and various braces for the ankle. Taping and bracing have been effective in reducing the incidence of clinically significant ankle injuries. Although it has the initial highest passive stability, taping loses up to 50% of its mechanical effectiveness after approximately 20 minutes of exercise. In addition, it is much more difficult to adjust the tape during a sporting event, and this method has been shown to be more time-consuming and expensive than stirrup soft lace-up or strap ankle braces.[9-12]

Tape and braces provide direct mechanical support for an unstable ankle, but it also has been suggested that the beneficial effect is explained by enhancement of proprioception through skin pressure. Preparticipation taping has been found to decrease peroneal reaction time and increase firing of the peroneus brevis (PB) during the swing phase of gait; however, taping does not significantly reduce talar tilt or anterior translation.

A recent study of sports such as gymnastics, judo, and dance that typically do not involve shoe wear showed that the benefits of bracing are not necessarily applicable. Most of the passive stability characteristics of stirrup-type semirigid ankle braces are lost when used by barefoot athletes.[12]

Although bracing is important, overall fitness, body mass, and prevention programs play important roles in preventing ankle injuries. In a randomized controlled study of 765 high school soccer and basketball athletes, a statistically significant decrease in ankle injuries was seen in the group that was randomized to a balance control program when compared with the group that performed only standard conditioning exercises.[13]

Studies showing decreased rates of ankle sprains by using a proactive, proprioceptive training regimen coincide nicely with evidence showing differences in muscle activation patterns in patients with chronic ankle instability. Patients with chronic ankle instability tend to recruit not only the muscles around their ankles later but also the muscles about the knee and hip.[14,15] This information may offer improved therapy and prevention techniques as the focus shifts from just the ankle to the entire lower extremity. It is important to understand that prevention can be instituted using a multidisciplinary approach, including bracing, balance training, rehabilitation, and muscle recruitment evaluation for the entire lower extremity.

Sequelae of Acute Ankle Sprains and Chronic Lateral Ligamentous Insufficiency

It has been reported in the literature that residual disability after ankle sprain is present in 32% to 76% of patients.[2,16-18] Disability usually presents as residual swelling, pain, instability, or a combination of these symptoms. Elucidating the cause of disability can be a complex and challenging process and can be determined using physical examination, stress radiography, CT, MRI, or ankle arthroscopy.

Multiple diagnoses need to be considered in the patient with dysfunction after a lateral ankle sprain, including missed injuries of the ankle and hindfoot, injury to the peroneal tendons, base of the fifth metatarsal fractures, lateral or posterior process of the talus fractures, anterior process of the calcaneus injuries, or a missed syndesmotic injury. Other potential causes of persistent pain include osteochondral lesions of the talus or plafond, osseous or fibrous impingement, bone bruises, calcific ossicles between the medial or lateral malleolus, peroneal tears or subluxation, degenerative joint disease, tarsal coalition, or symptomatic os subfibulare. Neurologic diagnoses, such as complex regional pain syndrome, superficial peroneal nerve entrapment, and tarsal tunnel syndrome must also be considered. Subtalar instability can be the culprit of lateral ankle injury. This instability is usually a result of injury to either the CFL, the lateral talocalcaneal ligament, the interosseous talocalcaneal ligament, or the cervical ligament.

A thorough physical examination is a critical starting point in evaluating these injuries. However, some injuries, such as lateral process of the talus or anterior process of the calcaneus injuries, are best seen with CT. For soft-tissue injuries, including ligaments and tendons, MRI is the modality of choice. However, as shown in recent studies, intra-articular pathology, most notably osteochondral lesions, fibrous or soft-tissue impingement, and anterior inferior tibiofibular ligament injuries, are often missed on MRI, with sensitivities of MRI ranging from 0% for soft-tissue impingement to 82.4% for distal tibiofibular ligament injuries. For these injuries, ankle arthroscopy has been found to be highly sensitive and very effective at diagnosing as well as treating these specific conditions.[1] Therefore, ankle arthroscopy should be considered if residual ankle pain and instability cannot be diagnosed using standard clinical examination techniques and radiographic imaging.

Treatment varies depending on the etiology of the residual disability after a lateral ankle sprain. It should be noted that in more than 90% of cases, a functional rehabilitation program with strengthening of the peroneal muscles and proprioceptive training, combined with the use of braces for high-risk activities, is successful in treating chronic instability and pain. This is especially true of functional instability without objective measurements of mechanical instability.

Chronic dysfunction associated with laxity of the medial or lateral ligamentous structures of the ankle is called mechanical instability. The pain or sensation of instability that results from intra-articular or periarticular changes without ligamentous laxity is called functional instability. The two conditions can occur in combination.

Mechanical instability is generally accepted as 10 mm of anterior translation of the talus on the tibia or a difference of greater than 3 mm compared with the contralateral side when performing the anterior drawer test. In addition, radiographs taken with the foot in

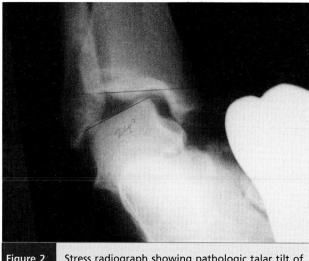

Figure 2 Stress radiograph showing pathologic talar tilt of 24° in relation to the plafond.

plantar flexion and the ankle subjected to an inversion stress showing greater than 9° of talar tilt or greater than 3° when compared with the contralateral extremity also indicates mechanical instability (**Figure 2**). If clinical examination, history, and radiologic evaluation are all consistent with functional instability and nonsurgical treatment fails, the standard of care is still an anatomic reconstruction of the CFL and ATFL known as the Gould modification of the Broström procedure (**Figures 3 and 4**). This procedure is described as an anatomic shortening of the ATFL and possibly the CFL, reinforced with the inferior extensor retinaculum. Follow-up results after 26 years have been published with this technique, showing excellent results for the treatment of chronic lateral ankle instability.[19]

Syndesmosis and Medial Ankle Sprains

Anatomy

The syndesmosis, continuous with the interosseous membrane proximally, is located at the level of the tibial plafond. It serves to maintain the relationship between the tibia and the fibula and is composed of four ligaments: the anteroinferior tibiofibular ligament (AITFL), the posteroinferior tibiofibular ligament (PITFL), the transverse tibiofibular ligament (TTFL), and the interosseous tibiofibular ligament (ITFL). The PITFL originates on the posterior aspect of the fibula and runs horizontally to the posterolateral distal tibia. This ligament has an approximate width of 18 mm and a thickness of 6 mm and is the strongest component of the syndesmosis. The AITFL originates from the anterior tibial tubercle and runs distally and laterally in an oblique fashion to insert onto the anteromedial distal fibula. This ligament has a width of approximately 18 mm and a thickness of 2 to 4 mm. An anomalous slip of the AITFL that can insert onto the distal anterior fibula is known as the Bassett ligament and can cause

3: Knee and Leg

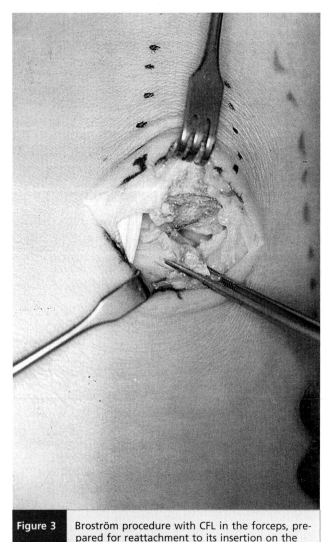

Figure 3   Broström procedure with CFL in the forceps, prepared for reattachment to its insertion on the fibula.

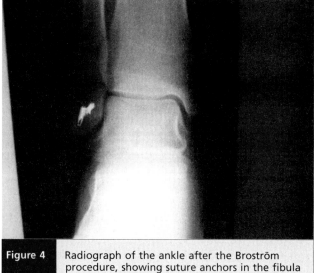

Figure 4   Radiograph of the ankle after the Broström procedure, showing suture anchors in the fibula and restoration of a normal tibiotalar relationship.

impingement with dorsiflexion. The TTFL is deep and inferior to the PITFL, extending over to the posterior aspect of the medial malleolus. The ITFL spans the space between the lateral tibia and medial fibula and is confluent with the proximal interosseous membrane. The ITFL is the main restraint to proximal migration of the talus between the tibia and the fibula.[20]

The deltoid ligament on the medial side of the ankle is composed of a superficial and deep layer. The superficial layer is a broad structure that originates from the anterior colliculus and fans out to insert into the navicular, neck of the talus, sustentaculum tali, and posteromedial talar tubercle. The tibiocalcaneal portion is the strongest component and resists eversion of the calcaneus. The deep portion of the deltoid is the primary medial stabilizer of the ankle joint. Unlike the superficial portion, it is organized into two short, thick, discrete bands: the anterior and posterior deep tibiotalar ligaments. Both of these ligaments are intra-articular but extrasynovial. The anterior portion arises from the anterior colliculus and attaches to the medial aspect of

the talus. The posterior band, the strongest of the entire deltoid complex, originates from the posterior colliculus and also inserts on the medial body of the talus.[21]

Mechanism of Injury

Although syndesmotic injuries have been reported to result from a variety of mechanisms, including inversion, and hyperplantar flexion, they most commonly result from a planted foot and a relative internal rotation of the leg and body with the foot planted. This position results in an external rotation of the talus in the mortise and thus an external rotatory force on the fibula, thereby separating it from the tibia and injuring the syndesmotic ligaments. Syndesmotic injuries tend to occur more frequently in sports that involve rigid immobilization of the ankle, such as hockey or skiing, as the ski or boot acts as a fulcrum by which the foot externally rotates in relation to the leg.[20]

Diagnosis

Syndesmotic ankle injuries or high ankle sprains are often underdiagnosed and difficult to detect. With the increased focus on these injuries as well as improved imaging methods, such as MRI, the ability to detect and treat these injuries is improving (**Figure 5**). However, even with recognition and treatment, it has been shown that syndesmosis involvement is the main predictor of chronic ankle dysfunction 6 months after ankle injury.[2]

Like with lateral ankle sprains, there is a spectrum of injuries ranging from severe injuries associated with fracture or gross diastasis as well as the more common subtle injuries without any abnormality of the distal tibiofibular relationship. It is the later injuries that are difficult to recognize and the choice of treatment may be controversial.

Patients with syndesmotic injuries typically have

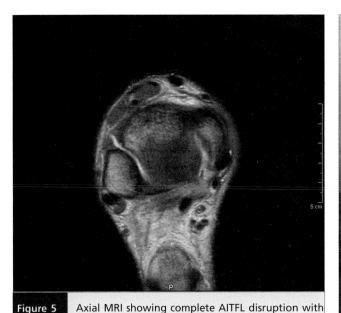

Figure 5 Axial MRI showing complete AITFL disruption with fluid extravasation through the injury.

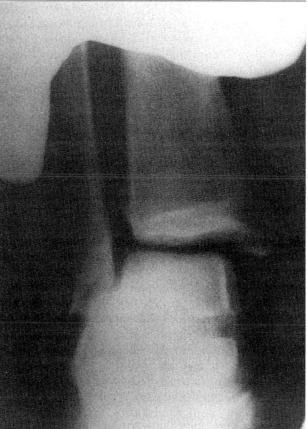

Figure 6 Stress radiograph showing a widened medial clear space and widening of the tibiofibular relationship, indicating that a syndesmotic injury has occurred.

point tenderness over the AITFL. In addition, there are several clinical tests designed to facilitate the diagnosis of these injuries, including the external rotation test, the squeeze test, the fibula translation test, and the Cotton test. In addition, a new test for syndesmosis injury that mimics the squeeze test, called the crossed-leg test, was described in a recent study.[25] This test is performed by having the sitting patient rest the mid tibia of the affected leg on the knee of the unaffected leg. A gentle downward force is applied to the medial side of the ankle; the test is positive if the patient experiences pain in the region of the syndesmosis.[22]

Imaging should begin with standard radiographs of the ankle to assess for fracture or gross diastases. Widening of more than 6 mm of the tibiofibular clear space on the AP radiograph is indicative of a syndesmotic injury (**Figure 6**). Many times, however, plain films are normal, so an MRI can be useful. In a study comparing MRI with diagnostic arthroscopy, MRI had a sensitivity of 100% and a specificity of 93% for diagnosis of an AITFL tear and sensitivity and specificity of 100% for diagnosis of PITFL tear.[23]

Nonsurgical Treatment

One of the more common classification systems used to describe syndesmotic injuries is called the West Point grading system.[2] Grade I indicates no instability, grade II indicates some evidence of instability, and grade III definite instability. Nonsurgical treatment is the treatment of choice for grade I injuries, and surgical treatment is generally preferred for grade III injuries, leaving much controversy without substantial literature regarding the optimal treatment of grade II injuries. Literature discussing nonsurgical or functional treatment of syndesmotic injuries share common themes in that the treatment is divided into stages. The first stage

involves protection of the injured joint and minimization of the inflammatory response including immobilization, ambulatory devices, nonsteroidal anti-inflammatory drugs, and ice. The extent of the injury will determine the extent of protection required. The second stage involves restoring mobility, strength, and function, with the primary goal of restoring a normal gait pattern with activities of daily living. The third stage is the gradual return to sports and continued therapy focused on strengthening and neuromuscular control so that the athlete can return to activities including jumping, pivoting, and twisting.

Surgical Treatment

Patients who have gross diastasis on plain radiographs, elite athletes with some evidence of instability, and those in whom prolonged functional rehabilitation fails are candidates for surgical treatment. Although there is debate on the optimal construct—two or three screws, metal or absorbable, three or four cortices—there is evidence that after the joint is stabilized, there can be a relatively rapid return to weight bearing and daily unrestricted activity within the first 2 to 3 weeks after surgical treatment. An aggressive rehabilitation program

3: Knee and Leg

instituted for West Point athletes allowed them to return to their sports in an average of 41 days (mean, 32 to 48 days).[24] Screw removal is advocated, and recommendations on when this should be done vary (from 6 weeks to 12 weeks after surgery). Four cortices allow medial side removal with broken hardware. One study showed that the foot position during fixation of the syndesmosis has no effect on postoperative range of motion.[25]

Haglund Deformity

Haglund deformity, or an enlarged posterolateral calcaneal tuberosity, is associated with various shoe types. Patients are typically women between ages 15 and 30 years. A simple pump bump is a chronic developing irritation of the adventitial bursa that causes thickening and pain and is aggravated by shoe wear. Pump bump often is accompanied by localized erythema and focal swelling.

Haglund deformity comprises a triad of retrocalcaneal bursitis, insertional Achilles tendinitis, and adventitial bursitis. An enlarged posterosuperior tuberosity of the calcaneus causes compression of the retrocalcaneal bursa against the Achilles tendon, with inflammation, thickening, and degeneration of the tendon occurring just proximally to its insertion. Subcutaneous thickening and swelling occur, along with palpable swelling anterior to the Achilles tendon. Nonsurgical treatment of Haglund deformity can relieve friction between the shoe counter, the adventitial bursa, the calcaneus, and the inflamed retrocalcaneal bursa. The patient should restrict activity, specifically hill running. Modifications should include relief of tight posterior heel counters, the use of heel lifts to decrease pressure on the retrocalcaneal bursa by decreasing the amount of dorsiflexion, and stretching and resultant lengthening of the Achilles tendon to decrease pressure on the bursa. Adjunctive treatment includes ice and anti-inflammatory medication.

Historically, surgical treatment was resection of the bony prominence and all of the surrounding inflamed bursal tissue. Both reinsertion of the tendon with drill holes and bone anchors have been effective. The key to a successful result is resection of an appropriate amount of bone. There are several methods for determining the amount of bony resection for surgical treatment of Haglund deformity. One such technique draws the calcaneal inclination line plantarly with a line paralleling this line, starting at the level of the base of the anterior process of the calcaneus and extending posteriorly. Then, a line is drawn with an angle of 50° to a point anterior to the Haglund deformity and resected posterior to this line. A recent prospective study has shown similar recovery times with fewer complications and improved cosmesis with endoscopic techniques than with open techniques.[26]

Posterior Tibial Tendon

The relevant anatomy of the medial ankle includes the posterior tibial tendon (PTT), the spring ligament, the deltoid ligament complex, and the articular relationship of the talonavicular and subtalar joints. The PTT has its origin on the posterior tibia, fibula, and interosseous membrane. It courses immediately posterior to the medial malleolus and inserts on the medial midfoot.[27]

In the athlete, injury to the PTT can occur with an eversion type injury or external rotation with a planted foot. The athlete will report medial pain and difficulty with push-off. Initial treatment includes rest in a cast or walking boot with medial longitudinal arch support. Physical therapy and strengthening of the tendon is important before return to sports to prevent chronic tendinitis.

In patients with chronic tendinitis, biomechanical overloading with push-off leads to chronic microtrauma in the tendon. With time, the tendon's elastic compliance decreases because of changes in collagen structure,[28] thus creating a pathologic sequence where tendon weakening results in failure of the static stabilizers of the arch. Poor blood supply may initiate this process or may prevent an adequate healing response, resulting in chronic inflammation, tenosynovitis, and tendinosis. In this setting, MRI is helpful to identify tearing of the tendon.

In the athlete without collapse of the longitudinal arch, surgical treatment with débridement of the synovium and direct repair of the tear are indicated. Return to sports is dependent on the amount of pathology but can take 4 to 6 months.

Accessory Navicular

In athletes with medial foot pain, especially skeletally immature elite athletes with an open physis, the accessory navicular should be included in the differential diagnosis. The diagnosis of an accessory navicular is based on careful physical examination and radiologic studies. Patients with an accessory navicular may present with point tenderness and erythema overlying the navicular tuberosity. Although they may have pain with resisted inversion, it is often not present during the physical examination because of the attachment of the PTT to the cuneiforms and the remainder of the navicular. When obtaining radiographs of the foot, it is always critical to order an oblique view because accessory naviculars can be missed on the AP and lateral views. When radiographs demonstrate an accessory navicular but it is not clear whether it is the source of pain, a bone scan or MRI can be helpful.

A type I accessory navicular is a sesamoid bone contained within the PTT that is rarely symptomatic. This type constitutes approximately 30% of all accessory naviculars. A type II accessory navicular, which is most commonly symptomatic, is an ossicle approximately 8

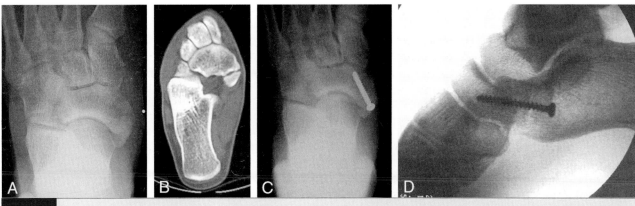

Figure 7 A large accessory navicular on a preoperative radiograph (**A**) and CT scan (**B**) fixed via open reduction and internal fixation on postoperative AP (**C**) and lateral (**D**) radiographs. *(Reproduced from Amendola A, Najibi S, Wasserman L: Athletic ankle injuries, in Garrick JG (ed): Orthopaedic Knowledge Update: Sports Medicine, ed 3. Rosemont, IL, American Academy of Orthopaedic Surgeons, 2004, pp 233-248.)*

to 12 mm adjacent to the parent navicular that is separated by an area of cartilage 1 to 3 mm thick. A type III accessory navicular is an ossicle united to the navicular by a bony bridge that forms a prominent navicular tuberosity.

Initial treatment of a symptomatic accessory navicular involves relieving the stress on the synchondrosis to allow healing, with modalities such as rest, anti-inflammatory medication, and soft shoe inserts. In young patients, these symptoms often will improve spontaneously with growth. In patients with a pronated foot, an orthotic and arch support with medial heel posting may be used and, once symptoms resolve, continued for a minimum of 6 months. Rigid orthotics increase pressure over the bony prominence of the accessory navicular and can worsen the symptoms. Cast treatment is reserved for patients with more severe symptoms; however, bony union between the accessory and primary navicular has been reported to be only between 10% and 14%.[29]

Patients who do not respond to nonsurgical treatment can be treated with surgery. Although smaller accessory naviculars can be excised,[33] larger fragments leave a sizable and unwanted defect in the PTT. In these cases, either fixation with a screw in skeletally mature patients or drilling percutaneously in patients with an open physis of the proximal phalanx of the great toe have both been shown to be effective[31,32] (**Figure 7**).

Flexor Hallucis Longus Tendon

The flexor hallucis longus (FHL) is a bipennate muscle that originates from the lower two thirds of the posterior aspect of the fibula and the interosseous membrane. Its tendinous portion begins high in the muscle belly; distally, the muscle extends low on the tendon. The FHL tendon runs on the posterior aspect of the tibia distally, lateral and posterior to the tibialis posterior and flexor digitorum longus (FDL) between the

medial and lateral talar tubercles. The lateral talar tubercle can ossify and form a synchondrosis known as the os trigonum. This can irritate the FHL tendon and become a source of pain in some patients. The FHL tendon then passes underneath the flexor retinaculum in the tarsal tunnel along with the tibialis posterior and FDL. Distally, it courses along the medial surface of the calcaneus in a fibro-osseous tunnel under the roof of the sustentaculum tali. Both the FHL and FDL tendons are bound to the vault of the arch by a common tendon sheath, the master knot of Henry. It is at the master knot of Henry, approximately 2 cm lateral to the navicular tuberosity, that the tendons cross. The FHL tendon progresses medially to the hallux, and the FDL tendon continues laterally to the lesser toes.

Stenosing tenosynovitis and or nodular tendinosis of the FHL tendon often is triggered by repetitive trauma. The repetitive and extreme plantar flexion experienced by ballet dancers makes them especially vulnerable to this condition. On physical examination, the patient may have pain anywhere along the course of the tendon from the base of the first metatarsal in between the sesamoids to the posteromedial ankle, although the most common area is behind the sustentaculum tali within its fibro-osseous tunnel. If a nodule is present in the tendon, full extension of the hallucal interphalangeal joint with the ankle in full dorsiflexion may be difficult or impossible because the nodular tendon cannot pass between the retinaculum spanning the medial and lateral tibial tubercles. The patient may also report triggering in this situation. Active plantar flexion of the hallux against resistance typically reproduces the pain. It is important to distinguish these symptoms from other entities seen in dancers, such as posterior impingement. This, in contrast, is exacerbated with extreme ankle plantar flexion, a maneuver that should not irritate FHL tenosynovitis. Finally, radiographs should be obtained to determine the presence of an os trigonum that may be irritating the FHL tendon. An

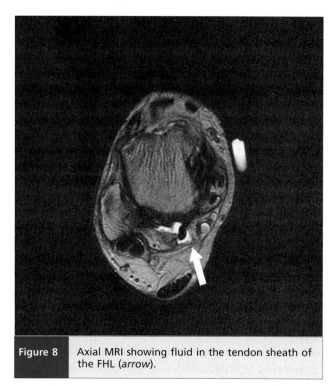

Figure 8 Axial MRI showing fluid in the tendon sheath of the FHL (*arrow*).

MRI will show fluid along the FHL tendon sheath (Figure 8).

Nonsurgical treatment should include a temporary reduction in activities and avoidance of jumping and point work during activity. In addition, a protocol of nonsteroidal anti-inflammatory drugs and physical therapy may provide relief. In patients who do not respond to nonsurgical treatment, surgical release of the fibro-osseous tunnel may be done.

Peroneal Tendons

Anatomy

The peroneals lie in the lateral compartment, originating from the lateral aspect of the fibula proximally. The PB has a muscle belly that extends further distally onto the tendon as it courses in the fibular groove. The PB is in direct contact with the posterior surface of the lateral malleolus and lies just anterior to the peroneus longus in a fibro-osseous tunnel bordered by the fibula and the superior retinaculum. This anterior position of the PB makes it more susceptible to attritional tears. The morphology of the posterior fibular retromalleolar groove is variable, with anywhere from 10% and 20% being flat or convex in shape.[33] The superior peroneal retinaculum inserts onto a fibrocartilaginous rim on the posterolateral fibula and can be seen on radiographs as an avulsion with acute peroneal dislocations. Although the PB follows a straightforward path to insert onto the base of the fifth metatarsal, the peroneus longus curves underneath the peroneal trochlea (a protuberance on the lateral aspect of the calcaneus) and then courses

through the cuboid tunnel to insert onto the base of the medial cuneiform as well as the first metatarsal.[21,34]

The peroneal tendons are the primary evertors of the foot and confer some stability to the lateral ankle. They can be injured either directly (usually a laceration), indirectly (repeated ankle sprains or calcaneus fracture), or through attrition (overuse, heel varus, entrapment, or chronic subluxation). Peroneal tenosynovitis, subluxation, dislocation, and tears have been reported in athletes and nonathletes.

Peroneal Tenosynovitis

Peroneal tenosynovitis can be caused by inversion injury to the ankle, anomalous extension of the PB tendon into the fibular groove, the presence of a large peroneal tubercle or os perineum, or acute trauma, such as an inversion injury or calcaneus fracture. Stenosing tenosynovitis is characterized by painful swelling with tenderness along the path of the peroneal tendons as they course behind the lateral malleolus, around the peroneal tubercle, and under the cuboid. This pain is often reproduced with forceful foot eversion. There is an association between lateral ankle instability and peroneal tenosynovitis. Coexisting peroneal tenosynovitis was present in 47 of 61 ankles undergoing surgery for chronic lateral ankle instability.[35]

Treatment of peroneal tenosynovitis should initially be nonsurgical. Nonsteroidal medications along with rest, shoe modifications such as a lateral heel wedge, and immobilization in a boot or cast are the first lines of treatment. A 6-week course of immobilization and nonsurgical treatment should be instituted before considering surgical treatment. Steroids should not be injected into the area because tendon rupture can occur. Surgical tenosynovectomy can be considered in patients with recalcitrant symptoms; however, it is important to recognize underlying pathology such as chronic ankle instability, calcaneus malunion, or varus hindfoot so that the underlying cause also can be treated surgically.

Peroneal Tendon Subluxation and Dislocation

Acute peroneal dislocations are commonly associated with trauma during athletic events such as skiing or football and are often accompanied by a palpable or audible snap. It is generally believed that a position of extreme dorsiflexion and inversion is responsible for this injury. The superior peroneal retinaculum is avulsed from the fibula and will commonly bring with it a piece of periosteum or cortical bone that can be seen on an oblique radiograph. On physical examination, there will be diffuse lateral swelling and ecchymosis with tenderness posteriorly along the course of the peroneal tendons. A key diagnostic examination is apprehension with resisted eversion testing of the foot. These injuries are commonly misdiagnosed as an acute lateral ankle sprain; however, the distinction should easily be made because ankle sprains have tenderness about the anterior lateral aspect of the fibula over the

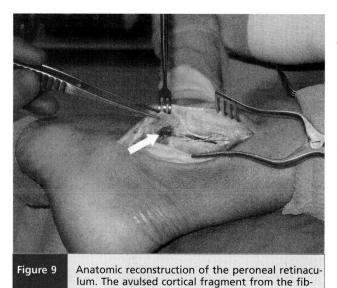

Figure 9 Anatomic reconstruction of the peroneal retinaculum. The avulsed cortical fragment from the fibula is seen (*arrow*).

ATFL and CFL and should not have tenderness over the peroneal tendons.

Although it has been shown that there is a greater than 50% success rate of nonsurgical treatment with casting for 6 weeks in slight plantar flexion, it is generally recommended that the young athlete have surgery for acute injury.[36] Surgery for an acute injury is less complicated than that for chronic injury. Generally, the avulsed cortical fragment or torn peroneal retinaculum is anatomically repaired and then plicated as necessary.

Chronic peroneal subluxation rarely responds to nonsurgical treatment. There are several different potential surgical procedures that can be used singly or in combination, including anatomic repair and plication of the peroneal retinaculum, deepening of the retrofibular peroneal groove, fibular osteotomy, or reconstruction of the peroneal retinaculum with autograft or allograft as needed (**Figure 9**).

Peroneal Tendon Tears

A peroneal tendon tear is commonly associated with preexisting pain and disability from a peroneal tenosynovitis. A partial tear should be considered in a patient with a presumed diagnosis of tenosynovitis in whom nonsurgical treatment is unsuccessful; in this instance, MRI is warranted. If MRI reveals a longitudinal attritional tear, then an initial course of nonsurgical treatment, similar to the course of treatment of tenosynovitis, is warranted. If nonsurgical treatment fails, then surgical treatment is needed. A complete rupture is an indication for surgical treatment. Complete tendon rupture can lead to recurrent ankle sprains and ankle instability.

The algorithm for surgical treatment of partial chronic complete, partial, or longitudinal tears of both peroneal tendons was outlined in a recent study.[37] Intraoperatively, if both tendons were grossly intact and the tears were repairable, then tendon débridement and

repair were performed. If one tendon was irreparable, then tenodesis to the intact tendon was performed. If neither tendon was salvageable, then a tendon graft (hamstring allograft) or a tendon transfer (FDL to PB) was performed. Any concurrent deformity as well as instability of the hindfoot or the ankle was corrected at the same time.[37]

Osteochondral Lesions of the Talus

Talar cartilage is distinctly different from other regions of the body in terms of its macroscopic properties and response to aging. Talar articular cartilage is thinner than that in the knee and hip. Biomechanical studies have shown that talar articular cartilage maintains its mechanical properties much more favorably as it ages.[38-40] The difference in mechanical properties may explain the higher incidence of nontraumatic arthritis in the knee than the ankle.

Athletes with cartilage damage to the talus will report swelling and medial or lateral ankle pain associated with training. An ankle sprain that has failed to completely heal by 8 weeks should raise suspicion of a talus cartilage injury. The patient may have a normal examination without evidence of instability; however, direct pressure over the talus with the ankle in plantar flexion will elicit tenderness.

The Berndt Harty radiographic system is commonly used to classify talus injuries.[41] A type I lesion is exemplified by subchondral compression; a type II lesion is a partially detached osteochondral fragment; a type III lesion is completely detached; and a type IV lesion is completely detached and displaced.[42] The advent of MRI and direct arthroscopic grading has increased understanding of cartilage lesions because many cartilage lesions are not seen on plain radiographs. The combined use of radiographs, MRI, and arthroscopy is essential to optimize the treatment of these lesions.

Medial lesions occur more frequently, and both medial and lateral lesions are more commonly located in the middle portion of the talar dome. Traumatic lesions occur on both the lateral and medial aspects of the talar dome.[43] The lateral injuries are more often delamination type injuries (**Figures 10 and 11**). The size of the lesion plays an important role for treatment because smaller lesions respond more effectively to simple curettage or microfracture.

The high failure rate with nonsurgical treatment of talar dome lesions has been documented.[7] According to a review of the literature, the success rate for nonsurgical treatment is 45%.[44] The long-term results of arthroscopic débridement, curettage, and drilling have been favorable, with successful outcomes in approximately 85% of patients.

For athletes, ankle arthroscopy is recommended, which is an effective means for diagnosis and treatment of lesions of the talus, with up to 85% of patients improving after arthroscopic drilling or curettage. Re-

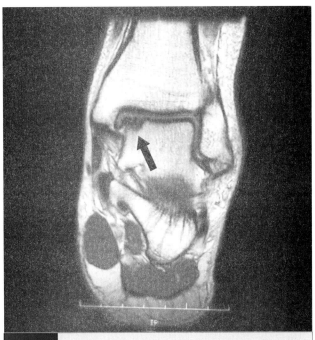

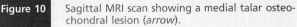

Figure 10 | Sagittal MRI scan showing a medial talar osteo-chondral lesion (*arrow*).

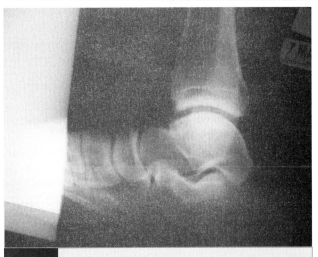

Figure 12 | Radiograph showing an osteophyte on the anterior node of the talus and anterior portion of the tibia, resulting in anterior impingement with dorsiflexion.

moval of damaged cartilage and treatment with microfracture rather than indirect, subchondral drilling will result in improved outcomes.[45] Larger lesions that fail to improve 6 months after arthroscopy should be considered for osteochondral grafting or autologous chondrocyte implantation. Osteochondral grafting (both autograft and allograft) of defects have yielded 91% to 94% good to excellent results; however, arthroscopic autologous chondrocyte implantation procedures using direct implantation or collagen scaffolds also have favorable results.

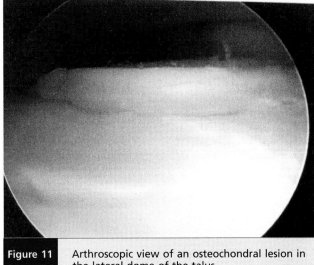

Figure 11 | Arthroscopic view of an osteochondral lesion in the lateral dome of the talus.

Ankle Impingement Syndrome

Anterior Bony Impingement

Both osseous and soft-tissue lesions can be responsible for anterior ankle pain associated with ankle dorsiflexion. When osseous lesions on the anterior portion of the tibia or talar neck are responsible, it is commonly referred to as footballer's (soccer player's) ankle (**Figure 12**). The term footballer's ankle was first used in the 1950s to describe the debilitating osteophytes of the distal tibia and talar neck found in up to 60% of football players. The characteristic locations are the medial aspect of the talar neck and lateral to the midline of the anterior distal tibia. Athletes will have a palpable ridge of bone at the medial or central distal tibia that can commonly be painful with palpation. These lesions may also cause pain with dorsiflexion and difficulty with cutting and push-off.

Lateral radiographs of the ankle may reveal osteophytes on the anterior tibia and talar neck. Although these spurs have been described as kissing osteophytes, studies of CT scans have shown that they in fact occur in different areas in relation to the midline and often do not contact one another with dorsiflexion, The anterior tibial spur tends to lie lateral to the midline, while the talar spur often lies medial to the midline. It is important to include oblique anteromedial radiographs because these osteophytes may not be visible on a true lateral radiograph. Chronic changes of the talar surface can occur from the osteophytes. Studies have described a divot sign of the talar neck and a tram track fissure of the talar dome articular cartilage surface corresponding to the offending spurs.[46,47]

The etiology of anterior impingement is likely a time-dependent exposure to football (soccer) and is represented by two theories. First, the spur formation could be caused by excessive stretching of the anterior capsule, resulting microtrauma, scar formation, and then ossification. The second, and more likely, theory is that direct trauma causes the inflammation and resultant spurring. A laboratory study of 150 kicking actions by 15 elite football players found that maximal plantar flexion and stretching of the capsule occurred in only 39% of the kicks, but direct trauma to the anteromedial tibia occurred in 76%.[48] A follow-up cadaver study showed that the anterior capsule inserts on average 1.5 cm from the distal tibia rather than the area where the spurring is located. Lateral instability can also contribute to spur formation. According to one study, spurs were 3.4 times more prevalent in patients undergoing a Broström procedure.[49]

Initial treatment can include rest, ice, and range-of-motion exercises for acute grade I injuries; however, arthroscopic treatment has been shown to be effective. According to one study, 90% of patients without joint space narrowing (grades I to III) and 73% of patients with pain for less than 2 years improved significantly.[50] These ankles are typically not osteoarthritic and therefore respond well to arthroscopic treatment with spur excision. Therefore, it is recommended that players with new symptoms and a positive examination undergo arthroscopic excision.

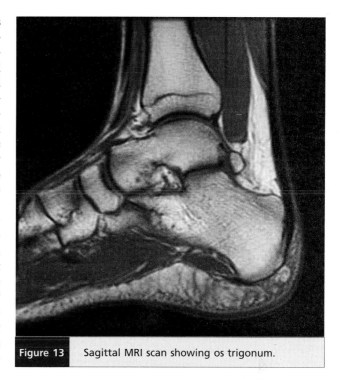

Figure 13   Sagittal MRI scan showing os trigonum.

Posterior Bony Impingement (Os Trigonum)

Chronic changes in the posterior aspect of the ankle can occur medially or laterally and include bony or soft-tissue pathology. Irritation or fracture of the os trigonum, which is an ununited lateral tubercle of the posterior talus, or an enlarged talar tubercle can occur from a hyperplantar flexion injury where the structures are pinched between the tibia and os calcis (**Figure 13**). This pain has classically been described as posterolateral pain, anterior to the Achilles tendon. This pain commonly occurs in dancers and can be distinguished from FHL tenosynovitis by pain reproduced with extreme plantar flexion. Fracture of the os or disruption of the synchondrosis can also be seen in other sports, such as soccer with kicking.[42,51] Work-up includes radiographs, which will commonly demonstrate evidence of the os trigonum or bony prominence. MRI can also be useful to assess for edema in or around the posterior talus or os trigonum. Initial treatment with rest and prevention of plantar flexion with bracing will be effective in 60% of athletes; however, continued symptoms respond well to open or arthroscopic excision. The open approach is just lateral to the Achilles tendon, taking care not to disturb the sural nerve.

Impingement of the soft tissues can occur both anteromedially and posteromedially. Stenosing tenosynovitis of the FHL, hypertrophy of the posterior capsule, and enlargement of the posterior intermalleolar ligament can lead to chronic posterior pain that necessitates surgical intervention. Rarely, anomalous muscles, such as an accessory soleus or peroneus quartus, can cause continued pain after a sprain. According to a recent study, excision is usually curative and allows a return to play.[52]

Soft-Tissue Impingement of the Ankle

Soft-tissue impingement of the ankle is common after repeated ankle sprains. Hemorrhage into the joint results in traumatic synovitis and scarring in the ligaments about the ankle. Although most of the time this tissue is resorbed, occasionally it becomes thickened and scarred, resulting in a synovial impingement lesion. The soft-tissue impingement lesions can involve the syndesmosis, the anterior and lateral gutters, or posteriorly in the syndesmosis or posterior gutter.

The most common area of impingement is anterolateral because of the mechanism of a lateral ankle sprain. This involves thickening of either the ATFL or the inferior portion of the AITFL and the surrounding tissues. This anterolateral impingement has been classically referred to as a meniscoid lesion, trapping a mass of hyalinized tissue between the fibula and talus[53] (**Figure 14**). Other etiologies to consider include the Bassett ligament, which is an anomalous band of the AITFL, as well as the extensor digitorum longus, which can cause symptoms by impinging on the anterolateral surface of the talar head. If the extensor digitorum longus is suspected as the source of the pain, a dynamic ultrasound is useful to confirm the diagnosis. Tenolysis of the tendon with exostectomy of the talar head has been shown to be very effective.

On physical examination, the patient will report vague anterior or anterolateral ankle pain. Patients will commonly have tenderness to palpation along the inferior syndesmosis as well as in the anterior gutter and along the ATFL. Radiographs are rarely helpful, but MRI has been shown to be useful.

Most patients with soft-tissue impingement of the anterior lateral ankle do not respond well to nonsurgi-

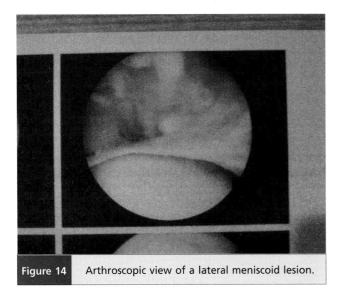

Figure 14 Arthroscopic view of a lateral meniscoid lesion.

cal treatment. Arthroscopy is the treatment of choice and has been shown to be very effective at relieving the symptoms, with good and excellent results seen in recent studies. Arthroscopic examination will reveal significant synovitis, scar tissue, and hemosiderin, whereas histologic examination will reveal chronic inflammation, synovial hyperplasia, and fibrosis.[54]

Summary

The most frequent ankle injury encountered in sports is a sprain of the lateral ligament complex. Proper postinjury rehabilitation and proprioceptive training remain the standard for nonsurgical treatment. Anatomic reconstruction of the lateral ligament complex is favored when surgical intervention is necessary. Recognition of medial ligament and syndesmosis injuries is important because these injuries can lead to increased time lost from athletic participation. Disorders of the Achilles, posterior tibial, and peroneal tendons require early detection and treatment to prevent progression to chronic tendinosis. Osteochondral lesions of the talus, as well as anterior/posterior impingement of the ankle, often result from chronic ankle instability and repetitive trauma. Because of the frequency of ankle injury in the athlete, a thorough understanding of the wide spectrum of pathology is needed.

Annotated References

1. Takao M, Uchio Y, Naito K, Fukazawa I, Ochi M: Arthroscopic assessment for intra-articular disorders in residual ankle disability after sprain. *Am J Sports Med* 2005;33:686-692.

    Ankle arthroscopy is a useful tool in identifying intra-articular disorders of the talocrural joint in cases of residual ankle disability after a sprain. The study results suggest that arthroscopy can be used to diagnose the cause of residual pain after an ankle sprain in most cases that are otherwise undiagnosable by clinical examination and imaging study. Level of evidence: II.

2. Gerber JP, Williams GN, Scoville CR, Arciero RA, Taylor CD: Persistent disability associated with ankle sprains: A prospective examination of an athletic population. *Foot Ankle Int* 1998;19:653-660.

3. Amendola A, Najibi S, Wasserman L: Athletic ankle injuries, in Garrick JG (ed): *Orthopaedic Knowledge Update: Sports Medicine*, ed 3. Rosemont, IL, American Academy of Orthopaedic Surgeons, 2004, pp 233-248.

    The anatomy of the lateral ankle is discussed.

4. Kofotolis ND, Kellis E, Vlachopoulos SP: Ankle sprain injuries and risk factors in amateur soccer players during a 2-year period. *Am J Sports Med* 2007;35:458-466.

    This study attempted to identify the incidence of ankle sprain injuries, associated time loss of participation, and risk factors during two consecutive seasons in amateur players. A total of 336 athletes were enrolled in the study; 312 male amateur soccer players were observed during a 2-year period. During the study, 208 ankle injuries were recorded, of which 139 were ankle sprains. These led to 975 sessions lost (on average, 7 lost sessions per injury). Most incidents (80.6%) were contact injuries, occurring mostly in defenders. Injury rates were equal between games and practices, whereas 61.1% of injuries were observed toward the end of each half of the game ($P < 0.05$). The injury incidence rate was higher during the first 2 months of the season as opposed to the last month ($P < 0.05$).

5. Kerkhoffs GMMJ, Rowe BH, Assendelft WJ, Kelly K, Struijs PA, van Dijk CN: Immobilization and functional treatment for acute lateral ankle injuries in adults. *Cochrane Database Syst Rev* 2002;3:CD003762.

6. Kerkhoffs GMMJ, Struijs PA, Marti RK, Assendelft WJ, Blankevoort L, van Dijk CN: Different functional treatment strategies for acute lateral ankle ligament injuries in adults. *Cochrane Database Syst Rev* 2002;3: CD002938.

7. Beynnon BD, Renström PA, Haugh L, Uh BS, Barker H: A prospective, randomized clinical investigation of the treatment of first-time ankle sprains. *Am J Sports Med* 2006;34:1401-1412.

    Treatment of grade I sprains with the Air-Stirrup brace combined with an elastic wrap returned subjects to normal walking and stair climbing in half the time required for those treated with the Air-Stirrup brace alone and in half the time required for those treated with an elastic wrap alone. Treatment of grade II sprains with the Air-Stirrup brace combined with the elastic wrap allowed patients to return to normal walking and stair climbing in the shortest time interval. Treatment of grade III sprains with the Air-Stirrup brace or a walking cast for 10 days followed by bracing returned subjects to normal walking and stair climbing in the same time intervals. The 6-month follow-up of each sprain severity group revealed no difference between the treatments of frequency of reinjury, ankle motion, and function. Level of evidence: I.

8. Haraguchi N, Toga H, Shiba N, Kato F: Avulsion fracture of the lateral ankle ligament complex in severe inversion injury. *Am J Sports Med* 2007;35:1144-1152.

A total of 169 consecutive patients with severe inversion injury were classified into a ligament rupture group or an avulsion fracture group on the basis of physical examination findings and ATFL and CFL radiographic views. Patients in both groups were treated with casting. Follow-up examinations of 152 patients included clinical assessment and functional evaluation based on the Karlsson system. Avulsion fracture was diagnosed in 44 (26%) of the 169 patients and was most common among children and patients older than 40 years. Sedentary level activity and low-energy injury were more common in the avulsion fracture group than in the ligament rupture group (77% compared with 37%, respectively, $P = 0.001$; 68% compared with 43%, respectively, $P = 0.004$). Nonsurgical treatment of avulsion fracture (mean Karlsson score, 89.1 points) yielded satisfactory results that were comparable with those of nonsurgical treatment of ligament rupture (mean Karlsson score, 88.4 points) ($P = 0.123$). Osseous union was achieved in 65% of the patients with avulsion fracture. Level of evidence: II.

9. Verhagen EA, van der Beek AJ, van Mechelen W: The effect of tape, braces and shoes on ankle range of motion. *Sports Med* 2001;31:667-677.

10. Metcalfe RC, Schlabach GA, Looney MA, Renehan EJ: A comparison of moleskin tape, linen tape, and lace-up brace on joint restriction and movement performance. *J Athl Train* 1997;32:136-140.

11. Pedowitz DI, Reddy S, Parekh SG, Huffman GR, Sennett BJ: Prophylactic bracing decreases ankle injuries in collegiate female volleyball players. *Am J Sports Med* 2008;36:324-327.

Injury data, preparticipation medical histories, and total exposure data were collected prospectively on female volleyball players from 1998 to 2005. Injuries and exposures were defined based on established National Collegiate Athletic Association (NCAA) Injury Surveillance System criteria. Injury rate was calculated as the number of injuries per 1000 exposures. The NCAA female volleyball injury data from 1998 to 2005 were used for comparison. During the study period, there were a total of 13,500 exposures and 1 injury, yielding an injury rate of 0.07 per 1,000 exposures. Nearly half of the athletes had a preparticipation history of ankle sprains, yet only 1 ankle injury occurred during all of the braced exposures. There were 811,710 exposures and 797 injuries in the NCAA comparison group, with an increased injury rate of 0.98 per 1,000 exposures ($P = 0.001$). Prophylactic use of a double-upright ankle brace significantly reduced the ankle injury rate compared with that reported by the NCAA. Level of evidence: IV.

12. Eils E, Imberge S, Völker K, Rosenbaum D: Passive stability characteristics of ankle braces and tape in simulated barefoot and shod conditions. *Am J Sports Med* 2007;35:282-287.

Twenty-five healthy subjects participated in the project (mean age, 26.2 ± 3.3 years; mean body mass, 71.2 ± 10.3 kg; mean height, 178 ± 7 cm). Passive range of motion measurements were performed with three different ankle stabilizers as well as two different shoe conditions. In the simulated barefoot condition, a significantly reduced stabilizing effect for inversion and eversion (19% and 29%, respectively) was found for the stirrup ankle brace. Small decreases were noted with the soft brace and tape, but these were not statistically significant. The passive stability characteristics of ankle braces depend to a great extent on being used in combination with a shoe. This is especially true for semirigid braces with a stirrup design. It is recommended that soft braces (such as the one tested in the present investigation) be used in barefoot sports for restricting passive range of motion of the foot and ankle complex.

13. McGuine TA, Keene JS: The effect of a balance training program on the risk of ankle sprains in high school athletes. *Am J Sports Med* 2006;34:1103-1111.

Seven hundred sixty-five high school soccer and basketball players (523 girls and 242 boys) were randomly assigned to either an intervention group (27 teams, 373 subjects) that participated in a balance training program or to a control group (28 teams, 392 subjects) that performed only standard conditioning exercises. On-site athletic trainers recorded athlete exposures and sprains. The rate of ankle sprains was significantly lower for subjects in the intervention group (6.1%, 1.13 of 1,000 exposures compared with 9.9%, 1.87 of 1,000 exposures; $P = 0.04$). Athletes with a history of an ankle sprain had a twofold increased risk of sustaining a sprain (risk ratio, 2.14), whereas athletes who performed the intervention program decreased their risk of a sprain by 50% (risk ratio, 0.56). The ankle sprain rate for athletes without previous sprains was 4.3% in the intervention group and 7.7% in the control group, but this difference was not significant ($P = 0.059$). A balance training program will significantly reduce the risk of ankle sprains in high school soccer and basketball players. Level of evidence: I.

14. Van Deun S, Staes FF, Stappaerts KH, Janssens L, Levin O, Peers K: Relationship of chronic ankle instability to muscle activation patterns during the transition from double-leg to single-leg stance. *Am J Sports Med* 2007;35:274-281.

Thirty control subjects and 10 subjects with chronic ankle instability participated in the study. The onset of muscle activity of 14 muscles of the lower limb and trunk was measured during the transition from a double-leg stance position to a single-leg stance position in eyes-open and eyes-closed test conditions. Subjects with chronic ankle instability showed significantly later onset times for the ankle, hip, and hamstring muscles compared with control subjects. Subjects with chronic ankle instability show less variability in muscle activation patterns between test conditions.

15. Larsen E, Lund PM: Peroneal muscle function in chronically unstable ankles. A prospective preoperative and postoperative electromyographic study. *Clin Orthop Relat Res* 1991;272:219-226.

16. Bosien WR, Staple OS, Russell SW: Residual disability following acute ankle sprains. *J Bone Joint Surg Am* 1955;37:1237-1243.

17. Jackson DW, Ashley RL, Powell JW: Ankle sprains in young athletes: Relation of severity and disability. *Clin Orthop Relat Res* 1974;101:201-215.

18. Lentell G, Baas B, Lopez D, McGuire L, Sarrels M, Snyder P: The contributions of proprioceptive deficits, muscle function, and anatomic laxity to functional instability of the ankle. *J Orthop Sports Phys Ther* 1995;21:206-215.

19. Bell SJ, Mologne TS, Sitler DF, Cox JS: Twenty-six-year results after Broström procedure for chronic lateral ankle instability. *Am J Sports Med* 2006;34:975-978.

    Thirty-one male patients (32 ankles) who underwent the Broström procedure for chronic lateral ankle instability while enrolled as students at the United States Naval Academy were identified. Each patient was mailed a questionnaire that included a functional outcome measure as described by Roos and associates, a score described by Good and associates, and a single-number ankle functional assessment. The mean age was 20.7 years (range, 18–23 years) at the time of the operation. A functional outcome score was completed on each patient, with a mean follow-up of 26.3 years (range, 24.6 to 27.9 years). The follow-up included 22 of the 31 original patients. The mean numeric score for overall ankle function was 91.2 of 100 (standard deviation, 10.2). The foot and ankle outcome score (described by Roos and associates) was 92.0 (92%; standard deviation, 12.8) averaged over five functional areas. Ninety-one percent of the patients described their ankle function as good or excellent using the scale devised by Good and associates. The long-term results of the Broström procedure for chronic lateral ankle instability were excellent with 26-year follow-up. Level of evidence: IV.

20. Williams GN, Jones MH, Amendola A: Syndesmotic ankle sprains in athletes. *Am J Sports Med* 2007;35:1197-1207.

    This article discusses the anatomy, mechanism of injury, diagnosis, and treatment of syndesmosis sprains of the ankle while identifying controversies in management and topics for future research.

21. De Asla RJ, Deland JT: Anatomy and biomechanics of the foot and ankle, in Thordarson DB (ed): *Foot and Ankle Orthopaedic Surgery Essentials.* Philadelphia, PA, Lippincott Williams and Wilkins, 2004, pp 8-9.

    The authors discuss foot and ankle anatomy and biomechanics.

22. Kiter E, Bozkurt M: The crossed-leg test for examination of ankle syndesmosis injuries. *Foot Ankle Int* 2005;26:187-188.

    The crossed-leg test is used to assess ankle syndesmosis injuries.

23. Takao M, Ochi M, Oae K, Naito K, Uchio Y: Diagnosis of a tear of the tibiofibular syndesmosis: The role of arthroscopy of the ankle. *J Bone Joint Surg Br* 2003;85:324-329.

    The authors compared the accuracy of standard AP radiographs, mortise radiographs, and MRI with arthroscopy of the ankle in 52 patients for the diagnosis of a tear of the tibiofibular syndesmosis. Because standard AP and mortise radiographs did not always provide a correct diagnosis and MRI resulted in two false-positive results, the authors suggest the use of arthroscopy for accurate diagnosis of ankle tears.

24. Taylor DC, Tenuta JJ, Uhorchak JM, Arciero RA: Aggressive surgical treatment and early return to sports in athletes with grade III syndesmosis sprains. *Am J Sports Med* 2007;35:1833-1838.

    A consecutive series of intercollegiate athletes treated surgically with 4.5-mm cortical screw fixation for grade III syndesmosis sprains was evaluated. At 1 week after surgery, patients were allowed to begin range-of-motion exercises, progressive weight bearing, and gradual return to full activity as tolerated. Outcome measures included time to return to full activity and, at final follow-up, the Sports Ankle Rating System scores. Six male intercollegiate college athletes met the inclusion criteria for this study. The average time for return to full activity was 41 days (range, 32 to 48 days), and there were no intraoperative complications or complications when resuming in-season sport activities with the screw in place. In selected cases, athletes can return to full activity as early as 6 weeks after internal fixation of grade III syndesmosis sprains. Level of evidence: IV.

25. Tornetta P III, Spoo JE, Reynolds FA, Lee C: Overtightening of the ankle syndesmosis: Is it really possible? *J Bone Joint Surg Am* 2001;83:489-492.

26. Leitze Z, Sella EJ, Aversa JM: Endoscopic decompression of the retrocalcaneal space. *J Bone Joint Surg Am* 2003;85:1488-1496.

    The authors concluded that endoscopic decompression is an efficient treatment for retrocalcaneal disorders, with results better than or the same as an open technique.

27. Sarrafian S: *Anatomy of the Foot and Ankle: Descriptive, Topographical,* ed 2. Philadelphia, PA, JB Lippincott, 1993.

28. Bare AA, Haddad SL: Tenosynovitis of the posterior tibial tendon. *Foot Ankle Clin* 2001;6:37-66.

29. Lawson JP, Ogden JA, Sella E, Barwick KW: The painful accessory navicular. *Skeletal Radiol* 1984;12:250-262.

30. Kidner FC: The pre-hallux (accessory scaphoid) in its relation to flatfoot. *J Bone Joint Surg* 1929;11:831-837.

31. Nakayama S, Sugimoto K, Takakura Y, Tanaka Y, Kasanami R: Percutaneous drilling of symptomatic accessory navicular in young athletes. *Am J Sports Med* 2005;33:531-535.

Thirty-one feet of 29 patients with type II accessory tarsal navicular treated by percutaneous drilling were reviewed. The outcome of treatment was assessed as excellent in 24 feet (77.4%), good in 6 (19.4%), and fair in 1 (3.2%). No feet were assessed as having a poor outcome. Bone union was obtained in 16 of the 20 feet (80%) when the proximal phalanx of the great toe was immature and in 2 of the 11 feet when it was mature. Percutaneous drilling of the synchondrosis was effective for a symptomatic type II accessory navicular, especially in patients with an immature proximal phalanx of the great toe. Level of evidence: IV.

32. Otsuka K, Takagishi K, Tomizawa S, Hasegawa A: Operative treatment of the accessory navicular in children . *J Jpn Pediatr Orthop Assoc* 2001;10:117-120.

33. Edwards ME: The relations of the peroneal tendons to the fibula, calcaneus, and cuboideum. *Am J Anat* 1928; 42:213-253.

34. Heckman DS, Reddy S, Pedowitz D, Wapner KL, Parekh SG: Operative treatment for peroneal tendon disorders. *J Bone Joint Surg Am* 2008;90:404-418.

Peroneal tendon subluxation is often treated with anatomic repair or reconstruction of the superior peroneal retinaculum with or without deepening of the retromalleolar groove. Surgical treatment of peroneal tendon tears is dependent on the amount of viable tendon that remains.

35. DiGiovanni BF, Fraga CJ, Cohen BE, Shereff MJ: Associated injuries found in chronic lateral ankle instability. *Foot Ankle Int* 2000;21:809-815.

36. Anderson RB, James WC III, Lee S: Athletic foot disorders, in Garrick JG: (ed): *Orthopaedic Knowledge Update: Sports Medicine*, ed 3. Rosemont, IL, American Academy of Orthopaedic Surgeons, 2004, pp 249-261.

Disorders of the hindfoot are discussed.

37. Redfern D, Myerson M: The management of concomitant tears of the peroneus longus and brevis tendons. *Foot Ankle Int* 2004;25:695-707.

The authors postoperatively studied 28 consecutive patients (29 feet) for a mean of 4.6 years. Study results indicate that patients with symptomatic concomitant tears of the peroneus longus or PB tendon are likely to have improved function with adequate surgical treatment.

38. Demirci S, Jubel A, Andermahr J, Koebke J: Chondral thickness and radii of curvature of the femoral condyles and talar trochlea. *Int J Sports Med* 2008;29:327-330.

Chondral thickness and the radii of curvature of femoral condyles and the talar trochlea were assessed to localize optimal donor regions for osteochondral graft transplantation.

39. Athanasiou KA, Niederauer GG, Schenck RC Jr: Biomechanical topography of human ankle cartilage. *Ann Biomed Eng* 1995;23:697-704.

40. Sugimoto K, Takakura Y, Tohno Y, Kumai T, Kawate K, Kadono K: Cartilage thickness of the talar dome. *Arthroscopy* 2005;21:401-404.

The authors determined the articular cartilage thickness of the talar dome where osteochondritis dissecans is common. Cartilage thickness varies according to gender, area, and individual.

41. Berndt AL, Harty M: Transchondral fractures (osteochondritis dissecans) of the talus. *J Bone Joint Surg Am* 1959;40:115-120.

42. Cannon LB, Hackney RG: Anterior tibiotalar impingement associated with chronic ankle instability. *J Foot Ankle Surg* 2000;39:383-386.

43. Robinson DE, Winson IG, Harries WJ, Kelly AJ: Arthroscopic treatment of osteochondral lesions of the talus. *J Bone Joint Surg Br* 2003;85:989-993.

The authors present the results of 65 patients who were treated with arthroscopy for osteochondral lesions of the talus. Mean follow-up was 3.5 years. At follow-up, results were good in 34 patients, fair in 17, and poor in 14. Of the 14 poor results, 13 involved medial lesions. Cystic lesions had a poor outcome in 53% of patients.

44. Tol JL, Struijs P, Bossuyt MM, Verhagen RA, Van Dijk CN: Treatment strategies in osteochondral defects of the talar dome: A systematic review. *Foot Ankle Int* 2000; 21:119-126.

45. Takao M, Uchio Y, Kakimaru H, Kumahashi N, Ochi M: Arthroscopic drilling with debridement of remaining cartilage for osteochondral lesions of the talar dome in unstable ankles. *Am J Sports Med* 2004;32:332-336.

Regenerative cartilage that appears after arthroscopic drilling for the treatment of osteochondral lesions of the talar dome does not always cover the cartilage defect sufficiently and may obstruct the healing of the articular cartilage. In this study, 39 patients had arthroscopic drilling that kept the remaining cartilage at the lesion (group A), and 30 patients had arthroscopic drilling that removed the remaining cartilage at the lesion (group B). Patients were evaluated 1 year after surgery. In group A, 11 patients had improved, 12 were unchanged, and 16 had deteriorated. In group B, 27 patients had improved, 2 were unchanged, and 1 was lost to follow-up. In treating osteochondral lesions of the talar dome, removing the remaining degenerative cartilage may be of some benefit.

46. Elias I, Zoga AC, Morrison WB, Besser MP, Schweitzer ME, Raikin SM: Osteochondral lesions of the talus: Localization and morphologic data from 424 patients using a novel anatomical grid scheme. *Foot Ankle Int* 2007;28:154-161.

The authors used MRI and a nine-zone anatomic grid system to evaluate the true incidence of osteochondral lesions on the talar dome by location and by morphologic characteristics.

47. Kim S, Ha K, Ahn J: Tram track lesion of the talar dome. *Arthroscopy* 1999;15:203-206.

3: Knee and Leg

48. Tol JL, Slim E, van Soest AJ, van Dijk CN: The relationship of the kicking action in soccer and anterior ankle impingement syndrome: A biomechanical analysis. *Am J Sports Med* 2002;30:45-50.

49. Scranton PE Jr, McDermott JE: Anterior tibiotalar spurs: A comparison of open versus arthroscopic debridement. *Foot Ankle* 1992;13:125-129.

50. van Dijk CN, Tol JL, Verheyen CC: A prospective study of prognostic factors concerning the outcome of arthroscopic surgery for anterior ankle impingement. *Am J Sports Med* 1997;25:737-745.

51. Hamilton WG, Geppert MJ, Thompson FM: Pain in the posterior aspect of the ankle in dancers: Differential diagnosis and operative treatment. *J Bone Joint Surg Am* 1996;78:1491-1500.

52. Best A, Giza E, Linklater J, Sullivan M: Posterior impingement of the ankle caused by anomalous muscles: A report of four cases. *J Bone Joint Surg Am* 2005;87: 2075-2079.

Anomalous muscles occur about the ankle. The peroneus quartus has been reported most frequently, with the prevalence of the muscle between 7% and 22%. The prevalence of other anomalous muscles has been reported to range between 1% and 8%. Most anomalous muscles are asymptomatic; however, they can cause tarsal tunnel syndrome or recalcitrant pain after an ankle sprain. This study included a report on three elite athlete with disabling posterior impingement that was treated successfully with resection of anomalous muscle-tendon units.

53. McCarroll JR, Schrader JW, Shelbourne KD, Rettig AC, Bisesi MA: Meniscoid lesions of the ankle in soccer players. *Am J Sports Med* 1987;15:255-257.

54. Meislin RJ, Rose DJ, Parisien JS, et al: Arthroscopic treatment of synovial impingement of the ankle. *Am J Sports Med* 1993;21:186-189.

Rehabilitation

SECTION EDITOR:
TODD S. ELLENBECKER, DPT, MS, SCS, OCS, CSCS

Chapter 18

Rehabilitation Principles Following Rotator Cuff and Superior Labral Repair

Todd S. Ellenbecker, DPT, MS, SCS, OCS, CSCS   George J. Davies, DPT, MEd, PT, SCS, ATC
Michael M. Reinold, PT, DPT, ATC, CSCS

Introduction

Injuries to the rotator cuff and superior labrum occur frequently in individuals involved in overhead functional activities. Advances in the surgical repair of these structures have led to enhanced rehabilitation and patient outcomes. Reduced tissue morbidity during arthroscopic treatment has led to early rehabilitation. Rehabilitation protocols based on basic science research are applied to safely restore range of motion and muscular strength and to optimize postsurgical function. The interventions contained in these protocols are based on basic science research to ensure safe application during appropriate time frames after surgery.

Rehabilitation Concepts Following Arthroscopic Rotator Cuff Repair

Range of Motion

Initial rehabilitation after surgery focuses on range of motion to prevent capsular adhesions while protecting the surgically repaired tissues. Some postsurgical rehabilitation protocols have specific range-of-motion limitations to be applied during the first 6 weeks of rehabilitation (**Table 1**). Several basic science studies have been published that provide a rationale for safe glenohumeral joint range of motion including the movements allowing joint excursion and capsular lengthening, and safe and protective inherent tensions produced in the repaired tendon. Supraspinatus tears measuring 1 cm x 2 cm were repaired in a cadaver model in a study of the effects of humeral rotation range of motion on tension in the supraspinatus in 30° of elevation in the coronal, scapular, and sagittal planes.[1] Results showed that compared with tension in a position of neutral rotation, there was a decrease in tension within the supraspinatus muscle tendon unit at 30° and 60° of external rotation. In contrast, tension was increased within the supraspinatus tendon at 30° and 60° of internal rotation. The intrinsic tensile load in the repaired supraspinatus tendon between the frontal or coronal plane, the scapular plane, and the sagittal planes was compared during humeral rotation. Significantly higher loading was present in the supraspinatus tendon during humeral rotation in the sagittal plane compared with both the frontal and scapular planes. Therefore, early passive range of motion can be performed the directions of both external and internal humeral rotation using the scapular plane position to minimize tensile loading in the repaired tendon.[1]

The effects of passive motion of the supraspinatus tendon during tensile loading in cadavers were compared in a recent study.[2] The authors found no significant increases in strain during the movement of cross-arm adduction in either the supraspinatus or infraspinatus tendons at 60° of elevation. However, internal rotation performed at 30° and 60° of elevation placed increased tension in the most inferior portion of the infraspinatus tendon over the resting or neutral position. This study provides additional guidance for the selection of safe range-of-motion positions following surgery. It is important to know the degree of tendon involvement and repair because posteriorly based rotator cuff repairs (those involving the infraspinatus and teres minor) may be subjected to increased tensile loads if early internal rotation is applied during postoperative rehabilitation. Therefore, communication between the surgeon and the treating therapist is of vital importance to ensure that range of motion is optimal following repair.

Active Assisted Exercise

The progression from passive range-of-motion applications to active assisted and active range of motion is an area of concern during the rehabilitation process after rotator cuff repair. One study provided clear delineation of the degree of muscular activation of the supraspinatus during supine assisted range of motion and seated elevation with the use of a pulley.[3] Although both activities arguably produce low levels of inherent muscular activation in the supraspinatus, the upright pulley activity produces significantly more muscular activity than the supine activities.

Table 1

Postoperative Rehabilitation Protocol for Arthroscopic Rotator Cuff Repair (Medium-Sized Tear)

General Guidelines

Progression of resistive exercise and ROM is dependent on patient tolerance.

Resistance exercise should not be performed with specific shoulder joint pain or pain over the incision site.

A sling is provided to the patient for support as needed with daily activities and to wear at night. The patient is weaned from the sling as tolerated.

Early home exercises are given to the patient following surgery, including stomach rubs, sawing, and gripping activity.

Progression to AROM against gravity and duration of sling use is predicated on the size of the rotator cuff tear, the quality of the tissue, and fixation.

Postoperative Weeks 1 and 2:

1. Early PROM to patient tolerance during the first 4 to 6 weeks:

   a. Flexion.

   b. Scapular and coronal plane abduction.

   c. IR/ER with 90° to 45° abduction.

2. Submaximal isometric IR/ER, flexion/extension, and adduction.

3. Mobilization of the glenohumeral joint and scapulothoracic joint. Passive stretching of elbow, forearm, and wrist to terminal ranges.

4. Sidelying scapular protraction/retraction resistance to encourage early serratus anterior and lower trapezius activation and endurance.

5. Home exercise instruction:

   a. Instruction in PROM and AAROM home exercises with T-bar, pulleys, or opposite arm assistance in supine position using ROM to patient tolerance.

   b. Weight-bearing (closed chain) Codman's exercise instruction over a ball or countertop/table.

   c. Resistive exercise putty for grip strength maintenance.

Postoperative Week 3:

1. Continue above shoulder ROM and isometric strength program to patient tolerance. Progress patient to AA ROM.

2. Add upper body ergometer if available.

3. Begin active scapular strengthening exercises and continue sidelying manual scapular stabilization exercise:

   a. Scapular retraction.

   b. Scapular retraction with depression.

4. Begin resistive exercise for total arm strength using positions with the glenohumeral joint completely supported, including

   a. Biceps curls.

   b. Triceps curls.

   c. Wrist curls—flexion, extension, radial and ulnar deviation.

5. Begin submaximal rhythmic stabilization using the balance point position (90° to 100° of elevation) in supine position to initiate dynamic stabilization.

Postoperative Weeks 5 and 6:

1. Initiate isotonic resistance exercise focusing on the following movements:

   a. Sidelying ER.

   b. Prone extension.

   c. Prone horizontal abduction (limited range to 45°).

   d. Supine IR.

   e. Flexion to 90°.

   A low resistance/high repetition (30 repetitions) format is recommended using no resistance initially (weight of the arm).

2. Progression to full PROM and AROM in all planes, including ER and IR, in neutral adduction progressing from the 90° abducted position used initially postoperatively.

3. External rotation oscillation (resisted ER with towel roll under axilla and oscillation device).

4. Home exercise program for strengthening the rotator cuff and scapular musculature with isotonic weights and/or elastic tubing.

Table 1

Postoperative Rehabilitation Protocol for Arthroscopic Rotator Cuff Repair (Medium- Sized Tear) (continued)

Postoperative Week 8:

1. Begin closed chain step-ups and quadruped rhythmic stabilization exercise.

2. Initiate upper extremity plyometric chest passes and functional two-hand rotation tennis groundstroke or golf swing simulation using small exercise ball and progressing to light medicine ball as tolerated.

Postoperative Week 10:

1. Initiation of submaximal isokinetic exercise for IR/ER in the modified neutral position. Criterion for progression to isokinetic exercise:

   a. Patient has IR/ER ROM greater than that used during the isokinetic exercise.

   b. Patient can complete isotonic exercise program pain-free with a 2- to 3-lb weight or medium resistance surgical tubing or elastic tubing.

2. Progression to 90° abducted rotational training in patients returning to overhead work or sport activity.

   a. Prone ER.

   b. Standing ER/IR with 90° abduction in the scapular plane.

   c. Statue of Liberty exercise (ER oscillation).

Postoperative Week 12 (3 Months):

1. Progression to maximal isokinetics in IR/ER and isokinetic testing to assess strength in modified base 30/30/30 position. Formal documentation of AROM, PROM, and administration of shoulder rating scales.

2. Begin interval return programs if criteria have been met:

   a. IR/ER strength minimum of 85% of contralateral extremity.

   b. ER/IR ratio 60% or higher.

   c. Pain-free range of motion.

   d. Negative impingement and instability signs during clinical examination and formal physical therapy to home program phase.

Postoperative Week 16 (4 Months):

1. Isokinetic re-evaluation, documentation of AROM, PROM, and shoulder rating scales.

2. Progression continues for return to full upper extremity sport activity (such as throwing, or serving in tennis)

3. Preparation for discharge from formal physical therapy to home program phase.

ROM = range of motion; AROM = assisted range of motion; AAROM = active assisted range of motion; PROM = passive range of motion; IR = internal rotation; ER = external rotation

In addition, levels of muscular activation during Codman's pendulum exercise have been quantified.[4] Minimal levels of muscular activation have been detected in the rotator cuff musculature during Codman's pendulum exercise; however, the exercise cannot be considered passive because the musculature is truly activated, especially in individuals with shoulder pathology. Muscular activity in the rotator cuff musculature was not changed between the performance of pendulum exercise with and without weight applied.[4] Pendulum exercises without weight applied have the same effect on muscular activity as weighted exercises, questioning the use of pendulum exercises in the early period after surgery when only passive movements may be indicated.

Rehabilitation in the first 2 to 4 weeks following rotator cuff repair typically consists of passive exercise as well as several minimally active or active assisted exer-cises for the rotator cuff (such as active assisted elevation, overhead pulleys, and pendulums). Additionally, the balance point position (90° of shoulder flexion) may be used while the patient is supine. The patient is queued to perform small active motions of flexion/extension from the 90° starting position to recruit rotator cuff and scapular muscular activity. These exercises, coupled with early scapular stabilization via manual resistance techniques emphasizing direct hand contacts on the scapula to bypass force application to the rotator cuff and optimize trapezius, rhomboid, and serratus anterior muscular activation, are recommended (Figure 1). Electromyogram quantification of low-level closed chain exercise such as weight-shifting on a rocker board was studied, and the low levels (< 10%) of activation of the rotator cuff and scapular musculature during application were highlighted.[5]

The effects of simulated active range of motion on the integrity of a cadaveric supraspinatus repair per-

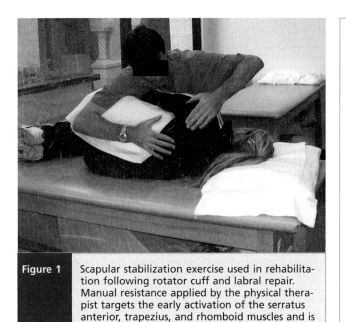

Figure 1 | Scapular stabilization exercise used in rehabilitation following rotator cuff and labral repair. Manual resistance applied by the physical therapist targets the early activation of the serratus anterior, trapezius, and rhomboid muscles and is used throughout the rehabilitation process.

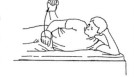

1. Sidelying External Rotation:
Lie on uninvolved side, with involved arm at side, with a small pillow between arm and body. Keeping elbow of involved arm bent and fixed to side, raise arm into external rotation. Slowly lower to starting position and repeat.

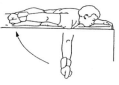

2. Shoulder Extension:
Lie on table on stomach, with involved arm hanging straight to the floor. With thumb pointed outward, raise arm straight back into extension toward your hip. Slowly lower arm and repeat.

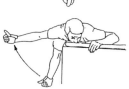

3. Prone Horizontal Abduction:
Lie on table on stomach, with involved arm hanging straight to the floor. With thumb pointed outward, raise arm out to the side, parallel to the floor. Slowly lower arm and repeat.

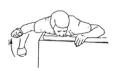

4. 90/90 External Rotation:
Lie on table on stomach, with shoulder abducted to 90° and arm supported on table, with elbow bent at 90°. Keeping the shoulder and elbow fixed, rotate arm into external rotation, slowly lower to start position, and repeat.

Figure 2 | Exercises applied to strengthen the rotator cuff based on electromyographic research.

formed using either transosseous tunnels or suture anchors has been studied.[6] Results showed no difference between repair constructs following repetitive loading, indicating the ability of an arthroscopically based suture anchor fixation model to withstand active loading in a manner similar to transosseous repair used during mini-open and open rotator cuff repair.

Resistive Exercise (Strengthening Progression)

The progression to resistive exercise for the rotator cuff and scapular musculature is variable, typically occurring approximately 6 weeks after surgery when early theoretic healing is assumed in the repaired tissues.[7-9] This progression is based on several factors, such as tear size, tear type, tissue quality, concomitant surgical procedures, patient health status, and age. Communication between the referring surgeon and the physical therapist is critical to share information regarding fixation limitations, tissue challenges, and/or other concomitant relative factors that would limit the progression of postoperative rehabilitation.

The clinical application of resistive exercise during this critical stage of rehabilitation is guided by the level of muscular activity within the individual muscles of the rotator cuff and scapular stabilizers as well as the patient's demonstrated exercise tolerance.[10-18] These factors help determine optimal exercise movement patterns to produce the desired level of muscular activation in the rotator cuff and scapular stabilizers (Figure 2). Repetitive low-resistance exercise is recommended both for safety and relative protection of the repaired tissues and to improve local muscular endurance. Multiple sets of 15 to 20 repetitions have been shown to improve muscular strength in the rotator cuff and scapular stabilizing musculature.[19-21] Exercise patterns using shorter lever arms and maintaining the gle-

nohumeral joint in positions less than 90° of elevation and anterior to the coronal plane of the body are theorized to reduce the risks of both compressive irritation and capsular loading/attenuation during performance.[22] Additionally, early focus on the rotator cuff and scapular stabilizers without emphasis on larger prime mover muscles such as the deltoid, pectorals, and upper trapezius is recommended to minimize unwanted joint shear and inappropriate arthrokinematics and optimize external/internal rotation muscle balance.[21,23,24] The inherent advantages of using low-resistance exercise strategies to target the infraspinatus during external rotation exercise have been studied.[24] External rotation exercise using a 40% maximum voluntary isometric contraction (MVIC) reportedly is superior to higher loads in preferentially recruiting the infraspinatus muscle over conditions with higher MVIC loading. Increased loading leads to a relative increase in the amount of middle deltoid muscle activation.

One specific exercise that has been described extensively in the literature is the empty can exercise (scapular plane elevation with an internally rotated [thumb down] extremity position). Although electromyographic studies have shown high levels of activation of the supraspinatus during the empty can exercise,[14,16,25] the combined movements of elevation and internal rotation have produced clinically disappointing results in practical application as well as the common occurrence of patterns of substitution and improper biomechanical execution in patients. These compensations have been objectively quantified, and increases in scapular internal rotation and anterior tilting have been shown when comparing the empty can to the full can exercise (scapular plane elevation with external rotation) using motion analysis.[26] Movement patterns characterized by scapular internal rotation and anterior tilting theoretically decrease the subacromial space and could jeopardize repetitive movement patterns required for strength acquisition during shoulder rehabilitation.[26]

Specific exercises for the scapular stabilizers focus on the lower trapezius and serratus anterior musculature.[5,27,28] Several studies have looked at upper extremity exercise movement patterns that elicit high levels of activation of these important force couple components responsible for scapular stabilization.[12,17,18] Progression from early manual resistive patterns to exercise patterns with elastic resistance bands and light dumbbells are important aspects of the rehabilitation protocol following rotator cuff and labral repair. Open and closed kinetic chain exercises to recruit key scapular stabilizers are recommended and applied throughout the rehabilitation process following surgical repair.[8,9] One study described improvements in muscular strength and positive changes in scapulohumeral rhythm following 6 weeks of training using elastic resistance exercise.[20] Resistive exercise patterns using scapular retraction and external humeral rotation are emphasized to optimize scapular stabilization and promote muscular balance during shoulder rehabilitation[29] (**Figure 3**).

Progression to Functional Activities

Progression of the patient to advanced strengthening exercises, including isokinetic training specifically emphasizing the movement of internal and external rotation, helps prepare the patient for the increased loading and faster joint angular movements inherent in most functional activities.[30,31] For most patients, the contralateral extremity serves as a baseline and allows meaningful comparison of postoperative range of motion and muscular strength. A return of 85% to 90% of rotational strength compared with the contralateral uninjured extremity and muscular balance represented via an external/internal rotation strength ratio of at least 60% (with 66% to 75% being the desired ratio)[30-32] is required before the patient resumes functional activities such as upper extremity sports and the aggressive activities of daily living. An absence of clinical impingement and signs of instability also is required before these higher level functional activities can be recommended.

The short-term follow-up of patients 12 weeks after both mini-open[33] and arthroscopic[34] rotator cuff repair shows the return of nearly full range of active and passive range of motion, with deficits in muscular strength ranging from 10% to 30% in internal and external rotation compared with the uninjured extremity. Greater deficits following both mini-open and arthroscopic rotator cuff repair have been reported in the posterior rotator cuff (external rotators) despite particular emphasis placed on these structures during postoperative rehabilitation.

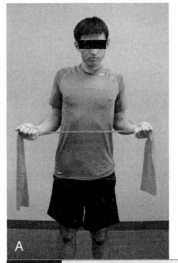
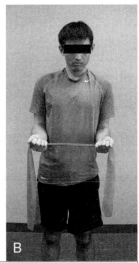

| Figure 3 | External rotation with scapular retraction exercise using elastic resistance band to target the lower trapezius. |

Rehabilitation Concepts Following Superior Labral Repair

Although many of the rehabilitation procedures following arthroscopic repair of superior labral injury resemble those used and recommended following rotator cuff repair, several specific modifications and additions are suggested (**Table 2**).

Range of Motion

In most protocols, early passive, active assisted, and active range of motion and glenohumeral joint mobilization are recommended following superior labral repair.[35,36] Although individual surgeon preference may vary, few limitations in the initial range of motion are typically recommended unless capsular plication or concomitant procedures were performed. The peelback mechanism (**Figure 4**) occurs with the glenohumeral joint in 90° of abduction and external rotation in which the biceps tendon force vector assumes a more vertical and posterior direction creating the "peelback" of the superior labrum.[37] In the first 6 weeks following surgery, this range of motion (external rotation in 90° of abduction) is limited (protected); no aggressive attempts at end range of motion are recommended to protect the superior labral repair and minimize any shear force applied via the biceps from range of motion in this position. Glenohumeral external rotation range of motion and stretching is initially performed in more neutrally abducted positions (0° to 45° of abduction) during the initial 6 to 8 weeks following superior labral repair.

Resistive Exercise (Strengthening Progression)

Repair of the labral lesion alone does not restore normal joint arthrokinematics and highlights the important role that dynamic stabilization plays in rehabilitation following superior labral repair. One specific issue pertaining to the strengthening sequences and rehabili-

4: Rehabilitation

Table 2

Arthroscopic Superior Labral Anterior and Posterior (SLAP) Repair: Postoperative Protocol

Note: Specific alterations in postoperative protocol if SLAP repair is combined with thermal capsulorrhaphy, capsular plication, rotator interval closure, or full-thickness rotator cuff repair.

Sling use as needed for precarious activities and to minimize biceps muscle activation during initial postoperative phase. Duration and degree of sling use determined by physician at postoperative recheck.

Early use of stomach rubs, sawing, and wax-on/wax-off exercise to stimulate home-based motion is recommended between therapy visits.

Phase I: Early Motion (Weeks 1 Through 3)
1. Passive ROM of the glenohumeral joint in movements of flexion, scapular and coronal plane abduction, cross-arm adduction, IR in multiple positions of elevation. ER performed primarily in the lower ranges of abduction (< 60°) to decrease the stress on the repair from the peelback mechanism. Cautious use of glenohumeral joint accessory mobilization unless specific joint hypomobility identified on initial postoperative examination. Use of pulleys and supine active assisted elevation using a cane applied based on patient tolerance to initial passive range of motion after surgery.
2. Patient to wear sling for comfort as needed.
3. ROM of elbow, forearm, and wrist.
4. Manual resistive exercise for scapular protraction and retraction minimizing stress to glenohumeral joint.
5. Initiation of submaximal IR and ER resistive exercise, progressing from manual resistance to very light isotonic and elastic resistance based on patient tolerance using a position with 10° to 20° of abduction in the scapular plane.
6. Manual resistance for elbow extension/flexion, forearm pronation/supination, and wrist flexion/extension and the use of resistive exercise putty or ball squeezes for grip strengthening. Note: No elbow flexion resistance or biceps activity for the first 6 weeks after surgery to protect the superior labral repair.
7. Modalities to control pain in shoulder as indicated.

Phase II: Progression of Strength and ROM (Weeks 4 Through 6)
1. Continue with above exercise guidelines.
2. Begin to progress gentle PROM of the glenohumeral joint with 90° of abduction to terminal ranges with full ER with 90° of abduction expected between 6 and 8 weeks after susrgery. All other motions continue with as in phase I, with continued use of both physiologic and accessory mobilization as indicated by the patient's underlying mobility status.
3. Initiate rotator cuff progression using movement patterns of sidelying ER, prone extension, and prone horizontal abduction using a lightweight and/or elastic resistance.
4. Initiate upper body ergometer for scapular and general upper body strengthening.
5. Rhythmic stabilization performed in 90° of shoulder elevation with limited flexion pressure application to protect SLAP repair.

Phase III: Total Arm Strength (Weeks 6 Through 10)
1. Initiation of elbow flexion (biceps) resistive exercise.
2. Initiate seated rowing variations for scapular strengthening.
3. Advance rotator cuff and scapular progressive resistive exercise using oscillation-based exercise to increase local muscular endurance. Initiation of 90° abducted exercise in scapular plane for IR and ER if patient is an overhead athlete or requires extensive overhead function at work.
4. Progression to closed chain exercises by week 8 including step-ups, quadruped rhythmic stabilization, and progressive weight bearing on an unstable surface.
5. Initiate upper extremity (two-arm) plyometric program, progressing from Swiss ball to weighted medicine balls as tolerated.

Phase IV: Advanced Strengthening (Weeks 10 Through 12; 12 Through 16)
1. Begin isokinetic exercise in the modified neutral position at intermediate and fast contractile velocities. Criterion for progression to isokinetics:
   a. Completion of isotonic exercise with a minimum of a 3-lb weight or medium resistance exercise bands or tubing.
   b. Pain-free ROM in the isokinetic training movement pattern.
2. Isokinetic test performed after two to three successful sessions of isokinetic exercise. Modified neutral test position.
3. Progression to 90° abducted isokinetic and functional plyometric strengthening exercises for the rotator cuff (shoulder IR/ER) based on patient tolerance.
4. Continue with scapular strengthening and ROM exercises listed in earlier stages.

Phase V: Return to Full Activity
Return to full activity is predicated based on the physician's evaluation, isokinetic strength parameters, functional ROM, and tolerance to interval sports return programs.

ROM = range of motion; PROM = passive range of motion; IR = internal rotation; ER = external rotation

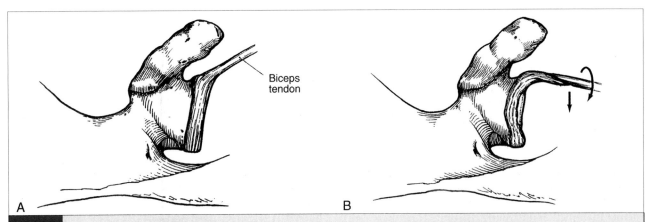

Figure 4 The peelback mechanism occurs with external rotation of the abducted shoulder. (*Reproduced with permission from Morgan CD, Burkhart SS: The peel-back mechanism: Its role in producing and extending posterior type II SLAP lesions and its effect on SLAP repair rehabilitation. Arthroscopy 1998;14:637-640.*)

tation protocol following superior labral repair is the protection of the biceps anchor during the initial period after surgery. Typically no resistive biceps exercise (elbow flexion or lifting) is used after surgery during the initial 6- to 8-week time frame. Exercises and activities that use the movement of shoulder flexion against gravity or during resistance can be gradually integrated. Studies have shown that the use of shoulder flexion initially in an active assisted role and then active and eventually resisted role is warranted.[38,39] Minimal levels (1.7% to 3.6% MVIC) of muscle activation of the long head of the biceps have been shown during multiple directions of shoulder movement, such as scapular plane elevation and glenohumeral rotational movements. Resistive exercise for the elbow flexors is delayed until 6 to 8 weeks after surgery and is applied in the form of rowing variations, upper body ergometry, and isolated elastic and isotonic resistance exercises.

The application of resistive exercise to strengthen the rotator cuff and scapular stabilizers is warranted during rehabilitation following superior labral repair. Progression from the initial patterns used to recruit high levels of rotator cuff and scapular muscle activation to positions at 90° of glenohumeral joint elevation in the scapular plane forms an important part of the end-stage strengthening before return to activities such as throwing and serving in the overhead position. Examples of these exercises include isokinetic training, which offers accommodative resistance at intermediate and fast functional training velocities from 120° to as much as 360° per second, as well as oscillation-based endurance exercises and medicine ball plyometrics in the 90/90 (90° external rotation, 90° abduction) position (**Figures 5** through **8**).

Research specifically outlining the return of rotator cuff strength after superior labral repair is sparse. Glenohumeral internal and external rotation strength was measured in 30 patients following superior labral repair.[36] Strength deficits of approximately 10% were found in the internal and external rotators 12 weeks after surgery following the strength progression outlined

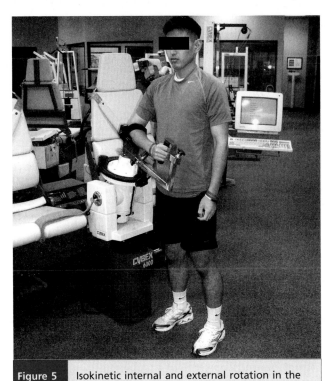

Figure 5 Isokinetic internal and external rotation in the scapular plane position with approximately 30° of glenohumeral joint elevation.

in **Table 2**. This finding shows that continued strengthening is needed even 12 weeks after surgery to facilitate a full functional recovery and safe progression to interval sport programs.[40]

Return-to-Sport Outcomes Following Rotator Cuff and Superior Labral Repairs

The final phase in the rehabilitation of a patient after repair of the rotator cuff and/or superior labrum is referred to as the return-to-activity phase. The goal of this

4: Rehabilitation

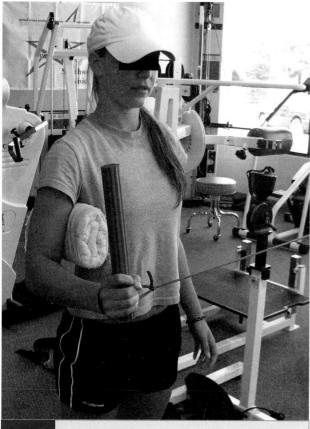

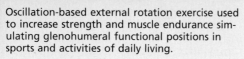

Figure 6 Oscillation-based external rotation exercise used to increase strength and muscle endurance simulating glenohumeral functional positions in sports and activities of daily living.

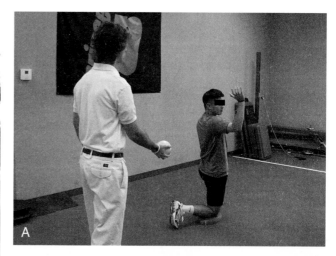

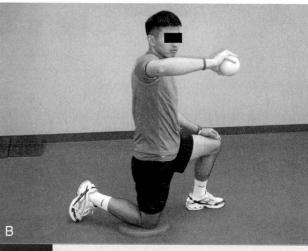

Figure 7 **A,** Plyometric 90/90 reverse catch exercise used to target the posterior rotator cuff and scapular musculature in end-stage rehabilitation following rotator cuff and labral repair (start position). **B,** After catching the ball, the patient accelerates the ball, keeping the shoulder at 90° of abduction, before throwing the ball backward to the partner (concentric external rotation).

phase is to gradually and progressively increase the functional demands on the shoulder to return the patient to full, unrestricted sports or daily activities. The criteria, goals, and progression during this phase are similar between rotator cuff and superior labrum anterior and posterior repair procedures. The criteria established before a patient's return to sports activities are a full functional range of motion, adequate static stability, satisfactory muscular strength and endurance, adequate dynamic stability, a satisfactory clinical examination, and an appropriate rehabilitation progression to this point. The last criterion is one of the most important and is often overlooked. Once these criteria are successfully met, the patient may initiate a gradual, controlled return to activity. The previously discussed healing constraints based on surgical technique and fixation, as well as the patient's tissue status, should be considered before a functional program can be initiated.

The final phase during rehabilitation often involves a gradual introduction to sport-specific activities in conjunction with high-level rehabilitative exercises. Interval sport programs refer to functional rehabilitation guidelines that simulate sport activities.[40] During this period, patients are instructed to continue performing their established rehabilitation program to facilitate the

progression of strength, power, endurance, and flexibility of the shoulder complex. Comprehensive total body flexibility and conditioning exercises are accelerated to ensure competitive sport-specific readiness.

The purpose of these interval programs is to progressively and systematically increase the demands placed on the shoulder complex while the patient is performing sport-specific activities. A gradual return to sports activities minimizes the risk of reinjury and allows progressive adaptation of tissue from the repetitive shoulder stresses. It is during this phase that timing, coordination, movement patterns, and synchronicity of muscle firing are reestablished to preinjury levels. The athlete completes a comprehensive total body flexibility and conditioning program in addition to strengthening and neuromuscular control drills. On the sport-specific training days, the athlete is encouraged to perform rehabilitative exercises as an active warm-up before the interval program. Because there is individual variability in all athletes, there is no set time table for completion of the program. Time to completion of the program will be based on the skill level, goals, and injury of each athlete. Highly competitive individuals who wish to return to competition quickly may have the tendency to increase the intensity of the interval sport program, possibly increasing the incidence of reinjury and retarding the rehabilitation process.

Summary

Surgical repair of the rotator cuff and superior labrum requires the application of a rehabilitation program based on the best available evidence to allow the safe return of range of motion without jeopardizing the surgical repair. The integration of basic science research enables clinicians to optimally progress range of motion and resistive exercise using an evidence-based approach. Communication between the orthopaedic surgeon and the physical therapist is essential to facilitate the rehabilitation following rotator cuff and labral repair.

Annotated References

1. Hatakeyama Y, Itoi E, Urayama M, Pradham RL, Sato K: Effect of superior capsule and coracohumeral ligament release on strain in the repaired rotator cuff tendon. *Am J Sports Med* 2001;29:633-640.

2. Muraki T, Aoki M, Uchiyama E, Murakami G, Miyamoto S: The effect of arm position on stretching of the supraspinatus, infraspinatus, and posterior portion of deltoid muscles: A cadaveric study. *Clin Biomech (Bristol, Avon)* 2006;21:474-480.

    This study examined the effect of rotational motion and cross-arm adduction on the supraspinatus and infraspinatus tendons. The authors report that internal rotation and cross-arm adduction at 60° of elevation do not increase strain on the infraspinatus tendon. This study has significant application for therapists designing ROM programs for use after rotator cuff repair.

3. McCann PD, Wooten ME, Kadaba MP, Bigliani LU: A kinematic and electromyographic study of shoulder rehabilitation exercises. *Clin Orthop Relat Res* 1993;288:179-188.

4. Ellsworth AA, Mullaney M, Tyler TF, McHugh M, Nicholas SJ: Electromyography of selected shoulder musculature during un-weighted and weighted pendulum exercises. *North Am J Sports Phys Ther* 2006;1:73-79.

    This study examined the muscle activity of the rotator cuff, deltoid, and scapular stabilizers during pendulum exercises with and without weights in various applications. They reported that pendulum exercises involve active muscle contractions of the rotator cuff, deltoid, and scapular muscles and cannot be prescribed as passive exercise.

5. Kibler WB, Livingston B, Bruce R: Current concepts in shoulder rehabilitation, in *Advances in Operative Orthopaedics*. St. Louis, MO, Mosby, 1995, vol 3, pp 249-297.

6. Tashjian RZ, Levanthal E, Spenciner DB, Green A, Fleming BC: Initial fixation strength of massive rotator cuff tears: In vitro comparison of single-row suture anchor and transosseous tunnel constructs. *Arthroscopy* 2007;23:710-716.

    This study provides fixation strength and gapping information for rotator cuff repairs and reports significant gapping under repeated loads based on levels meant to simulate active elevation of the shoulder. No difference in gapping was noted between constructs; however, both repair techniques showed significant gapping during experimental testing.

7. Bigiliani LU, Kimmel J, McCann PD, Wolf I: Repair of rotator cuff tears in tennis players. *Am J Sports Med* 1992;20:112-117.

8. Wilk KE, Arrigo C: Current concepts in the rehabilitation of the athletic shoulder. *J Orthop Sports Phys Ther* 1993;18:365-378.

9. Ellenbecker TS, Bailie DS, Kibler WB: Rehabilitation following rotator cuff repair, in Manske R (ed): *Postoperative Rehabilitation of the Knee and Shoulder*. Philadelphia, PA, Elsevier Science, 2005.

    This chapter presents an overview of the methods for rehabilitation after rotator cuff repair and discusses resistive exercise progressions and range of motion based on basic science research along with rehabilitation protocols after rotator cuff repair.

10. Ballantyne BT, O'Hare SJ, Paschall JL, et al: Electromyographic activity of selected shoulder muscles in commonly used therapeutic exercises. *Phys Ther* 1993;73:668-677

11. Blackburn TA, McLeod WD, White B, et al: EMG analysis of posterior rotator cuff exercises. *Athletic Training* 1990;25:40.

12. Moseley JB Jr, Jobe FW, Pink M, Perry J, Tibone J: EMG analysis of the scapular muscles during a shoulder rehabilitation program. *Am J Sports Med* 1992;20:128-134.

13. Reinold MM, Wilk KE, Fleisig GS, et al: Electromyographic analysis of the rotator cuff and deltoid musculature during common shoulder external rotation exercises. *J Orthop Sports Phys Ther* 2004;34:385-394.

This study measured muscle activity of the rotator cuff and deltoid during exercises used in rehabilitation, including internal and external rotation in multiple positions and shoulder elevation. High levels of muscle activity were noted for specific rotator cuff exercises and are recommended for inclusion in rehabilitation.

14. Townsend H, Jobe FW, Pink M, et al: Electromyographic analysis of the glenohumeral muscles during a baseball rehabilitation program. *Am J Sports Med* 1991;19:264-272.

15. Reinold MM, Macrina LC, Wilk KE, et al: Electromyographic analysis of the supraspinatus and deltoid muscles during 3 common rehabilitation exercises. *J Athletic Training* 2007;42:464-469.

    This study demonstrates the muscle activity of the supraspinatus and deltoid muscles during three exercises and gives specific guidance on which exercise maximally recruits the supraspinatus during rehabilitation. The activity during the empty can and full can exercise is discussed.

16. Malanga GA, Jemp YN, Growney E, An K: EMG analysis of shoulder positioning in testing and strengthening the supraspinatus. *Med Sci Sports Exerc* 1996;28:661-664.

17. Decker MJ, Hintermeister RA, Faber KJ, Hawkins RJ: Serratus anterior muscle activity during selected rehabilitation exercises. *Am J Sports Med* 1999;27:784-791.

18. Ekstrom RA, Donatelli RA, Soderberg GL: Surface electromyographic analysis of exercises for the trapezius and serratus anterior muscles. *J Orthop Sports Phys Ther* 2003;33:247-258.

    This study carefully profiles muscle activity during rehabilitation exercise for the scapular stabilizers. It confirms earlier work for serratus anterior activation, emphasizing the importance of a protracted scapular position to recruit the serratus anterior.

19. Moncrief SA, Lau JD, Gale JR, Scott SA: Effect of rotator cuff exercise on humeral rotation torque in healthy individuals. *J Strength Cond Res* 2002;16:262-270.

20. Wang CH, McClure P, Pratt NE, Nobilini R: Stretching and strengthening exercises: Their effect on three-dimensional scapular kinematics. *Arch Phys Med Rehabil* 1999;80:923-929.

21. Giannakopoulos K, Beneka A, Lalliou P, Godolias G: Isolated vs. complex exercise in strengthening the rotator cuff muscle group. *J Strength Cond Res* 2004;18:144-148.

    This study compared the effects of an isolated exercise that specifically recruits the rotator cuff to an exercise that uses multiple muscle groups (complex) exercise movement. Greater overall strength gains were found in the complex exercise training group, but isolated exercise plays a role in early rehabilitation to target a specific muscle, such as the rotator cuff.

22. Ellenbecker TS: *Shoulder Rehabilitation: Nonoperative Treatment*. New York, NY, Thieme, 2006.

    This book comprises multiple chapters on nonsurgical shoulder rehabilitation and includes evidence-based guidelines for rehabilitation of impingement, instability, and scapular dysfunction and provides information on taping and exercise modifications for the shoulder.

23. Lee SB, An KN: Dynamic glenohumeral stability provided by three heads of the deltoid muscle. *Clin Orthop Relat Res* 2002;400:40-47.

24. Bitter NL, Clisby EF, Jones MA, Magarey ME, Jaberzadeh S, Sandow MJ: Relative contributions of infraspinatus and deltoid during external rotation in healthy shoulders. *J Shoulder Elbow Surg* 2007;16:563-568.

    This study compares the relative activation of the rotator cuff and deltoid during external rotation exercises at different levels of MVIC. The significant findings of this study show that external rotation exercise should be performed at a level of 40% to optimally recruit and use the infraspinatus muscle over the deltoid muscle. This study provides guidance for using low-resistance, high-repetition training programs recommended in shoulder rehabilitation.

25. Kelly BT, Kadrmas WH, Speer KP: The manual muscle examination for rotator cuff strength. An electromyographic investigation. *Am J Sports Med* 1996;24:581-588.

26. Thigpen CA, Padua DA, Morgan N, Kreps C, Karas SG: Scapular kinematics during supraspinatus rehabilitation exercise: A comparison of full-can versus empty can techniques. *Am J Sports Med* 2006;34:644-652.

    This study compared the full-can shoulder elevation exercise to the empty can exercise to specifically study scapular mechanics. The findings support use of the full-can exercise with its external humeral rotation position because of improved scapular kinematics compared with the empty can exercise.

27. Kibler WB: The role of the scapula in athletic shoulder function. *Am J Sports Med* 1998;26:325-337.

28. Bagg SD, Forrest WJ: A biomechanical analysis of scapular rotation during arm abduction in the scapular plane. *Arch Phys Med Rehabil* 1988;67:238-245.

29. McCabe RA, Orishimo KF, McHugh MP, Nicholas SJ: Surface electromyographic analysis of the lower trapezius muscle during exercises performed below ninety degrees of shoulder elevation in healthy subject. *North Am J Sports Phys Ther* 2007;2:34-43.

    This study provides detailed information on commonly used scapular stabilization exercises and gives objective measures of muscle activity in the lower trapezius muscle. One exercise combining external rotation with scapular retraction inherently recruited the lower trapezius muscle at high levels.

30. Davies GJ: *A Compendium of Isokinetics in Clinical Usage and Rehabilitation Techniques,* ed 4. Onalaska, WI, S & S Publishing, 1992.

31. Ellenbecker TS, Davies GJ: The application of isokinetics in testing and rehabilitation of the shoulder complex. *J Athletic Training* 2000;35:338-350.

32. Ivey FM, Calhoun JH, Rusche K, Bierschenk J: Isokinetic testing of shoulder strength: Normal values. *Arch Phys Med Rehabil* 1985;66:384-386.

33. Ellenbecker TS, Elmore E, Bailie DS: Descriptive report of shoulder ROM and rotational strength 6 and 12 weeks following rotator cuff repair using a mini-open deltoid splitting technique. *J Orthop Sports Phys Ther* 2006;36:326-335.

    This study reported on the short-term outcome of patients after mini-open rotator cuff repair. Isokinetic strength testing showed greater deficits in external rotation on the injured extremity compared with the uninjured extremity deficits in internal rotation. Range of motion significantly improved between 6 and 12 weeks after surgery using a standardized rehabilitation protocol.

34. Ellenbecker TS, Fischer DJ, Zeman D: Glenohumeral joint range of motion, rotational isokinetic strength, and functional self-report measures following all-arthroscopic rotator cuff repair. *J Orthop Sports Phys Ther* 2006;36:A68.

    The authors studied patients following arthroscopic superior labral repair, measuring range of motion at 6 and 12 weeks and isokinetic rotational strength 12 weeks after surgery. Findings showed minimal deficits in glenohumeral joint range of motion when compared with the contralateral side at 12 weeks following repair and minor deficiencies in rotator cuff strength. This study shows institution of a rehabilitation program following SLAP repair can lead to a nearly full return of strength and range of motion. A protocol for rehabilitation following SLAP repair based on the current evidence is included in this study.

35. Wilk KE, Reinold MM, Dugas JR, Arrigo CA, Moser MW, Andrews JR: Current concepts in the recognition and treatment of superior labral (SLAP) lesions. *J Orthop Sports Phys Ther* 2005;35:273-291.

    This article provides an overview of superior labral injury and a protocol outlining the steps and progressions for rehabilitation after superior labral repair.

36. Ellenbecker TS, Sueyoshi T, Winters M, Zeman D: Descriptive report of shoulder range of motion and rotational strength 6 and 12 weeks following arthroscopic rotator cuff repair. *North Am J Sports Phys Ther* 2008; 3:95-106.

    This study reports patient range of motion and isokinetic strength data after superior labral repair. At 12 weeks after surgery, minor strength deficits were measured in rotational strength, and almost complete range of motion was present when a standardized rehabilitation protocol is followed.

37. Morgan CD, Burkhart SS: The peel-back mechanism: Its role in producing and extending posterior type II SLAP lesions and its effect on SLAP repair rehabilitation. Technical note. *Arthroscopy* 1998;14:637-640.

38. Yamaguchi K, Riew DK, Galatz LM, Syme JA, Neviaser RJ: Biceps activity during shoulder motion: An electromyographic analysis. *Clin Orthop Relat Res* 1997; 336:122-129.

39. Levy AS, Kelly BT, Lintner SA, Osbahr DC, Speer KP: Function of the long head of the biceps at the shoulder: Electromyographic analysis. *J Shoulder Elbow Surg* 2001;10:250-255.

40. Reinold MM, Wilk KE, Reed J, Crenshaw K, Andrews JR: Internal sport programs: Guidelines for baseball, tennis, and golf. *J Orthop Sports Phys Ther* 2002; 32:293-298.

4: Rehabilitation

Chapter 19

Rehabilitation of the Overhead Athlete's Elbow

Kevin E. Wilk, PT, DPT   Todd S. Ellenbecker, DPT, MS, SCS, OCS, CSCS

Introduction

The act of the overhead throw, especially pitching, produces high levels of forces at the elbow joint. Rehabilitation following injury or surgery to the throwing elbow is vital to fully restore normal function and return the athlete to competition as quickly and safely as possible. Rehabilitation of the elbow, whether postinjury or postsurgical, must follow a progressive and sequential order to ensure that healing tissues have not been compromised. Emphasis is placed on restoring full motion, muscular strength, and neuromuscular control, and gradually applying loads to healing tissue to allow for a return to full upper extremity function. A total arm or total extremity approach to rehabilitation of the patient with an injured elbow is required.[1]

General Rehabilitation Guidelines

Rehabilitation following elbow injury or elbow surgery follows a sequential and progressive multiphased approach. The ultimate goal of elbow rehabilitation is to return the athlete to his or her previous functional level as quickly and safely as possible. An overview of the rehabilitation process following elbow injury and surgery is presented in **Tables 1** and **and 2**; rehabilitation protocols for specific pathologies are discussed in the following sections.

Phase I: Immediate Motion Phase

The goals of phase I are to minimize the effects of immobilization, reestablish painless range of motion (ROM), decrease pain and inflammation, and retard muscular atrophy.

Early ROM activities are performed to nourish the articular cartilage and assist in the synthesis, alignment, and organization of collagen tissue.[2] ROM activities are performed for all planes of elbow and wrist motions to prevent the formation of scar tissue and adhesions. Active-assisted and passive ROM exercises are performed to restore flexion/extension to the humeroulnar joint as well as to restore supination/pronation to the humeroradial and radioulnar joints. Reestablish-

ing full elbow extension, or preinjury motion, is the primary goal of early ROM activities to minimize the occurrence of elbow flexion contractures. Preoperative elbow motion must be carefully assessed and recorded using a goniometer to most accurately provide a baseline reference value.[3,4]

Postoperative ROM is often related to preoperative motion, especially in the case of ulnar collateral ligament (UCL) reconstruction. The loss of motion can be a deleterious side effect for the overhead athlete. The elbow is predisposed to flexion contractures because of the intimate congruency of the joint articulations, the tightness of the joint capsule, and the tendency for the development of adhesions in the anterior capsule following injury.[2] The brachialis muscle also attaches to the capsule and crosses the elbow joint before becoming a tendinous structure. Injury to the elbow may cause excessive scar tissue formation of the brachialis muscle as well as functional splinting of the elbow.[2]

In addition to ROM exercises, joint mobilizations may be performed as tolerated to minimize the occurrence of joint contractures. Posterior glides with oscillations are performed at end ROM to assist in restoring full elbow extension. Joint mobilization must include the radiocapitellar and radioulnar joints.

If the patient continues to have difficulty achieving full extension using ROM and mobilization techniques, a low load, long duration stretch may produce a deformation (creep) of the collagen tissue, resulting in tissue elongation. The patient lies supine with a towel roll or foam placed under the distal brachium to act as a cushion and fulcrum. Light resistance exercise tubing is applied to the patient's wrist and secured to the table or a dumbbell on the ground (**Figure 1**). The patient is instructed to relax as much as possible for 10 to 15 minutes per treatment. The amount of resistance applied should be of low magnitude to enable the patient to perform the stretch for the entire duration without pain or muscle spasm, this technique should impart a low load but a long duration stretch. Patients are instructed to perform these stretches several times each day (15-minute stretch, 4 times per day), equaling 60 minutes of total end range time.

The aggressiveness of stretching and mobilization techniques is dictated based on the healing constraints

Table 1

Nonsurgical Rehabilitation Program for Elbow Injuries

I. Acute Phase (Week 1)

Goals: Improve motion, diminish pain and inflammation, retard muscle atrophy
Exercises and Therapies
1. Stretching for wrist and elbow joint, stretches for shoulder joint
2. Strengthening exercise isometrics for wrist, elbow, and shoulder musculature
3. Pain and inflammation control cryotherapy, high-voltage galvanic stimulation, ultrasound, and whirlpool

II. Subacute Phase (Weeks 2 to 4)

Goals: Normalize motion; improve muscular strength, power, and endurance
Week 2
1. Initiate isotonic strengthening for wrist and elbow muscles
2. Initiate exercise tubing exercises for shoulder
3. Continue use of cryotherapy, and so forth
Week 3
1. Initiate rhythmic stabilization drills for elbow and shoulder joint
2. Progress isotonic strengthening for entire upper extremity
3. Initiate isokinetic strengthening exercises for elbow flexion/extension
Week 4
1. Initiate Throwers' Ten program
2. Emphasize eccentric biceps work, concentric triceps and wrist flexor work
3. Program endurance training
4. Initiate light plyometric drills
5. Initiate swinging drills

III. Advanced Phase (Weeks 4 to 6)

Goals: Preparation of athlete for return to functional activities
Criteria to progress to Advanced Phase:
1. Full painless ROM
2. No pain or tenderness
3. Satisfactory isokinetic test
4. Satisfactory clinical examination
Weeks 4 to 5
1. Continue strengthening exercises, endurance drills, and flexibility exercises daily
2. Thrower's Ten program
3. Progress plyometric drills
4. Emphasize maintenance program based on pathology
5. Progress swinging drills (for example, hitting)
Weeks 6 to 8
1. Initiate interval sport program once determined by physician (phase I program)

IV. Return to Activity Phase (Weeks 6 to 9)

Return to play depends on athlete's condition and progress; the physician will determine when it is safe.
1. Continue strengthening program and Thrower's Ten program
2. Continue flexibility program
3. Progress functional drills to unrestricted play

Table 2

Postoperative Rehabilitative Protocol for Elbow Arthroscopy

I. Initial Phase (Week 1)

Goals: Full wrist and elbow ROM, decrease swelling, decrease pain, retardation or muscle atrophy

A. Day of surgery

 Begin gently moving elbow in bulky dressing

B. Postoperative day 1 and 2

 1. Remove bulky dressing and replace with elastic bandages

 2. Immediate postoperative hand, wrist, and elbow exercises

 a. Putty/grip strengthening

 b. Wrist flexor stretching

 c. Wrist extensor stretching

 d. Wrist curls

 e. Reverse wrist curls

 f. Neutral wrist curls

 g. Pronation/supination

 h. Active-assisted ROM/passive ROM elbow flexion/extension

C. Postoperative day 3 through 7

 1. Postoperative ROM elbow ext1flex (motion to tolerance)

 2. Begin progressive resistive exercises with 1-lb weight

 a. Wrist curls

 b. Reverse wrist curls

 c. Neutral wrist curls

 d. Pronation/supination

 e. Broomstick roll-up

II. Intermediate Phase (Weeks 2 to 4)

Goal: Improve muscular strength and endurance; normalize joint arthrokinematics

A. Week 2 ROM exercises (overpressure into extension)

 1. Addition of biceps curl and triceps extension

 2. Continue to progress progressive resistive exercise, weight and repetitions as tolerable

B. Week 3

 1 . Initiate biceps and biceps eccentric exercise program

 2. Initiate rotator cuff exercises program

 a. External rotators

 b. Internal rotators

 c. Deltoid

 d. Supraspinatus

 e. Scapulothoracic strengthening

III. Advanced Phase (Weeks 4 to 8)

Goals: Preparation of athlete for return to functional activities

Criteria to progress to advanced phase:

 1. Full painless ROM

 2. No pain or tenderness

 3. Isokinetic test that fulfills criteria to throw

 4. Satisfactory clinical examination

A. Weeks 4 through 6

 1. Continue maintenance program, emphasizing muscular strength, endurance, and flexibility

 2. Initiate interval throwing program

ROM = range of motion

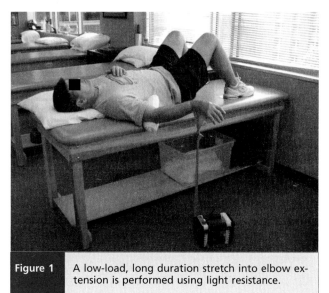

Figure 1 A low-load, long duration stretch into elbow extension is performed using light resistance.

of involved tissues, specific pathology/surgery, and the amount of motion and end feel. If the patient has decreased motion and hard end feel without pain, aggressive stretching and mobilization techniques may be used. Conversely, a patient exhibiting pain before resistance or with empty end feel should undergo gentle stretching.

Another goal of this phase is to decrease the patient's pain and inflammation. Cryotherapy and high-voltage stimulation may be performed as required to further assist in reducing pain and inflammation. Once the acute inflammatory response has subsided, moist heat, warm whirlpool, and ultrasound may be used at the onset of treatment to prepare the tissue for stretching and improve the extensibility of the capsule and musculotendinous structures.

The early phases of rehabilitation also focus on voluntary activation of muscle and retarding muscular atrophy. Subpainful and submaximal isometrics are performed initially for the elbow flexor and extensor, as well as the wrist flexor, extensor, pronator, and supinator muscle groups. Shoulder isometrics also may be performed during this phase, with caution against internal and external rotation exercises if painful. Alternating rhythmic stabilization drills for shoulder flexion/extension/horizontal abduction/adduction, shoulder internal/external rotation, and elbow flexion/extension/supination/pronation are performed to reestablish proprioception and neuromuscular control of the upper extremity.

Phase II: Intermediate Phase

Phase II is initiated when the patient exhibits full ROM, minimal pain and tenderness, and a good (4/5) manual muscle test of the elbow flexor and extensor musculature. The emphasis during this phase includes enhancing elbow and upper extremity mobility, improving muscular strength and endurance, and reestab-

lishing neuromuscular control of the elbow complex.

Stretching exercises are continued to maintain full elbow and wrist ROM. Flexibility is progressed during this phase to focus on wrist flexion, extension, pronation, and supination. Particular emphasis is placed on elbow extension and forearm pronation flexibility for throwing athletes to perform efficiently. Shoulder flexibility also is maintained, with emphasis on external and internal rotation at 90° of abduction, flexion and horizontal adduction, and particularly, shoulder external rotation at 90° abduction; loss of external rotation may result in increased strain on the medial elbow structures during the overhead throwing motion.

Strengthening exercises are progressed during this phase to include isotonic contractions, beginning with concentric and progressing to include eccentric contractions. Emphasis is placed on elbow flexion and extension, wrist flexion and extension, and a progressive resistance program during the later stages of this phase. Emphasis is placed on strengthening the shoulder external rotators and scapular muscles. A complete upper extremity strengthening program, such as the Thrower's Ten, may be instituted (**Figure 2**).

Neuromuscular control exercises are initiated in this phase to enhance the muscles' ability to control the elbow joint during athletic activities. These exercises include proprioceptive neuromuscular facilitation exercises with rhythmic stabilizations (**Figure 3**) and slow reversal manual resistance elbow/wrist flexion drills (**Figure 4**).

Phase III: Advanced Strengthening Phase

The goals of this phase are to gradually increase strength, power, endurance, and neuromuscular control to prepare for a gradual return to sport. A progression of activities prepare the athlete for sports participation. Specific criteria that must be met before entering this phase include full painless ROM, no pain or tenderness, and strength that is 70% of the contralateral extremity.

Advanced strengthening activities during this phase include exercises emphasizing higher resistance, functional movements, eccentric contraction and plyometric activities. Elbow flexion exercises are progressed to emphasize eccentric control. The biceps muscle is an important stabilizer during the follow-through phase of overhead throwing; it eccentrically controls the deceleration of the elbow, preventing pathologic abutting of the olecranon within the fossa. Elbow flexion can be performed with elastic tubing to emphasize slow and fast concentric and eccentric contractions. Isokinetic exercise also can produce high-speed muscular training. Aggressive strengthening exercises with weight machines (for example, bench press, seated rowing, and front latissimus dorsi pulldowns) also are incorporated during this phase. The triceps are primarily exercised with a concentric contraction because of the acceleration activity of the muscle during the acceleration phase of throwing.

Exercises for neuromuscular control are progressed

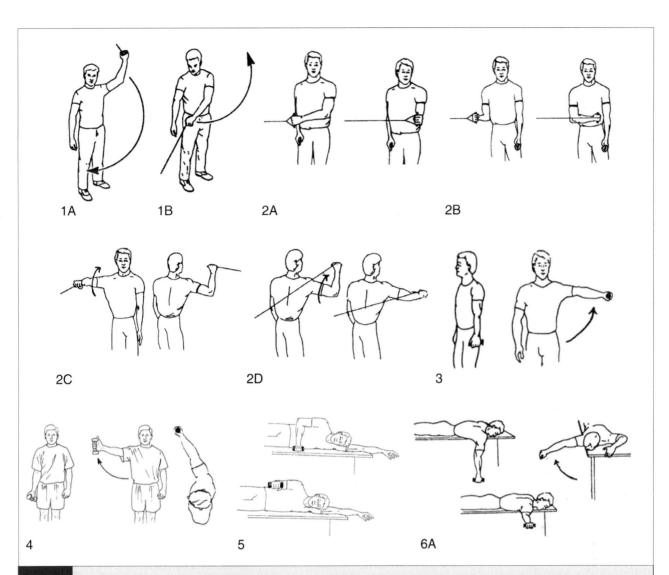

Figure 2	Thrower's Ten Program. **1A. Diagonal Pattern D2 Extension:** Involved hand will grip tubing handle overhead and out to the side. Pull tubing down and across your body to the opposite side of leg. During the motion, lead with your thumb. Perform __ sets of __ repetitions __ daily. **1B. Diagonal Pattern D2 Flexion:** Gripping tubing handle in hand of involved arm, begin with arm out from side 45° and palm facing backward. After turning palm forward, proceed to flex elbow and bring arm up and over involved shoulder. Turn palm down and reverse to take arm to starting position. Exercise should be performed __ sets of __ repetitions __ daily. **2A. External Rotation at 0° Abduction:** Stand with involved elbow fixed at side, elbow at 90° and involved arm across front of body. Grip tubing handle while the other end of tubing is fixed. Pull out arm, keeping elbow at side. Return tubing slowly with controlled motion. Perform __ sets of __ repetitions __ times daily. **2B. Internal Rotation at 0° Abduction:** Standing with elbow at side fixed at 90° and shoulder rotated out. Grip tubing handle while other end of tubing is fixed. Pull arm across body keeping elbow at side. Return tubing slowly with controlled motion. Perform __ sets of __ repetitions __ times daily. **2C. (Optional) External Rotation at 90° Abduction:** Stand with shoulder abducted 90°. Grip tubing handle while the other end is fixed straight ahead, slightly lower than the shoulder. Keeping shoulder abducted, rotate shoulder back, keeping elbow at 90°. Return tubing and hand to start position. I. Slow Speed Sets: (Slow and Controlled) Perform __ sets of __ repetitions __ times daily. II. Fast Speed Sets: Perform __ sets of __ repetitions __ times daily. **2D. (Optional) Internal Rotation at 90° Abduction:** Stand with shoulder abducted to 90°, and elbow bent to 90°. Keeping shoulder abducted, rotate shoulder forward, keeping elbow bent at 90°. Return tubing and hand to start position. Slow and fast speed sets: same as 2C. **3. Shoulder Abduction to 90°:** Stand with arm at side, elbow straight, and palm down, until arm reaches 90° (shoulder level). Perform __ sets of __ repetitions __ times daily. **4. Scaption, External Rotation:** Stand with elbow straight and thumb up. Raise arm to shoulder level at 30° angle in front of body. Do not go above shoulder height. Hold 2 seconds and lower slowly. Perform __ sets of __ repetitions __ times daily. **5. Sidelying External Rotation:** Lie on uninvolved side, with involved arm at side of body and elbow bent to 90°. Keeping the elbow of involved arm fixed to side, raise arm. Hold 2 seconds and lower slowly. Perform __ sets of __ repetitions __ times daily. **6A. Prone Horizontal Abduction (Neutral):** Lie on table, face down, with involved arm hanging straight to the floor, and palm facing down. Raise arm out to the side, parallel to the floor. Hold 2 seconds and lower slowly. Perform __ sets of __ repetitions __ times daily.

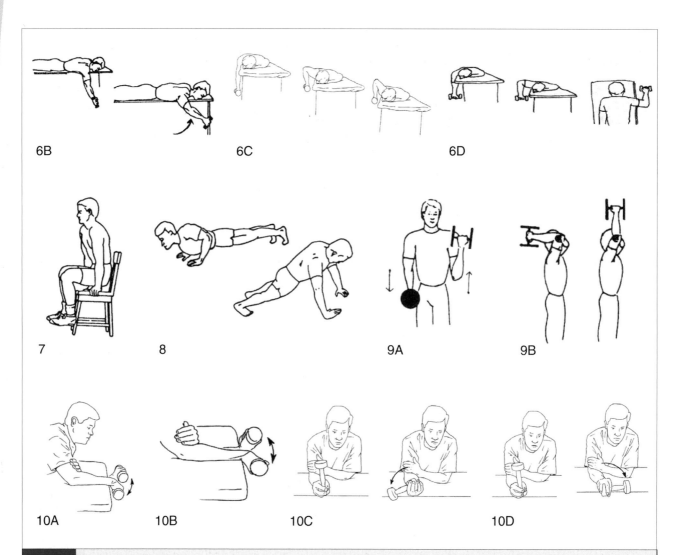

6B   6C   6D

7   8   9A   9B

10A   10B   10C   10D

Figure 2   Thrower's Ten Program (continued). **6B. Prone Horizontal Abduction (Full External Rotation, 100° Abduction):** Lie on table face down, with involved arm hanging straight to the floor and thumb rotated up (hitchhiker). Raise arm out to the side with arm slightly in front of shoulder, parallel to the floor. Hold 2 seconds and lower slowly. Perform __ sets of __repetitions __ times daily. **6C. Prone Rowing:** Lying on your stomach with your involved arm hanging over the side of the table, dumbbell in hand and elbow straight. Slowly raise arm, bending elbow, and bring dumbbell as high as possible. Hold at the top for 2 seconds, then slowly lower. Perform __ sets of __ repetitions __ times daily. **6D. Prone Rowing into External Rotation:** Lying on your stomach with your involved arm hanging over the side of the table, dumbbell in hand and elbow straight. Slowly raise arm, bending elbow, up to the level of the table. Pause 1 second. Then rotate shoulder upward until dumbbell is even with the table, keeping elbow at 90°. Hold at the top for 2 seconds, then slowly lower taking 2 to 3 seconds. Perform __ sets of __ repetitions __ times daily. **7. Press-ups:** Seated on a chair or table, place both hands firmly on the sides of the chair or table, palm down and fingers pointed outward. Hands should be placed equal with shoulders. Slowly push downward through the hands to elevate your body. Hold the elevated position for 2 seconds and lower body slowly. Perform __ sets of __ repetitions __ times daily. **8. Push-ups:** Start in the down position with arms in a comfortable position. Place hands no more than shoulder width apart. Push up as high as possible, rolling shoulders forward after elbows are straight. Start with a push-up into wall. Gradually progress to tabletop and eventually to floor as tolerable. Perform __ sets of __ repetitions __ times daily. **9A. Elbow Flexion:** Standing with arm against side and palm facing inward, bend elbow upward, turning palm up as you progress. Hold 2 seconds and lower slowly. Perform __ sets of __ repetitions __ times daily. **9B. Elbow Extension (Abduction):** Raise involved arm overhead. Provide support at elbow from uninvolved hand. Straighten arm overhead. Hold 2 seconds and lower slowly. Perform __ sets of __ repetitions __ times daily. **10A. Wrist Extension:** Supporting the forearm and with palm facing downward, raise weight in hand as far as possible. Hold 2 seconds and lower slowly. Perform __ sets of __ repetitions __ times daily. **10B. Wrist Flexion:** Supporting the forearm and with palm facing upward, lower a weight in hand as far as possible and then curl it up as high as possible. Hold for 2 seconds and lower slowly. **10C. Supination:** Forearm is supported on table with wrist in neutral position. Using a weight or hammer, roll wrist, taking palm up. Hold for a 2 count and return to starting position. Perform __ sets of __ repetitions __ times daily. **10D. Pronation:** Forearm should be supported on a table with wrist in neutral position. Using a weight or hammer, roll wrist, taking palm down. Hold for a 2 count and return to starting position. Perform __ sets of __ repetitions __ times daily. *(Reproduced with permission from The Advanced Continuing Education Institute, LLC, Winchester, MA, 2004.)*

4: Rehabilitation

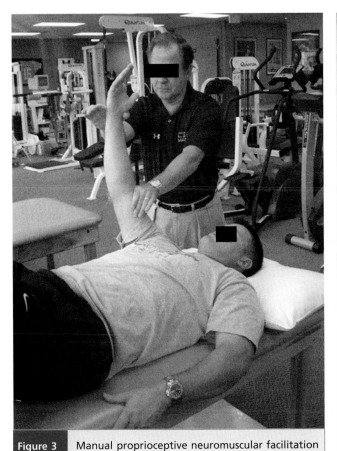

Figure 3 | Manual proprioceptive neuromuscular facilitation upper extremity D2 patterns with rhythmic stabilization.

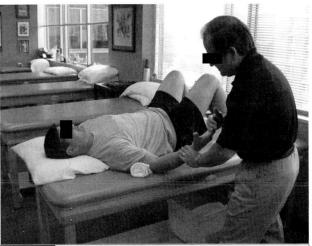

Figure 4 | Manual concentric and eccentric resistance exercise for the elbow flexors and wrist flexor-pronators.

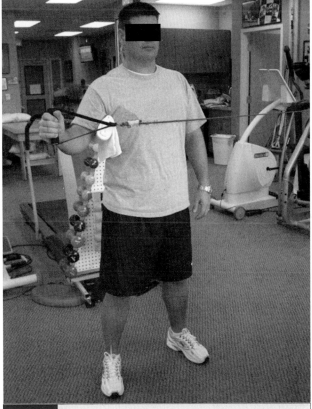

Figure 5 | External rotation at 90° abduction with exercise tubing, manual resistance, and rhythmic stabilizations.

to include sidelying external rotation with manual resistance. Concentric and eccentric external rotation is performed against the clinician's resistance with the addition of rhythmic stabilizations. This manual resistance exercise may be progressed to standing external rotation with exercise tubing at 0° and finally at 90° (Figure 5).

Plyometric drills can be an extremely beneficial form of functional exercise for training the elbow in overhead athletes.[2,5] Plyometric exercises are performed using a weighted medicine ball during the later stages of this phase to train the shoulder and elbow to develop and withstand high levels of stress. Plyometric exercises are initially performed with two hands performing a chest pass, side-to-side throw, and overhead soccer throw. These exercises may later include one-hand activities such as 90/90 throws (90° of abduction and 90° of elbow flexion; Figure 6), external and internal rotation throws at 0° of abduction (Figure 7), and wall dribbles. Specific plyometric drills for the forearm musculature include wrist flexion flips, wrist flexion snaps, and extension grips. The plyometric drills are an important component to an elbow rehabilitation program, emphasizing the forearm and hand musculature.

Phase IV: Return to Activity Phase

The final phase of elbow rehabilitation, the return to activity phase, allows the athlete to progressively return to full competition using an interval return-to-throwing program.

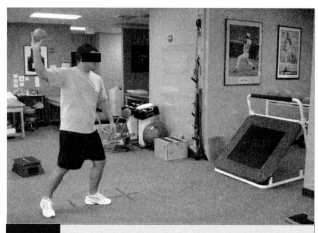

Figure 6 | Plyometric internal rotation throws at 90° abduction.

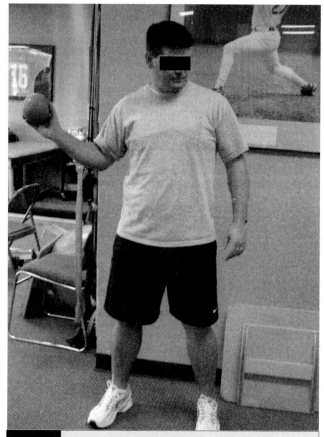

Figure 7 | Plyometric internal rotation throws at 0° abduction.

Before an athlete is allowed to begin this phase, the athlete must exhibit full ROM, no pain or tenderness, a satisfactory isokinetic test, and a satisfactory clinical examination. Isokinetic testing may be used to help determine the readiness of the athlete to begin an interval sport program.[6,7]

Upon achieving the previously mentioned criteria to return to sports participation, these patients are placed on an interval sport program.[6] For the overhead thrower, a long-toss interval throwing program is initiated, beginning at 45 ft and gradually progressing to 120 or 180 ft (**Table 3**).[6] Throwing should be performed without pain or a significant increase in symptoms. It is important for the overhead athlete to stretch and go through an abbreviated strengthening program before and after performing the interval sport program. Typically, overhead throwers warm up, stretch, and perform one set of their exercise program before throwing, followed by two additional sets of exercises proceeding throwing.[6] This is adequate warm-up, but the regimen also ensures maintenance of necessary ROM and flexibility of the shoulder joint. The following day, the thrower will exercise the scapular muscles and external rotators, and perform a core stabilization program.

After completion of a long toss program, pitchers will progress to phase II of the throwing program, throwing off a mound[6] (**Table 4**). In phase II the number of throws, intensity, and type of pitch are progressed to gradually increase stress on the elbow and shoulder joints.[6] The pitcher usually begins at 50% intensity and gradually progresses to 75%, 90%, and 100% intensity over 4 to 6 weeks. Breaking balls are initiated once the pitcher can throw 40 to 50 pitches at a minimum intensity of 80%.

Two other important aspects of the return to sport activity are the continued application of resistive exercise and the modification or evaluation of the patient's equipment. Continuation of the total arm strength rehabilitation exercises using elastic resistance, medicine balls, and isotonic or isokinetic resistance is important to continue to enhance not only strength but also muscular endurance.[8]

Specific Nonsurgical Rehabilitation Guidelines

Medial Epicondylitis and Flexor-Pronator Tendinitis

Medial epicondylitis occurs as a result of changes within the flexor-pronator musculotendinous unit. Associated ulnar neuropathy has been reported in 25% to 60% of patients with medial epicondylitis.[9] The underlying pathology is a microscopic or macroscopic tear within the flexor carpi radialis or pronator teres near the origin on the medial epicondyle. Overhead throwers who exhibit flexor-pronator tendinitis may have an associated UCL injury. The tendinitis may develop as a secondary pathology or a false symptom. Patients with long histories of medial epicondylitis may exhibit tendinosis, not tendinitis. Conversely, patients with first-time episodes probably exhibit paratendinitis and tendinitis. The treatment is significantly different for both.

The treatment of tendinitis typically is focused on reducing inflammation and pain by limiting activity, and

Table 3

Interval Throwing Program for Baseball Players: Phase I

45 Ft* Phase	60 Ft* Phase	90 Ft* Phase
Step 1:	Step 3:	Step 5:
A) Warm-up throwing	A) Warm-up throwing	A) Warm-up throwing
B) 45 ft (25 throws)	B) 60 ft (25 throws)	B) 90 Ft (25 throws)
C) Rest 5 to 10 min	C) Rest 5 to 10 min	C) Rest 5 to10 min
D) Warm-up throwing	D) Warm-up throwing	D) Warm-up throwing
E) 45 ft (25 throws)	E) 60 ft (25 throws)	E) 90 Ft (25 throws)
Step 2:	Step 4:	Step 6:
A) Warm-up throwing	A) Warm-up throwing	A) Warm-up throwing
B) 45 ft (25 throws)	B) 60 ft (25 throws)	B) 90 Ft (25 throws)
C) Rest 5 to 10 min	C) Rest 5 to 10 min	C) Rest 5 to 10 min
D) Warm-up throwing	D) Warm-up throwing	D) Warm-up throwing
E) 45 ft (25 throws)	E) 60 ft (25 throws)	E) 90 Ft (25 throws)
F) Rest 5 to 10 min.	F) Rest 5 to 10 min	F) Rest 5 to 10 min
G) Warm-up throwing	G) Warm-up throwing	G) Warm-up throwing
H) 45 ft (25 throws)	H) 60 ft (25 throws)	H) 90 Ft (25 throws)

120 Ft* Phase	150 Ft* Phase	180 Ft* Phase
Step 7:	Step 9:	Step 11:
A) Warm-up throwing	A) Warm-up throwing	A) Warm-up throwing
B)120 ft (25 throws)	B) 150 ft (25 throws)	B) 180 ft (25 throws)
C) Rest 5 to 10 min	C) Rest 5 to 10 min	C) Rest 5 to 10 min
D) Warm-up throwing	D) Warm-up throwing	D) Warm-up throwing
E) 120 ft (25 throws)	E) 150 ft (25 throws)	E) 180 ft (25 throws)
Step 8:	Step 10:	Step 12:
A) Warm-up throwing	A) Warm-up throwing	A) Warm-up throwing
B) 120 ft (25 throws)	B) 150 ft (25 throws)	B) 180 ft (25 throws)
C) Rest 5 to 10 min	C) Rest 5 to 10 min	C) Rest 5 to 10 min
D) Warm-up throwing	D) Warm-up throwing	D) Warm-up throwing
E) 120 ft (25 throws)	E) 150 ft (25 throws)	E) 180 ft (25 throws)
F) Rest 5 to 10 min	F) Rest 5 to 10 min	F) Rest 5 to 10 min
G) Warm-up throwing	G) Warm-up throwing	G) Warm-up throwing
H) 120 ft (25 throws)	H) 150 ft (25 throws)	H) 180 ft (25 throws)

*45 ft = 13.7 m; 60 ft = 18.3 m; 90 ft = 27.4 m; 120 ft = 36.6 m; 150 ft = 45.7 m; 180 ft = 54.8 m

using anti-inflammatory medications, cryotherapy, iontophoresis, light exercise, and stretching.

Conversely, the treatment of tendinosis focuses on increasing circulation to promote collagen synthesis and collagen organization. The treatment modalities include heat, ultrasound, stretching, eccentrics, laser therapy, transverse massage, and soft-tissue mobilization.

The nonsurgical treatment of epicondylitis (tendinitis and/or paratendinitis) (Table 5) focuses on diminishing associated pain and inflammation and then gradually improving muscular strength. The primary goals of rehabilitation are to control the applied loads and create an environment for healing. The initial treatment consists of warm whirlpool baths, iontophoresis, stretching exercises, and light strengthening exercises to stimulate a repair response. A disposable iontophoresis patch has

4: Rehabilitation

Table 3

Interval Throwing Program for Baseball Players: Phase I (continued)

180 Ft* Phase

Step 13:

A) Warm-up throwing

B) 180 Ft (25 throws)

C) Rest 5 to 10 min

D) Warm-up throwing

E) 180 Ft (25 throws)

F) Rest 5 to 10 min

G) Warm-up throwing

H) 180 Ft (20 throws)

I) Rest 5 to 10 min

J) Warm-up throwing

K) 15 throws

Return to respective position or progress to step 14 below.

All throws should be on an arc with a crow-hop.

Warm-up throws consist of 10 to 20 throws at approximately 30 ft.

Throwing program should be performed every other day, 3 times per week unless otherwise specified by your physician or rehabilitation specialist.

Perform each step ___ times before progressing to next step.

Flat Ground Throwing for Baseball Pitchers

Step 14:	Step 15:
A) Warm-up throwing	A) Warm-up throwing
B) Throw 60 ft (10 to 15 throws)	B) Throw 60 ft (10 to 15 throws)
C) Throw 90 ft (10 throws)	C) Throw 90 ft (10 throws)
D) Throw 120 ft (10 throws)	D) Throw 120 ft (10 throws)
E) Throw 60 ft (flat ground) using pitching mechanics (20 to 30 throws)	E) Throw 60 ft (flat ground) using pitching mechanics (20 to 30 throws)
	F) Throw 60 to 90 ft (10 to 15 throws)
	G) Throw 60 ft (flat ground) using pitching mechanics (20 throws)

Progress to phase II—Throwing Off the Mound

*45 ft = 13.7 m; 60 ft = 18.3 m; 90 ft = 27.4 m; 120 ft = 36.6 m; 150 ft = 45.7 m; 180 ft = 54.8 m

Table 4

Interval Throwing Program for Baseball Players: Phase II—Throwing Off the Mound

Stage One: Fastballs Only

Step 1: Interval throwing
15 throws off mound 50%*†

Step 2: Interval throwing
30 throws off mound 50%†

Step 3: Interval throwing
45 throws off mound 50%†

Step 4: Interval throwing
60 throws off mound 50%†

Step 5: Interval throwing
70 throws off mound 50%

Step 6: 45 throws off mound 50%
30 throws off mound 75%

Step 7: 30 throws off mound 50%
45 throws off mound 75%

Step 8: 10 throws off mound 50%
65 throws off mound 75%

Stage Two: Fastballs Only

Step 9: 60 throws off mound 75%
15 throws in batting practice

Step 10: 50 to 60 throws off mound 75%
30 throws in batting practice

Step 11: 45 to 50 throws off mound 75%
45 throws in batting practice

Stage Three

Step 12: 30 throws off mound, 75% warm-up
15 throws off mound, 50% begin breaking balls
45 to 60 throws in batting practice (fastball only)

Step 13: 30 throws off mound 75%
30 breaking balls 75%
30 throws in batting practice

Step 14: 30 throws off mound 75%
60 to 90 throws in batting practice (gradually increase breaking balls)

Step 15: Simulated game: Progress by 15 throws per workout (pitch count)

All throwing off the mound should be done in the presence of a pitching coach or sport biomechanist to stress proper throwing mechanics. (A speed gun should be used to aid in effort control.)

* Percentage effort

† Use Interval Throwing 120 ft (36.6 m) phase as warm-up.

---

been used to treat tendinitis. The patch is worn for 20 to 24 h with dexamethasone applied. High-voltage stimulation and cryotherapy are used to alleviate pain and postexercise inflammation. Few published studies are presently available regarding the identification of an optimal modality or modality sequence to assist with the initial phase of pain diminution. Modalities used during the early stage of nonsurgical treatment have been critically reviewed.[10] Continued research

Table 5

Epicondylitis Rehabilitation Protocol

Phase I: Acute Phase

Goals: Decrease inflammation, promote tissue healing, retard muscular atrophy

Cryotherapy

Whirlpool

Stretching to increase wrist flexibility; elbow extension/flexion; forearm extension/flexion; supination/pronation

Wrist isometrics; elbow extension/flexion; forearm extension/flexion; supination/pronation

High-voltage galvanic stimulation

Phonophoresis

Friction massage

Iontophoresis (with anti-inflammatory medication; for example, dexamethasone)

Avoid painful movements (such as gripping)

Phase II: Subacute Phase

Goals: Improve flexibility, increase muscle strength/endurance; increase functional activities/return to function

Emphasize concentric/eccentric strengthening

Concentration on involved muscle group

Wrist extension/flexion

Forearm pronation/supination

Elbow flexion/extension

Initiate shoulder strengthening (if deficiencies are noted)

Continue flexibility exercises

May use counterforce brace

Continue use of cryotherapy after exercise/function

Gradual return to stressful activities

Gradually reinitiate activity once painful movements subside

Phase III: Chronic Phase

Goals: Improve muscular strength and endurance; maintain or enhance flexibility; gradual return to sports, high-level activities

Continue strengthening exercises (emphasize eccentric/concentric)

Continue to emphasize deficiencies in shoulder and elbow strength

Continue flexibility exercises

Gradually decrease use of counterforce brace

Use cryotherapy as needed

Gradual return to sport activity

Equipment modification (grip size, string tension, playing surface)

Emphasize maintenance program

highlighting prospective randomized models will assist in the identification of preferred treatment methods for this phase of rehabilitation of overuse tendon injury.

Patients with tendinosis can be treated with transverse friction massage, stretching, a focus on eccentric strengthening[11] with gradually progressing loads, and warm packs or ultrasound to promote tendon regeneration.

Once the patient's symptoms have subsided, aggressive stretching and a high load, low repetition strengthening program with emphasis on eccentric contractions are initiated. Wrist flexion and extension activities should be performed initially with the elbow flexed 30° to 45°. A gradual progression through plyometric and throwing activities precedes the initiation of the interval throwing program. Because poor mechanics are often a cause of this condition, an analysis of sport mechanics and proper supervision through the interval throwing program are critical. If nonsurgical treatment fails, surgical débridement of the necrosection tissue can be done.

Ulnar Neuropathy

Numerous theories exist regarding the cause of ulnar neuropathy of the elbow in throwing athletes. Ulnar nerve changes can result from tensile forces, compressive forces, or nerve instability. Any one or a combination of these mechanisms may be responsible for ulnar nerve symptoms.

A leading mechanism for tensile force on the ulnar nerve is valgus stress, which may be coupled with an external rotation-supination stress overload mechanism. The traction forces are further magnified when underlying valgus instability from UCL injuries is present. Ulnar neuropathy is often a secondary pathology of UCL insufficiency. Compression of the ulnar nerve is often caused by hypertrophy of the surrounding soft tissues or the presence of scar tissue. The nerve also may be trapped between the two heads of the flexor carpi ulnaris. Repetitive flexion and extension of the elbow with an unstable nerve can irritate or inflame the nerve. The nerve may subluxate or rest on the medial epicondyle, rendering it vulnerable to direct trauma.

The first stage of ulnar neuropathy includes an acute onset of radicular symptoms. The second stage is manifested by a recurrence of symptoms as the athlete attempts to return to competition. The third stage is associated with persistent motor weakness and sensory changes. Once the athlete enters the third stage of injury, nonsurgical treatment may not be effective.

The nonsurgical treatment of ulnar neuropathy focuses on diminishing ulnar nerve irritation, enhancing dynamic medial joint stability, and gradually returning the athlete to competition. Often nonsteroidal anti-inflammatory drugs are prescribed, and rehabilitation includes iontophoresis with a disposable patch and cryotherapy. Following the diagnosis of ulnar neuropathy, throwing athletes are instructed to discontinue throwing activities for at least 4 weeks, depending on the severity and chronicity of symptoms. The athlete progresses through the immediate motion and intermediate phases over the course of 4 to 6 weeks with emphasis placed on eccentric and dynamic stabilization drills. Plyometric exercises are used to facilitate further dynamic stabilization of the medial elbow. The athlete is allowed to begin an interval throwing program when full painless ROM and muscle performance is exhibited without neurologic symptoms. The athlete may gradu-

ally return to play if progression through the interval throwing program does not reveal neurologic symptoms.

Valgus Extension Overload

Valgus extension overload can occur during repetitive sport activities such as throwing, or during the acceleration or deceleration phase as the olecranon wedges against the medial olecranon fossa during elbow extension. This mechanism may result in osteophyte formation and potentially loose bodies. Repetitive extension stress from the triceps may further contribute to this injury. There is often a certain degree of underlying valgus laxity of the elbow in these athletes, further facilitating osteophyte formation through compression of the radiocapitellar joint and the posteromedial elbow. Overhead athletes typically present with pain at the posteromedial aspect of the elbow that is exacerbated with forced extension and valgus stress.

Nonsurgical treatment is often attempted before surgical intervention is considered. Initial treatment involves relieving posterior elbow pain and inflammation. As symptoms subside and ROM normalizes, dynamic stabilization and strengthening exercises are initiated. Emphasis is placed on improving eccentric strength of the elbow flexors in an attempt to control the rapid extension that occurs at the elbow during athletics. Forceful triceps extension, especially performed rapidly, is progressively integrated. Manual resistance exercises of concentric and eccentric elbow flexion are performed as well as elbow flexion with exercise tubing. The athlete's throwing mechanics should be carefully assessed to determine if mechanical faults are causing symptoms of valgus extension overload.

Ulnar Collateral Ligament Injury

Injuries to the UCL are becoming increasingly more common in overhead throwing athletes, although the higher incidence of injury may be a result of an increase in the diagnosis of these injuries. The elbow experiences a tremendous amount of valgus stress during overhead throwing that approaches the ultimate failure load of the ligament with each throw. The repetitive nature of overhead throwing activities such as baseball pitching, javelin throwing, and football passing further increase the susceptibility of UCL injury by exposing the ligament to repetitive microtraumatic forces. The stresses on the UCL are greater with specific types of pitches, such as the slider and split-fingered pitch.

Conservative treatment is attempted with partial tears and sprains of the UCL, although surgical reconstruction may be warranted for complete tears or if nonsurgical treatment is unsuccessful. A nonsurgical rehabilitation program is outlined in **Table 6**. ROM is initially permitted in a nonpainful arc of motion, usually from 10° to 100°, to allow for a decrease in inflammation and the alignment of collagen tissue. A brace may be used to restrict motion and prevent valgus loading. Furthermore, it may be beneficial to rest the UCL

Table 6

Conservative Treatment Following Ulnar Collateral Sprains of the Elbow

I. Immediate Motion Phase (Weeks 0 through 2)

Goals: Increase range of motion (ROM); promote healing of ulnar collateral ligament; retard muscle atrophy; decrease pain and inflammation

1. ROM:

Brace (optional) nonpainful ROM (20° to 90°)

Active-assisted ROM, passive ROM elbow and wrist (nonpainful range)

2. Exercises:

Isometrics—wrist and elbow musculature

Shoulder strengthening (no external rotation strengthening)

3. Ice and compression

II. Intermediate Phase (Weeks 3 through 6)

Goals: Increase ROM; improve strength/endurance; decrease pain and inflammation; promote stability

1. ROM:

Gradually increase motion 0° to 135° (increase flexion 10° per week)

2. Exercises:

Initiate isotonic exercises, wrist curls, wrist extensions, pronation/supination, biceps/triceps dumbbells, external rotation, deltoid, supraspinatus, rhomboids, internal rotation

3. Ice and compression

III. Advanced Phase (Weeks 6 and 7 through 12 and 14)

Criteria to progress

1. Full ROM

2. No pain or tenderness

3. No increase in laxity

4. Strength 4/5 of elbow flexor/extensor

Goals: Increase strength, power, and endurance; improve neuromuscular control; initiate high-speed drills

1. Exercises:

Initiate exercise tubing, shoulder program (Thrower's Ten program, biceps/triceps program), supination/pronation, wrist extension/flexion, plyometrics throwing drills

IV. Return to Activity Phase (Weeks 12 through 14)

Criteria to progress to return to throwing:

1. Full painless ROM

2. No increase in laxity

3. Isokinetic test fulfills criteria

4. Satisfactory clinical examination

1. Exercises:

Initiate interval throwing

Continue Thrower's Ten program

Continue plyometrics

immediately following the initial painful episode of throwing to prevent additionally deleterious stresses on the injured UCL. Isometric exercises are performed for the shoulder, elbow, and wrist to prevent muscular atrophy. Ice and anti-inflammatory medications are prescribed to control pain and inflammation.

ROM of both flexion and extension is gradually increased by 5° to 10° per week during the second phase of treatment or as tolerated. Full ROM should be achieved by at least 3 to 4 weeks. Elbow flexion/extension motion is encouraged. Rhythmic stabilization exercises are initiated to develop dynamic stabilization and neuromuscular control of the upper extremity. As dynamic stability is advanced, isotonic exercises are incorporated for the entire upper extremity.

The advanced strengthening phase is usually initiated at 6 to 7 weeks postinjury. During this phase, the athlete is progressed to the Thrower's Ten isotonic strengthening program, and plyometric exercises are slowly initiated. An interval return-to-throwing program is initiated once the athlete regains full motion, adequate strength, and dynamic stability of the elbow. The athlete is allowed to return to competition following the asymptomatic completion of the interval sport program. If symptoms recur during the interval throwing program, it is usually with throwing at longer distances or greater intensities or with off-the-mound throwing. If symptoms continue to persist, surgical intervention is considered.

Little League Elbow

Pain in the medial elbow is common in adolescent throwers. The medial epicondyle physis is subject to repetitive tensile and valgus forces during the arm-cocking and acceleration phases of throwing. These forces may result in microtraumatic injury to the physis with potential fragmentation, hypertrophy, separation of the epiphysis, or avulsion of the medial epicondyle. Treatment varies based on the extent of injury.

In the absence of an avulsion, a rehabilitation program similar to that of the nonsurgical UCL program is initiated. Emphasis is placed initially on reducing pain and inflammation and restoring motion and strength. Strengthening exercises are performed in a gradual fashion. Isometric exercises are performed first, followed by light isotonic exercises. No heavy lifting is permitted for 12 to 14 weeks. An interval throwing program is initiated as tolerated when symptoms subside.

In the presence of a nondisplaced or minimally displaced avulsion, a brief period of immobilization for approximately 7 days is encouraged, followed by a gradual progression of ROM, flexibility, and strengthening exercises. An interval throwing program is usually allowed at weeks 6 to 8. If the avulsion is displaced, an open reduction, internal fixation procedure may be required.

Specific Postoperative Rehabilitation Guidelines

Ulnar Nerve Transposition

Transposition of the ulnar nerve usually is performed in a subcutaneous fashion using fascial slings. Caution is taken to avoid overstressing the soft-tissue structures involved with relocating the nerve while healing occurs.[2] The rehabilitation protocol following an ulnar nerve transposition is outlined in **Table 7**. A posterior splint at 90° of elbow flexion is used for the first week postoperatively to prevent excessive extension ROM and tension on the nerve. The splint is removed at the beginning of week 2 for exercise and bathing, and light ROM activities are initiated. Full ROM is usually restored by weeks 3 to 4. Gentle isotonic strengthening is begun during week 4 and progressed to the full Thrower's Ten program by 6 weeks following surgery. Aggressive strengthening including eccentric and plyometric training is incorporated by weeks 7 to 8, and an interval throwing program at weeks 8 to 9, if all previously outlined criteria are met. A return to competition usually occurs between weeks 12 and 16 postoperatively.

Posterior Olecranon Osteophyte Excision

Surgical excision of posterior olecranon osteophytes is performed arthroscopically using an osteotome or motorized burr. The rehabilitation program following arthroscopic posterior olecranon osteophyte excision is slightly more conservative in restoring full elbow extension secondary to postsurgical pain. ROM is progressed within the patient's tolerance; by 10 days after surgery, the patient should exhibit at least 15° to 110° of ROM, and 5° to 115° of ROM by day 14. Full ROM (≤145°) is typically restored by days 20 to 25 postsurgery. The rate of ROM progression is most often limited by osseous pain and synovial joint inflammation, usually located at the top of the olecranon.

The strengthening program is similar to the previously discussed progression. Isometric exercises are performed for the first 10 to 14 days and isotonic strengthening exercises from weeks 2 to 6. Initially, especially during the first 2 weeks, forceful triceps contractions may produce posterior elbow pain; the force produced by the triceps muscle should be avoided or reduced. The full Thrower's Ten program is initiated by week 6. An interval throwing program is included by weeks 10 to 12. The rehabilitation focus is similar to the nonsurgical treatment of valgus extension overload. Emphasis is placed on eccentric control of the elbow flexors and dynamic stabilization of the medial elbow.[12]

Ulnar Collateral Ligament Reconstruction

Surgical reconstruction of the UCL attempts to restore the stabilizing functions of the anterior bundle of the UCL. The palmaris longus or gracilis graft source is taken and passed in a figure-of-8 pattern through drill holes in the sublime tubercle of the ulna and the medial epicondyle. A subcutaneous ulnar nerve transposition is performed at the time of reconstruction. Some surgeons

Table 7

Postoperative Rehabilitation Following Ulnar Nerve Transposition

Phase I: Immediate Postoperative Phase (Weeks 0 to 1)

Goals: Allow soft-tissue healing of relocated nerve; decrease pain and inflammation; retard muscle atrophy

A. Week 1
1. Posterior splint at 90° elbow flexion with wrist free for motion (sling for comfort)
2. Compression dressing
3. Exercises such as gripping exercises, wrist ROM, shoulder isometrics

B. Week 2
1. Remove posterior splint for exercise and bathing
2. Progress elbow ROM (postoperative ROM 15° to 120°)
3. Initiate elbow and wrist isometrics
4. Continue shoulder isometrics

Phase II: Intermediate Phase (Weeks 3 to 7)

Goals: Restore full painless ROM; improve strength, power, and endurance of upper extremity musculature; gradually increase functional demands

A. Week 3
1. Discontinue posterior splint
2. Progress elbow ROM, emphasize full extension
3. Initiate flexibility exercise for wrist extension/flexion, forearm supination/pronation, and elbow extension/flexion
4. Initiate strengthening exercises for wrist extension/flexion, forearm supination/pronation, elbow extensors/flexors, and a shoulder program

B. Week 6
1. Continue all exercises listed above
2. Initiate light sports activities

Phase III: Advanced Strengthening Phase (Weeks 8 to 12)

Goals: Increase strength, power, and endurance; gradually initiate sports activity
1. Initiate eccentric exercise program
2. Initiate plyometric exercise drills
3. Continue shoulder and elbow strengthening and flexibility exercises
4. Initiate interval throwing program

Phase IV: Return to Activity Phase (Weeks 12 to 16)

Goals: Gradually return to sports activities
1. Return to competitive throwing
2. Continue Thrower's Ten exercise program

ROM = range of motion

are performing UCL reconstruction using the docking procedure.[13] The rehabilitation program following UCL reconstruction is based on the specific surgical procedure (Table 8). The athlete is placed in a posterior splint, with the elbow immobilized at 90° of flexion for the first 7 days postoperatively to allow adequate healing of the UCL graft and soft-tissue slings involved in the nerve transposition. The patient is allowed to per-

4: Rehabilitation

Table 8

Postoperative Rehabilitation Following Chronic Ulnar Collateral Ligament Reconstruction Using Autogenous Graft

Phase I: Immediate Postoperative Phase (0 to 3 Weeks)

Goals: Protect healing tissue, decrease pain/inflammation, retard muscle atrophy
A. Postoperative week 1
   1. Posterior splint at 90° elbow flexion
   2. Wrist active ROM extension/flexion
   3. Elbow compression dressing (2 to 3 days)
   4. Exercises such as gripping exercises, wrist ROM, shoulder isometrics (except shoulder external rotation), biceps isometrics
   5. Cryotherapy
B . Postoperative week 2
   1. Application of functional brace to allow 30° to 100° of flexion
   2. Initiate wrist isometrics
   3. Initiate elbow flexion/extension isometrics
   4. Continue all exercises listed above
C. Postoperative week 3
   1. Advance brace 15° to 110° (gradually increase ROM; 5° of extension and 10° of flexion per week)

Phase II: Intermediate Phase (Weeks 4 to 8)

Goals: Gradual increase in range of motion, promote healing of repaired tissue, regain and improve muscle strength
A. Week 4
   1. Functional brace set (10° to 120°)
   2. Begin light resistance exercises for arm (1 lb) wrist curls, extensions pronation/supination elbow extension/flexion
   3. Progress shoulder program emphasizes rotator cuff strengthening (avoid external rotation until sixth week)
B. Week 6
   1. Functional brace set (0° to 130°); active ROM 0° to 145° (without brace)
   2. Progress elbow strengthening exercises
   3. Initiate shoulder external rotation strengthening
   4. Progress shoulder program

Phase III: Advanced Strengthening Phase (Weeks 9 to 13)

Goals: Increase strength, power and endurance; maintain full elbow ROM; gradually initiate sports activity
A. Week 9
   1. Initiate eccentric elbow flexion/extension
   2. Continue isotonic program; forearm and wrist
   3. Continue shoulder program—Thrower's Ten program
   4. Manual resistance diagonal patterns
   5. Initiate plyometric exercise program
B. Week 11
   1. Continue all exercises listed above
   2. May begin light sport activities (such as golf or swimming)

Phase IV: Return to Activity Phase (Weeks 14 to 26)

Goals: Continue to increase strength, power, and endurance of upper extremity musculature; gradual return to sport activities
A. Week 14
   1. Initiate interval throwing program (phase 1)
   2. Continue strengthening program
   3. Emphasis on elbow and wrist strengthening and flexibility exercises
B. Weeks 22 through 26
   1. Return to competitive throwing

ROM = range of motion

form wrist ROM and gripping and submaximal isometric exercises for the wrist and elbow. The patient is progressed from the posterior splint to an elbow ROM brace, which is adjusted to allow approximately postoperative ROM from approximately 30° to 100° of flexion. Motion is increased by 5° of extension and 10° of flexion thereafter to restore full ROM (≤145°) by the end of week 6. The brace is discontinued by weeks 5 to 6.

Isometric exercises are progressed to include light resistance isotonic exercises at week 4 and the full Thrower's Ten program by week 6. Progressive resistance exercises are incorporated at weeks 8 to 9. Focus is again placed on developing dynamic stabilization of the medial elbow. Because of the anatomic orientation of the flexor carpi ulnaris and flexor digitorum superficialis overlying the UCL, isotonic and stabilization activities for these muscles may assist the UCL in stabilizing valgus stress at the medial elbow. Thus, concentric strengthening of these muscles is performed.[12,14]

Aggressive exercises involving eccentric and plyometric contractions are included in the advanced phase, usually weeks 12 through 16. Two-hand plyometric drills are performed at weeks 10 to 12, and one-hand drills at weeks 13 to 14. An interval throwing program is allowed at postoperative week 16. In most instances, throwing from a mound is progressed within 4 to 6 weeks following the initiation of an interval throwing program and a return to competitive throwing at approximately 9 months following surgery.

The rehabilitation program following UCL reconstruction using the docking procedure is slightly different. An elbow brace with ROM from 30° to 90° is used for 6 weeks. During the first 6 weeks, light exercise is allowed. Light tossing is permitted at 4 months, pitching at 9 months, and a return to competition at 12 months.

Summary

The elbow joint is a common site of injury in athletes, particularly the overhead athlete. Elbow injury in the overhead athlete usually is caused by repetitive microtraumatic injuries observed during the act of throwing. In other athletes, such as those who participate in collision sports such as football, wrestling, soccer, or gymnastics, the elbow injury often is caused by macrotraumatic forces during fractures, dislocations, and ligamentous injuries. Rehabilitation of the elbow, whether postinjury or postoperatively, must follow a progressive and sequential order to ensure that healing tissues are not overstressed. The rehabilitation program should limit immobilization and achieve full ROM early, especially elbow extension. Furthermore, the rehabilitation program should progressively restore strength and neuromuscular control; gradually incorporating sport specific activities is essential to successfully returning the athlete to his or her previous level of competition as quickly and safely as possible. The rehabilitation of the elbow must include rehabilitation for the entire kinetic chain (scapula, shoulder, hand, core/hips and legs) to ensure the athlete's return to high-level sports participation.

Annotated References

1. Werner SL, Fleisig GS, Dillman CJ, Andrews JR: Biomechanics of the elbow during baseball pitching. *J Orthop Sports Phys Ther* 1993;17:274-278.

2. Wilk KE, Arrigo C, Andrews JR: Rehabilitation of the elbow in the throwing athlete. *J Orthop Sports Phys Ther* 1993;17:305-317.

3. Wright RW, Steger-May K, Wasserlauf BL, O'Neal ME, Weinberg BW, Paletta GA: Elbow range of motion in professional baseball pitchers. *Am J Sports Med* 2006; 34:190-193.

   This study measured elbow ROM in 33 professional baseball pitchers using a goniometer. Results of this study showed an 8° flexion contracture on the dominant elbow on average with a 5.5° loss of elbow flexion on the dominant side. This study portrays normal ROM variations and adaptations in the elite level throwing athlete.

4. Ellenbecker TS, Mattalino AJ, Elam EA, Caplinger RA: Medial elbow laxity in professional baseball pitchers: A bilateral comparison using stress radiography. *Am J Sports Med* 1998;26:420-424.

5. Wilk KE, Voight M, Keirns MD, et al: Plyometrics for the upper extremities: Theory and clinical application. *J Orthop Sports Phys Ther* 1993;17:225-239.

6. Reinold MM, Wilk KE, Reed J, Crenshaw K, Andrews JR: Internal sport programs: Guidelines for baseball, tennis, and golf. *J Orthop Sports Phys Ther* 2002; 32:293-298.

7. Wilk KE, Arrigo CA: Rehabilitation of elbow injuries, in Andrews JR, Harrelson GL, Wilk KE (eds): *Physical Rehabilitation of the Injured Athlete*, ed 3. Philadelphia, PA, WB Saunders Company, 2004, pp 590-618.

   This chapter provides an overview of the rehabilitation strategies for the elbow, with an emphasis on humeral epicondylitis and UCL injury. Protocols are included for rehabilitation.

8. Nirschl R, Sobel J: Conservative treatment of tennis elbow. *Phys Sportsmed* 1981;9:43-54.

9. Gabel GT, Morrey BF: Medial epicondylitis: Surgical management, influence of ulnar neuropathy. *J Shoulder Elbow Surg* 1994;3:511-516.

10. Boyer MI, Hastings H II: Lateral tennis elbow: Is there any science out there? *J Shoulder Elbow Surg* 1999;8: 481-491.

4: Rehabilitation

11. Svernlov B, Adolfsson L: Non-operative treatment regime including eccentric training for lateral humeral epicondylalgia. *Scand J Med Sci Sports* 2001;11: 328-334.

12. Wilk KE, Reinhold MM, Andrews JR: Rehabilitation of the thrower's elbow. *Sports Med Arthroscopy Rev* 2003; 11:79-95.

    This article presents an overview of the rehabilitation program for the throwing athlete with elbow dysfunction. It includes most of the common elbow injuries and specific aspects of each rehabilitation program. The return to throwing recommendations as well as ROM and strengthening progressions are included.

13. Rohrbough JT, Altchek DW, Hyman-Williams RJ, Botts JD: Medial collateral ligament reconstruction of the elbow using the docking procedure. *Am J Sports Med* 2002;30:541-548.

14. Wilk KE, Reinold MM, Andrews JR: Rehabilitation of the thrower's elbow. *Clin Sports Med* 2004;23:765-801.

    This article provides rehabilitation strategies for the thrower's elbow including an overview of proximal strengthening of the shoulder and the interval throwing program used in the later stages of rehabilitation.

Chapter 20

Anterior Cruciate Ligament Reconstruction: Rehabilitation Concepts

Robert C. Manske, PT, DPT, MEd, SCS, ATC   Mark DeCarlo, PT, MHS, SCS, ATC
George J. Davies, DPT, MEd, PT, FAPTA, SCS, ATC   Mark Paterno, PT, MS, MBA, SCS, ATC

General Principles

Patient Education

After anterior cruciate ligament (ACL) reconstruction, the patient should be aware of key issues. The patient should have a general overview of the rehabilitation process, which should include expectations for the subsequent rehabilitation and proposed outcomes. Concomitant procedures done at the time of surgery (meniscus procedures, chondroplasty, or other articular cartilage procedures) should be discussed as they relate to the existing protocol. Other factors of concern include range of motion (ROM) and weight-bearing limitations or progressions. Time frames during which graft necrosis and weakness occur, which is when patients notice substantial improvement in overall symptoms, should be discussed. Although a rare occurrence, redness or drainage caused by infection at incision sites should be discussed because of the possible devastating consequences.

Pain

Pain is always present after an invasive surgical procedure and can impede quadriceps firing and ROM. Cryotherapy and electrical stimulation can be used to alleviate pain. Cryotherapy decreases nerve conduction velocity[1] and releases endogenous opiates.[2]

Swelling

Swelling has detrimental effects on intra-articular structures such as articular cartilage and synovium. Intra-articular effusion affects muscle recruitment by causing quadriceps muscle inhibition. Impairments related to knee effusion can be treated with several available therapeutic modalities, such as cryotherapy. Recent evidence supports the dis-inhibition effect of cryotherapy on the quadriceps muscles.[3,4] In a randomized controlled trial, patients were placed into one of four treatment groups: a cooling pad filled with water at 40° to 50°F, a cooling pad filled with water at 70° to 80°F, a

bag filled with crushed ice, and no cold therapy. A significant decrease in knee temperature was achieved with the different cooling methods, although no difference in objective outcomes such as length of hospital stay, knee ROM, and the use of intramuscular and oral pain medication was found. Other commonly used methods are compressive wrappings and high-voltage galvanic electrical stimulation (HVGS). When HVGS was used immediately after injury (within the first hour), edema formation was decreased.[5]

Range of Motion

Because prolonged joint immobilization will result in the loss of ground substance along with dehydration and approximation of embedded fibers in the extracellular matrix,[6,7] early immediate motion is warranted. These changes contribute to fibrous adhesions and increased friction between soft-tissue fibers.[8-10] Controlled remobilization after injury and surgery can reverse the effects of immobilization by stimulating collagen synthesis and optimizing alignment.[11-13]

Immediate motion is more beneficial to a healing graft than delayed motion. In early prospective randomized controlled trials on the effects of immediate ROM, patients donned a dorsal plaster splint immediately after surgery and were randomly assigned to either continue wearing a plaster hinged splint, or to continue wearing an ordinary cylinder splint that restricted motion.[14,15] Immobilization lasted 4 weeks, but outcomes were gathered 1 year after surgery. The immobilized group had marked atrophy of the vastus lateralis and slow twitch muscle fibers, whereas there was no change in cross-sectional area of slow or fast twitch muscle fibers in those wearing the hinged splint.

In another study, patients undergoing ACL rehabilitation were placed into continuous passive motion (CPM) devices either on the second or seventh postoperative day.[16] Patients in whom CPM was delayed until postoperative day 7 also were immediately placed in a brace locked at 10° of knee flexion until CPM was started. Objective outcomes, including joint effusion, hemarthrosis, soft-tissue swelling, flexion and extension limits of ROM, and length of hospital stay, were found to be similar for each group. Immediate passive ROM via CPM did not endanger the graft.

The efficacy of early active ROM, CPM, or a combination of both was studied after bone-patellar tendon-bone (BPTB) reconstructions.[17] Patients placed in the early active ROM group had similar outcomes for ROM and ligament laxity as the other groups. It was reported that CPM during the first 4 to 14 days following ACL reconstruction resulted in favorable knee motion and limb girth.[18] In one study, patients were randomly placed into either a cast immobilization group or an early ROM training group in a brace.[19] All performed similar exercises except for the initial ROM limitations during the first 5 weeks. At 2-year follow-up, the early ROM in the brace did not increase knee laxity nor hinder ROM or subjective knee function and activity level in comparison with plaster cast immobilization for 5 weeks.

Early ROM after ACL reconstruction is not detrimental to the graft source. Additionally, early ROM may be beneficial by reducing pain, lessening adverse changes in articular cartilage, and preventing early scar formation and capsular contractions that can limit motion. Because there is evidence to support early ROM no matter which graft source is used, immediate, full, passive, terminal extension of the knee is required. Although knee flexion losses are rarely incurred, knee extension loss is one of the more common complications after reconstruction. Abnormal tibiofemoral joint arthrokinematics can cause patellofemoral and tibiofemoral joint contact pressures to increase, resulting in reflex pain inhibition to the quadriceps femoris.[20,21] These forces appear to increase at angles of knee flexion beyond 15°.[22] Another reason for obtaining full knee extension is to ensure that the intracondylar notch does not allow infiltration of scar tissue that can block full knee extension ROM. Full extensions can be unachievable if the intracondylar notch is allowed to proliferate with scar tissue, resulting in a cyclops lesion. Preoperative indicators of loss of knee extension were studied in 102 patients within 2 weeks of ACL reconstruction surgery and 6 months afterward.[23] Patients with loss of knee extension ROM before surgery (in comparison with the contralateral knee) were more likely to have limited knee extension after surgery. For optimal outcomes following ACL reconstruction, prerehabilitation may be needed before surgery in select patients with limited knee extension motion.

Therefore, the first postoperative goal is to regain symmetric full terminal knee extension. The goal is to achieve 0° of extension during the first postoperative visit regardless of the timing (day 2 versus week 2). This goal may be achieved initially at the expense of flexion motion. Unlike knee extension limitations, knee flexion limitations usually are resolved without complications. Impediments to full knee extension are pain

and swelling, which can be treated with electrical stimulation. An acute surgical hemarthrosis must be treated. Specific therapeutic exercises for regaining knee extension motion include manual passive ROM exercise into hyperextension, supine hangs with a towel roll under the heel, prone hangs, and knee thunks.[24,25] Hangs can be done with the patient supine or sitting with the foot in another chair or on a stool. Overpressure can be applied by a therapist or with a 5- to 10-lb weight. Using a weight for an extended period is a way to induce a prolonged, low-load, long-duration stretch to the tissues in an attempt to gain a more plastic deformation.

Patellofemoral complications are common after ACL reconstruction, especially with BPTB repair.[26] The loss of patellar mobility, also known as infrapatellar contracture syndrome, may be a fate worse than if the ACL had not been replaced.[27,28] This loss of patellar mobility is caused by intra-articular medial and lateral gutter scar formation. Scarring may proliferate during immobilization, enticing scar adhesions to form along the incision following harvest of the patellar tendon or the hamstring grafts. Scarring also may occur along the smaller portal incision sites. These areas of potential scar proliferation should be treated with immediate scar mobilization around the periphery of the incisions. Mobilizations should be performed medial to lateral and in the superior–inferior direction (**Figure 1**). Of most importance to extensor mechanism alignment are the superior-inferior patellofemoral joint mobilizations. Superior glide joint mobilizations assist with knee extension and inferior glide mobilizations assist with knee flexion. Patients are instructed to perform these mobilizations as part of their home exercise program.

Muscle Recruitment

Multiple studies have proven that electrical muscle stimulation after ACL reconstruction is warranted. Volitional exercises combined with neuromuscular electrical stimulation result in more normal gait parameters and better restoration of extensor strength than rehabilitation with volitional exercises alone.[29] Quadriceps isometric strength measurements in a group of patients who performed voluntary contraction of the quadriceps muscle were compared with those of a group who received electrical muscle stimulation superimposed on the voluntary contraction. After 6 weeks of treatment, the group that performed voluntary contraction alone had a significant decrease in isometric muscle force production compared with those who received electrical stimulation.[30] Applying neuromuscular electrical stimulation to the hamstrings and quadriceps in a patient 6 weeks after ACL reconstruction elicited increases in knee flexion and extension torque.[31] In a study of five groups of ACL reconstruction patients, the group that used neuromuscular electrical stimulation did not have a reduction in atrophy according to girth measurements around the quadriceps.[32] Loss of strength in the neuromuscular electrical stimulation

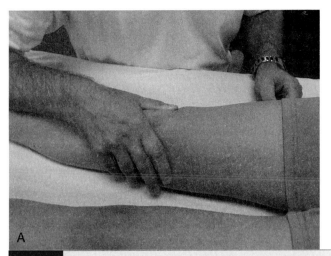
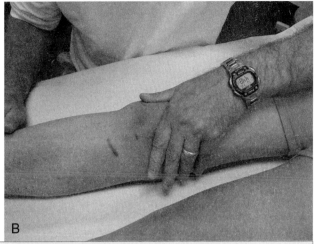

Figure 1 | **A,** Superior patellar glide joint mobilization. **B,** Inferior patellar glide joint mobilization.

group was minimized in comparison with the other four groups, in which a transcutaneous electrical nerve stimulation unit, immobilization in flexion, immobilization in extension, and CPM were implemented. The neuromuscular electrical stimulation group also noticed a substantial decrease in patellofemoral crepitus. In another study, 20 ACL reconstruction patients were placed into one of two groups.[33] One group received neuromuscular electrical stimulation and volitional exercises for the quadriceps and the other received volitional exercises alone. After 4 weeks of treatment, less strength was lost in the electrical stimulation and volitional exercises group than the group that performed volitional exercises alone. The stimulation and volitional group additionally had significant improvements in functional performance parameters such as gait cadence, walking velocity, stance time of the involved limb, and flexion-extension of the knee during stance phase. In a larger study, 110 patients were randomly assigned to one of several groups: high-intensity neuromuscular stimulation, high-level volitional exercises, low-intensity neuromuscular stimulation, or a combined high- and low-intensity neuromuscular stimulation group.[34] Isometric quadriceps strength was assessed after 4 weeks of treatment. Quadriceps strength averaged 70% or greater (in comparison with the uninvolved knee) in the two groups that received high-intensity electrical stimulation, while averaging only 57% and 51%, respectively, in the groups receiving high-level volitional exercises and low-intensity neuromuscular stimulation.

It appears that the most appropriate use of neuromuscular electrical stimulation is in conjunction with volitional contraction of both the quadriceps and hamstring musculature. Empirically, it appears that the best results clinically are seen when neuromuscular electrical stimulation is done while in a weight-bearing, dependent position (**Figure 2**). This upright position may reflexively facilitate normal motor firing patterns called

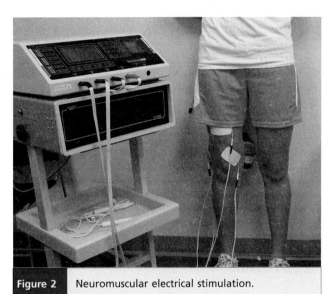

Figure 2 | Neuromuscular electrical stimulation.

upon during weight-bearing activities. Electrical muscle stimulation is used early, within the first few days after surgery, when muscle inhibition caused by swelling and pain is most evident. Muscle stimulation techniques also can be done during isometric activities such as the straight leg raise, quadriceps sets, and isometric knee extension exercises performed within safe ranges of knee flexion (90° to 45°). Once the patient is able to actively fire the quadriceps, the addition of biofeedback may be helpful to allow motivation for the enhancement of quadriceps muscle firing and recruitment.

Weight Bearing

One of the advancements of most accelerated protocols following ACL reconstruction is the initiation of weight bearing as tolerated to full weight-bearing status immediately after surgery. Before the advent of accelerated rehabilitation, weight bearing was limited initially because of concerns about graft strain or impairment of graft-

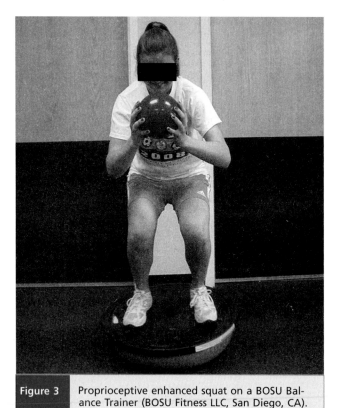

Figure 3 Proprioceptive enhanced squat on a BOSU Balance Trainer (BOSU Fitness LLC, San Diego, CA).

tunnel healing. Animal studies have shown that grafts that allow for bone-to-bone healing, such as the BPTB graft, heal faster (in 6 weeks), whereas soft-tissue grafts require tendon-to-bone healing and healing occurs in up to 12 weeks.[35,36] Although animal studies cannot be extrapolated exactly to humans, early graft-tunnel healing is desirable for subsequent rehabilitation. Exact time frames of graft incorporation in the human model are not yet known. In most instances, a high-strength graft that has judicious fixation is used, allowing early and immediate weight bearing. Some protocols still limit weight bearing after soft-tissue fixation methods, such as hamstring-gracilis tendon reconstructions. Because of excellent fixation from the bony construct in the BPTB graft, full weight bearing immediately after the surgical reconstruction is common.

Partial weight bearing should begin initially to ensure that proper gait sequence and cadence can be performed. Pain should be under control to allow normal progression to full weight bearing. If pain continues, medication should be given to help control reflex inhibition of the quadriceps muscle. Immediate full-knee extension is important to facilitate a normal heel-toe gait cycle to avoid a flexed knee gait pattern, which can place significant stress on the anterior knee and the extensor mechanism.

Rehabilitation with immediate weight bearing was compared with weight bearing delayed for 2 weeks.[37] At a mean time of 7.3 months, there were no differences between weight-bearing status with regard to ROM, vastus medialis oblique function, and knee lax-

ity. Immediate weight bearing resulted in a decreased incidence of anterior knee pain.

It appears that immediate weight bearing is indicated after ACL reconstruction because it appears that fixation problems or excessive loads that can harm or deform the graft are avoided. One instance where this may not be the case is with the hamstring-gracilis ACL reconstruction. Because this graft construct uses soft tissue to bone fixation, some patients are required to avoid full weight bearing until 4 to 6 weeks after the procedure.

Proprioceptive Control

It is well established that proprioceptive sense is lost and bilateral proprioceptive deficits occur after ACL reconstruction.[38-41] An increased focus is placed on restoring lost proprioception, dynamic knee stability, and neuromuscular control, including recruitment and timing. Neuromuscular training is done to improve the nervous system's ability to generate a fast and optimal muscle firing pattern, to increase dynamic joint stability, to decrease joint forces, and to relearn movement patterns and skills so that muscles achieve a state of "readiness" to respond to joint forces resulting in enhanced motor control.[42-44]

Basic proprioceptive exercises are begun the first day after surgery and are not dependent on weight-bearing status. If other concomitant procedures do not allow early, full weight bearing, basic proprioceptive drills (such as sitting on the edge of a table with the foot on a ball or Dynadisk [Exertools, Vavato, CA], moving the foot and knee through gentle motions, progressing to standing partial weight bearing on the disk) are performed submaximally in a partial weight-bearing position.

Once full weight bearing is allowed, closed kinetic chain weight-bearing shifting exercises are instituted. Beginning on level ground, patients will shift their weight into anterior/posterior, medial/lateral, and diagonal directions. Once these exercises are mastered on level surfaces, patients progress to exercising in more dynamic situations, such as incorporation of the Kinesthetic Ability Trainer (KAT; Breg, Vista, CA) or any of the various force platform systems. Partial squats or "minisquats" can begin through a safe range (0°-30°) of knee flexion, initially progressing to up to 45° as technique improves. Patients may have trouble with proper squatting technique after surgery; therefore, it is useful to demonstrate proper form or to have patients exercise while looking at themselves in a mirror until proper form is achieved. Exercise progression continues to a more labile surface, such as a piece of foam, a disk, or KAT for minisquats (**Figure 3**).

Weight-bearing, closed kinetic chain exercises were believed to create stabilization of the knee and minimize strain on the healing ACL graft.[43-45] The effect of weight-bearing and non–weight-bearing exercises on strain behavior of the normal ACL during squatting and active flexion-extension motions was studied in humans.[46] The strain values on the ACL during squatting were not different from those obtained during active flexion-extension exercises. Additionally, increasing the resistance torque across the knee joint in an effort to increase the magnitude of the muscle force during an open kinetic chain exercise will further increase the peak ACL strain. A similar increase in resistance will not produce this result in the closed kinetic chain exercise.[47] These studies suggest that the compressive load of body weight and muscle co-contraction may attenuate peak ACL strain values.[48,49] ACL strain was assessed after rehabilitation weight-bearing exercise; step-up, step-down, lunge, and one-legged sit-to-stand exercises did not produce greater strain on the ACL than the traditional two-legged squat,[48] possibly because increases in hamstring muscle activity decrease strains on the ACL.[50] The lunge and the one-legged sit-to-stand exercises are typically done in deeper ranges of knee flexion, which may assist in increased control and firing of the hamstring muscles.[44,51]

Once full weight bearing is achieved, single-leg balance exercises are initiated. These exercises are begun on level ground and sometimes near a rack that can be grasped for patient safety. These functional balance training exercises should be done at 30° of knee flexion to facilitate co-contraction of quadriceps/hamstring muscle synergy. The patient may start by standing on the affected leg, then moving the opposite leg in small increments in multiple directions. Once small oscillations are mastered, larger movements can begin. Further progression of single-limb balance can be done by adding or instituting movements of the upper extremities through straight and then diagonal movements and then by having the patient stand on a piece of foam or a disk. Throwing and catching a medicine ball of various weights is done in an attempt to move the center of gravity to stimulate neuromuscular control and stabilization.

In the later stages of rehabilitation, perturbation training can be instituted. Perturbation training involves the application of support surface perturbations through the use of rollerboards, rockerboards, and rollerboards with stationary platforms. During perturbation training, the goal is to induce dynamic knee stability through activities that challenge knee stability, allowing patients to develop their own compensation strategies to maintain stability.[52] Various techniques exist, including resisting the force of a perturbation or attempting to regain a balanced position after an application of perturbation.[53] Disruption of the patients' conscious thought during activities can be done by tossing a ball to catch or having them kick a soccer ball while attempting to balance on a single leg.

Return to Sports Participation After ACL Reconstruction

Current recommendations regarding the optimal means to advance an athlete through the final steps of rehabilitation and objectively determine their readiness to safely return to play lack concensus.[54,55] Some authors rely on objective measures of strength to drive the decision to return to sports participation, whereas others rely on functional performance testing, such as hop testing. No single test has proved sufficient to objectively make this clinical determination. As a result, widespread disagreement persists between practitioners regarding the safest and optimal time to return to sports participation.

The controversy regarding the optimal time to return to sports participation following ACL reconstruction is complex. Current ACL reconstruction protocols specify exercises and criteria to progress in the initial stages of rehabilitation;[56,57] however, many fail to describe exercise prescriptions and detailed progressions at the end stages of rehabilitation before return to sports participation. Therefore, there is less guidance in creating optimal end stage rehabilitation programs, which is a cause for concern considering recent evidence that as many as one in four patients undergoing an ACL reconstruction will have a second ACL injury within 10 years after reconstruction.[58] Despite rehabilitation, these patients may have ongoing neuromuscular risk factors, which have been shown to be modifiable in an uninjured population.[59,60] If the incidence of reinjury after ACL reconstruction remains high, and modifiable risk factors persist following the completion of rehabilitation,[61,62] then current rehabilitation programs may be failing to address these factors in the end stages of rehabilitation.

A second deficit in existing ACL reconstruction protocols is a lack of appropriate objective measures to accurately determine an athlete's readiness to safely return to sports participation. Current evidence suggests that measures such as isokinetic strength, functional hop performance, or temporal guidelines typically are used to determine readiness to return to sports participation.[54] However, these measures have limitations when used in isolation. Recommendations regarding return to sports participation based solely on temporal guidelines are highly variable in the medical community,[63] and do not consider individual patient variability in healing as well as the progression of impairments and function. Open kinetic chain assessments, such as isokinetic strength deficits, have historically shown moderate correlations to functional tasks,[64] and these deficits may persists up to 24 months after ACL reconstruction.[62,65] Conversely, closed kinetic chain assessments may fail to elucidate isolated quadriceps weaknesses because of the development of compensatory muscle recruitment patterns.[66] Furthermore, when assessed on more dynamic tasks, such as a drop vertical jump maneuver,[67] subjects demonstrated persistent at-risk deficits for as long as 2 years after ACL reconstruction, despite participating in athletic tasks.[61] Considering this current evidence, future research should focus on investigating what cluster of objective assessments could potentially provide better information

4: Rehabilitation

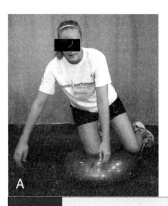
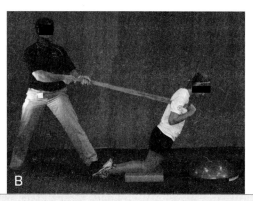
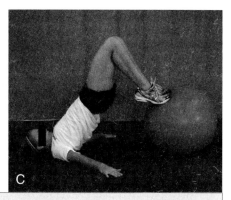

Figure 4 **A,** Core strengthening on a BOSU Balance Trainer. **B,** Eccentric hamstring strengthening. **C,** Swiss ball hamstring strengthening. (*A and C reproduced with permission from Myer GD, Chu DA, Brent JL, Hewett TE: Trunk and hip control neuromuscular training for the prevention of knee joint injury. Clin Sports Med 2008;27:425-428.*)

regarding an athlete's readiness to return to sports activity at the previous level of function, with minimal risk of reinjury.

Attempts have been made to specifically address the lack of objectivity in rehabilitation progression, optimal timing to release to activity, and the absence of a criteria-based progression.[55,68] A program was created that targets specific neuromuscular imbalances believed to increase risk for ACL injury.[69] An initial model of a criteria-based progression of end stage rehabilitation[68] as well as an algorithmic approach to navigating this progression with the ultimate criteria determining readiness to return to sports participation also was developed.[55] The intent was to introduce principles of ACL prevention to the end stages of rehabilitation with the goal of addressing neuromuscular imbalances and potentially reducing the risk of future ACL injury.[59,60] The program included specific rehabilitation phases targeting core stability, functional strength, power development, and sports performance symmetry[68] (**Figure 4**). Each phase was designed to specifically target a neuromuscular imbalance previously identified as a potential risk factor for ACL injury.[69,70] The program attempted to use the best current available evidence and supplemented any deficits in the literature with expert clinical opinion. The final outcome was designed as a template and may stimulate future research for developing more rigorous treatment progressions designed for the end stages of rehabilitation in addition to designing validated, reliable, and objective means to determine an athlete's readiness to successfully and safely return to sport with minimal risk of reinjury.

Summary

Since the inception of ACL reconstruction, rehabilitation has been and will remain an evolving process. As advancements continue to be made in the science of ACL reconstruction and the subsequent rehabilitation, changes will be made for the benefit of athletes in an attempt to allow a safe and expedient return to compe-

tition. Parameters for return to sports participation and specific points regarding optimal exercise dosage as it relates to the patient after ACL reconstruction are key to successful rehabilitation.

Annotated References

1. Ohkoshi Y, Ohkoshi M, Nagasaki S, Ono A, Hashimoto T, Yamane S: The effect of cryotherapy on intra-articular temperature and postoperative care after anterior cruciate ligament reconstruction. *Am J Sports Med* 1999;27:357-362.

2. Washington LL, Gibson SH, Helme RD: Age-related differences in the endogenous analgesic response to repeated cold water immersion in human volunteers. *Pain* 2000;89:89-96.

3. Hopkins JT, Ingersoll CD, Edwards JE, Cordova ML: Effect of knee joint effusion on quadriceps and soleus motoneuron pool excitability. *Med Sci Sports Exerc* 2001;33:123-126.

4. Konrath GA, Lock T, Goitz HT, Scheidler J: The use of cold therapy after anterior cruciate ligament reconstruction: A prospective, randomized study and literature review. *Am J Sports Med* 1996;24:629-639.

5. Thornton R, Mendel F, Fish D: Effects of electrical stimulation on edema formation in different strains of rats. *Phys Ther* 1998;78:386-394.

6. Vailas AC, Tipton CM, Matthes RD, Gart M: Physical activity and its influence on the repair process of medial collateral ligaments. *Connect Tissue Res* 1981;9:25-31.

7. Noyes FR: Functional properties of knee ligaments and alterations induced by immobilization: A correlative biomechanical and histological study in primates. *Clin Orthop Relat Res* 1977;123:210-242.

8. Culav EM, Clark CH, Merrilees MJ: Connective tissues: Matrix composition and its relevance to physical therapy. *Phys Ther* 1999;79:308-319.

9. Woo SL, Gomez MA, Sites TJ, Newton PO, Orlando CA, Akeson WH: The biomechanical and morphological changes in the medial collateral ligament of the rabbit after immobilization and remobilization. *J Bone Joint Surg Am* 1987;69:1200-1211.

10. Amiel D, Woo SL, Harwood FL, Akeson WH: The effect of immobilization on collagen turnover in connective tissue: A biochemical-biomechanical correlation. *Acta Orthop Scand* 1982;53:325-332.

11. Noyes FR, Torvik PJ, Hyde WB, DeLucas JL: Biomechanics of ligament failure: II. An analysis of immobilization, exercise, and reconditioning effects in primates. *J Bone Joint Surg Am* 1974;56:1406-1418.

12. Tipton CM, Vailas AC, Matthes RD: Experimental studies on the influences of physical activity on ligaments, tendons, and joints: A brief review. *Acta Med Scand Suppl* 1986;771:157-168.

13. Buckwalter JA, Grodzinsky AJ: The effects of loading on healing bone, fibrous tissue and muscle: Clinical implications. *J Am Acad Orthop Surg* 1999;7:291-299.

14. Eriksson E: Reconstruction of the anterior cruciate ligament. *Orthop Clin North Am* 1976;7:167.

15. Haggmark T, Eriksson E: Cylinder or mobile cast brace after knee ligament surgery: A clinical analysis and morphological and enzymatic study of changes in quadriceps muscle. *Am J Sports Med* 1979;7:48-56.

16. Noyes FR, Mangine RE, Barber S: Early knee motion after open and arthroscopic anterior cruciate ligament reconstruction. *Am J Sports Med* 1987;15:149-160.

17. Rosen MA, Jackson DW, Atwell EA: The efficacy of continuous passive motion in the rehabilitation of anterior cruciate ligament reconstruction. *Am J Sports Med* 1992;20:122-127.

18. Richmond JC, Gladstone J, MacGillivray J: Continuous passive motion after arthroscopically assisted anterior cruciate ligament reconstruction: Comparison of short-versus long-term use. *Arthroscopy* 1991;7:39-44.

19. Henricksson M, Rockborn R, Good L: Range of motion training in brace vs. plaster immobilization after anterior cruciate ligament reconstruction: A prospective randomized comparison with a 2-year follow-up. *Scand J Med Sci Sports* 2002;12:73-80.

20. Benum P: Operative mobilization of stiff knees after surgical treatment of knee injuries and posttraumatic conditions. *Acta Orthop Scand* 1982;53:625-631.

21. Perry J, Antonelli D, Ford W: Analysis of knee-joint forces during flexed-knee stance. *J Bone Joint Surg Am* 1975;57:961-967.

22. Waters RL: Energy expenditure, in Perry J (ed): *Gait Analysis: Normal and Pathological Function*. Thorofare, NJ, SLACK, 1992.

23. McHugh MP, Tyler TF, Gleim GW, Nicholas SJ: Preoperative indicators of motion loss and weakness following anterior cruciate ligament reconstruction. *J Orthop Sports Phys Ther* 1998;27:407-411.

24. Manske RC, Prohaska D, Livermore R: Anterior cruciate ligament reconstruction using the hamstring-gracilis tendon autograft, in Manske RC (ed): *Postsurgical Orthopedic Sports Rehabilitation: Knee and Shoulder*. St. Louis, Mosby, 2006, pp 189-206.
This chapter describes surgical considerations and specifics related to postoperative rehabilitation of the ACL after a hamstring-gracilis tendon autograft reconstruction technique.

25. Shelbourne KD, DeCarlo MS, Henne TD: Rehabilitation after anterior cruciate ligament reconstruction with a contralateral patellar tendon graft: Philosophy, protocol and addressing problems, in Manske RC (ed): *Postsurgical Orthopedic Sports Rehabilitation: Knee and Shoulder*. St. Louis, Mosby, 2006, pp 175-187.
This chapter describes specifies related to postoperative rehabilitation of the ACL after a contralateral patellar tendon graft reconstruction technique.

26. Sachs R, Daniel DM, Stone ML, Garfein RF: Patellofemoral problems after anterior cruciate ligament reconstruction. *Am J Sports Med* 1989;17:760-765.

27. Paulos LE, Rosenberg TD, Drawbar J, Manning J, Abbott P: Infrapatellar contracture syndrome: An unrecognized cause of knee stiffness with patella entrapment and patella infera. *Am J Sports Med* 1987;15:331-341.

28. Paulos LE, Wnorowski DC, Greenwald AE: Infrapatellar contracture syndrome: Diagnosis, treatment, and long-term follow-up. *Am J Sports Med* 1994;22:440-449.

29. Beynnon BD, Johnson RJ, Abate JA, Fleming BC, Nichols CE: Treatment of anterior cruciate ligament injuries, Part 2. *Am J Sports Med* 2005;33:1751-1767.
This article is second in a two-part series discussing surgical treatment of ACL injuries. It includes the technical aspects of ACL surgery bone tunnel widening; graft healing; rehabilitation; and the effect of age, sex, and activity level on the outcome of surgery.

30. Wigerstad-Lossing I, Grimby G, Jonsson T, Morelli B, Peterson L, Renström P: Effects of electrical muscle stimulation combined with voluntary contractions after knee ligament surgery. *Med Sci Sports Exerc* 1988;20:93-98.

31. Delitto A, McKowen JM, McCarthy JA, Shively RA, Rose SJ: Electrically elicited co-contraction of thigh musculature after anterior cruciate ligament surgery: A description and single-case experiment. *Phys Ther* 1988;68:45-50.

4: Rehabilitation

32. Anderson AF, Lipscomb B: Analysis of rehabilitation techniques after anterior cruciate reconstruction. *Am J Sports Med* 1989;17:154-160.

33. Snyder-Mackler L, Ladin Z, Schepsis AA, Young JC: Electrical stimulation of the thigh muscles after reconstruction of the anterior cruciate ligament: Effects of electrically elicited contraction of the quadriceps femoris and hamstring muscles on gait and on strength of the thigh muscles. *J Bone Joint Surg Am* 1991;73:1025-1036.

34. Snyder-Mackler L, DeLitto A, Bailey SL, Stralka SW: Strength of the quadriceps femoris muscle and functional recovery after reconstruction of the anterior cruciate ligament. *J Bone Joint Surg Am* 1995;77:1166-1172.

35. Gulotta LV, Rodeo SA: Biology of autograft and allograft healing in anterior cruciate ligament reconstruction. *Clin J Sports Med* 2007;26:509-524.

   This descriptive article presents the various graft options and different healing characteristics and potential after ACL reconstruction.

36. Rodeo SA, Arnoczky SP, Torzili PA, Hidaka C, Warren RF: Tendon-healing in a bone tunnel: A biological and histological study in the dog. *J Bone Joint Surg Am* 1993;75:1795-1803.

37. Tyler TF, Mcugh MP, Gleim GW, Nicholas SJ: The effect of immediate weight bearing after anterior cruciate ligament reconstruction. *Clin Orthop Relat Res* 1998;357:141-148.

38. Barrett DS: Proprioception and function after anterior cruciate reconstruction. *J Bone Joint Surg Br* 1991;73:833-837.

39. Lephart SM, Mininder SK, Fu FH, Borsa PA, Harner CD: Proprioception following anterior cruciate ligament reconstruction. *J Sport Rehabil* 1992;1:188-196.

40. MacDonald PB, Hedden D, Pacin O, Sutherland K: Proprioception in anterior cruciate ligament-deficient and reconstructed knees. *Am J Sports Med* 1996;24:774-778.

41. Roberts D, Friden T, Stomberg A, Lindstrand A, Moritz U: Bilateral proprioceptive deficits in patients with a unilateral anterior cruciate ligament reconstruction: A comparison between patients and healthy individuals. *J Orthop Res* 2000;18:565-571.

42. Risberg MA, Mork M, Jenssen HK, Holm I: Design and implementation of a neuromuscular training program following anterior cruciate ligament reconstruction. *J Orthop Sports Phys Ther* 2001;31:620-623.

43. Escamilla RF, Fleisig GS, Zheng N, Barrentine SW, Wilk KE, Andrews JA: Biomechanics of the knee during closed kinetic chain and open kinetic chain exercises. *Med Sci Sports Exerc* 1998;30:556-569.

44. Ohkoshi YK, Yasuda K, Kaneda K, Wada T, Yamanaka M: Biomechanical analysis of rehabilitation in the standing position. *Am J Sports Med* 1991;19:605-611.

45. Wilk KE, Andrews JR: Current concepts in the treatment of anterior cruciate ligament disruption. *J Orthop Sports Phys Ther* 1992;6:279-293.

46. Beynnon BD, Johnson RJ, Fleming BC, Stankewich CJ, Renstrom PA, Nichols CE: The strain behavior of the anterior cruciate ligament during squatting and active flexion-extension: A comparison of an open and a closed kinetic chain exercise. *Am J Sports Med* 1997;25:823-829.

47. Fleming BC, Ohlen G, Renstrom PA, Peura GD, Beynnon BD, Badger GJ: The effects of compressive load and knee joint torque on peak anterior cruciate ligament strains. *Am J Sports Med* 2003;31:701-707.

   This controlled laboratory study evaluated the effects of a compressive load and knee joint torque on ACL strain. An increase in resistance produced an increase in peak ACL strain for extensor exercise when no compressive load was applied. When using knee flexors without a compressive load, an increase in resistance produced a decrease in peak strain. During the extensor exercise, peak anterior strain was not reduced with a compressive force.

48. Heijne A, Fleming BC, Renstrom PA, Peura GD, Beynnon BD, Werner S: Strain on the anterior cruciate ligament during closed kinetic chain exercises. *Med Sci Sports Exerc* 2004;36:935-941.

   This study investigated ACL strains produced during several closed kinetic chain exercises. Exercises included the step-up, the step-down, the lunge, and the single leg sit-to-stand. It was determined that no differences were found in peak ACL strain values between exercises. There was a significant increase in ACL strain as the knee was extended for each exercise.

49. Beynnon BD, Fleming BC: Anterior cruciate ligament strain in vivo: A review of previous work. *J Biomech* 1998;31:519-525.

50. Solomonow M, Baratta R, Zhou BH, et al: The synergistic action of the anterior cruciate ligament and thigh muscles in maintaining joint stability. *Am J Sports Med* 1987;3:207-213.

51. Palmiter RA, An KN, Scott SG, Chao EY: Kinetic chain exercises in knee rehabilitation. *Sports Med* 1991;11:402-413.

52. Rudolph KS, Axe MJ, Buchanan TS, Scholz JP, Snyder-Mackler L: Dynamic stability in the anterior cruciate ligament deficient knee. *Knee Surg Sports Traumatol Arthrosc* 2001;9:62-71.

53. Chmielewski TL, Rudolph KS, Snyder-Mackler L: Development of dynamic knee stability after acute ACL injury. *J Electromyogr Kinesiol* 2002;12:267-274.

54. Kvist J: Rehabilitation following anterior cruciate ligament injury: Current recommendations for sports participation. *Sports Med* 2004;34:269-280.

This article describes rehabilitation after ACL reconstruction.

55. Myer GD, Paterno MV, Ford KR, Quatman CE, Hewett TE: Rehabilitation after anterior cruciate ligament reconstruction: Criteria based progression through the return to sport phase. *J Orthop Sports Phys Ther* 2006;36:385-402.

This article describes a criteria-based progression through the return to sport phase following ACL reconstruction. This progression uses objective criteria such as baseline limb strength, patient-reported outcomes, functional knee stability, postural control, power, endurance, agility, and the performance of sport-specific tasks.

56. Shelbourne KD, Nitz P: Accelerated rehabilitation after anterior cruciate ligament reconstruction. *Am J Sports Med* 1990;18:292-299.

57. Wilk KE, Reinold MM, Hooks TR: Recent advances in the rehabilitation of isolated and combined anterior cruciate ligament injuries. *Orthop Clin North Am* 2003;34:107-137.

This article discusses the rehabilitation of ACL injuries.

58. Pinczewski LA, Lyman J, Salmon LJ, Russell VJ, Roe J, Linklater J: A 10-year comparison of anterior cruciate ligament reconstructions with hamstring tendon and patellar tendon autograft: A controlled, prospective trial. *Am J Sports Med* 2007;35:564-574.

The authors present the results of a 10-year study comparing hamstring with patellar tendon ACL reconstructions. One hundred eighty patients entered the study: 90 patellar tendon and 90 hamstring reconstructions. The outcomes studied included graft rupture rates, laxity, function, and osteoarthritis. It was concluded that both graft sources can achieve excellent results. However, hamstring reconstruction is recommended because of decreased harvest site pain and osteoarthritis.

59. Myer GD, Ford KR, McLean SG, Hewett TE: The effects of plyometric versus dynamic stabilization and balance training on lower extremity biomechanics. *Am J Sports Med* 2006;34:445-455.

This study assessed two groups of patients: a plyometric training group and a balance training group. A three-dimensional motion analysis technique was used to determine lower extremity kinematics before and after 7 weeks of training for the drop vertical jump and medial jump landing. Both plyometric and balance training can reduce lower extremity valgus measures.

60. Myer GD, Ford KR, Palumbo JP, Hewett TE: Neuromuscular training improves performance and lower-extremity biomechanics in female athletes. *J Strength Cond Res* 2005;19:51-60.

This study examined the effects of a comprehensive neuromuscular training program on measures of performance and lower-extremity movement biomechanics in female athletes. Forty-one female athletes underwent 6 weeks of training, including plyometrics, core strengthening, balance, resistance, and speed training. Training had a positive effect on all measures. The results support a combination of multiple-injury prevention-training components into a comprehensive program to improve measures of performance and movement biomechanics.

61. Paterno MV, Ford KR, Myer GD, Heyl R, Hewett TE: Limb asymmetries in landing and jumping 2 years following anterior cruciate ligament reconstruction. *Clin J Sport Med* 2007;17:258-262.

This study assessed lower limb asymmetries in landing and takeoff force after ACL reconstruction in 14 female athletes and compared them to those of 18 healthy female athletes. A drop vertical jump task onto two force plates was assessed in these individuals. Females who had undergone ACL reconstruction had increased vertical ground reaction forces and loading rates on the uninvolved limb during landing when compared to the involved limb and the control group. During takeoff, the involved limb showed significantly less ability to generate force than the uninvolved limb and the control subjects. These limb asymmetries may remain for more than 2 years.

62. Mattacola CG, Perrin DH, Gansneder BM, Gieck JH, Saliba EN, McCue FC III: Strength, functional outcome, and postural stability after anterior cruciate ligament reconstruction. *J Athl Train* 2002;37:262-268.

63. Harner CD, Fu FH, Irrgang JJ, Vogrin TM: Anterior and posterior cruciate ligament reconstruction in the new millennium: A global perspective. *Knee Surg Sports Traumatol Arthrosc* 2001;9:330-336.

64. Greenberger HB, Paterno MV: Relationship of knee extensor strength and hopping test performance in the assessment of lower extremity function. *J Orthop Sports Phys Ther* 1995;22:202-206.

65. Kobayashi A, Terauchi M, Kobayashi F, Kimura M, Takagishi K: Muscle performance after anterior cruciate ligament reconstruction. *Int Orthop* 2004;28:48-51.

This study assessed quadriceps and hamstring strength after a BPTB ACL reconstruction. Quadriceps and hamstring strength was measured at 60° and 180° per second at 1, 6, 12, and 24 months after surgery. It took the quadriceps approximately 24 months to obtain 90% of the strength of the contralateral side; the hamstrings needed 6 months to recover 90% strength.

66. Ernst GP, Saliba E, Diduch DR, Hurwitz SR, Ball DW: Lower extremity compensations following anterior cruciate ligament reconstruction. *Phys Ther* 2000;80:251-260.

67. Ford KR, Myer GD, Hewett TE: Valgus knee motion during landing in high school female and male basketball players. *Med Sci Sports Exerc* 2003;35:1745-1750.

Motion analysis was used to determine if gender differences exist in knee valgus kinematics in high school basketball athletes when performing a landing maneuver.

Study participants were 47 females and 34 males. Outcome was assessment of a drop vertical jump and calculation of knee varus/valgus angulation. Females landed with greater total valgus knee motion and a greater maximum valgus knee angle than males. Females also had significant differences between their dominant and nondominant side in maximal valgus knee angles.

68. Myer GD, Paterno MV, Ford KR, Hewett TE: Neuromuscular training techniques to target deficits prior to return to sport following anterior cruciate ligament reconstruction. *J Strength Cond Res* 2008;22:987-1014.

This review article describes a return-to-sport program that targets measured deficits of neuromuscular control, strength, power, and functional symmetry that are rehabilitative landmarks after ACL reconstruction. The authors suggest that this algorithmic approach may improve the potential for athletes to return to sport after ACL reconstruction at optimal levels, thus minimizing the risk of injury.

69. Hewett TE, Paterno MV, Myer GD: Strategies for enhancing proprioception and neuromuscular control of the knee. *Clin Orthop Relat Res* 2002;402:76-94.

70. Hewett TE, Myer GD, Ford KR, et al: Biomechanical measures of neuromuscular control and valgus loading of the knee predict anterior cruciate ligament injury risk in female athletes: A prospective study. *Am J Sports Med* 2005;33:492-501.

In this study, 205 female athletes participating in high-risk sports were prospectively measured for neuromuscular control using motion analysis during a jump-landing task. Nine of the premeasured athletes incurred an ACL injury and demonstrated significantly different knee posture and loading than the 196 who did not have an ACL rupture. Knee abduction angle was greater at landing, knee abduction moment was 2.5 times higher, and there was a 20% higher ground reaction force in the patients with ACL injury. It also was determined that stance time was shorter, thus increased motion, force, and moments occurred much faster.

Chapter 21

Rehabilitation Following Osteochondral Injury to the Knee

Timothy F. Tyler, MS, PT, ATC   Christopher Johnson, MPT, MCMT   Walter L. Jenkins, PT, DHS, ATC

Introduction

Articular cartilage pathology can affect several joints in the human body, although it is more prevalent in the lower extremity. Of the weight-bearing joints, the knee is particularly vulnerable to articular cartilage lesions given its role in the kinetic chain, its unique biomechanical design, and the demands it is subjected to during activities of daily living and sport. Ulcerated cartilage poses a significant challenge to the orthopaedic surgeon and physical therapist largely because without intervention, articular cartilage lesions have minimal to no potential of healing with normal hyaline cartilage. Articular cartilage lesions have a high prevalence. According to a retrospective review of more than 31,000 knee arthroscopies, chondral lesions were found in 63% of patients, with an average of 2.7 lesions per knee.[1] Another study of 993 consecutive knee arthroscopies showed that 66% of patients had articular cartilage pathology, with 11% of these knees exhibiting full-thickness articular cartilage lesions.[2]

Focal chondral and osteochondral defects of loading surfaces often cause symptoms such as pain, swelling, catching, and instability. Of even greater concern is that such lesions may result in early degenerative changes and decreased function. Various surgical techniques including débridement, drilling of the defect, microfracture, and abrasion arthroplasty have been described to treat articular cartilage pathology. Although these techniques have resulted in improved function for some patients, they fail to restore the biomechanical characteristics of the native hyaline cartilage. Over the past two decades, however, reconstructive procedures designed to restore hyaline or hyalinelike cartilage have been developed. The most common of these procedures are osteochondral autograft transplantation (OAT), or mosaicplasty, and autologous chondrocyte implantation (ACI). Microfracture has been used arthroscopically to treat chondral defects.

Osteochondral Autograft Transplantation

OAT involves the transplantation of bone plugs with overlying articular cartilage; these bone plugs are harvested from non–weight-bearing areas of the knee to restore damaged articular cartilage. This technique, however, is limited by the amount of donor tissue available. The ideal indications for OAT include symptomatic, distal femoral condyle articular lesions with intact menisci and tibial cartilage in a nondegenerative joint with proper mechanical alignment.[3] Although reports of treating large lesions with this technique exist, the ideal lesion is between 1 to 4 cm^2. Furthermore, lesions deeper than 10 mm are not amenable to OAT alone because bone plugs may not be long enough for adequate fixation. The peripheral parts of both femoral condyles at the level of the patellofemoral joint can serve as donor sites. Notch area grafts are also available but less favorable because of the concave hyaline cartilage surface.[4]

Postoperative Rehabilitation Guidelines

In contrast to marrow stimulation procedures (microfracture and chondroplasty), which result in fibrocartilaginous tissue, the goal of OAT is to restore type II or hyaline cartilage. By attempting to re-create the native articular cartilage, the biomechanical strength and resiliency of the tissues should in turn prevent the early onset of degenerative changes.

Exposing the knee joint to a controlled amount of force without overstressing the healing tissue is the guiding principle of postoperative rehabilitation. The lesion, the patient, and the surgery dictate the speed of rehabilitation. A more cautious progression is encouraged when numerous bone plugs have been harvested because of possible joint incongruence. For the initial 2 weeks after surgery, weight bearing is strictly avoided because a 44% reduction in push-in and pullout strength has been documented 1 week after surgery.[5] Partial weight bearing is allowed between weeks 2 and 4 based on the lesion size and the number of transplanted bone plugs. Research has demonstrated that by 6 weeks after surgery, full subchondral integration has occurred. Despite integration, a 63% decrease in graft stiffness has been reported 6 weeks after surgery. Weight bearing is gradually progressed from weeks 6 to 8, at which time full weight bearing can resume because fibrocartilage,

Table 1

Rehabilitation Considerations Following OAT

Assistive Devices	Crutches and hinged knee orthosis locked in full extension for all lesions.
Weight bearing	Condylar lesions: NWB initial 2 weeks unless lesion is > 5 cm², then delay up to 4 weeks; PWB at 6 weeks, and FWB at 8 weeks. Patellofemoral lesions: Immediate TTWB unless physician directs otherwise; PWB by 6 weeks; and FWB at 8 weeks.
CPM	Immediate; perform 6 to 8 h/day starting 0°-60°, progressing 5°-10°/day except for patellofemoral lesions > 6 cm², then 0°-40°. If no CPM, then perform wall slides—500 repetitions, 3 times/day.
Range of Motion	Condylar lesions Patellofemoral lesions Week 2: 90° Week 3: 90° Week 3: 105° Week 4: 105° Week 4: 115° Week 6: 120° Week 6: 125°
Strengthening	Weeks 0 to 6: QS, SLRs: four-way, active knee extensions 90°-40° for condylar lesions but not permitted for patellar/trochlear lesions. Weeks 6 to 12: Condylar lesions: active knee extensions 0°-90°, mini squats (0°-60°) at 8 weeks, leg press at 10 weeks (0°-90°). Patellar/trochlear lesions: mini squats (0°-45°) at 8 weeks, leg press at 10 weeks (0°-60°), active knee extensions (0°-30°) at 12 weeks. Weeks 12 to 26: Leg press, unilateral step-ups, hip PREs; progress active knee extensions, advance stationary cycling, stair stepper and elliptical machines. Weeks 26 to 52+: Progress resistance as tolerated, impact loading customized to patient's needs, initiate light agility work and directional changes at 5 months per physician clearance. Interval sport programs implemented at 6 to 8 months.

NWB = no weight bearing; PWB = partial weight bearing; FWB = full weight bearing; TTWB = toe-touch weight bearing; CPM = continuous passive motion; SLRs = straight leg raises; PRE = progressive resistive exercise

which seals the recipient and donor site hyaline cartilage, exists on the surface. Immediate weight bearing is permitted for patients with patellofemoral lesions; a drop-lock knee orthosis is used, and full weight bearing without the brace is allowed 6 to 8 weeks after surgery.

Rehabilitation Progression

There are several key factors to consider when designing a rehabilitation program related to OAT and mosaicplasty (Table 1). The location of the lesion is one such factor. Lesions involving a weight-bearing region of the femoral condyle should be protected from compressive forces; lesions on the trochlea or retropatellar surfaces should be protected against shearing forces. Size, depth, and containment of the lesion(s) also are of great importance because some patients with larger, deeper, and more poorly contained lesions should progress at a slower pace during rehabilitation. The rate of progression during the rehabilitation process is governed by the four biologic phases of cartilage maturation: proliferation, transitional, remodeling, and maturation. In describing components of the rehabilitation program, the stages can be categorized as early (0 to 6 weeks), intermediate (6 to 12 weeks), late (12 to 26 weeks), and return to full function (26 to 52 weeks) and correlate with the biologic phases of healing tissue.[6]

Autologous Chondrocyte Implantation

ACI is a two-phase procedure that involves the implantation of healthy cartilage cells harvested from a non–weight-bearing area of the knee to treat areas with damaged cartilage. During the first phase, an arthroscopy is performed, and the healthy cartilage cells are collected, usually from the femoral condyle. During the second phase, an open surgical procedure is performed to implant the cultured cells, and the chondral defect is débrided back to healthy tissue.

Postoperative Rehabilitation Guidelines

After ACI surgery, an intensive rehabilitation program must be followed to achieve maximal results. Early motion stimulates the growth of healthy cartilage; however, the motion must provide minimal pressure to avoid damaging the transplant. If ACI has been used to treat a cartilage defect in the patella or the trochlea groove, motion must be limited for 2 months. Continuous passive motion (CPM) is used for 4 to 6 hours every day for the first 4 to 6 weeks. Weight bearing is minimal for approximately 2 months. A gradual load to the knee will be applied for approximately 6 to 8 weeks (Table 2). After 3 months, the patient can return to light impact activities such as driving, walking, and swimming; after 6 months, more intensive activities usually can be initi-

Table 2

Rehabilitation Considerations Following ACI

Assistive Devices	Crutches and hinged knee orthosis locked in full extension for all lesions.
Weight Bearing	Condylar lesions: TTWB for initial 6 weeks. Patellar/trochlear lesions: TTWB initial 2 weeks then progressed to 50% by week 3, 75% by week 4 to 5, and FWB at week 6. Wean off crutches by week 8 for all lesions unless otherwise directed by surgeon
CPM	4 to 6 h/day starting 0°-40° and advancing 5° to 10°/day
Range of Motion	Passive knee flexion of 90° by 2 weeks, 120° by 4 weeks, and full PROM by 8 weeks.
Strengthening	Weeks 0 to 6: QS, SLRs: four-way, ankle PREs, stationary bike when 100° of knee flexion achieved, water walking at 4 weeks in waist-high water, isometric leg press at 4 weeks, active knee extension 90° to 40° without resistance for condylar lesions; not permitted for patellar/trochlear lesions. Weeks 6 to 12: Mini squats 0°-45°, leg press, wall sits, TKEs, calf raises, treadmill walking, aquatic treadmill/pool walking program. Femoral condyle lesions: open chain knee extensions and front/lateral step-ups. Patellar/trochlear lesions: no knee extensions, leg press 0°-60°, front/lateral step-ups at week 8. Weeks 12 to 26: leg press 0°-90°, squats 0°-60°, front/lateral step-ups, hip stabilizer strengthening, walking program, bicycle, elliptical machine, stair stepper machine. Femoral condyle lesions: forward lunges and open chain knee extension 0°-90°. Patellar/trochlear lesions: backward lunges and open chain knee extension (initiate 0°-30°) Light running can be initiated for all lesions at 24 to 26 weeks per physician clearance. Weeks 26 to 52+: • 6 months: golf, swimming, skating/blading • 8 to 9 months: jogging, running, aerobics • 12 months: tennis, basketball, football, baseball

For all surgeries:
Establish full passive extension immediately postoperatively.
Assistive devices discontinued when the following criteria are met:
- Full knee extension
- Knee flexion = 100°
- No extensor lag
- Ambulate pain free without gait abnormalities

FWB = full weight bearing; TTWB = toe-touch weight bearing; CPM = continuous passive motion; SLRs = straight leg raises; PROM = passive range of motion; QS = quadriceps sets; PRE = progressive resistive exercise; TKEs = terminal knee extensions

ated. The patient should not participate in heavy load activities such as jogging and tennis for 1 year after surgery; otherwise, the outcome might be compromised. These guidelines depend on the size, severity, and location of the cartilage injury.

Microfracture

Marrow stimulation techniques, such as drilling of the subchondral bone to allow the hole to be filled with fibrocartilage, have been described previously for the treatment of osteoarthritis of the knee. Microfracture, which has been used arthroscopically to treat chondral defects, was developed and first used in the 1980s to provide an appropriate environment to enhance the body's own healing capacities for tissue repair.[7]

Postoperative Rehabilitation Guidelines
The time period for chondral defect healing is not well established in humans; there is typically a restricted or non–weight-bearing phase to protect the repair tissue. However, chondral defect healing after microfracture has been investigated in primates. In one study, 12 primates underwent microfracture of the medial and lateral femoral condyles and trochlear groove of each knee. Results demonstrated limited repair of the chondral tissue at 6 weeks with resorption of subchondral bone. By 12 weeks, the bone demonstrated improved bone repair and hyalinelike cartilage that was more mature. These findings suggest that restrictions in weight bearing and protection of the defect site may be warranted for more than 6 weeks to allow the tissue repair to adapt to increased stress.[8] After microfracture surgery, the rehabilitation program proceeds in accordance with the anatomic location and size of the chondral defect.[9] Other factors such as age, body mass index, and activity level also must be considered when developing a treatment plan.[10] Two different guidelines have been developed to treat lesions for both the femoral condyles and patellofemoral region.

Table 3

Rehabilitation Considerations Following Microfracture

Assistive Devices	Crutches for all lesions. Bracing not typically performed except for patellar/trochlear lesions, in which case orthosis prescribed for initial 8 weeks with ROM restricted 0°-20°.
Weight bearing	Condylar lesions: TTWB with crutches during initial 6 to 8 weeks then progressed to WBAT. Patellar/trochlear lesions: PWB progressed to WBAT after 2 weeks although in orthosis.
CPM	Condylar lesions: Immediately 6 to 8 h/day, starting from 30° to 70° and advancing 10° to 20°/day until reaching full PROM. Patellar/trochlear lesions: Per above but starting 0°-50° If no CPM, then peform wall slides—500 repetitions, 3 times per day.
Range of Motion	Unloaded PROM exercsises in ranges tolerated, initially starting in CPM per above guidelines.
Strengthening	Weeks 0 to 8: QS, SLRs: four-way, wall slides, ankle pumps, core stability training.
	Weeks 8 to 12: Gait training initially emphasized. Treadmill, elliptical machine, stationary bike with resistance, interval pool workouts in waist-high water allowed when patient is walking independently, carpet drags (high repetitions with good eccentric control).
	Weeks 12 to 16: Four-way hip PREs in standing, sidestepping, and forward/backward walking, cardiovascular program advanced to 75%.
	Weeks 16+: Functional sporting loads, moderate weight training; that is, leg press 0°-90°, leg curls/extensions, squats, lunges (maintaining good frontal plane control), light agility work.

TTWB = toe-touch weight bearing; WBAT = weight bearing as tolerated; PWB = partial weight bearing; CPM = continuous passive motion; SLRs = straight leg raises; PROM = passive range of motion; PRE = progressive resistive exercise; QS = quadriceps sets

Rehabilitation for Defects on the Condyles of the Femur or Tibial Plateau

Phase I: 0 to 8 Weeks

The initial goals of phase I include protecting the site of repair, restoring normal quadriceps function and patellar mobility, and decreasing swelling of the joint. Restrictions are placed on the amount of weight a patient is allowed to place on the involved lower extremity. In most instances, touchdown weight bearing with assistance of crutches is allowed during the first 6 to 8 weeks, although this can change depending on the size of the lesion (**Table 3**). Bracing of the knee is not typically performed with femoral condyle or tibial plateau lesions.

Immediately after surgery, the patient is placed in a CPM machine for 6 to 8 hours per day. Range of motion (ROM) is started from 30° to 70° and gradually progressed by 10° to 20° based on patient tolerance until full passive ROM is reached. The use of CPM after microfracture has been shown to improve cartilage lesion grades in patients with full-thickness chondral defects. Of 77 patients who participated in the study, 46 used CPM and 31 did not.[11] The average duration of CPM use was 7.83 weeks. Improvements in articular cartilage in those patients who used CPM was significantly greater ($P = 0.003$) than no CPM when measured using second-look arthroscopy. Additionally, these improvements were the same regardless of patient age or lesion location.

Exercises in phase I include quadriceps sets, straight leg raises in all four directions, wall slides, ankle pumps, and core stabilization training. Emphasis is placed on patellar mobilizations in the medial, lateral, superior, and inferior directions to decrease the risk of arthrofibrosis. The patient is also taught self-mobilizations to be performed at home three to four times per day. Cryotherapy is used for pain and inflammation and is continued until signs and symptoms are under control. After 1 to 2 weeks, stationary bike riding with no resistance and aquatic exercises in deep water are initiated. The goals of phase I are to decrease swelling, increase ROM, protect the site of healing, and improve quadriceps function.

Phase II: 8 to 12 Weeks

Gait training is emphasized as the patient completes phase I and enters phase II. Weight-bearing status is progressed as the patient is weaned from the crutches and allowed to bear weight as tolerated. Instructions for correct gait mechanics are given to the patient and reiterated as the normal gait pattern is restored. More aggressive activities, such as incline treadmill walking, interval pool workouts, elliptical exercise, and stationary bike riding with resistance, are acceptable once gait is normalized and pain free. Exercises in this phase shift from early protection of the surgical site to concentrating on muscle endurance of the quadriceps, the hamstrings, the gastrocnemius-soleus complex, and the gluteal muscles with a continued focus on core stability. Patients are instructed to perform high repetitions of exercises for these muscle groups, using good eccentric control with each exercise to protect the site. As the muscle endurance base is established, strength gains can be made in later phases. The goals of this phase include protecting the surgical site, increasing muscle endurance and proximal stability, and reestablishing proprioception and kinesthesia of the knee and lower extremity.

Phase III: 12 to 16 Weeks

In the third phase of rehabilitation, the cardiovascular aspect is intensified over the ensuing 4-week period with the stationary bike and elliptical machine while focusing on the importance of low-impact joint loading. Agility exercises are initiated on soft surfaces while focusing on controlling the forces going through the knee by using correct form and using the muscles for shock absorption. The key focus of this phase is teaching the patient to protect the joint surface by eccentrically loading the muscles during functional activities. The initial step is to teach the patient how to control the knee in all three cardinal planes of motion. Decreased core and hip strength have been implicated as factors contributing to lower extremity alignment during functional activities. Weakness of the hip extensors can lead to quadriceps overuse and increased compression and shearing at the knee joint.

Phase IV: 16 Weeks to Return to Sport

Exercises are structured such that functional sport loads are applied to the joint in preparation for return to sport. Based on the performance demands of the sport, rehabilitation at this stage should attempt to re-create an environment similar to that encountered on the field of play. Modified weight training also is begun at this point. Leg presses above 90°, leg curls, short arc leg extensions, and squats can be performed with high repetitions and low weights if the patient uses good control with a neutral spine. Agility drills are progressed to full speed or 100% throughout this phase. Soft surfaces are still encouraged while reminding the patient to absorb the forces through the muscles. Outdoor activities such as biking and golfing also are performed during this phase. Resumption of running, skiing, basketball, soccer, and football is considered between 6 to 9 months. Typically, sports that demand jumping, cutting, or twisting may require a longer rehabilitation period before full return. Determination of readiness for return to play, however, is dependent on the size and location of the lesion, the healing of the microfracture site, and the ability of the patient to efficiently use the muscles to absorb forces encountered during these activities.

Rehabilitation for Defects on the Trochlear Groove or Patella

There are a few differences in the rehabilitation of defects on the trochlear groove or patella compared with tibiofemoral lesions. After surgery, patients with defects on the trochlear groove or patella are placed in a brace with ROM restricted from 0° to 20°. The brace is worn for the first 8 weeks after surgery to prevent the median ridge of the patella from engaging the trochlear groove and potentially causing compression and shear forces at the site of repair during knee flexion. At 8 weeks, the patient is gradually weaned from the brace. Partial weight bearing on the affected extremity is allowed after surgery and progressed after 2 weeks to weight bearing as tolerated while wearing the brace. Immediately after surgery, CPM is started from 0° to 50° and progressed according to the same parameters for tibiofemoral lesions. For most patients, full passive ROM after surgery is allowed unless there are multiple defects, the size of the defect is significant, or kissing lesions are present. With kissing lesions, ROM limits are adjusted accordingly. Apart from bracing, weight-bearing, and ROM restrictions, the initial 8 weeks of the rehabilitation process follow the same guidelines as that of the tibiofemoral lesion. During the remainder of the rehabilitation process, careful attention is given to the joint angles encountered during strengthening exercises. To prevent joint compression and/or shearing forces at the repair site, the angle at which the patella engages the trochlear groove is avoided for the first 4 to 6 months during strengthening exercises. Otherwise, progression of rehabilitation follows the same standards as described for microfracture in the femur and tibia.

Summary

Rehabilitation following OAT, ACI, or microfracture is premised on exposing the knee to a controlled force without overstressing healing tissues and while gradually restoring full function. Through the cooperative efforts of the surgeon, therapist, and patient, restoration of a smooth gliding knee is possible in the face of articular cartilage pathology.

Annotated References

1. Curl WW, Krome J, Gordon ES, Rushing J, Smith BP, Poehling GG: Cartilage injuries: A review of 31,516 knee arthroscopies. *Arthroscopy* 1997;13: 456-460.

2. Aroen A, Loken S, Heir S, et al: Articular cartilage lesions in 993 consecutive knee arthroscopies. *Am J Sports Med* 2004;32:211-215.

   Nine hundred ninety-three consecutive knee arthroscopies in patients with a median age of 35 years were consecutively evaluated. Preoperative radiographs demonstrated degenerative changes in 13% of the knees. Articular cartilage pathology was found in 66% of knees, and a localized cartilage defect was found in 20%. Eleven percent of all knee arthroscopies showed cartilage defects that may be suitable for cartilage repair procedures. Level of evidence: IV.

3. Marcacci M, Kon E, Zaffagnini S, et al: Multiple osteochondral arthroscopic grafting (mosaicplasty) for cartilage defects of the knee: Prospective study results at 2-year follow-up. *Arthroscopy* 2005;21:462-470.

   This study prospectively evaluated mosaicplasty for the treatment of femoral condyle cartilage lesions less than 2.5 cm² in young active patients. Thirty-seven patients with full-thickness knee chondral lesions were treated with arthroscopic mosaicplasty. At follow-up, 78.3% reported clinically satisfactory results. This arthroscopic surgery appears to be a valid solution for the treatment of cartilage defects not more than 2.5 cm². Level of evidence: IV.

4. Gudas R, Kalesinskas RJ, Kimtys V, et al: A prospective randomized clinical study of mosaic osteochondral autologous transplantation versus microfracture for the treatment of osteochondral defects in the knee joint in young athletes. *Arthroscopy* 2005;21:1066-1075.

    A randomized comparison of OAT and microfracture procedures for the treatment of the articular cartilage defects of the knee joint in 60 athletes with a mean age of 24.3 years is presented. At an average of 37.1 months follow-up, the data showed that OAT is superior over microfracture for the repair of articular cartilage defects in the knee. Level of evidence: I.

5. Whiteside RA, Bryant JT, Jakob RP, Mainil-Varlet P, Wyss UP: Short term load bearing capacity of osteochondral autografts implanted by the mosaicplasty technique: An in vitro porcine model. *J Biomech* 2003;36: 1203-1208.

    This study examined a live tissue in vitro model to assess short-term fixation strength of mosaicplasty autografts immediately after and 1 week after graft implantation. Immediately after the surgical procedure, graft push-in and pullout strength tests as well as indentation tests to determine modulus of the surrounding cancellous bone were performed on 50% of the specimens from the distal femurs of each animal. The other 50% were used as matched control specimens. The in vitro results demonstrate a substantial deterioration of short-term fixation strength of mosaicplasty grafts from the immediate postoperative state. Such a reduction in short-term graft load-bearing capacity may pose a threat to the surgically established articular surface congruency and blood vessels formed during the early stages of the healing response. Level of evidence: IV.

6. Lahav A, Burks RT, Greis PE, Chapman AW, Ford GM, Fink BP: Clinical outcomes following osteochondral autologous transplantation (OATS). *J Knee Surg* 2006;19: 169-173.

    This study evaluated the clinical outcome in 21 patients undergoing OAT over a 5-year period. On subjective questionnaire, the average preoperative grade given was 3.1, with an improvement at the most recent follow-up to a grade of 8.0 ($P < 0.01$). Eighty-six percent of patients reported that they would have the surgery again.

7. Steadman JR, Rodkey WG, Briggs KK, Rodrigo JJ: The microfracture procedure: Rationale, technique, and clinical observations for treatment of articular cartilage defects. *J Sports Traumatol Rel Res* 1998;20(2):61-70.

8. Gill TJ, McCulloch PC, Glasson SS, Blanchet T, Morris EA: Chondral defect repair after the microfracture procedure: A nonhuman primate model. *Am J Sports Med* 2005;33:680-685.

    Evaluation of the status of chondral defect repair at different time points after microfracture in a primate model may provide a rationale for postoperative activity recommendations. Full-thickness chondral defects created on the femoral condyles and trochlea of 12 cynomolgus macaques were treated with microfracture and evaluated by gross and histologic examination at 6 and 12 weeks. At 6 weeks, there was limited chondral repair and ongoing resorption of subchondral bone. By 12 weeks, the defects were completely filled and showed more mature cartilage and bone repair. Postoperative weight bearing and activity restrictions in patients after microfracture are supported by this study to protect immature repair tissue. Level of evidence: IV.

9. Mithoefer K, Williams RJ III, Warren RF, Wickiewicz TL, Marx RG: High-impact athletics after knee articular cartilage repair: A prospective evaluation of the microfracture technique. *Am J Sports Med* 2006;34: 1413-1418.

    Thirty-two athletes who regularly participated in high-impact, pivoting sports before articular cartilage injury were treated with microfracture for single articular cartilage lesions of the knee. At 2-year follow-up, 66% of athletes reported good or excellent results. Activities of daily living, Marx activity rating scale, and Tegner activity scores increased significantly after microfracture. Microfracture is an effective first-line treatment for young athletes with short symptomatic intervals and small articular cartilage lesions of the knee who wish to return to high-impact athletic activity. Level of evidence: IV.

10. Kreuz PC, Erggelet C, Steinwachs MR, et al: Is microfracture of chondral defects in the knee associated with different results in patients aged 40 years or younger? *Arthroscopy* 2006;22:1180-1186.

    This prospective study was performed to determine age-dependent differences in the results after microfracture over 36 months. The clinical results after microfracture of full-thickness cartilage lesions in the knee are age dependent. Deterioration begins 18 months after surgery and is significantly pronounced in patients older than age 40 years. The best prognostic factor was a patient age of 40 years or younger with defects on the femoral condyles. Level of evidence: IV.

11. Rodrigo JJ, Steadman JR, Silliman JF, Fulstone HA: Improvement of full-thickness chondral defect healing in the human knee after debridement and microfracture using continuous passive motion. *Am J Knee Surg* 1994; 7:109-116.

Chapter 22

Core Stabilization

Carl DeRosa, PT, PhD   Cory Manton, PT, DPT, OCS, CSCS

Introduction

Core training and core exercises are terms used by patients and the general public but often with diverse and different intended meanings. The use of core stabilization exercises is varied and diverse. Core stabilization exercises are often an intervention of choice in the rehabilitation of patients with low back pain or who have had low back surgery. An athlete may be instructed to participate in rigorous training or exercise classes such as Pilates or yoga to strengthen and properly stabilize their core to improve athletic performance. Core training exercises can be used in the injured, deconditioned individual and in the individual incorporating core training to reach an even higher level of athletic performance.

Description of the Core and the Concept of Stabilization

Terms such as core training, core strengthening, lumbar stabilization, dynamic stabilization, neuromuscular retraining, neutral spine control, core control, muscular fusion, and trunk stabilization describe core stabilization. Similarly, there is no single term to describe the intended region of the body targeted for core exercises. The core may refer to the lumbar spine, the lumbopelvic complex including or not including the hips, the shoulder girdle, or all of these regions combined. The musculoskeletal core has been described as consisting of the spine, the hips and pelvis, the proximal lower limb, and abdominal structures.[1] The word core also has been used as a synonym for trunk, but there is confusion when the hips and shoulder girdle are included in this description.

Stabilization implies training of the neuromotor system associated with the spine and pelvis to generate the optimum forces necessary to counter imparted loads, provide a stable platform from which the extremities can function, and sufficiently generate the necessary torque over the spine from which the momentum achieved can be transferred and used efficiently by the extremities.

Core stabilization and core training are best defined as a broad spectrum of exercises that strengthen multiple muscles of the trunk, including superficial and deep muscles that act directly on the spine or exert control to the spine through specific anatomic linkages, as well as the shoulder girdle and the pelvic girdle musculature. This extensive array of muscles contributing to the core has resulted in attempts to subclassify the muscles to better describe their role. Global muscles include large, torque-producing muscles that act on the spine, shoulder girdle, and pelvic girdle.[2] Local muscles are those considered to act directly on the spine and include the transversus abdominis acting through the thoracolumbar fascia, the multifidus, and the intersegmental muscles.[2] These muscles attach directly to the lumbar vertebrae and provide segmental stability.

Low Back Pain and Core Stabilization Concepts

Segmental instability of the lumbar spine is a clinical condition suggested as a possible mechanism for low back pain. Segmental instability is usually considered to occur when a lumbar vertebral body translates or rotates to a greater degree than that found in a normal lumbar spine, with clinical findings including mild to severe low back pain, aberrant motion during active movement of the lumbar spine, and differences in vertebral position as palpated in supine and prone positions. Instability may be the result of intervertebral disk or apophyseal joint degeneration.

With instability serving as a potential framework for some mechanical disorders of the lumbar spine, attention to the muscular training necessary to help stabilize the spine evolved much in the same manner as attention to strength considerations of the unstable shoulder or knee surfaced in the sports medicine literature. Likewise, it became apparent that it was a combination of the nervous system and the muscular system that together influenced stability of the trunk. Core stability was thus defined as the "restoration or augmentation of the ability of the neuromuscular system to control and protect the spine from injury or reinjury."[3] It is suggested that core stabilization exercises can be used to improve lumbopelvic control and can be divided into two groups: "those that aim to restore the coordination and control of the trunk muscles to improve control of the lumbar spine and pelvis, and those that aim to restore the capacity (strength and endurance) of the trunk muscles to meet the demands of control."[3]

Core Stabilization Exercises Across the Spectrum of Injury and Performance

Concurrent with the paradigm shift of managing patients with mechanical spine pain through exercise and functional training strategies has been a shift in attention to the role of the trunk in sport and how it is effectively, efficiently, and safely trained. Numerous strategies exist to rapidly return an injured athlete to activity as well as improve sport performance by emphasizing improvements in the neuromuscular efficiency of the trunk. Core stabilization requires elements of strength training, endurance training, coordination development, and, perhaps most importantly, motor learning. Training programs for nearly every professional sport include attention to optimizing neuromotor function of the trunk. Optimal function of the trunk serves as the keystone allowing precise function and explosive motion of the extremities for the complex and coordinated activities performed during sports participation.

Numerous studies have attempted to precisely identify the contributions of specific muscles to spinal postures; for the most part, many muscles simultaneously contribute to spinal stability, and these contributions ultimately depend on such factors as task, load imparted to the spine or extremities, posture required, and direction of movement.[4] Based on afferent information received, the central nervous system must then coordinate the muscle activity via programmed muscle sequencing to counter the internal and external forces to which the spine is subjected. The actions of the central nervous system can be in direct response to forces placed over the spine, or the response can be anticipatory.

There are several unique biomechanical considerations relating to how the lumbar spine normally attenuates loads and how core stabilization exercises should be prescribed. The lumbar apophyseal joints are oriented in the sagittal plane and serve as restraints to lumbar rotation and anterior shear but allow more freedom of motion in flexion and extension. Consequently, the design of core stabilization exercises and trunk functional progression programs must be such that the rate and amplitude of lumbar rotation and torsion are controlled. Unchecked rotary stresses increase the compressive load to the facet joint contralateral to the rotated side and result in a potential compression injury to these joints.

Extension of the lumbar spine also increases facet joint compression and results in increased compressive loading between the inferior articular process and the lamina of the subjacent vertebrae. This compression can cause damage to the pars interarticularis that can contribute to the development of lumbar spondylolisthesis. Extension and rotation compound the loading to the lumbar facets, with the facet joint on the contralateral side rotated toward having the greatest compressive load. Although the bone-disk interface is built to withstand compressive loads, the facet joints have limited capacity to tolerate such compressive loading. Positions or movements in exercise that adversely load these facet joints in compression should be avoided.

The biomechanics of the disk are such that the anulus fibrosus is particularly vulnerable to excessive tensile loads. Flexion and rotation of the lumbar spine place an increased tensile load on the posterior annular rings, resulting in two potential problems. First, there is a loss of stability between adjacent vertebral bodies because of the annular damage resulting in increased translation between adjacent vertebrae. Few muscles are oriented to directly control translation because most muscles are oriented perpendicular to the translational plane. Coordinated contraction of the diaphragm and the transversus abdominis and pelvic floor muscles helps stiffen the spine and may help to control translation.[5] This concept often is incorporated in the initial training for core stabilization exercises. Second, and perhaps even more crucial, the altered anulus fibrosus cannot exert an equal and opposite force against the pressure of the nucleus pulposus. This condition can result in the nucleus pulposus "leaking" through defects in the anulus fibrosus and into the spinal canal where irritation to the thecal sac and nerve root complex occurs, causing signs and symptoms of nerve root irritation. Because the erector spinae group and the psoas major span the lumbar column, contraction of these muscles further increases intradiskal pressure. Many of the core stabilization exercises can result in increased intradiskal pressure and therefore may not be the best choice of treatment initially, especially in the presence of nerve root irritation.

Selection and Progression of Exercises

A comprehensive program typically starts with training at the motor learning level and consists of teaching postural positions and lumbopelvic motion and positions and sequencing of muscle contractions during simulated tasks. Stabilization exercises are then progressed to more dynamic movements often involving progressive resistance loading of the trunk, hip, and shoulder girdle. These exercises often are used for conditions occurring during preseason conditioning, maintenance of optimum trunk function within the season, and rehabilitation if injury has occurred.

The key muscles of the trunk that are essential to core stability are the abdominal muscles, the superficial and deep erector spinae muscles, the multifidus muscles, and the deep intersegmental muscles; both the local and global muscles are included. Most core training exercises place demands over both groups of muscles simultaneously, because no single muscle predominates in terms of stability of the lumbar spine.

Most advanced core strengthening programs consist of analyzing movement and subsequently training motor patterns that use well coordinated, synchronous activation of axial and appendicular skeletal muscles.[6,7] The ideal exercises are those that provide overload to the neuromuscular system and stimulate the necessary anatomic, biochemical, and neurologic changes while sparing joint loading over the region. The most important principle to recognize is that the trunk serves as a stable yet dynamic platform for extremity motion, and attention to spine posture and motion during extremity motion should serve as the focus of core strengthening. Initial stabilization exercises for the trunk focus on training the individual to satisfactorily contract the abdominal mechanism while maintaining proper breathing patterns regardless of the activity, taking advantage of the orientation of the transversus abdominis muscle. Contraction of the transversus abdominis muscle results in a "hollowing" of the abdominal wall that increases tension to the thoracolumbar and abdominal fascia mechanisms and initiates stabilization of the lumbar spine.

The progression of core exercises is from simple to complex and from minimal weight-bearing postures to full weight-bearing dynamic activities. The lumbar spine has less compressive and shear loading in the supine, prone, and sidelying positions; these positions can be starting points for core stabilization exercises. Progression to antigravity postures is important because it challenges the core to adapt to increasing loading conditions and best prepares the individual for functional and sports-related activities.

The second stage of exercises develops a sense of proprioceptive and kinesthetic awareness of the lumbopelvic region, along with neuromotor control over motion, velocity, and position of the spine, and maintains safe positions of the spine during movement of the extremities. An example is the quadruped lumbopelvic flexion and extension exercise that progresses to a neutral position of the spine while alternately moving the extremities (Figure 1). The inability to maintain neutral position of the spine while raising the extremities provides a good indication of weakness of the

trunk muscles that stabilize the spine in the important horizontal plane.

The initial group of core exercises also can include plank positioning, which requires strong contraction of the trunk muscles but avoids loading the apophyseal joints and the bone-disk-bone interface in compression (Figure 2). In the side plank position, the lateral abdominal muscles and erector spinae are contracting to stabilize the spine against movement into rotation and sidebending, whereas the front plank position requires strong abdominal muscle contraction to minimize spine movement toward end range extension.

A bilateral leg lowering exercise can be used in high-level athletes. This exercise requires a very strong trunk platform to minimize shear and torsional loading to the lumbar spine. Bilateral diagonal leg lowering is performed from the supine position and requires a strong, coordinated concentric, isometric, and eccentric contraction of the anterior abdominal, lateral abdominal, and hip musculature. From the elevated straight leg

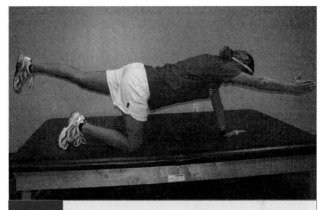

Figure 1 Quadruped position. The individual is raising the arm and the contralateral lower extremity while attempting to maintain the neutral position of the spine.

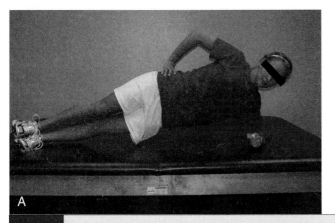
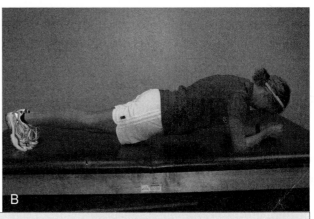

Figure 2 **A,** The side plank position requires a strong contraction of the lateral abdominals and the erector spinae muscles. **B,** The front plank position requires strong abdominal muscle contraction to prevent movement of the spine into extension.

4: Rehabilitation

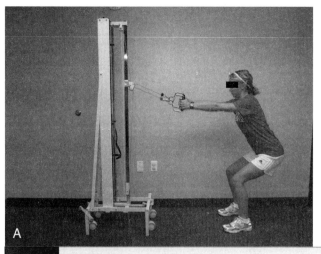
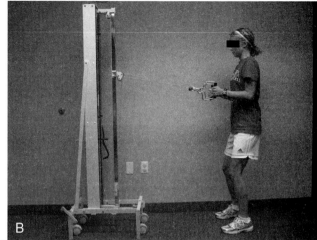

Figure 3 **A** and **B**, Bilateral upright rowing activity.

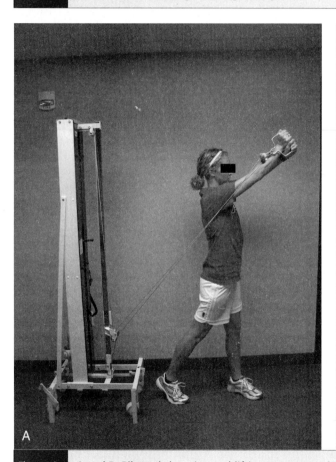
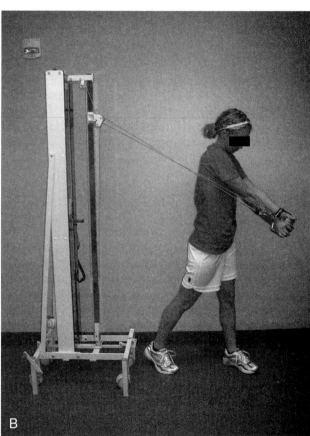

Figure 4 **A** and **B**, Bilateral chopping and lifting patterns against resistance.

raise position, the lower extremities are then lowered in a slightly diagonal position, resulting in a precisely controlled rotary motion of the pelvis under the lumbar spine.

Progression of core stabilization exercise to standing and dynamic postures is essential because these positions mimic those of sports and daily activities. One progression is the standing upright bilateral rowing exercises against resistance (**Figure 3**). In this exercise the

individual flexes the hip and knees while controlling how the weight pulls the upper extremities and trunk forward and strongly pulls the arms back against the weight as they rise to the standing position. This complex movement illustrates the muscle coordination necessary between the shoulder girdle, the hips, and the lumbopelvic regions. A pulley machine provides great variability in exercise design because it can be used to provide resistance for chopping and lifting patterns that

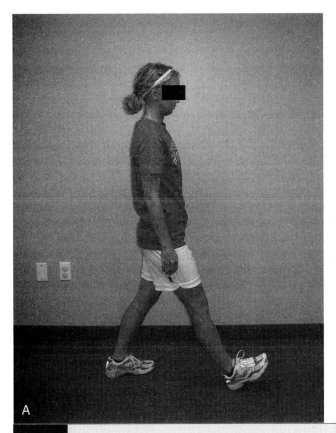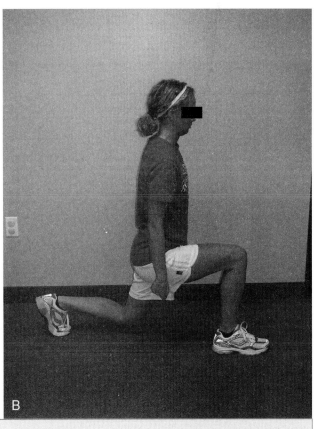

| Figure 5 | **A** and **B**, Walking lunges. This complex exercise provides overload to the hip and trunk musculature. In particular, the spinal extensors are challenged to control the flexion and rotary moments being generated. |

challenge the synchronous movement of the hips, the shoulder girdle, and the lumbopelvic regions (**Figure 4**).

Advanced core exercises can be used for athletes who seek to improve performance in addition to recovery from injury. The walking lunge is an example of an advanced core strengthening exercise that includes the upright posture but also a significant dynamic component. A walking lunge requires a strong extensor mechanism to effectively balance the trunk and the ability of the abdominal mechanism to control lumbopelvic posture and movement, especially to minimize excessive rotary forces across the spine. Strength of the hip and knee extensor mechanisms also are required. The correct technique for this important exercise is as follows (**Figure 5**):

1. Step out with one leg, keeping the spine upright and shoulders retracted.
2. The lunge foot should strike the ground with the heel.
3. Upon striking with the heel, the foot should immediately move to the foot flat position.
4. At foot flat, the pelvis descends straight down by simultaneous extension of the low back, flexion of the hip, and flexion of the knee.

Walking lunges with controlled rotations using a medicine ball are an excellent complex core exercise, especially for the higher level athlete (**Figure 5**). Exercise training focus is placed on the spinal extensors rather than the abdominal mechanism. With the medicine ball held out in front of the body, a flexion and rotary moment is introduced to the lumbar spine and the hips over this long lever arm. This moment must be countered by a strong contraction of the trunk extensors, the hip extensors, and the lateral abdominal muscles. An increase in the weight of the object held in front of the body increases the potential torque over the spine and hips, requiring an even stronger contraction of the spinal extensors and the hip extensors.

Further progression might include simulated "over the shoulder" weight toss (**Figure 6**). With a medicine ball (or free weight) held in front of the spine, a flexion moment over the lumbar spine is created (as described in the previous paragraph) that must be countered by a strong contraction of the spinal extensor mechanism. From this starting position, the individual is asked to descend into a squat position, keeping the heels on the ground. Then by pushing through the heels, the individual rapidly rises from the squat position and simultaneously brings the ball overhead as if throwing it overhead and behind. This results in a vigorous contraction of the spinal extensor mechanism that powerfully moves the spine from a flexed to an extended posture, and simultaneously provides a stable spinal platform for the shoulder girdle activity. Numerous variables of the exercise can be modified to increase or

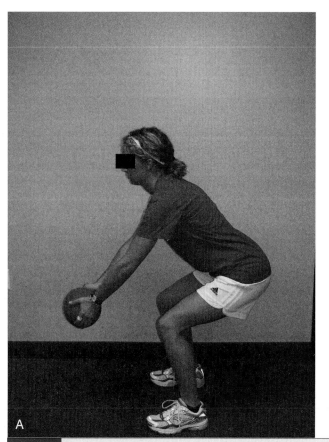 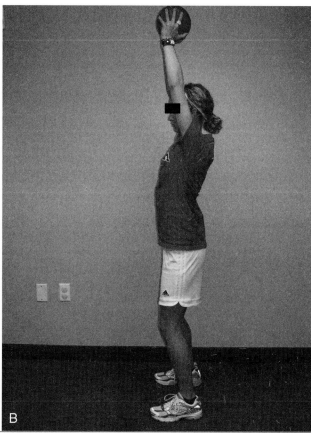

Figure 6 | **A** and **B,** Simulated weight toss with a medicine ball emphasizing strong hip and trunk extension.

decrease the demand on the muscles, including the weight itself, the depth of the squat maneuver, and the distance the weight is held in front of the body.

The final example of core stabilization exercises is perturbation training. The force causing a perturbation can be expected or unexpected. Balance boards used for such training can have a side-to-side range of motion, whereas other balance boards use a full range of motion that increases the proprioceptive challenges. Two examples of exercises that can be performed over these unstable surfaces are the body weight squat and the cable pull on either a balance board or balance disk. Cable pulls from a balance board simultaneously challenge the upper extremities, the lower extremities, and trunk and can be further modified into high pull, mid pull, and low pull actions. The intent of such activity is to further develop an individual's proprioceptive and kinesthetic trunk sense with the goal of rapid reflexive response when needed for sports activity or other dynamic conditions.

Low Back Pain and Outcomes

The effectiveness of classification-based physical therapy was compared with that of therapy based on clinical practice guidelines for patients with acute, work-related

low back pain by randomly assigning 78 subjects to one of the treatment groups, including stabilization.[8,9] The subjects assigned to the clinical practice guidelines physical therapy group were educated about the prognosis of patients with low back pain and participated in low-stress aerobic exercises and general muscle reconditioning exercises. In the classification-based physical therapy group, subjects were placed into one of four treatment classifications (manipulation, stabilization, specific exercise, or traction) based on their signs and symptoms. The results suggest that the classification-based approach resulted in improved disability and return-to-work status after 4 weeks for patients with acute, work-related back pain.

The outcomes of patients with low back pain that were generalized and the same for all within the group or were individualized based on clinical presentation were assessed in a recent study.[10] The patients who received treatment that matched their clinical presentation had a greater change in their Oswestry scores after 4 weeks of treatment and at 1 year.

A clinical prediction rule was developed to determine which patients with low back pain will respond to a stabilization exercise program.[11] The prediction rule for success with stabilization exercise was composed of four variables: positive prone instability test, aberrant movements present, average straight leg raising greater than 91°, and age younger than 40 years. Four variables that were associated with failure of stabilization exercise were negative prone instability test, aberrant movement absent, a Fear Avoidance Belief Questionnaire physical activity subscale greater than 9, and no hypermobility with lumbar spring testing.[11]

It has been suggested that specific stabilizing exercises were more effective than other treatment programs in patients with chronically symptomatic spondylolysis or spondylolistheses.[12] The stabilizing exercises in this study involved specific training of the internal oblique, transversus abdominis, and lumbar multifidus muscles, with progression of these exercises to previously aggravating postures and functional activities. The patients in this study performed the stabilizing exercises under the supervision of a physical therapist on a weekly basis, and at home on a daily basis, for 10 weeks. The stabilization exercises were specific to the local muscles of the spine. The patients were encouraged to activate these muscles regularly during daily activities, with the purpose of dynamically stabilizing the lumbar spine. The patients in the specific exercise group maintained their reduction in pain intensity and functional disability levels at a 30-month follow-up.

The effects of stabilization exercises in patients during their first episode of low back pain have been studied.[13] The specific stabilization exercises used in this study activated and trained the isometric holding function of the multifidus in co-contraction with the transversus abdominis muscle. The patients who participated in the specific stabilizing exercise group had a recurrence rate of 30% at 1 year, whereas patients in the control group had a recurrence rate of 84% at 1 year. Specific core stabilization exercises may be an effective, early intervention in the treatment of acute low back pain.

The cost effectiveness of spinal stabilization programs and other forms of therapy for the treatment of low back conditions were investigated in a 2007 study.[14] Spinal stabilization exercises were found to have outcomes similar to individual physical therapy and a pain management program. All three groups improved in disability measures and in other outcome measures as measured at 6 months, 12 months, and 18 months from the baseline assessment.

Rehabilitation, Injury Prevention, and Performance Enhancement Research

The effects of a treatment program, consisting of agility and trunk stabilization exercises, for acute hamstring strain were evaluated in a 2004 study.[15] The athletes who participated in the agility and trunk stabilization exercise program returned to sports activity sooner and had a lower reinjury rate than athletes who participated in a static stretching and strengthening program. The trunk stabilization exercises included in this study were bridging while supine, prone, and sidelying and push-up stabilization with trunk rotation. The athletes in this group also performed a single-leg stand windmill touch. This exercise trains the local and global muscles of the trunk and promotes the eccentric contraction of the gluteus maximus and hamstring muscles.

The effects of trunk stability training on vertical takeoff velocity (defining trunk stability as "the ability to maintain active control of spinal and pelvic posture during dynamic loading and movement conditions") were studied.[16] The exercises used in the trunk stability program trained local and global stability muscles while emphasizing a neutral spine posture. Results suggest that trunk stability training was similar in effectiveness to leg strength training or the combination of trunk stability and leg strength training in improving vertical takeoff velocity. The authors concluded that "trunk stability training may optimize the ability of the leg muscles to produce force by providing a stable base from which those muscles can contract or by enhancing the neural drive to the leg muscles."[16]

It has been suggested that core stability has an important role in injury prevention.[17] The authors of this 2004 study defined the core as consisting of the lumbopelvic musculature. Athletes who did not sustain a lower extremity injury during the season were noted to have stronger hip abduction and hip external rotation. The athletes who participated in this study were collegiate basketball and track and field athletes. The hip abductors and external rotators may play an important role in controlling the position of the trunk and lower extremity during functional movement, especially because the hip musculature exerts powerful forces over the pelvis when the lower extremity is weight bearing and the foot is fixed to the ground.

According to a 2007 study, factors related to core stability predicted risk of athletic knee, ligament, and anterior cruciate ligament injuries with high sensitivity and moderate specificity in female, but not male, athletes.[18] It was noted that "inadequate neuromuscular control of the body's trunk or 'core' may compromise dynamic stability of the lower extremity and result in increased abduction torque at the knee, which may increase strain on knee ligaments and lead to injury."[18] Core stability was defined as "the body's ability to maintain or resume an equilibrium position of the trunk after perturbation."[18] The position of the trunk over the lower extremity during functional movement can change the vector of the center of mass and ground reaction force acting on the joints of the lower extremity and can lead to lower extremity injuries. An athlete's ability to dynamically control the trunk over the lower extremity may decrease the risk of lower extremity injury.

Summary

Significant advances have been made in understanding the anatomy and biomechanics of the trunk. Similar advances have been made in developing the necessary

4: Rehabilitation

strategies to train the neuromotor mechanisms of trunk control and dynamic movement. From its roots as isometric stabilization of the lumbar spine, core training has evolved to include complex, coordinated, multiplanar motion of the shoulder girdle, the spine, and the pelvic girdle with an understanding that the central nervous system plays a key role in assuring optimal function. Current research is focused on not only identifying the most advantageous exercises and exercise strategies but also the subgroup of individuals, whether they be patients or elite athletes, who will be the best responders to specific exercises.

Annotated References

1. Kibler WB, Press J, Sciascia A: The role of core stability in athletic function. *Sports Med* 2006;36:189-198.

   The authors provide a comprehensive review of core stability and its relation to athletic performance.

2. Danneels LA, Vanderstraeten GG, Cambier DC, Witvrouw EE, Stevens VK, DeCuyper HJ: A functional subdivision of hip, abdominal, and back muscles during asymmetric lifting. *Spine* 2001;26:E114-E121.

3. Hodges PW: Core stability exercise in chronic low back pain. *Orthop Clin North Am* 2003;34:245-254.

   The application of core stability exercises in the management of chronic low back pain is discussed.

4. Granata KP, Marras WS: Cost benefit of muscle cocontraction in protecting against spinal instability. *Spine* 2000;25:1398-1404.

5. Hodges PW, Eriksson AE, Shirley D, Gandevia SC: Intra-abdominal pressure increases stiffness of the lumbar spine. *J Biomech* 2005;38:1873-1880.

   The increase in spinal stiffness was positively correlated with the amount of intra-abdominal pressure increase. Intra-abdominal pressure increased stiffness at the L2 and L4 levels. The results provide evidence that stiffness of the lumbar spine is increased when intra-abdominal pressure is elevated.

6. Cholewicki J, McGill SM: Mechanical stability of the in vivo spine: Implications for injury and chronic low back pain. *Clin Biomech (Bristol, Avon)* 1996;11:1-15.

7. Kavic N, Grenier S, McGill SM: Determining the stabilizing role of individual torso muscles during rehabilitation exercises. *Spine* 2004;29:1254-1263.

   Stabilization exercises are believed to train muscle patterns that ensure spine stability; however, little quantification and no consensus exist as to which muscles contribute to stability.

8. Fritz JM, Cleland JA, Childs JD: Subgrouping patients with low back pain: Evolution of a classification approach to physical therapy. *J Orthop Sports Phys Ther* 2007;37:290-302.

The authors provide an update on a classification approach to the physical therapy treatment of patients with low back pain. Current evidence, as well as examination and management considerations, are presented for each classification area, including manipulation, stabilization, specific exercise, and traction.

9. Fritz JM, Delitto A, Erhard RE: Comparison of classification-based physical therapy with therapy based on clinical practice guidelines for patients with acute low back pain: A randomized clinical trial. *Spine* 2003; 28:1363-1372.

   The authors assessed the effects of a classification-based physical therapy versus the effects of therapy based on clinical practice guidelines based on the Agency for Health Care Policy and Research guidelines. Seventy-eight subjects who had low back pain of less than 3 weeks' duration were randomly assigned to one of the treatment groups. Outcome measurements were completed at the initial evaluation, after 4 weeks, and after 1 year. Subjects in the classification-based therapy group showed greater changes on the Oswestry scale at 4 weeks and after 1 year.

10. Brennan GP, Fritz JM, Hunter SJ, Thackeray A, Delitto A, Erhard R: Identifying subgroups of patients with acute/subacute "nonspecific" low back pain: Results of a randomized clinical trial. *Spine* 2006;31:623-631.

    The 123 subjects who participated in this study had low back pain of less than 90 days duration. They were evaluated and assigned to one of three groups (manipulation, specific exercise, and or stabilization exercise). The subjects were randomly assigned to one of the above treatment groups. The authors compared the outcomes, after 4 weeks and 1 year, of patients who were matched or unmatched to the treatment received. Patients who were matched demonstrated a reduction in the Oswestry score at 4 weeks and 1 year.

11. Hicks GE, Fritz JM, Delitto A, McGill SM: Preliminary development of a clinical prediction rule for determining which patients with low back pain will respond to a stabilization exercise program. *Arch Phys Med Rehabil* 2005;86:1753-1762.

    All the subjects in this study received stabilization exercises as a treatment of nonradicular low back pain. A preliminary clinical prediction rule was developed based on common factors among subjects who had a successful outcome.

12. O'Sullivan PB, Phyty GD, Twomey LT, Allison GT: Evaluation of specific stabilizing exercise in the treatment of chronic low back pain with radiologic diagnosis of spondylolysis or spondylolisthesis. *Spine* 1997;22: 2959-2967.

13. Hides JA, Jull GA, Richardson CA: Long-term effects of specific stabilizing exercises for first-episode low back pain. *Spine* 2001;26:E243-E248.

14. Critchley DJ, Ratcliffe J, Noonan S, Jones RH, Hurley MV: Effectiveness and cost-effectiveness of three types of physiotherapy used to reduce chronic low back pain disability: A pragmatic randomized trial with eco-

nomic evaluation. *Spine* 2007;32:1474-1481.

The authors compared the effectiveness of traditional outpatient physiotherapy, physiotherapist-led pain management classes, and spinal stabilization classes. Two hundred twelve patients were randomly assigned to one of the above treatment groups. Outcome measures were completed at the initial evaluation, 6 months after, 12 months after, and 18 months after. All groups showed improvement in disability, pain, quality of life, and time off work with no between-group difference.

15. Sherry MA, Best TM: A comparison of 2 rehabilitation programs in the treatment of acute hamstring strains. *J Orthop Sports Phys Ther* 2004;34:116-125.

Twenty-four athletes were randomly assigned to either a hamstring stretching and strengthening group or a progressive agility and trunk stabilization group. The authors compared the time to return to sport, injury recurrence, and lower extremity functional evaluation. Athletes who participated in the progressive agility and trunk stabilization exercise group returned to sports activity sooner and had a decreased rate of recurrence of hamstring strain.

16. Butcher SJ, Craven BR, Chilibeck PD, Spink KS, Grona SL, Sprigings EJ: The effect of trunk stability training on vertical takeoff velocity. *J Orthop Sports Phys Ther* 2007;37:223-231.

The authors compared the effects of four training programs on vertical takeoff velocity. The four groups were trunk stability, leg strength, trunk stability and leg strength, and control. Fifty-five athletes participated in this study. After 9 weeks of training, all three training groups had a greater takeoff velocity than the control group, with no between-group difference.

17. Leetun DT, Ireland ML, Willson JD, Ballantyne BT, Davis IM: Core stability measures as risk factors for lower extremity injury in athletes. *Med Sci Sports Exerc* 2004;36:926-934.

Core stability measures, including hip abduction and external rotation strength, abdominal muscle function, and back extensor and quadratus lumborum endurance, were collected for 80 female and 60 male athletes. The core stability measures were compared for athletes who sustained an injury during the following season and those who did not sustain an injury. Hip abduction and external rotation strength were greater in athletes who were not injured.

18. Zazulak BT, Hewett TE, Reeves NP, Goldberg B, Cholewicki J: Deficits in neuromuscular control of the trunk predict knee injury risk: A prospective biomechanical-epidemiologic study. *Am J Sports Med* 2007;35:1123-1129.

The authors of this study tested 277 collegiate athletes for trunk displacement after a sudden force release. Knee injury data were collected for these athletes. The authors identified factors related to core stability that predicted knee injury risk. Trunk displacement was greater in athletes with knee, ligament, and anterior cruciate ligament injuries than in uninjured athletes. A history of low back pain was also found to be a predictor of injury risk.

4: Rehabilitation

Chapter 23

Hip Arthroscopy Rehabilitation: Evidence-Based Practice

Michael Wahoff, PT   Karen K. Briggs, MPH   *Marc J. Philippon, MD

Introduction

Arthroscopic management of intra-articular hip pathology has greatly improved over the past decade because of advances in diagnostic evaluation and arthroscopic instrumentation. Enhanced descriptions of the proper patient indications and surgical candidates, as well as detailed and streamlined physical therapy, continue to improve patient outcomes after arthroscopy.[1,2] Rehabilitation after hip arthroscopy is critical; however, there are few data or little evidence-based research to support any specific rehabilitation guidelines or current trends. This chapter describes a four-phase rehabilitation protocol based on current intra-articular diagnosis and arthroscopic surgical techniques, known hip biomechanics (for a mechanical foundation), and consideration of soft-tissue healing constraints (for a basic science foundation). Each phase of the protocol can be individualized to the patient's age, fitness level, previous surgeries, or other extra-articular pathologies that may be present (for example, sports hernia or snapping hip).

Hip Biomechanics and Neuromuscular Control Considerations

The goals of hip surgery are the correction of bony, chondral, labral, and capsular abnormalities; the restoration of abnormal joint mechanics; and pain relief.[3-5] The goals of postsurgical rehabilitation are control of swelling and pain, prevention of muscle inhibition, protection of the surgical repair, recovery of neuromuscular control and strength, correction of muscle imbalance, restoration of normal functional activity (such as walking, running, and skating), and return to previous level of function or sports activity.[6] An understanding of hip biomechanics and the healing constraints of the

surgical repair are required to develop an appropriate physical therapy protocol.

Osseous Structures

Cam type femoroacetabular impingement is described as the lack of femoral head-neck offset, which contributes to irregular and repetitive abutment at the anterosuperior acetabular rim and results in early chondral delamination and labral dysfunction.[3-5,7-9] Pincer-type femoroacetabular impingement is a decrease in acetabular anteversion (known as acetabular retroversion), where the anterior wall superiorly impedes the posterior wall or coxa profundus (deep socket) and can contribute to preemptive chondrolabral dysfunction.[4,5,7-9] The normal acetabular coverage measured as the center edge angle is anywhere from 20° to 25° or greater.[10] Patients with less than 20° in the center edge angle are considered dysplastic.

Rehabilitation of the hip considering the osseous structures involves several factors. The cam and pincer effects must be completely eliminated. Attempts at regaining full motion may stress the labrum and the labral repair. If a nonsurgical treatment approach is taken, then end range of motion and aggressive stretching should be avoided to prevent pathologic impingement. Patients with developmental dysplasia of the hip may require more protection to allow longer soft-tissue healing times as they rely more on soft tissue for stability. It should also be stressed to these patients that end range of motion and aggressive stretching should be avoided. The superior and anterior aspects of the femur are exposed in neutral, and maximal articular congruence occurs at 90° of flexion, slight abduction, and slight external rotation (Figure 1). The quadruped (hands and knees) position is good for bony congruence with minimal stress on articular cartilage (Figure 2).

Capsule and Ligamentous Structures

The capsule of the hip joint is dense, strong, and fibrous.[11] Longitudinal superficial fibers and circular deep fibers form the zona orbicularis or collar around the femoral neck. The capsule is thick anterosuperiorly and loose and thin posteroinferiorly. During rehabilitation of the hip in consideration of the ligamentous

*Marc J. Philippon, MD or the department with which he is affiliated has received research or institutional support, miscellaneous nonincome support, commercially derived honoraria, or other nonresearch-related funding from Smith & Nephew and is a consultant for or an employee of Smith & Nephew.

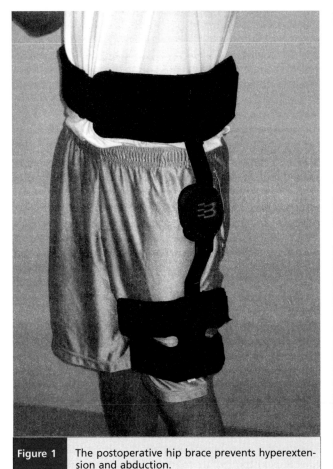

Figure 1   The postoperative hip brace prevents hyperextension and abduction.

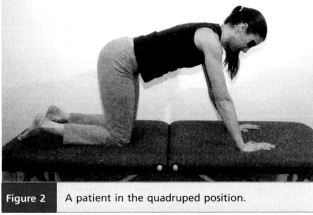

Figure 2   A patient in the quadruped position.

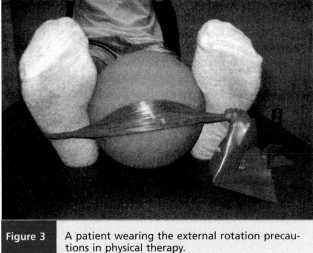

Figure 3   A patient wearing the external rotation precautions in physical therapy.

structures, the pubofemoral ligament blends with the pectineus muscle at the anterior pubic rami. Differentiating medial capsular tightness from muscle tendinitis is difficult postoperatively in this region. The ischiofemoral ligament is continuous with the zona orbicularis and the tendon of the obturator externus muscle. Limits should be placed on external rotation and extension to allow healing time for the iliofemoral ligament following resection or plication (**Figure 3**). Ligamentous structures provide hip stability. During standing, the body's center of gravity lies just posterior to the axis of the hip in the sagittal plane, causing the pelvis to tilt posteriorly on the femoral head. This force is opposed by the tensile forces of the stretched anterior capsule and ligaments. If the anterior capsule is too tight, the center of gravity through the hip may be altered. A capsule that is too loose may prevent the counterforces needed during standing and require too much muscle support.

Neuromuscular Control
The hip does not rely solely on the correct bony geometry and labrum for normal hip stabilization. The ligamentous structures, along with the muscles that cross the joint, contribute to the congruency of the femoroacetabular complex by checking motions and providing a

stabilization effect. Muscles that cross the joint may act as prime movers or as stabilizers throughout a wide range of motions. To act as stabilizers, muscle stiffness must be regulated through a neural feedback control system, including regulation by muscle fiber recruitment, the sarcomere length–tension relationship, and the passive sarcomere length–tension relationship. The muscle force and moment are regulated by skeletal muscle architecture.[12]

The more superficial muscles, including the gluteus maximus, the gluteus medius, the gluteus minimus, and the iliopsoas, have been studied for their ability to generate support during the stance phase of gait.[13] The gluteus medius, the gluteus maximus, and the gluteus minimus provided most of the support in 0% to 30% of stance.[8] From foot flat to contralateral toe-off (10% to 50%), the gluteus maximus and the posterior medius and minimus make significant contributions.[13] With assistance from joints and bones to gravity, the anterior and posterior gluteus medius and gluteus minimus generated all the support evident in midstance. The posterior portion contributed throughout midstance, whereas the anterior contributed only toward the end of midstance. The iliopsoas developed substantial forces during late stance but did not make substantial contributions to support.[13] The muscle action of the gluteus medius and the gluteus minimus depends strongly on body positions. For rehabilitation of the hip considering the neuromuscular system, abnormal femoral, pelvic, or lumbar positions may alter the muscle's moment arms across the hip and cause abnormal forces in these or other muscles. Emphasis must be placed on correct alignment and body position as patients are progressed through rehabilitation. Exercises need to be monitored as they become more challenging; otherwise, abnormal body positions may facilitate abnormal force production in the muscles and cause extra-articular pathologies such as tendinitis, iliotibial band syndrome, and low back pain.

The lumbar spine-pelvis-hip relationship is critical to consider because of the structures' close proximity to each other and the location of muscle origins and insertions that cross and control the hip. Core stability will allow proper position of the pelvis throughout functional movements. The inability to control the pelvis will alter muscle moment arms because of abnormal pelvic positions and the potential to incur altered force production or length tension relationships in the muscles during functional movements.

A common pattern noted is a flexor dominance with weakness of the core muscle groups (transverse abdominus) and gluteal muscle (deep rotators and gluteus maximus) group with abnormally shortened and tight hip flexor group (iliopsoas) and lumbar group (quadratus lumborum). The following scenario is a hip to shoulder comparison to consider: the pelvis acts as the scapula of the shoulder with its position critical in the normal function of the muscle groups. The core muscles act as the scapular stabilizers to position the pelvis. The deep rotator muscles act as stabilizers during movements of the hip. The combined actions of the two-joint muscles produce coordinated movements of the lower extremity. The single-joint muscles produce speed, power, and stability. The conjoined abdominal and adductor tendons at the pelvis and the effect a weakened abdominal wall or tight adductors may have in this area also should be considered.

<h2>Intra-articular Diagnosis and Surgical Techniques Considerations</h2>

Rehabilitation Considerations After Osteoplasty and/or Rim Trimming

Passive range of motion has no limits. Full and consistent (two or three times per day) passive range of motion is stressed because of the increased bleeding from the removal of the bone. Passive range of motion will help prevent adhesions, especially between the acetabular rim and the attachment of the capsule. Passive range of motion is performed up to the limits of pain and stiffness. Passive circumduction at 70° and neutral is also stressed to prevent adhesions between the circular fibers of the zona obicularis and the femoral neck. Foot flat weight bearing should be instituted for 2 weeks because a stress fracture of the femoral neck may occur. Two weeks of reduced weight bearing also will help bring about faster reduction of joint inflammation. Foot flat weight bearing, described as 20% body weight and the avoidance of heel strike, is used to prevent excessive use of the hip flexor and shearing force at heel strike. Because impingement is caused by a bony abnormality, no preventive measure is known. Proper maintenance of core strength and muscle balance and the avoidance of aggressive stretching of the hip may help protect the soft tissues of the joint. Early diagnosis and treatment of femoroacetabular impingement may reduce the risk of extensive damage to the labrum and cartilage surfaces.

Rehabilitation Considerations After Chondroplasty or Microfracture

After a chondroplasty, the patient can bear weight as tolerated; after microfracture, 8 weeks of foot flat weight bearing should be instituted.[14,15] The patient should undergo continuous passive motion (CPM) for 2 weeks for 4 hours per day following a chondroplasty, and 8 weeks for 6 to 8 hours per day following a microfracture. The patient should lie prone at least 2 hours per day to stretch the hip flexor muscles after CPM to avoid flexor contracture. Passive range of motion in all planes should be instituted for 6 to 8 weeks after chondroplasty or microfracture.

Rehabilitation Considerations After Labral Débridement or Repair

Because of a lack of muscle attachment directly onto the labrum, no specific active range of motion limits exist; because of the depth of the joint through all the soft tissues, limiting the volume of active motion is highly recommended. Passive range of motion is recommended to prevent adhesions between the capsule and the labrum. Flexion is not limited. Abduction beyond 45° is not allowed until after 10 to 21 days. No weight-bearing restrictions are required. Proper maintenance of core strength and muscle balance in and around the hip is critical in protecting the joint from injury. In patients with femoroacetabular impingement, forceful stretching is contraindicated because excessive forces are placed on the labrum. Early treatment of femoroacetabular impingement may prevent or limit the extent of the damage to the labrum.

Rehabilitation Considerations After Capsular Plication and/or Capsulorrhaphy

Limits of external rotation and extension are considered for 14 to 21 days. Because of the frequency in which hip flexor contracture occurs, neutral extension is recommended by the end of week 1. No weight bearing restrictions are required. Proper maintenance of core strength and muscle balance in and around the hip is critical to reduce excessive stresses on the capsule, especially in the presence of a labral tear.

Four-Phase Rehabilitation Protocol

The four-phase rehabilitation protocol is described under the following considerations: the overall goal of rehabilitation is return to preinjury level of function, and the healing constraints of the surgical repair and normal hip biomechanics are understood.

The first phase, mobility and protection, is most reliant on soft-tissue healing constraints and preventing the effects of immobilization; therefore, this phase is continued for a time frame of 6 to 8 weeks. The other three phases are more reliant on the patient's ability to reach the goals of each phase and meet the criteria to advance to the next phase. The progression through exercises listed for the last three phases are therefore more dependent on the individual patient, using such factors as patient age, fitness level, prior surgeries, or other conditions. The time frames are those expected in a young, healthy patient without previous surgeries or complications.

Early stabilization exercises are critical in the prevention of muscle inhibition, atrophy, and regaining the normal mechanics of the lumbar-pelvic-hip complex. Early stabilization exercises can be performed while maintaining the precautions for the surgical repairs. When the gait restrictions are removed, the second section of phase 2 is initiated to include gait training and weight shifting. Mobility continues throughout this period. Stabilization exercises are advanced to include more functional movements. The third section of phase 2 is for high school and professional athletes who participate in sports such as running, skating, dance, or golf. There are no more surgical precautions at this time, so phase 1 is complete.

Strengthening is not initiated until the goals of phase 2 and the criteria to advance to phase 3 have been achieved. The ability of the patient to perform a series of functional movements, including normal gait, single leg bridges, side planks, symmetrical lunges, single leg stance, single knee bends, and trunk rotation with good stabilization and no compensation is required.

Phase 4 is return to sport or activities of choice. For high school, elite, and professional level athletes, training for return to competition can begin with no restrictions once they have passed the sport test (Table 1). The precautions, goals, and criteria to advance through each phase are outlined in the following sections.

Phase 1: Mobility and Protection
Precautions
Foot flat weight bearing should be maintained for 2 weeks in patients without a microfracture and for 8 weeks for those with a microfracture. A CPM machine is used for 2 weeks, 4 hours per day for the patient without a microfracture and for 8 weeks, 6 to 8 hours per day for the patient with a microfracture. Range of motion in the CPM machine is 30° to 70° at onset and increased per patient tolerance. The patient lies prone for a minimum of 2 hours per day to stretch the hip flexor and prevent a flexion contracture. Passive range of motion is full flexion and abduction to 45° by the end of week 1 with no external rotation for 14 to 21 days. Limits of external rotation exist to allow adequate healing of the capsule in the presence of a capsulorrhaphy, plication, or even nonclosure of the capsule during surgery.[16] The patient should not push through pain or pinching with passive range of motion. External rotation boots are used while the patient is lying supine to prevent external rotation for the first 14 to 21 days. A hinged hip brace locked from 0° to 105° is used for the first 14 to 21 days. This brace can be fitted to adjust for the amount of abduction the surgeon would prefer when more protection and better bony congruency are required.

Goals and Criteria to Advance
The goals to achieve during phase 1 are to protect the integrity of the repaired tissues, restore passive range of motion within restrictions, lessen the patient's pain and inflammation, and prevent muscular inhibition. Stabilization exercises of phase 2 will begin simultaneously with phase 1 exercises during week 2 and continued to maintain precautions.

Phase 2: Stabilization and Gait
Precautions
Divided into three sections, the first section of phase 2 (neuromuscular control) overlaps phase 1; therefore, the precautions are the same. The second section of phase 2 is gait; therefore, patients without a microfracture can be weaned from crutches after 2 weeks and patients with a microfracture after 8 weeks. Advancement of stabilization exercises throughout this section should continue to challenge the patient without any indication of hip flexor, adductor, or piriformis irritation. The third section of phase 2 includes starting the functional aspect of the individual patient's sport for high school through professional athletes. Running for all field and court sports, skating for all ice sports, and dance movements for dancers can be initiated. The treadmill (including underwater treadmills) should never be used by the patient from this point forward because of the secondary shearing forces across the anterior hip joint as a result of the moving tread. All surgical precautions at this point are unnecessary; however, the patient's ability to demonstrate good stabilization and control with movements and a normal gait pattern is recommended. A gradual progression through the functional aspect of the patient's sport should be applied (Tables 2 through 5). Golf swings can also be started with chipping and putting, progressing to high irons.

Goals and Criteria to Advance
The goals of phase 1 should be continued, in addition to correcting muscle imbalances and gait abnormalities and early initiation of functional activities. Before advancing to the next phase, the patient should have no pain, full range of motion, and normal gait.

Table 1

Rehabilitation Phase Timelines

Non-Mfx Level 1	Mfx Level 1	Non-Mfx Level 2	Mfx Level 2
Phase 1 (Mobility): weeks 1-6	Phase 1 (Mobility): weeks 1-8	Phase 1 (Mobility): weeks 1-6	Phase 1 (Mobility): weeks 1-8
Phase 2 (Core): weeks 2-8	Phase 2 (Core): weeks 2-12	Phase 2 (Core): week 2-8	Phase 2 (Core): week 2-16
Week 2+ core exercises	Week 2 + core exercises	Week 2 + core exercises	Week 2 + core exercises
Week 7 + functional exercises (skate/run/dance positions)	Week 9 + gait exercises	Week 3 + gait exercises	Week 3 + gait exercises
Phase 3 (Strength): week 9-11	Week 11 + functional exercises (skate/run/dance positions)	Week 7+ functional exercises (walking/hiking/biking)	Week 7 + functional exercises (walking/hiking/biking)
Phase 4 (Sport-specific training): week 12 +	Phase 3 (Strength): week 13-15	Phase 3 (Strength): week 13-15	Phase 3 (Strength): week 15-19
	Phase 4 (Sport-specific training): week 16 +	Phase 4 (Return to function): week 16 +	Phase 4 (Return to function): week 20 +

Level 1 = accelerated; Level 2 = normal (nonathlete and/or prior surgery); Mfx = microfracture

Table 2

Running Progression*

Stage	Walk/ Run Ratio	Sets and Total Time	Frequency
R1	4 min/1 min	4 sets = 20 min	3 times/ week
R2	3 min/2 min	4 sets = 20 min	3 times/ week
R3	2 min/3 min	4 sets = 20 min	3 times/ week
R4	1 min/4 min	4 sets = 20 min	3 times/ week
R5	5 min jog	2 sets = 10 min	3 times/ week

From 10-min jogging, increase as tolerated to build a base. Speed and power drills after a base is developed
*No treadmill. Use softer surface or grass to start.

Table 3

Skating Progression

Stage	Skating Progression*	Time	Frequency
S1	Skate no pads forward and back with crossover	20 min	2 times/ week
S2	Skate using pads with change of direction, stop/start	30 min	3 times/ week
S3	Sport-specific drills	45 min	4 times/ week
S4	Sport test (for participation clearance)		Week 10 of protocol
S5	Full contact: Practice with team		After passing sport test

*The goalie should refrain from using pads an extra week.

Phase 3: Strengthening

Precautions
Strengthening should be initiated when the patient is able to demonstrate excellent stabilization and control with functional movements. The "functional movement test" can include gait, single leg bridge, planks in all positions, and single knee bends. These maneuvers should all be performed without compensation in any plane.

Goals and Criteria to Advance
The goals of phase 3 are progression of the patient's functional activity to be able to initiate training, and muscle strength that is 100% that of the nonoperated leg. Before the patient can advance to the next phase, he or she should pass the sport test. Patients not attempting to return to a higher level of athletic function do not need to complete the sport test and would continue to progress with their normal daily activities as tolerated.

Sport Test
The sport test is a functional test that comprises four exercises with a 20-point scoring system to test the patient's ability to demonstrate endurance and functional strength in the lower extremity; good explosion (the ability to dynamically push off in a quick and controlled manner with 70° of knee flexion) off and absorption (the ability to land in a soft, controlled man-

4: Rehabilitation

ner) onto the involved lower extremity in a lateral and a rotational direction; and the ability to flex and extend into a lunge position without pain, fatigue, or compensation. The four tests are the single knee bends, side-to-side lateral movement, diagonal side-to-side movement, and forward box lunges (Figure 4). The single knee bends with cord resistance are performed for 3 minutes at a pace of 1 second down and 1 second up without any pelvic obliquity or corkscrewing (medial rotation/adduction) of the lower extremity (Figure 4, A). For the first test, 1 point is given for every 30 seconds for a total of 6 points. The lateral side-to-side movement is performed with a cord attached to the waist on the involved side (Figure 4, B). The patient pushes (explodes) off the involved side against the resistance of the cord and returns onto the involved leg with good absorption described as landing in a soft and controlled manner to 70° of knee flexion. The patient performs this movement for 100 seconds without any of the above compensations (medial rotation/adduction). For the second test, 1 point is given for each 20 seconds performed correctly and without pain for a total of 5 points. The third test is similar to the second; however, it is performed at a 45° angle forward and 45° angle backward from the frontal plane (Figure 4, C). It is also performed for 100 seconds and scored the same as the previous test. The final test is a forward box lunge onto a box set at the height of the patient's knee (Figure 4, D) to assess the ability of the hip to flex and extend without pain. It is performed for 2 minutes with cord resistance and scored 1 point for each 30 seconds performed without pain or compensation for a total of 4 points. A score of 17 points or higher is considered a passing score. The sport test is used as a presurgery functional examination as well as a functional test for return to training or play. Once the patient has passed the sport test, training may commence before actual return to play.

The sport test is an important adjunct to the patient's clinical examination and subjective impressions because it helps quantify the patient's functional level. A maintenance program, including core stabilization exercises, deep external rotator strengthening, maintenance of proper muscle balance around the hip, and avoidance of deep squats greater than 70°, is recommended after the patient has been cleared for sports participation and has returned to his or her prior level of activity.

Table 4

Golf Progression

Stage	Golf Progression*	Volume	Frequency
G1	Putt, chip, half swing only	1 bucket	1 to 2 weeks
G2	8- or 9-irons, three-quarter swing only	1 bucket	2 weeks
G3	All irons, use cart, full swing	9 holes	2 weeks
G4	Full play, walking 18 holes	18 holes	

*The athlete should not carry the golf bag or pull the golf cart.

Summary

Rehabilitation after hip arthroscopy to repair or correct labral tears, femoroacetabular impingement, chondral defects, and instability is critical. Protocols protecting the repaired tissues and focusing on mobility in the early phases of rehabilitation; emphasizing stabilization in the second phase; and strengthening during the third

Table 5

Dance Progression

Stage	Dance Progression*	
D1—Week 2	Four-way ankle strength with elastic band	
D2—Week 4	Bar work: stabilization on operated leg and progress turn out (complete movements with legs rotated outward)	Single leg balance (tendus) and turned out bridges on ball (with legs rotated outward)
D3—Week 5	Multiplane muscle stretching	Including pike and V stretching, progress to splits over 4 weeks; duration approximately 8 weeks
D4—Week 5	Double knee bends = Plie	
D5—Week 6	Multiplane muscle, single-leg activities/moves	External rotation leg lift (when short lever hip flexion is pain free)
D6	Sport test	
D7	Jumps	D5 after passing sport test

*In ballet or dance, the athlete may incorporate stages D1 through D5 as part of phase 2 exercises. Frequency: four to five times per week

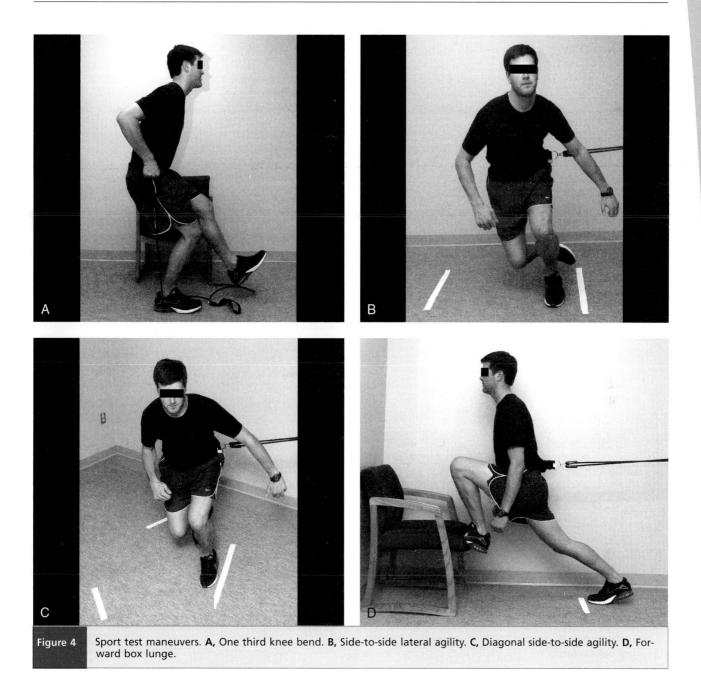

Figure 4   Sport test maneuvers. **A,** One third knee bend. **B,** Side-to-side lateral agility. **C,** Diagonal side-to-side agility. **D,** Forward box lunge.

phase has shown positive outcomes. Continued research is important to achieve a better understanding of the function of the muscles surrounding the hip and healing constraints of surgical repairs.

Annotated References

1. Philippon M, Schenker M, Briggs K, Kuppersmith D: Femoroacetabular impingement in 45 professional athletes: Associated pathologies and return to sport following arthroscopic decompression. *Knee Surg Sports Traumatol Arthrosc* 2007;15:908-914.

   The purpose of this study was to define associated pathologies and determine if an arthroscopic approach to

treating femoroacetabular impingement will allow professional athletes to return to high-level sports. In 45 professional athletes who had hip arthroscopy for the decompression of femoroacetabular impingement, 93% returned to professional competition after arthroscopic decompression. Athletes who did not return to sports competition had diffuse osteoarthritis.

2. Farjo LA, Glick JM, Sampson TG: Hip arthroscopy for acetabular labral tears. *Arthroscopy* 1999;15:132-137.

3. Beck M, Kalhor M, Leunig M, Ganz R: Hip morphology influences the pattern of damage to the articular cartilage: Femoroacetabular impingement as a cause of early osteoarthritis of the hip. *J Bone Joint Surg Br* 2005;87:1012-1018.

Cam and pincer femoroacetabular impingement and its progression to osteoarthritis of the hip were studied. Twenty-six patients with isolated cam impingement and 16 with isolated pincer impingement were studied. The authors documented the mechanisms behind the damage involving both types of impingement, including the location of chondral damage and the presence of labral tears.

4. Ganz R, Parvizi J, Beck M, Leunig M, Nötzli H, Siebenrock KA: Femoroacetabular impingement: A cause for osteoarthritis of the hip. *Clin Orthop Relat Res* 2003; 417:112-120.

This article establishes possible causes of idiopathic osteoarthritis in the hip. The authors propose femoroacetabular impingement as a mechanism leading to early osteoarthritis in nondysplastic hips. Clinical, radiographic and intraoperative information is used to confirm accurate diagnoses. The authors suggest that early surgical intervention for the treatment of femoroacetabular impingement may decelerate the progression of the degenerative process in the hip.

5. Philippon MJ, Stubbs AJ, Schenker ML, Maxwell RB, Ganz R, Leunig M: Arthroscopic management of femoroacetabular impingement: Osteoplasty technique and literature review. *Am J Sports Med* 2007;35:1571-1580.

This study presents a discussion of pertinent literature and the arthroscopic surgical approach associated with femoroacetabular impingement is described. Specific anatomic abnormalities are documented and subsequent patterns of injury are explained. Surgical intervention for the treatment of femoroacetabular impingement is particularly relevant to high-demand patients, specifically athletes who wish to return to high-level sports participation.

6. Stalzer S, Wahoff M, Scanlan M: Rehabilitation following hip arthroscopy. *Clin Sports Med* 2006;25:337-357.

As the techniques of arthroscopic hip surgery have evolved and advanced, the protocols for postoperative rehabilitation should follow accordingly. The focus of this article was to develop a set of rehabilitation guidelines that should be used to achieve consistent outcomes after hip surgery.

7. Johnston TL, Schenker ML, Briggs KK, Philippon MJ: Relationship between offset angle alpha and hip chondral injury in femoroacetabular impingement. *Arthroscopy* 2008;24:669-675.

This study examined the relationship between the size of cam lesions and the presence of cartilage damage, labral damage, and changes in the range of motion of hips with signs and symptoms of femoroacetabular impingement. The authors had access to cross-table lateral radiographs of 85 patients; cam-type femoroacebular impingement, as measured by an increased offset alpha angle, was correlated with increased chondral damage, labral injury, and decreased range of motion.

8. Philippon MJ, Maxwell RB, Johnston TL, Schenker M, Briggs KK: Clinical presentation of femoroacetabular impingement. *Knee Surg Sports Traumatol Arthrosc* 2007;15:1041-1047.

This study identified 301 arthroscopic hip surgeries for femoroacetabular impingement and investigated the relationship between objective findings and the patient's subjective complaints. The authors found that the most common complaint was groin pain, and the ability to perform activities of daily living and participate in sports was decreased in these patients. Furthermore, significant decreases in hip range of motion were observed in surgically treated hips.

9. Philippon MJ, Schenker ML: Arthroscopy for the treatment of femoroacetabular impingement in the athlete. *Clin Sports Med* 2006;25:299-308.

This article examined the role of femoroacetabular impingement and its association with hip pain, labral and chondral pathology, early arthritis, and decreased athletic performance. The classic open surgical treatment has led to open trauma and delayed return to sports activity in some patients, leading to the development of an arthroscopic approach to treatment. The authors describe arthroscopic treatment of cam and pincer hip impingement.

10. Armfield DR, Towers JD, Robertson DD: Radiographic and MR imaging of the athletic hip. *Clin Sports Med* 2006;25:211-239.

Clinical imaging practices for the hip were studied. High resolution direct magnetic resonance arthrography is an effective means of evaluating intra-articular pathology, and radiography is important for the diagnosis of subtle bony irregularities associated with femoroacetabular impingement.

11. Shindle MK, Ranawat AS, Kelly BT: Diagnosis and management of traumatic and atraumatic hip instability in the athletic patient. *Clin Sports Med* 2006;25:309-326.

Hip instability as a source of significant disability in the athletic patient was studied. The authors attempt to define a treatment plan for hip instability caused by traumatic and atraumatic events among high-level athletes by reviewing the literature and discussing relevant anatomy, history, physical examination findings, and imaging studies.

12. Torry MR, Schenker ML, Martin HD, Hogoboom D, Philippon MJ: Neuromuscular hip biomechanics and pathology in the athlete. *Clin Sports Med* 2006;25: 179-197.

Osseous and ligamentous support as well as neuromuscular control associated with the hip joint was studied. The probable mechanisms of injury in sports activities most often associated with hip injury also are discussed.

13. Anderson FC, Pandy MG: Individual muscle contributions to support in normal walking. *Gait Posture* 2003; 17:159-169.

The specific contributions made by individual muscles that support the entire body during normal gait were analyzed. A three-dimensional muscle-actuated model of the body and a dynamic optimization solution for normal walking made this analysis possible. The study documented the multiple stages of walking and the individual muscles associated with each action.

14. Crawford K, Philippon MJ, Sekiya JK, Rodkey WG, Steadman JR: Microfracture of the hip in athletes. *Clin Sports Med* 2006;25:327-335.

    The indications and outcomes for hip microfracture were investigated in athletes. The microfracture technique for the treatment of chondral injuries in the knee has evolved and has recently been expanded to treat lesions in the hip, which are common in athletes. Early results after hip microfracture have been encouraging.

15. Philippon MJ, Briggs KK, Kuppersmith DA, et al: Outcomes following hip arthroscopy with microfracture. *Arthroscopy* 2007;23:211.

    The 1-year outcomes of patients who had hip arthroscopy with microfracture were documented. Indications for this procedure included a full-thickness loss of articular cartilage in the weight-bearing region of the hip between the femur and the acetabulum. Between March 2005 and June 2005, 19 hips underwent hip arthroscopy with microfracture. Modified Harris hip scores improved from an average of 58 before surgery to an average of 74 after surgery; an average of 8.6 of 10 patients were satisfied with the outcome.

16. Philippon MJ: New frontiers in hip arthroscopy: The role of arthroscopic hip labral repair and capsulorrhaphy in the treatment of hip disorders. *Instr Course Lect* 2006;55:309-316.

    The pathologies that commonly underlie hip pain were investigated. For example, a labral tear can be a source of hip pain and can also cause other mechanical symptoms and is treated with débridement and suture anchor repair. To maintain function within the hip joint, capsular laxity is commonly treated with thermal capsulorrhaphy or capsular plication to reduce capsular redundancy and avoid premature arthritis.

Head and Neck

SECTION EDITOR:

STANLEY A. HERRING, MD

Chapter 24

Assessment and Return to Play Following Sports-Related Concussion

Kevin M. Guskiewicz, PhD, ATC   *Ruben J. Echemendia, PhD   Robert C. Cantu, MD, FACS, FACSM

Introduction

Sports-related concussions are occurring more frequently, creating a much-needed awareness of this often puzzling injury. Despite an increased volume of published research over the past decade, misconceptions exist about concussions and how best to manage such injuries.

Cerebral concussion is a common condition, comprising almost 10% of all athletic injuries.[1,2] It is perhaps the most puzzling and mismanaged neurologic condition described in the sports medicine literature. Although identification and diagnosis of the injury can be a challenge, the pathophysiology of cerebral concussion and the brain's unsystematic course of recovery is a mystery. New knowledge in this area has led to significant discussions among international experts and consensus groups, which has resulted in several recent articles on the topic of sports-related concussion.[3-6]

The most recent scientific and clinical-based literature on sports-related concussion presents the current state of the art and science of the assessment and management of athletes who are at risk for injury.

Defining the Injury

Cerebral concussion can best be classified as a mild diffuse brain injury that is often referred to as mild traumatic brain injury (MTBI). MTBI occurs as a result of a blow to the head or other part of the body, causing an acceleration or deceleration of the brain inside the skull. Typical symptoms include headache, nausea, vomiting, dizziness, balance problems, feeling "slowed down," fatigue, trouble sleeping, drowsiness, sensitivity to light or noise, loss of consciousness, blurred vision, difficulty remembering, or difficulty concentrating.[3,7] It is often reported that there is no universal agreement on a definition of concussion; however, agreement does exist on several features that incorporate clinical, pathologic, and biomechanical factors associated with MTBI:

(1) Concussion is caused by a direct blow to the head or elsewhere on the body resulting in a sudden mechanical loading of the head that generates turbulent rotatory and linear movements of the cerebral hemispheres.

(2) These collisions or impacts between the cortex and bony walls of the skull typically cause an immediate and short-lived impairment of neurologic function involving a potpourri of symptoms; these symptoms are sometimes long-lasting and result in a condition known as postconcussion syndrome.

(3) Concussion may cause neuropathologic changes or temporary deformation of tissue; however, the acute clinical symptoms primarily reflect a functional metabolic disturbance rather than a structural injury.

(4) Concussion may cause a gradient of clinical syndromes that may or may not involve loss of consciousness (LOC). Resolution of the clinical and cognitive symptoms often follows a sequential course but is dependent on several factors, including magnitude of the impact and the individual's concussion history.

(5) Concussion is most often associated with normal results on conventional neuroimaging studies.[3,4,8,9]

Athletes who sustain a blow or ding to the head often experience a state of stunned confusion that resolves within minutes. Unfortunately, the term 'ding' trivializes the importance of this initial confusional state because the evolving signs and symptoms of a concussion are often not evident until several minutes to hours after the blow.[4] Although it is important for clinicians to recognize and eventually classify the concussive injury, it is equally important for the athlete to understand the signs and symptoms of a concussion, as well as the potential negative consequences (for example, second-impact syndrome, predisposition to future

*Ruben J. Echemendia, PhD or the department with which he is affiliated has received research or institutional support from the National Operating Committee on Standards for Athletic Equipment.

5: Head and Neck

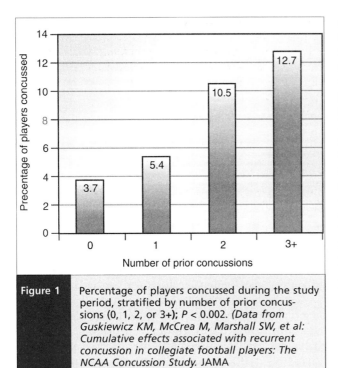

Figure 1 Percentage of players concussed during the study period, stratified by number of prior concussions (0, 1, 2, or 3+); P < 0.002. *(Data from Guskiewicz KM, McCrea M, Marshall SW, et al: Cumulative effects associated with recurrent concussion in collegiate football players: The NCAA Concussion Study. JAMA 2003;290:2549-2555.)*

concussions, and postconcussion syndrome) of not reporting a concussive injury. Once the athlete understands the injury, he or she can provide a more accurate report of factors associated with the concussion. Creating this awareness is of vital importance in the global management of the injury. One point of widespread agreement is that the immediate management of the head-injured athlete varies according to the nature and severity of the injury. It is important for clinicians to recognize that concussions are rarely associated with macroscopic abnormalities on neuroimaging because MTBI most often results in select neurons being rendered temporarily dysfunctional but not destroyed. Although concussion is often referred to as a diffuse axonal injury; MTBI does not usually appear to result in the shearing of axons but rather in a stretching, twisting, and (in some instances) a separation of dendritic branches. This process typically occurs in a very small number of axons within the region of insult, and most axons initially affected recover over a short period of time. The pathophysiologic sequence that occurs following traumatic brain injury, even in the mildest form, is best described as a process, not an event.[8,10]

Once an athlete has suffered a concussion, he or she is at increased risk for subsequent head injuries. Studies found that collegiate athletes had a threefold greater risk of suffering a concussion if they had sustained three or more previous concussions in a 7-year-period, and players with two or more previous concussions required a longer time for total symptom resolution after subsequent injuries[11,12] (**Figure 1**). Players also had a threefold greater risk for subsequent concussions in the same season, whereas recurrent, in-season injuries oc-

curred within 10 days of the initial injury 92% of the time.[11] Another similar study of high school athletes found that athletes with three or more prior concussions were at an increased risk of experiencing LOC (eightfold greater risk), anterograde amnesia (5.5-fold greater risk), and confusion (5.1-fold greater risk) after subsequent concussion.[13] Despite the increasing body of literature, debate still surrounds the question of how many concussions are enough to recommend ending the player's career. Some research suggests that three concussions in a career may be enough to permanently end a player's participation in sports.[11,13] However, other studies suggest that the total number of concussions is not related to decreased neurocognitive functioning.[14,15] In light of these contradictory findings, an individualized approach to concussion management appears to be the most appropriate because concussions present in varying degrees of severity, and all athletes do not respond in the same way to this injury. Emerging human as well as animal data suggest that an athlete's age is an important consideration in the management of concussion. Younger athletes tend to have more severe symptoms that last longer than those of older athletes.[16-18]

The increased risk of recurrent injury, as well as the slower recovery often seen after subsequent concussions, may be indicative of increased neuronal vulnerability after recurrent concussive injuries. Animal studies have described an acute neurometabolic cascade involving accelerated glycolysis, and increased lactate production immediately after concussion.[10] The increased lactate is believed to leave neurons more vulnerable to secondary ischemic injury and has been considered a possible predisposition to recurrent injury.[10] Later steps in this physiologic cascade involve increased intracellular calcium, mitochondrial dysfunction, impaired oxidative metabolism, decreased glycolysis, axonal disconnection, neurotransmitter disturbances, and delayed cell death. Decreased cerebral blood flow has been reported to last approximately 10 days following concussive injuries in animal models,[10] which is consistent with the finding of an apparent 7- to 10-day period of increased susceptibility to recurrent injury.

Clinical Evaluation

A thorough clinical examination conducted on the field of play is critical for the identification and management of sports concussions. This initial evaluation or series of evaluations should include a thorough history (including number and severity of previous head injuries), observation (including pupil responses), palpation, and special tests (including simple tests of memory, concentration, motor coordination, and cranial nerve functioning). The primary goal of the on-field assessment is to identify any life-threatening conditions such as a developing intracranial bleed. When the athlete's symptomatology is worsening, especially if there is deterioration to a stuporous, semicomatose, or comatose state of consciousness, the situation must be treated as a medical emergency.

In most instances, the athlete will be medically stable, so the assessment progresses to a secondary level with the intent of determining the developing signs and symptoms of the concussion. An emerging model of sports concussion assessment involves the use of brief screening tools to evaluate postconcussion signs and symptoms, cognitive functioning, and postural stability on the sidelines immediately after a concussion, as well as more sophisticated neuropsychological evaluation to track recovery well after the time of injury. The results from the neuropsychological tests, coupled with the physical examination and other aspects of the injury evaluation, assist the clinician and other sports medicine professionals in making a safe and informed decision about return to play (RTP).

Postconcussion Symptom Assessment

Several concussion symptom checklists[19-22] and scales[17,23,24] have been used in both research and clinical settings. A symptom checklist, which is composed of a list of concussion-related symptoms, allows the athlete to report whether the symptom is present or not by responding either "yes" (experiencing the symptom) or "no" (not experiencing the symptom). A symptom scale is a summative measure that allows the athlete to describe the extent to which he or she is experiencing the symptom. These instruments commonly incorporate a Likert-type scale that allows the athlete to rate the presence and severity of postconcussion symptoms. These scores are then summed to form a composite score that yields a quantitative measure of overall injury severity and a benchmark against which to track postinjury symptom recovery. Initial evidence has been provided for the structural validity for a self-report concussion symptom scale. The symptoms contained in these checklists are not specific to concussion. Thus, obtaining a baseline symptom score is helpful to establish the type and frequency of any preexisting symptoms that are attributable to factors other than the head injury (for example, illness, fatigue, menstruation, somatization). Serial administration of the graded symptom checklist is recommended for tracking symptom resolution over time (Table 1). Although very useful in assessing and managing concussive injuries, the symptom checklist is important to underscore that athletes are motivated to return to play and may consciously or unconsciously minimize their symptoms to return to the playing field.[5,25]

Objective Concussion Assessment Tools

Comprehensive assessment of concussion is best accomplished within the context of a multidisciplinary sports medicine team that has access to a variety of assessment techniques. In addition to sideline assessment and medical evaluation, neuropsychological testing and assessment of postural stability are important tools.

Neuropsychological Testing

Although the advent of neuropsychological testing in sports is relatively new, neuropsychological techniques have been used to assess traumatic brain injury for many years. Neurophysiological testing in the assessment of MTBI involves identification of a patient's functional and cognitive limitations as a result of the injury.

In order for neuropsychologists to infer the presence of pathology through deficit measurement, postinjury test scores must be compared with estimates of premorbid or preinjury measurement. Unlike most other populations, athletes can be evaluated before sustaining a MTBI to create baseline data than can be used to accurately compare preinjury and postinjury functioning. Using baseline testing among college football players, studies have demonstrated that neurocognitive deficits were apparent in athletes 24 hours after injury and 5 days after concussion. Cognitive functioning gradually improved over a period of time, with most but not all athletes having complete recovery by 10 days after injury. One study used retrospective analyses of college football players and found that athletes with a history of two or more concussions had poorer baseline performance on measures of information processing speed and executive functioning than athletes with no prior history of concussion.[26] Athletes in the study sample with a history of learning disability, coupled with a history of multiple concussions, had even poorer baseline functioning than those athletes without learning disabilities. Another study examined a multisport college population and found that a limited battery of neuropsychological measures could reliably differentiate athletes with concussion from uninjured control athletes as soon as 2 hours after injury.[20] The athletes with concussions scored significantly lower than control subjects at 2 hours after and 48 hours after injury, and group differences were also evident 1 week following injury. No differences were found between the groups at 1 month after injury. These data were interesting because they revealed that athletes with a concussion were unable to benefit from prior exposure to the test battery (practice effect) at the same level as the control subjects, largely because the concussed athletes were unable to use semantic clustering techniques during verbal learning and memory tasks.[20] This study underscored the dynamic nature of recovery following concussion because these athletes' neuropsychological performance declined from 2 hours to 48 hours after injury, whereas the control subjects improved during the same time frame. More importantly, although neuropsychological test scores could statistically differentiate between athletes with and without concussion at 48 hours, postconcussion symptoms, as measured by the standard Postconcussion Symptom Scale, could not distinguish the two groups. This finding is noteworthy because it helped to expose problems with relying exclusively on symptoms to determine RTP.

Table 1

Graded Symptom Checklist

Symptom	Time of Injury	2 to 3 Hours Postinjury	24 Hours Postinjury	48 Hours Postinjury	72 Hours Postinjury
Blurred vision					
Dizziness					
Drowsiness					
Excess sleep					
Easily distracted					
Fatigue					
Feel "in a fog"					
Feel "slowed down"					
Headache					
Inappropriate emotions					
Irritability					
Loss of consciousness					
Loss of orientation					
Memory problems					
Nausea					
Nervousness					
Personality change					
Poor balance/coordination					
Poor concentration					
Ringing in ears					
Sadness					
Seeing stars					
Sensitivity to light					
Sensitivity to noise					
Sleep disturbance					
Vacant stare/ glassy eyed					
Vomiting					

Note: The graded symptom checklist should be used not only for the initial evaluation but for each subsequent follow-up assessment until all signs and symptoms have cleared at rest and during physical exertion. In lieu of simply checking each symptom present, the health care provider can ask the athlete to grade or score the severity of the symptom on a scale of 0 to 6, where 0 = not present, 1 = mild, 3 = moderate, and 6 = most severe.

A sideline cognitive screening instrument, the Standardized Assessment of Concussion (SAC), was used in combination with selected traditional neuropsychological measures in college students.[27] The SAC scores of athletes with a concussion were significantly lower than baseline when compared with uninjured athletes. In contrast with studies using more comprehensive neuropsychologic measures that showed typical recovery by 10 days after injury, scores on the SAC returned to baseline within 48 hours of injury. These findings highlight the complementary nature of brief screening instruments and the more comprehensive batteries of tests. Brief screening instruments such as the SAC have been useful on the sidelines and during the acute phase of recovery (initial 48 hours after injury), whereas neuropsychological test batteries are more effective in identifying enduring neurocognitive deficits.[28]

The development of computerized test platforms provided a paradigm shift for neuropsychological assessment in sports. Four major computerized platforms have been used in sports concussion management: ImPACT (Immediate Post Concussion Assessment and Cognitive Testing),[29] CogSport,[30] HeadMinder Concussion Resolution Index,[31] and the Automated Neuropsychological Assessment Metrics Sports Medicine Battery (ANAM-SMB).[32] These batteries allow for groups of athletes to be assessed in a standardized manner and allow immediate access to test scores. Although different in their content, each of these batteries allows for a thorough assessment of simple and complex information processing speed, which has been shown to be a key deficit following concussion. Although these batteries have extended the use of neuropsychological measurement to a much larger number of athletes in a cost-effective manner, they also have drawbacks: (1) they do not fully assess memory functioning because they are only capable of examining recognition memory; (2) they minimize the interaction between the athlete and the neuropsychologist, thereby reducing qualitative observations of performance; (3) player motivation and effort is less effectively assessed and managed using group administration formats; and (4) they limit the ability to examine the process by which injured athletes solve problems and learn and remember information, which has been shown to be useful in the assessment of athletes with a concussion.

Using ImPACT, a recent study examined on-field predictors of neuropsychological functioning in a large sample of concussed high school and college athletes.[33] At 3 days after injury, athletes with poor outcomes were 10 times more likely to have had on-field retrograde amnesia and 4 times more likely to have had on-field posttraumatic amnesia. No effect was found for loss of consciousness. In another study using the HeadMinder Concussion Resolution Index computer battery, cognitive impairment at initial postconcussion assessment (when compared with baseline levels) is a significant predictor of the duration of postconcussion symptoms.[21] The findings of a 2001 study[20] were replicated in a recent study using the ANAM-SMB, measuring impairment in cognitive function in a 14-day period in concussed athletes compared with control subjects.[34] The differences between the groups were not necessarily caused by a decrement in functioning but rather an absent or restricted practice effect in the concussion group when compared with the control group.[34] Interestingly, the same pattern was observed when injured athletes with a history of concussion were compared with those with no history of concussion. Control subjects and injured athletes with no history of concussion revealed practice effects, whereas athletes with a history of previous concussions did not.[32]

There is a high degree of agreeement that neuropsychological testing is an integral part of the assessment plan after concussion. However, there is still some disagreement as to the most appropriate timing and frequency of these postinjury assessments. Many clinical research protocols[5,17,20-2,26,35] have used daily serial testing, regardless of the presence of symptoms,

whereas others have recommended that testing be conducted once an athlete is reportedly symptom-free.[5] Future studies should consider using a controlled, randomized design to better answer this important clinical question.

Postural Stability Assessment

Recent results of studies involving postural stability testing following concussion have helped substantiate the use of clinical balance tests in the sports medicine setting.[22] A growing body of literature suggests that areas of the brain disrupted as a result of head injury are responsible for the maintenance of postural equilibrium.[22,36] Clinicians have long evaluated head injuries with the Romberg test, which assesses balance based on sensory input. This is an easy and effective test to perform on the sidelines, but there is more to posture control than just balance and sensory input, especially when assessing athletes with head injuries.[37,38]

Systems such as the Smart Balance Master (NeuroCom International, Inc, Clackamas, OR) and the Chattecx Balance System (Chattecx, Division of Chattanooga Group Inc, Hixson, TN) can provide an easy and practical method of quantitatively assessing functional postural stability. These systems can assess athletes with mild head injuries, as well as identify possible abnormalities that might be associated with concussion, and develop a recovery curve based on quantitative measures for determining readiness to return to activity. Force platform systems have recently been developed for quantitatively assessing both static and dynamic balance. Their use has gained acceptance in clinical practice; however, they are expensive and therefore not readily available to many clinicians in high schools. The use of a clinical balance test, the Balance Error Scoring System (BESS), was developed as a valid and reliable low-tech assessment tool for managing sports-related concussion.[22,39]

Several studies have identified balance deficits during the initial 3 to 5 days after concussion; however, there is limited explanation as to why some concussed athletes demonstrate these deficits and others do not.[22,35-37] One study identified postural stability deficits lasting up to 3 days after injury in 36 collegiate athletes recovering from mild head injury when assessed using both the Smart Balance Master and the BESS.[22] The BESS is recommended over the standard Romberg test to assess balance. The BESS was developed to provide clinicians with a rapid, cost-effective method of objectively assessing postural stability in athletes on the sidelines or training room after a concussion. Three different stances (double, single, and tandem) are completed twice, once while on a firm surface and once while on a piece of medium density foam (Airex, Inc) for a total of six trials (**Figure 2**). The test has been described in the literature.[22,28,39]

5: Head and Neck

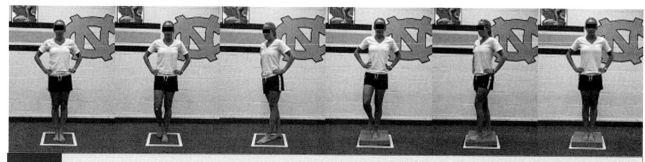

Figure 2 Patient using the BESS to assess balance. The patient completes three different stances twice, once on a firm surface and again while standing on a piece of medium-density foam.

Table 2

Cantu Evidence-Based Grading System for Concussion

Grade 1 (mild)	No LOC, PTA < 30 minutes, PCSS < 24 hours
Grade 2 (moderate)	LOC < 1 minute or PTA > 30 minutes < 24 hours or PCSS > 24 hours < 7 days
Grade 3 (severe)	LOC ≥ 1 minute or PTA ≥ 24 hours or PCSS > 7 days

LOC = loss of consciousness; PTA = posttraumatic amnesia (anterograde/retrograde); PCSS = postconcussion signs/symptoms other than amnesia

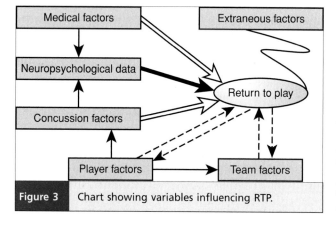

Figure 3 Chart showing variables influencing RTP.

Determining Injury Severity

At present, all concussion severity guidelines, with the exception of the evidence-based revised Cantu guidelines[19] (**Table 2**), grade concussion severity on the day of injury. Most grading scales have placed emphasis on the presence or absence of loss of consciousness and amnesia. Some prospective studies[13,17,21] have shown that memory dysfunction correlates with abnormal neuropsychological test scores 48 hours after an injury, but no studies have identified loss of consciousness as a predictor of such deficits. A recent study of collegiate and professional athletes has shown that concussed athletes with symptoms lasting longer than 7 days may have poorer overall outcome, which further validates symptom duration as a key factor in grading concussive injury.[11] Therefore, it is important to monitor all postconcussion symptoms that the athlete may experience; final grading of the severity should be deferred until the symptoms have cleared. It is this belief that gave rise to the grading scale shown in **Table 2**, in which posttraumatic amnesia symptoms in most mild grades of concussion resolve within 30 minutes; other symptoms resolve within 24 hours with no loss of consciousness. An intermediate concussion is defined as loss of consciousness for less than 1 minute, posttraumatic amnesia of greater than 30 minutes but less than 24 hours, or other postconcussion symptoms that last longer than 24 hours but less than 7 days. A severe concussion occurs when consciousness is lost for more than 1 minute, posttraumatic amnesia lasts for more than 24 hours, or other postconcussion symptoms last longer than 7 days.

It is certainly possible to manage concussions without grading severity. Several consensus statements have done just that, because of a lack of agreement on how to grade severity. Grading concussion severity is meaningful, especially in regard to how future concussions may be managed. Although the concussion grade will have no implications for the management of the current concussion, it can provide a concise descriptor of concussion history when managing subsequent concussions. For example, a more conservative approach would seem appropriate for an athlete with multiple, severe concussions with signs and symptoms lasting weeks rather than an athlete with multiple minor concussions with signs and symptoms lasting less than 24 hours.

Return to Play: The Management of Concussion

The RTP decision is a dynamic process involving the inclusion of many variables into relatively complex cost-

5: Head and Neck

benefit equations (**Figure 3**). The question raised most often regarding concussion grading and RTP systems is one of practicality in the sports setting. Many clinicians believe the RTP guidelines are too conservative and, therefore, choose to base decisions on clinical judgment of individual cases rather than on general recommendations. It has been reported that 30% of all high school and collegiate football players with concussions return to competition on the same day of injury; the remaining 70% average 4 days of rest before returning to participation.[11] Some RTP guidelines call for the athlete to be asymptomatic for at least 7 days before returning to participation after a grade 1 or 2 concussion.[40] Although many clinicians deviate from these recommendations and are more liberal in making RTP decisions, recent studies suggest that perhaps the 7-day waiting period can minimize the risk of recurrent injury.[11,28] On average, athletes required 7 days to fully recover after concussion. Same-season recurrent injuries typically take place within a short window of time, 7 to 10 days after the first concussion,[11] supporting the concept that there may be increased neuronal vulnerability or changes in blood flow during that time.

The sports medicine clinician now has an array of techniques and measurement instruments that can and should be used, either individually or in combination, in the management of concussion. Although differences exist, several studies have arrived at a consensus that emphasizes an individualized, graded RTP following a return to baseline of postconcussion signs and symptoms.[3-5] All signs and symptoms should be evaluated using a graded symptom scale or checklist when performing follow-up assessments and should be evaluated both at rest and after exertional maneuvers such as biking, jogging, sit-ups, and push-ups. Baseline measurements of neuropsychological and postural stability are strongly recommended for comparison with postinjury measurements. Postural stability and neurocognitive function should return to baseline levels, allowing for changes because of practice effects and measurement error. The need for cognitive rest in addition to physical rest is emphasized in the literature.[5] In general, a graded progression of physical and cognitive exertion is implemented following a period of being asymptomatic (usually 24 hours). Light aerobic exercise is followed by sport-specific training and noncontact training drills. For the basketball player, this may include shooting baskets or participating in walk-throughs; for the soccer player, this may include dribbling or shooting drills (but no heading) or other sport-specific activities, followed by full contact drills and then RTP. Progression from one level of exertion to the next is predicated on the absence of postconcussion signs and symptoms at the previous level. At no time before release for full contact should a player be placed in a situation where he or she is at risk for a head injury. The amount of time spent at each level of activity may vary depending on player history of concussion. For example, a player with a history of multiple concussions or a particularly severe concussion can be held at a level of exertion or activity for 72 hours, rather than just 24 hours. Conversely, a player with a relatively minor concussion may be progressed more rapidly.

It is strongly recommended that after recurrent injury, especially within-season repeat injuries, the athlete be withheld from participation for an extended period of time (approximately 7 days) after symptoms have resolved.

When to Disqualify an Athlete From Participation

Previous RTP guidelines have suggested that athletes who sustain a suspected head injury, but whose symptoms resolve within 15 to 20 minutes, may return to participation on the same day of injury. Athletes who are symptomatic at rest and after exertion for at least 20 minutes should be disqualified from returning to participation on the day of the injury. Exertional exercises should include sideline jogging followed by sprinting, sit-ups, push-ups, and any sport-specific, noncontact activities (or positions or stances) the athlete might need to perform when returning to participation. When symptoms resolve quickly (within 20 minutes) and the athlete remains asymptomatic following exertional activities, the question becomes whether or not he or she is at risk for another concussion or even a catastrophic injury if returned to participation immediately. Several factors should be considered, including the athlete's age and concussion history. If the athlete is age 18 years or younger or has had a concussion, he or she should refrain from sports participation on the same day. In the rare instances when the clinician decides to return the athlete to participation on the same day, the clinician should be certain that the athlete is not only asymptomatic but also demonstrates normal (at baseline or better) neuropsychological and postural stability functioning. Additionally, the athlete should be monitored closely after returning to play and during the 48 hours after injury to identify any delayed onset of symptoms.

Athletes who experience LOC or amnesia should be disqualified from participating on the day of the injury. The decision to disqualify from further participation on the day of a concussion should be based on a comprehensive physical examination, assessment of self-reported postconcussion signs and symptoms, functional impairments, and the athlete's past history of concussions. If assessment tools such as the SAC, the BESS, the neuropsychological test battery, and the symptom checklist are not used, a 7-day, symptom-free wait period before returning to participation is recommended.

Although not based on prospective studies, many clinicians believe that three mild concussions in one season should terminate participation in that season. Similarly, some believe that two moderate or severe concussions should also terminate a season. Although definitive recommendations cannot be made because of the lack of empirical evidence, clinical experience suggests that terminating a player's season because of multiple concussions should be considered. If the season is terminated, it is recommended that a sufficient amount of time (for example, 3 months) with the player free of symptoms at rest and following exertion should elapse before returning to play. Retirement from contact or collision sports participation should be seriously considered if a player's neurologic examination has not returned to normal, or if any postconcussion signs or symptoms are present at rest or during exertion. Additional criteria that might well preclude return to competition would be a neuropsychological test battery that has not returned to baseline or above or imaging studies that show a lesion, placing the athlete at increased risk of future head injury.

Additional criteria that may be used in disqualifying an athlete from further contact or collision sport participation, especially athletes with a history of more than three concussions, is when the duration of postconcussion symptoms progressively increases with subsequent concussions, especially when such postconcussion symptoms last 3 months or longer. Also, the severity of the blow that produced the concussion is used to determine whether or not an athlete should consider retirement. Mild, indirect blows where the head is not struck directly or impulsive loading of acceleration forces to the brain from a blow to another body part that produces prolonged postconcussive symptoms are worrisome findings that would possibly lead to an athlete's retirement from a contact or collision sport.

The long-term consequences of repeated concussions were examined in a 2005 study.[41] Retired professional football players with three or more reported concussions had a fivefold prevalence of mild cognitive impairment. Additionally, retired players with three or more concussions had a threefold prevalence of reported significant memory problems in comparison with retirees who did not have a history of concussion. Other recent studies have suggested a link between recurrent concussion and clinical depression in retired professional football players.[42-44] These findings suggest that the histopathologic features of dementia-related syndromes, as well as depression, may be initiated by repetitive cerebral concussions in professional football players These findings may suggest early disqualification for those with recurrent concussion. Further studies will be helpful.

Annotated References

1. Centers for Disease Control: NEISS-AIP Data. Washington, DC, CDC, 2002.

2. Powell JW, Barber-Foss KD: Traumatic brain injury in high school athletes. *JAMA* 1999;282:958-963.

3. Aubry M, Cantu R, Dvorak J, et al: Summary and agreement statement of the First International Conference on Concussion in Sport, Vienna 2001: Recommendations for the improvement of safety and health of athletes who suffer concussive injuries. *Br J Sports Med* 2002;36:6-10.

4. Guskiewicz KM, Bruce SL, Cantu RC, et al: National Athletic Trainer's Association position statement: Management of sport-related concussion. *J Athl Train* 2004;39:280-297.

   The authors review the literature pertaining to concussion assessment and recommend a multifaceted approach to concussion evaluation, including clinical evaluation, symptom assessment, balance assessment, and neurocognitive assessment.

5. McCrory P, Johnston K, Meeuwisse W, et al: Summary and agreement statement of the 2nd international conference on concussion in sport, Prague 2004. *Br J Sports Med* 2005;39:196-204.

   The authors make recommendations based on agreement from an international conference on concussion in sport. These recommendations include a comprehensive assessment of concussion and a distinction between simple and complex concussive injuries.

6. Medicine and Science in Sports and Exercise: Concussion (mild traumatic brain injury) and the team physician: A consensus statement. *Med Sci Sports Exerc* 2006;38:395-399.

   A group of six professional organizations provide a consensus regarding concussion with the goal of assisting team physicians in the care of athletes with a concussion by providing guidelines for a multifaceted evaluation process for concussion.

7. Webbe F: Definition, physiology, and severity of cerebral concussion, in Echemendia RJ (ed): *Sports Neuropsychology: Assessment and Management of Traumatic Brain Injury*. New York, NY, Guilford Publications, 2006, pp 45-70.

   The author presents a historical perspective of the definition, physiology, and severity of cerebral concussion and concludes that no unitary account for concussion and its phenomena exists.

8. Iverson GL: Outcome from mild traumatic brain injury. *Curr Opin Psychiatry* 2005;18:301-317.

   The author presents a review of the literature related to traumatic brain injury with the conclusion that athletes typically return to preinjury status in 2 to 14 days. Trauma patients often take longer to return to preinjury functioning.

9. Shaw NA: The neurophysiology of concussion. *Prog Neurobiol* 2002;67:281-344.

10. Giza CC, Hovda DA: The neurometabolic cascade of concussion. *J Athl Train* 2001;36:228-235.

11. Guskiewicz KM, McCrea M, Marshall SW, et al: Cumulative effects associated with recurrent concussion in collegiate football players: The NCAA Concussion

Study. *JAMA* 2003;290:2549-2555.

The authors examine repeat concussions in collegiate football players and suggest that individuals with a history of three or more concussions took longer to recover after subsequent injuries and were more likely to suffer a recurrent injury in the same season.

12. Guskiewicz KM, Weaver NL, Padua DA, Garrett WE Jr: Epidemiology of concussion in collegiate and high school football players. *Am J Sports Med* 2000;28: 643-650.

13. Collins MW, Lovell MR, Iverson GL, Cantu RC, Maroon JC, Field M: Cumulative effects of concussion in high school athletes. *Neurosurgery* 2002;51:1175-1179.

14. Collie A, McCrory P, Makdissi M: Does history of concussion affect current cognitive status? *Br J Sports Med* 2006;40:550-551.

The authors examined the effect of concussion history on cognitive status using CogSport. The study used Australian rules football players and concluded that the number of previous reported concussive episodes did not affect current cognitive state.

15. McCrory P: The eighth wonder of the world: The mythology of concussion management. *Br J Sports Med* 1999;33:136-137.

16. Field M, Collins MW, Lovell MR, Maroon J: Does age play a role in recovery from sports-related concussion? A comparison of high school and collegiate athletes. *J Pediatr* 2003;142:546-553.

The authors examined the effect of age on recovery following concussion and concluded that high school athletes may take longer to recover after injury than college athletes.

17. Lovell MR, Collins MW, Iverson GL, et al: Recovery from mild concussion in high school athletes. *J Neurosurg* 2003;98:296-301.

The authors examined recovery following concussion in high school athletes and concluded that athletes with a mild concussion showed significant declines on memory performance at days 4 and 7 postinjury compared with matched control subjects. An additional conclusion was that on-field mental status appears to be a predictor of recovery time.

18. Moser RS, Schatz P: Enduring effects of concussion in youth athletes. *Arch Clin Neuropsychol* 2002;17: 91-100.

19. Cantu RC: Posttraumatic retrograde and anterograde amnesia: Pathophysiology and implications in grading and safe return to play. *J Athl Train* 2001;36:244-248.

20. Echemendia RJ, Putukian M, Mackin RS, Julian L, Shoss N: Neuropsychological test performance prior to and following sports-related mild traumatic brain injury. *Clin J Sport Med* 2001;11:23-31.

21. Erlanger D, Kaushik T, Cantu R, et al: Symptom-based assessment of the severity of concussion. *J Neurosurg* 2003;98:477-484.

The authors examine the role of symptom assessment in predicting concussion severity and conclude that self-reported memory problems were significantly related to concussion severity. Brief loss of consciousness and a history of concussion were not useful predictors of severity.

22. Guskiewicz KM, Ross SE, Marshall SW: Postural stability and neuropsychological deficits following concussion in collegiate athletes. *J Athl Train* 2001;36:263-273.

23. Maroon JC, Lovell MR, Norwig J, Podell K, Powell JW, Hartl R: Cerebral concussion in athletes: Evaluation and neuropsychological testing. *Neurosurgery* 2000;47: 659-669.

24. McCrea M, Kelly JP, Randolph C: *Standardized Assessment of Concussion (SAC): Manual for Administration, Scoring and Interpretation*, ed 2. Waukesha, WI, 2000, pp 1-3.

25. Barth JT, Brashek DK, Freeman JR: A new frontier for neuropsychology, in Echemendia RJ (ed): *Sports Neuropsychology: Assessment and Management of Traumatic Brain Injury*. New York, NY, Guilford Publications, 2006, pp 3-16.

26. Collins MW, Grindel SH, Lovell MR: Relationship between concussion and neuropsychological performance in college football players. *JAMA* 1999;282:964-970.

27. McCrea M, Kelly JP, Randolph C, Cisler R, Berger L: Immediate neurocognitive effects of concussion. *Neurosurgery* 2002;50:1032-1042.

28. McCrea M, Guskiewicz KM, Marshall SW, et al: Acute effects and recovery time following concussion in collegiate football players: The NCAA Concussion Study. *JAMA* 2003;290:2556-2563.

The authors examine acute effects and recovery time in collegiate football athletes and conclude that a gradual recovery of symptoms, neurocognition, and balance typically occurs between 5 and 7 days after injury.

29. Lovell M: The ImPACT neuropsychological test battery, in Echemendia RJ (ed): *Sports Neuropsychology: Assessment and Management of Traumatic Brain Injury*. New York, NY, Guilford Publications, 2006, pp 193-215.

The authors present a review of the literature pertaining to ImPACT and its usefulness in the assessment of sports-related concussion.

30. Collie A, Maruff P, Makdissi M, et al: CogSport: Reliability and correlation with conventional cognitive tests used in postconcussion medical evaluations. *Clin J Sport Med* 2003;13:28-32.

The authors examine the reliability of the CogSport test and the correlation between CogSport measures and other commonly used neuropsychological tests with the conclusion that CogSport is highly reliable when used to assess healthy young adults and is highly correlated with other neuropsychological tests.

31. Kaushik TE: The HeadMinder concussion resolution index, in Echemendia RJ (ed): *Sports Neuropsychology: Assessment and Management of Traumatic Brain Injury.* New York, NY, Guilford Publications, 2006, pp 216-239.

    The authors present a review of the literature pertaining to the HeadMinder Concussion Resolution Index and its usefulness in the assessment of sports-related concussion.

32. Bleiberg J, Cernich A, Reeves D: Sports concussion applications of the Automated Neuropsychological Assessment Metrics Sports Medicine Battery, in Echemendia RJ (ed): *Sports Neuropsychology: Assessment and Management of Traumatic Brain Injury.* New York, NY, Guilford Publications, 2006, pp 263-283.

    The authors present a review of the literature pertaining to the ANAM-SMB and its usefulness in the assessment of sports-related concussion.

33. Collins MW, Iverson GL, Lovell MR, et al: On-field predictors of neuropsychological and symptoms deficit following sports-related concussion. *Clin J Sport Med* 2003;13:222-229.

    The authors examine the association between on-field markers of severity and cognitive deficits after concussion and concluded that athletes with poor clinical measures scores at day 2 postinjury were 10 times more likely to have experienced on-field retrograde amnesia and were more than 4 times more likely to have exhibited posttraumatic amnesia and at least 5 minutes of mental status change.

34. Bleiberg J, Cernich NN, Cameron KL, et al: Duration of cognitive impiarment following sports concussion. *Neurosurgery* 2004;54:1073-1078.

    The authors investigate the duration of impaired cognition after concussion and conclude that most cognitive impairments after injury last from 3 to 7 days.

35. Guskiewicz KM, Riemann D, Perrin DH, Nashner LM: Alternative approaches to the assessment of mild head injury in athletes. *Med Sci Sports Exerc* 1997;29: S213-S221.

36. Guskiewicz KM: Postural stability assessment following concussion: One piece of the puzzle. *Clin J Sport Med* 2001;11:182-189.

37. Guskiewicz KM, Perrin D: Effect of mild head injury on cognition and postural stability. *J Athl Train* 1998; 33:S8.

38. Ingersoll CD, Armstrong CW: The effects of closed-head injury on postural sway. *Med Sci Sports Exerc* 1992;24:739-742.

39. Riemann BL, Guskiewicz KM: Objective assessment of mild head injury using a clinical battery of postural stability tests. *J Athl Train* 2000;35:19-25.

40. Kelly JP: Loss of consciousness: Pathophysiology and implications in grading and safe return to play. *J Athl Train* 2001;36:249-252.

41. Guskiewicz KM, Marshall SW, Bailes J, et al: Association between recurrent concussion and late-life cognitive impairment in retired professional football players. *Neurosurgery* 2005;57:719-726.

    The authors examine the association between multiple concussions and cognitive impairment and conclude that the onset of dementia-related issues in professional football players later in life may be related to repeated concussions during the playing career.

42. Guskiewicz KM, Marshall SW, Bailes J, et al: Recurrent concussion and risk of depression in retired professional football players. *Med Sci Sports Exerc* 2007;39:903-909.

    The authors investigate the association between previous concussion history and risk of clinical depression and suggest a possible link between recurrent concussion and clinical depression.

43. Omalu BI, DeKosky ST, Minster RL, Kamboh MI, Hamilton RL, Wecht CH: Chronic traumatic encephalopathy in a National Football League player. *Neurosurgery* 2006;59:1086-1092.

    The authors present the first of two case studies of a professional football player with chronic traumatic encephalopathy and suggest potential long-term neurodegenerative outcomes related to repeated mild traumatic brain injury sustained while playing professional football.

44. Omalu BI, DeKosky ST, Hamilton RL, et al : Chronic traumatic encephalopathy in a national football league player: Part II. *Neurosurgery* 2006;59:1092-1093.

    The authors present the second of two case studies of a professional football player with chronic traumatic encephalopathy and conclude that more research should be conducted on the neuropathological cascades of the condition.

Chapter 25

Cervical Spine

Mark A. Harrast, MD   Stuart M. Weinstein, MD

Introduction

Cervical spine trauma in athletes can result in several different pathologic entities, including vertebral fracture and dislocation, ligamentous instability, acute disk herniation, spinal cord injury, disk degeneration, radiculopathy and cervical strains. There has been new research and information about transient quadriparesis and stingers. In addition, as rehabilitation strategies for many musculoskeletal and neurologic disorders become better defined, a basic rehabilitation treatment strategy for the athlete with neck pain and dysfunction can be implemented, along with appropriate return-to-competition guidelines.

Transient Quadriparesis

Ten percent of all cervical spine injuries in the United States occur during sports activity.[1] Most spinal cord injuries sustained during sports participation occur in the cervical spine. The incidence of transient quadriparesis in National Collegiate Athletic Association (NCAA) football players is 7.3 per 10,000 players, which can be subdivided to 1.3 per 10,000 players with transient weakness and paresthesias and 6.0 per 10,000 players with transient paresthesias alone.[2] Although transient quadriparesis is most commonly seen in athletes who participate in traditional contact sports such as football, wrestling, and ice hockey, it is also seen in athletes who participate in other sports during which collisions occur, such as soccer, gymnastics, and basketball.

Transient quadriparesis has been referred to as a neurapraxia of the cervical cord because sensory dysfunction may occur without loss of motor function. These terms imply a self-limited phenomenon, with signs and symptoms typically lasting no more than 24 hours; a more prolonged recovery lasting greater than 24 hours can occur.[3] There have been instances, and some unpublished reports, of athletes with episodes of transient quadriparesis without initial MRI findings to suggest any overt long-term neurologic compromise who later are found to have imaging signs of significant trauma to the cervical cord, including high signal within the cord.[4] For this reason, the term "spinal cord concussion" may be a more appropriate name for this injury involving the cervical cord, which has distinct initial symptoms that seem to resolve but may still be associated with long-term sequelae because of the initial injury.[4]

Transient quadriparesis is quite distinct from stingers, which are peripheral nerve injuries, and always affects more than one limb—typically all four. However, a common, single presenting symptom in athletes is burning sensation in the hands, which the athlete may not recognize as originating from a cervical source. This symptom in both hands is typical of central cord syndrome, an injury affecting the central corticospinal and spinothalamic tracts. Because of the stratification of these tracts, the clinical manifestations are noted in the upper limbs more than in the lower limbs.

Mechanism of Injury

The two chief mechanisms of cervical cord injury in sports are hyperextension and axial loading. Cervical hyperextension creates functional spinal stenosis with infolding of the ligamentum flavum. This is called the pincer mechanism, whereby cervical extension leads to compression of the spinal cord between the posteroinferior portion of one vertebral body and the lamina of the vertebra below[5] (Figure 1). Dynamic cord compression occurs more readily in a person with preexisting spinal stenosis. In nonathletes, premorbid spinal stenosis is a significant risk factor for permanent spinal cord injury with cervical hyperextension injuries.

The axial loading mechanism occurs after a direct axial load to a slightly flexed cervical spine or in a spine with loss of the usual cervical lordosis (straight spine), also termed spear tackler's spine. Two possible injuries can result from axial loading in this manner. The first injury results in fracture-dislocation from a strong axial load as the inherent shock-absorbing capacity of the cervical spine is diminished when cervical lordosis is lost or reversed. Usually, some degree of permanent spinal cord injury results. The second injury occurs in the presence of a central disk herniation or disk-osteophyte complex, where transient compression of the anterior cervical cord and anterior spinal artery can result in cord ischemia and subsequent myelopathic symptoms and signs that may be temporary or potentially less transient and more severe. Since 1976, when the NCAA banned head-first tackling, the incidence of permanent quadriparesis has decreased. Educating coaches and younger athletes on proper tackling tech-

5: Head and Neck

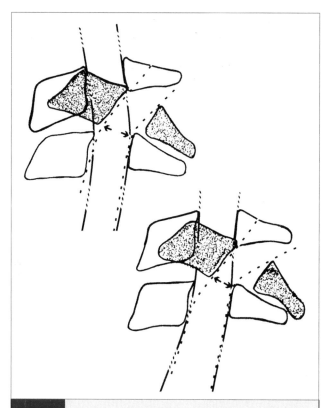

Figure 1 The pincer mechanism, as described by Penning, occurs when the distance between the postero-inferior margins of the superior vertebral body and the anterosuperior aspect of the spinolaminar line of the subjacent vertebra decrease with hyperextension; compression of the spinal cord occurs. With hyperflexion, the anterosuperior aspect of the spinolaminar line of the superior vertebra and the posterior margin of the inferior vertebra would be the pincers. *(Reproduced with permission from Penning L: Some aspects of plain radiography of the cervical spine in chronic myelopathy. Neurology 1962;12:513-519.)*

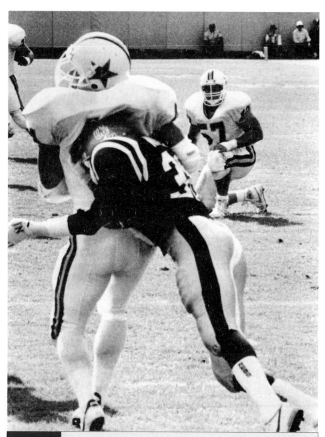

Figure 2 A college defensive back (dark jersey) is shown ramming an opposing ball carrier with his head, resulting in severe axial loading of the cervical spine. The defensive player suffered fractures of C4, C5, and C6 and was rendered quadriplegic. *(Reproduced with permission from Torg JS, Sennett B, Pavlov H, Leventhal MR, Glasgow SG: Spear tackler's spine: An entity precluding participation in tackle football and collision activities that expose the cervical spine to axial energy inputs. Am J Sports Med 1993;21:640-649.)*

niques has thus far been the most effective intervention in reducing cervical spinal cord injuries in football (**Figure 2**). Similar education in the sport of hockey also has been effective in reducing catastrophic cervical injuries. Checking an opposing player from behind can cause the checked athlete to hit the boards headfirst. Because rules have been adopted that prohibit checking from behind and from checking a player who is no longer in control of the puck, major cervical spine traumatic injuries in hockey players have been effectively reduced.[6]

Clinical Presentation

The athlete with transient quadriparesis may experience a variety of symptoms affecting two to four limbs. A common presentation is burning dysesthesias in the hands, which suggests a central cord syndrome. However, the sensory symptoms can range from burning dysesthesia to numbness and/or tingling. Motor symptoms also can be variable, from no motor deficit to mild quad-

riparesis to complete quadriplegia; the greater the motor loss, the less likely the injury will manifest as a transient insult.

Assessment and Initial Management

If a cervical spinal cord injury is not considered and if the athlete is improperly handled initially, further catastrophic injury is possible; therefore, appropriate on-field management is necessary for recognition, early treatment, and avoidance of injury progression. The initial on-field treatment of an athlete with a suspected cervical cord injury should follow appropriate Advanced Trauma Life Support (ATLS) guidelines. An adequate airway should be established and maintained. Full spine precautions, including cervical immobilization, are to be maintained. The helmet should be left in place and taped to the backboard, and the facemask should be removed to gain airway access. Once spontaneous respirations and a pulse are noted, neurologic status can be evaluated.

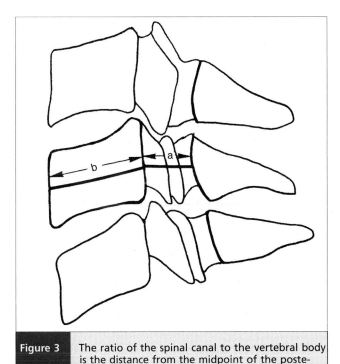

| Figure 3 | The ratio of the spinal canal to the vertebral body is the distance from the midpoint of the posterior aspect of the vertebral body to the nearest point on the corresponding spinolaminar line (a) divided by the anteroposterior width of the vertebral body (b). *(Reproduced with permission from Torg JS, Pavlov H, Genuario SE, et al: Neurapraxia of the cervical spinal cord with transient quadriplegia. J Bone Joint Surg Am 1986;68:1354-1370.)* |

Diagnostic Imaging

In the controlled environment of an emergency department, additional diagnostic evaluation can be completed, with imaging as a key element. Plain radiographs are performed initially to determine the integrity of the bony elements. First, a lateral cervical spine radiograph is obtained with the helmet left in place.[7] However, lower cervical spine imaging with plain radiography may be compromised by the shoulder pads, and CT of the cervical spine with the helmet left in place may be the optimal imaging modality in an athlete with an acute injury. Once the helmet can be safely removed, a full cervical spine series can be performed, potentially to include active flexion and extension views if the athlete is neurologically stable. Advanced imaging, typically with MRI, allows a more detailed evaluation of the spinal canal to identify a compressing soft-tissue lesion, such as a disk herniation, a hard disk, or a bony spur, as well as to evaluate the shape of the spinal cord and the amount of cerebrospinal fluid surrounding the cord, also known as the functional reserve. Dynamic MRI, which evaluates the spine in cervical extension, neutral, and flexion, is now available and may provide more insight into the source of transient quadriparesis by evaluating functional stenosis, or dynamic compression that may only occur in cervical extension, and thus may not be readily apparent in

neutral positioning. Conceptually, dynamic MRI appears to be quite promising in this regard; however, its definite clinical usefulness has yet to be determined

Before the widespread availability of MRI, a plain radiographic measure of the cervical spine was used to indirectly assess for cervical stenosis. The so-called Torg ratio compares the sagittal diameter of the spinal canal as measured from the back of the vertebral body to the spinolaminar line (the numerator), to the AP diameter of the corresponding vertebral body (the denominator)[2] (**Figure 3**). A ratio of less than 0.8 reportedly was indicative of significant spinal stenosis. Although the Torg ratio has a relatively high sensitivity, it has a low positive predictive value, particularly in mature football players, in whom a large vertebral body size will decrease the ratio even if the spinal canal size is within a normal range. MRI has supplanted the Torg ratio and is the most appropriate modality for determining the presence of true cervical stenosis because spinal canal size can be assessed directly and the presence of a soft-tissue compressing lesion, such as a disk herniation, can be determined. Further, MRI is also useful to determine the functional reserve of the spinal canal.

Return to Competition

The time to return to competition after transient quadriparesis is controversial. The sports medicine physician must provide accurate and contemporary medical information to the athlete, family, and coach to allow the most informed decision. In a study of 110 athletes with reported transient quadriparesis, 57% returned to competition. Of those returning to play, 56% sustained at least one more episode of transient quadriparesis, but none had any permanent deficits.[3] There was a noted correlation with a smaller canal size (spinal stenosis) and recurrent episodes of transient quadriparesis; however, MRI was not done on all athletes; thus, the true relationship between spinal stenosis and recurrence of transient quadriparesis cannot be determined by this study. Also, the follow-up period was on average 3.3 years; therefore, these results cannot be extrapolated to long-term outcome.

Recent case series highlight the controversy over when to return to competition. In a case series of 10 athletes with transient quadriparesis lasting 15 minutes to 48 hours, all athletes had some degree of stenosis on cross-sectional imaging (cervical canal diameter of 7 to 12 mm at three or more levels), but none was treated surgically.[8] The three athletes who had diminished functional reserve (lack of cerebrospinal fluid signal) retired from collision sports. Four of the remaining seven athletes who had attenuation but preservation of some cerebrospinal fluid signal returned to competition and did not report any further instances of transient quadriparesis during the mean follow-up period of 36 months.

In another report, five elite football players were evaluated, three after a first episode of transient

5: Head and Neck

quadriparesis and two after two episodes of transient quadriparesis.[9] All cases were evaluated by MRI, which showed cord impingement caused by osseous and discogenic material. All athletes had anterior cervical diskectomy and fusion. The athletes returned to football from 9 weeks to 8 months postoperatively. Recurrent disk herniations (one above and the other below the level of fusion), developed in two players, both of whom subsequently discontinued football. The other three continued to play at the professional level for at least 2 to 3 years without additional or recurrent symptoms.

General return-to-play guidelines are not entirely uniformly accepted. The ultimate goal is to best identify those athletes who are at an increased risk of further injury after an episode of transient quadriparesis. However, there are few data to accurately determine the factors that may increase the risk of further injury after an episode of transient quadriparesis. It is generally accepted that an athlete who is fully asymptomatic with a normal neurologic examination after an episode of transient quadriparesis, who also has a normal MRI without stenosis, other disk disease, or instability, and who has a normal spinal curvature should not be restricted from competition. However, others may caution the asymptomatic athlete that a risk of further injury remains, even with a normal physical examination and imaging studies. This scenario may be considered a relative contraindication to return to play. More defined scenarios for relative contraindications to return to play are described, such as an episode of transient quadriparesis in athletes who are found to have spinal stenosis, intervertebral disk disease, and/or cord deformation on MRI.[10] An episode of transient quadriparesis with ligamentous instability, a cord defect or edema, symptoms persisting for 36 hours or longer, and/or more than one episode of transient quadriparesis are absolute contraindications.[10] According to one study, acute or chronic cervical disk herniation and functional spinal stenosis are considered absolute contraindications in the athlete with a single episode of transient quadriparesis.[11] The athlete with transient quadriparesis must understand that the injury is not benign, and a small risk of recurrent injury with permanent neurologic sequelae exists.[8] It is accepted that cervical stenosis is a risk factor for transient quadriparesis, but whether it is a risk factor for permanent neurologic impairment is unknown. The risk of a second episode of transient quadriparesis may be as high as 56%.[3] Determining if an athlete can or should return to competition after an episode of transient quadriparesis involves multiple factors, including medical and nonmedical issues.

Spinal Cord Resuscitation and Neuroprotection
There has been a recent, well-publicized report of using hypothermia when treating a professional athlete with an acute cervical spinal cord injury.[12] There has been a resurgence in research evaluating the effects of induced hypothermia in traumatic spinal cord injury.[13] The use of hypothermia fell out of favor in the 1980s because of adverse effects, in particular cardiac arrhythmias, hypotension, coagulopathies, and electrolyte disturbances.[14] Mild hypothermia is purported to limit the secondary hypoxic injury and metabolic response to the initial trauma, which is likely a significant factor in permanent neurologic impairment. The standard measures of resuscitation after spinal cord injury include supporting the patient's respiratory and hemodynamic function to facilitate spinal cord perfusion, intravenous corticosteroids, and early spinal reduction and stabilization. Following cardiac arrest caused by ventricular fibrillation, mild hypothermia to 32°C is more commonly used because of improved clinical survival outcomes.[15] For spinal cord injury, experimental animal data for hypothermia have had promising results over the years; however, clinical application of therapeutic hypothermia cannot yet be recommended for routine use in neurotrauma.[16,17]

Stingers

The stinger, also known as a burner, is probably one of the most common but least understood peripheral nerve injuries that occurs in sports. A stinger should not be confused with burning hands syndrome, which is the residual of a central cord syndrome. Stingers are nerve injuries that occur within the peripheral neural axis at a specific but variable point from the nerve root to the brachial plexus. The true incidence of stingers is unknown; however, it is estimated that more than 50% of collegiate football players sustain a stinger each year.[18]

Mechanism of Injury
There is a great deal of controversy regarding the pathomechanics and pathoanatomy of stingers. The symptoms may result from a tensile (stretch) or compressive injury to the cervical nerve root or brachial plexus. Because of its anatomy, the cervical nerve root appears to be at greater risk for both tensile and compressive injury than the brachial plexus. In particular, the C5 root is most vulnerable to injury because it is the shortest root and is in direct alignment with the upper trunk of the brachial plexus. The ventral (motor) root is also susceptible to injury because it does not contain the dorsal root ganglion, which can have a dampening effect on injury of the dorsal root. This is why motor impairment (particularly in the deltoid and biceps, that is, the C5 myotome) is the most common residual neurologic symptom of an athlete with a stinger.

The literature slightly favors brachial plexus tensile overload[18-24] over nerve root stretch,[25-27] nerve root compression,[28-30] and direct brachial plexus compression[31,32] as the primary mechanism of injury in stingers.

The differing pathomechanics likely occur because of the age and experience of the athlete and the specific sport. Tensile injuries typically occur in the less experienced younger athlete with weaker neck and shoulder girdle musculature, which decreases the ability to withstand sudden or forceful neck lateral bending to the contralateral side while the ipsilateral shoulder and arm are depressed. Cervical root compression is likely to occur in the older, stronger, and more experienced athlete during forceful cervical extension and rotation, which narrows the neuroforamen, as is more commonly seen in professional football defensive backs and offensive lineman. A compressive blow to the brachial plexus is the least common injury and may be related to equipment issues such as padding.

Clinical Presentation

The classic symptoms of the athlete with a stinger include the sudden onset of lancinating, burning pain in one upper limb after a traumatic event. Typically, the symptoms follow a single dermatomal distribution, most commonly in a C5, C6, or C7 pattern. The pain usually lasts seconds to minutes, with the sensory disturbance usually resolving quickly, while the weakness sometimes is more persistent. Simultaneous, bilateral stingers are an uncommon occurrence; any athlete who reports bilateral upper limb paresthesias or dysesthesias should be evaluated for a spinal cord injury and not given a diagnosis of bilateral stingers. With the first occurrence of a stinger, these symptoms generally resolve rather quickly, and thus the stinger is often not reported by the athlete. Recurrence can be frequent; with each subsequent event, more distinct neurologic sequelae, including persistent motor weakness, may result.

The athlete with a stinger typically exits the playing field unaided while holding the affected limb motionless against the abdomen in a slinglike position. The arm position may be similar to a shoulder dislocation, making appropriate evaluation necessary for an accurate diagnosis. The physician should determine the specific mechanism of injury and the precise distribution and duration of symptoms during the initial sideline evaluation. The sideline physical examination includes active cervical range of motion to assess pain provocation and rigidity, palpation to determine specific bony tenderness and/or paraspinal muscle spasm, and a detailed neurologic examination with close attention to the C5-C7 myotomes.

All athletes with suspected stingers must be carefully monitored for persistence of symptoms and signs because this injury will impact return-to-play decisions. Most first-time stingers resolve very quickly, sometimes even before the athlete reaches the sideline. However, the duration of any given episode may vary from seconds to hours, much less commonly lasting for days or longer. Serial assessment of the athlete, initially in the locker room and then in the training room or team physician's office, is important. If symptoms progressively worsen over the first few days, or weakness persists for more than 10 to 14 days, additional ancillary testing and specialty consultation would be reasonable and necessary to precisely determine the site of injury and the degree of axonal damage.

Diagnostic Evaluation

Ancillary testing in the evaluation of an athlete with a stinger includes imaging of the cervical spine and potentially the shoulder girdle to assess pathoanatomy and electrodiagnostic testing of the cervical nerve roots and brachial plexus to assess neural dysfunction. These studies often complement each other.

If the athlete's symptoms resolve within seconds to minutes and the physical examination (including full pain-free cervical range of motion) reveals no abnormality, then no additional testing may be necessary. However, persistent symptoms or signs and recurrent stingers are indications for further diagnostic testing. Although the relative value of plain radiographs is limited in this setting, they may reveal clues to pathoanatomy contributing to the symptoms, including degenerative changes, uncovertebral or zygapophyseal joint arthropathy leading to neuroforaminal narrowing, ligamentous instability and hypermobility, and postural dysfunction with a loss of normal cervical lordosis. The cervical plain radiographic examination includes an AP view, lateral view in neutral as well as flexion and extension, and bilateral oblique views to examine the foramen.

In the past, the Torg ratio has been adapted to assist in the evaluation of stingers, although it was originally described as a simple radiographic screening tool for the presence of central cervical spinal stenosis. However, the Torg ratio was never meant to define relative risk to the peripheral nerves (the location of neuropathology in stingers). Abnormalities of the Torg ratio have reportedly been correlated with an increased risk of a complicated clinical course after a stinger.[33] An increased risk of a complicated clinical course may be the case because of the higher incidence of degenerative changes (creating central canal and neuroforaminal stenosis concomitantly) in more experienced athletes with stingers.[34] In a cohort of football players with chronic stingers, 93% had significant cervical disk disease or neural foraminal narrowing.[34] The lateral canal and foraminal degenerative changes contributing to root level neuropathology are likely created by the same degenerative processes that contribute to central stenosis.

Advanced imaging with MRI or CT is the most definitive approach when evaluating the pathoanatomic sources of neurologic symptoms such as stingers. MRI and CT can more directly demonstrate neuroforaminal stenosis, disk abnormalities, and other degenerative changes. Advanced imaging is imperative if an athlete experiences severe, unrelenting pain, persistent symptoms, or significant neurologic examination abnormalities such as weakness.

Electrodiagnostic testing is complementary to imaging studies when evaluating the athlete with a stinger to quantify the neural dysfunction. Electrodiagnostic testing is most useful in the athlete with persistent or progressive weakness beyond 2 weeks after injury or in the setting of recurrent stingers. Generally, a minimum of 7 to 10 days is required for the axonal damage to manifest on electromyography (EMG); therefore, this test should not be used immediately after injury. Furthermore, it may be difficult to detect milder injury because a minimum of 30% of the axons need to be affected for the EMG abnormalities to be present.[35] In the evaluation of recurrent stingers, EMG testing helps distinguish old and new injuries and helps quantify the amount of reinnervation that has occurred after an old injury. Finally, EMG testing can help to differentiate the site of nerve injury between the brachial plexus and cervical nerve root by identifying abnormalities in the cervical paraspinals (radiculopathy) or a reduction in the distal sensory amplitudes (plexopathy).

Treatment

Management of the athlete with a stinger includes controlling pain and inflammation, rehabilitating strength deficits from the initial neurologic injury but also rehabilitating postural faults and muscle imbalances that may have contributed to the athlete's risk of sustaining the stinger as well as recurrent stingers, and equipment modification for preventing recurrent injury.

The first stage of treatment to control pain and inflammation is rest to eliminate the overload forces that caused the initial injury. Oral anti-inflammatory agents and other analgesics as well as physical therapy modalities, such as thermal agents, gentle stretching, and manual traction, may be useful if pain does not resolve quickly. Because the painful dysesthesias generally resolve rather quickly, it would be uncommon to use different treatments to control pain or inflammation. Infrequently, depending on the age of the athlete and the level of competition, persistent symptoms may be treated with fluoroscopically guided transforaminal epidural steroid injections after MRI confirms the pathologic site as the nerve root and not the plexus. A transforaminal epidural steroid injection can effectively place a localized dose of corticosteroid along an inflamed nerve root. Even less commonly required, surgical decompression of neuroforaminal stenosis may be indicated if there is progressive motor loss, which would be quite rare after a stinger.

The second stage of treatment is rehabilitation. The general goals of this phase of treatment include pain-free range of motion and full strength, as well as prevention of future recurrences by closely examining the athlete's posture and taking into account other mechanical factors, such as muscular imbalances, and devising an appropriate rehabilitation strategy that addresses these issues. Equipment modification is generally used for the prevention of stingers, although research is lacking to support its effectiveness. Evaluation for proper shoulder pad fit and using shoulder pad lifters to limit terminal range lateral bending is a common intervention. A cervical roll can be used to prevent cervical hyperextension. The use of any motion-restricting device must be considered in the context of interfering with an athlete's performance as well as positioning the cervical spine in relative flexion, which may increase the risk of traumatic spinal cord injury. Despite the widespread use of these devices, they cannot replace a comprehensive rehabilitation program.

Return to Competition

Following a stinger, return-to-competition decisions are based on a combination of clinical, imaging, and electrodiagnostic findings. The clinical factors in determining the time course of return to play include assessment of any neurologic deficit, persistent pain, range-of-motion deficits; whether the stinger is the first or recurrent; and how the athlete has progressed through the key components of a comprehensive rehabilitation program.

The number of previous stingers that the athlete has had is important information in guiding return-to-play decisions because more severe and persistent motor deficits occur in athletes who have experienced recurrent stingers. Because well-established return-to-competition guidelines do not exist for stingers, the following is a general guide based on a combination of clinical experience, neurophysiologic principles, and extrapolation of information from other peripheral nerve injuries. Following an initial stinger, if full recovery is demonstrated within 15 minutes, return to same-game competition is allowed. If full recovery occurs within 1 week after the initial stinger, then return to competition the next week is allowed. Even though prolonged recovery is rare after the first stinger, a limited rehabilitation program to address postural dysfunction and relative weaknesses should be prescribed during the in-season strength and conditioning program and definitely in a more comprehensive fashion during the off-season. If the athlete has sustained recurrent stingers, a general rule is to prohibit competition for the number of weeks that corresponds to the number of stingers sustained in a given season (for example, two weeks for a second stinger). If more than three stingers occur in a season, consideration should be given to ending that season, particularly if there is significant weakness, notable EMG findings suggestive of significant axonopathy, and focal disk herniation or significant foraminal stenosis noted on MRI. These recommendations should be considered as guidelines only. As with any athletic injury, other medical and nonmedical factors contribute to the decision-making process of an athlete returning to play.

Rehabilitation of the Athlete With Cervical Pain and Associated Symptoms

A general template of a comprehensive rehabilitation program of any athlete recovering from injury includes

Table 1

Biomechanics of Forward Head Posture

Postural Components	Muscular Components	
	Shortened Muscles	Lengthened Muscles
Exaggerated thoracic kyphosis	Capital extensors	Capital flexors
Excessive scapular protraction	Cervical extensors	Cervical flexors
Glenohumeral internal rotation	Sternocleidomastoid	Middle trapezius
Lower cervical and upper thoracic segmental hyperflexion	Upper trapezius	Lower trapezius
Upper cervical spine segmental hyperextension	Levator scapulae	Rhomboids
	Pectorals	Thoracic extensors
	Anterior deltoid	Latissimus dorsi
	Subscapularis	
	Serratus anterior	
	Anterior scalenes	

relative rest, control of pain and inflammation, restoration of pain-free range of motion and strength, appropriate neuromuscular recruitment patterning, proprioception, appropriate functioning within the kinetic chain of motion for the athlete's sport, and agility and power restoration. Applying these components to the rehabilitation program of an athlete with cervical dysfunction entails a systematic approach. Postural abnormalities of the cervicothoracic spine and shoulder girdle are the most common conditions in cervical pain syndromes that can be directly rehabilitated. These postural conditions result in forward head posture. This forward head posture is noted radiographically as reduction or absence of the normal cervical lordosis on cervical plain radiographs. There are many sources for this common postural fault noted in the general population, including acute muscle spasm; however, this finding is more commonly chronic in duration and cannot solely be attributed to focal muscle spasm. In the athletic population in particular, the usual cause is strength and flexibility imbalances about the cervical and thoracic spine and shoulder girdle (Table 1).

The chronic forward head posture accompanied by a loss of cervical lordosis results in a relative maldistribution of segmental motion with stiffness in the upper cervical and upper thoracic regions and thus compensatory increased motion in the mid and lower cervical regions. This relative hypermobility may lead to a greater degree of degenerative changes typically found in the mid and lower cervical segments.

The specific segmental spinal and myofascial abnormalities that contribute to this forward head posture include an exaggerated thoracic kyphosis, excessive scapular protraction with glenohumeral internal rotation, segmental hyperflexion of the lower cervical and upper thoracic spine (with relative restrictions of the zygapophyseal joints at these levels), segmental hyperextension of the upper cervical spine with compensa-

tory relative hypermobility of the mid cervical segments, and weakening of many muscle groups controlling head and neck motion because of an alteration of their normal length-tension relationship. Because of this chronic posturing and the segmental abnormalities that develop, some muscles become shortened (and relatively weak), whereas other muscles become lengthened (and also relatively weak). The shortened muscles are the capital and cervical extensors, the sternocleidomastoid, the upper trapezius, the levator scapulae, the pectoralis minor and major, the anterior deltoid, the subscapularis, the serratus anterior, and the anterior scalene. The lengthened muscles are the capital and cervical flexors, the middle and lower trapezius, the rhomboids, thoracic extensors, and the latissimus dorsi.

A rehabilitation program can be formulated based on an understanding of this complex arrangement of segmental spinal and myofascial components that contribute to the forward head posture. The goal of such a comprehensive rehabilitation program is to lessen the joint and muscle imbalances contributing to the maladaptive posture with the eventual hope of preventing future injury to the cervical-thoracic-shoulder girdle complex when returning to sport. Manual therapy is an initial component of a postural corrective rehabilitation program. Manual therapeutic techniques, including joint and soft-tissue mobilization, are used to restore normal spinal mechanics as much as possible. This includes joint mobilization techniques to the hypomobile zygapophyseal joints first (particularly the upper cervical, lower cervical, and upper thoracic segments). However, forceful manipulation (the highest grade of mobilization) in the presence of significant degenerative disease (such as neuroforaminal stenosis) can be aggravating and/or damaging to the nerve root. Regaining segmental mobility first with hands-on treatments will eventually allow the athlete to work independently on regaining more gross mobility next, such as with a foam roll to regain thoracic extension.

In addition to joint mobilization, myofascial techniques are also an important component of the rehabilitation program. Stretching with myofascial release and massage can be used to lengthen the shortened muscles in preparation for the next step of strengthening. Improved soft-tissue extensibility will also improve segmental motion at the hypomobile levels.

The strength training component of this rehabilitation program includes directed strengthening of the paraspinals, local postural control muscles (upper thoracic and scapular stabilizers), global postural control muscles (trunk and core musculature), and targeted strengthening of the muscles that may have been weakened as a result of any inciting neural injury such as a stinger. The rate of exercise progression is based primarily on the persistence of symptoms. Generally, exercise starts safely with well-protected isometric strengthening of the paraspinal musculature in neutral spine posture, advancing as possible to multiplanar, functional exercises emphasizing strength, agility, balance, and endurance throughout the entire kinetic chain of motion. Finally, sport and position specific training completes the rehabilitation program.

Summary

Cervical spine injuries in sports are common. Neurologic injuries affecting the cervical spine can range from self-limited stingers to catastrophic spinal cord injury. Transient quadriparesis, a serious injury to the spinal cord, is typically a self-limited phenomenon; however, some patients have experienced long-term sequelae. Appropriate assessment, management, and return-to-competition guidelines are necessary for all sports injuries, and are even more important for cervical spine injuries, given the potential for long-term neurologic effects if not treated appropriately. Rehabilitation of the athlete with neck pain and dysfunction requires attention to posture and a kinetic chain approach, and a thorough understanding of the connection between the cervical spine, the thoracic spine, and the shoulder girdle complex.

Annotated References

1. Maroon JC, Bailes JE: Athletes with cervical spine injury. *Spine* 1996;21:2294-2299.

2. Torg JS, Pavlov H, Genuario SE, et al: Neurapraxia of the cervical spinal cord with transient quadriplegia. *J Bone Joint Surg Am* 1986;68:1354-1370.

3. Torg JS, Corcoran TA, Thibault LE, et al: Cervical cord neurapraxia: Classification, pathomechanics, morbidity, and management guidelines. *J Neurosurg* 1997;87: 843-850.

4. Brigham CD, Adamson TE: Permanent partial cervical spinal cord injury in a professional football player who had only congenital stenosis: A case report. *J Bone Joint Surg Am* 2003;85:1553-1556.

   An important case report of a professional football player who developed four-limb paresthesias with neck flexion with congenital stenosis as the only finding on MRI. He was allowed to play knowing that he may be at risk for transient quadriparesis; 2 years later a permanent partial spinal cord injury developed during a tackle. Level of evidence: III.

5. Penning L: Some aspects of plain radiography of the cervical spine in chronic myelopathy. *Neurology* 1962;12: 513-519.

6. Tator CH, Carson JD, Edmonds VE: Spinal injuries in ice hockey. *Clin Sports Med* 1998;17:183-194.

7. Waninger KN: Management of the helmeted athlete with suspected cervical spine injury. *Am J Sports Med* 2004;32:1331-1350.

   The published evidence on cervical management in the helmeted athlete with a suspected spinal injury is reviewed. Level of evidence: II-3.

8. Bailes JE: Experience with cervical stenosis and temporary paralysis in athletes. *J Neurosurg Spine* 2005;2: 11-16.

   In this descriptive case series, the clinical course and return-to-sport experience of 10 athletes with transient quadriparesis was discussed. Level of evidence: III.

9. Maroon JC, El-Kadi H, Abla AA, et al: Cervical neurapraxia in elite athletes: Evaluation and surgical treatment: Report of five cases. *J Neurosurg Spine* 2007;6: 356-363.

   A descriptive case series of five elite football players with transient quadriparesis who underwent surgical decompression is presented.

10. Torg JS, Guille JT, Jaffe S: Injuries to the cervical spine in American football players. *J Bone Joint Surg Am* 2002;84-A:112-122.

11. Cantu RV, Cantu RC: Current thinking: Return to play and transient quadriplegia. *Curr Sports Med Rep* 2005; 4:27-32.

    This review article with case reports highlights a reasonable return-to-competition strategy after transient quadriparesis. Level of evidence: III.

12. Garza M: "Cool" new treatment: NFL uses hypothermia for spinal cord injury. *JEMS* 2007;32:20.

    A case presentation of an elite football player with a spinal cord injury who was treated with hypothermia is discussed. Level of evidence: III.

13. Kwon BK, Mann C, Sohn HM, et al: Hypothermia for spinal cord injury. *Spine J* 2008;8:859-874.

    This article presents a comprehensive review of hypothermia for the initial treatment of spinal cord injury. Although there is a biologic rationale for using hypothermia, animal studies have not supported a consistent neuroprotective effect, and no human studies have been published for more than two decades. Level of evidence: II.

14. Inamasu J, Nakamura Y, Ichikizaki K: Induced hypothermia in experimental traumatic spinal cord injury: An update. *J Neurol Sci* 2003;209:55-60.

    This article presents a comprehensive review of the use of hypothermia to treat experimental traumatic animal spinal cord injury, noting that there may be a role for hypothermia in improving functional outcome in mild to moderate spinal cord injury but not for severe injury. Level of evidence: II-3.

15. Hypothermia After Cardiac Arrest Study Group: Mild therapeutic hypothermia to improve the neurologic outcome after cardiac arrest. *N Engl J Med* 2002;346: 549-556.

16. Fu ES, Tummala RP: Neuroprotection in brain and spinal cord trauma. *Curr Opin Anaesthesiol* 2005;18: 181-187.

    A comprehensive review of neuroprotective strategies in limiting secondary injury after traumatic brain and spinal cord injury is presented. Although there is still much research underway, no pharmacologic agents or other strategies (hypothermia) definitively provide neuroprotection after traumatic brain injury and spinal cord injury. Level of evidence: II-3.

17. Yoshitake A, Mori A, Shimizu H, et al: Use of an epidural cooling catheter with a closed countercurrent lumen to protect against ischemic spinal cord injury in pigs. *J Thorac Cardiovasc Surg* 2007;134:1220-1226.

    This basic science study demonstrates the positive neuroprotective effect of cooling the spinal cord directly over systemic hypothermia to protect against ischemic spinal cord injury. Level of evidence: II.

18. Clancy WG Jr, Brand RL, Bergfield JA: Upper trunk brachial plexus injuries in contact sports. *Am J Sports Med* 1977;5:209-216.

19. Archmbault J: Brachial plexus stretch injury. *J Am Coll Health* 1983;31:256-260.

20. Funk FJ, Wells RE: Injuries of the cervical spine in football. *Clin Orthop Relat Res* 1975;109:50-58.

21. Hunter C: Injuries to the brachial plexus: Experience of a private sports medicine clinic. *J Am Osteopath Assoc* 1982;81:757-760.

22. Jackson DW, Lohr FT: Cervical spine injuries. *Clin Sports Med* 1986;5:373-386.

23. Robertson WC Jr, Eichman PL, Clancy WG: Upper trunk brachial plexopathy in football players. *JAMA* 1979;241:1480-1482.

24. Wroble RR, Albright JP: Neck and low back injuries in wrestling. *Clin Sports Med* 1986;5:295-325.

25. Chrisman OD, Snook GA, Stanitis JM, Keedy VA: Lateral-flexion neck injuries in athletic competition. *JAMA* 1965;192:613-615.

26. Marshall TM: Nerve pinch injuries in football. *J Ky Med Assoc* 1970;68:648-649.

27. Speer KP, Bassett FH III: The prolonged burner syndrome. *Am J Sports Med* 1990;18:591-594.

28. Poindexter DP, Johnson EW: Football shoulder and neck injury: A study of the "stinger." *Arch Phys Med Rehabil* 1984;65:601-602.

29. Rockett FX: Observations on the "burner": Traumatic cervical radiculopathy. *Clin Orthop Relat Res* 1982; 164:18-19.

30. Watkins RG: Neck injuries in football players. *Clin Sports Med* 1986;5:215-246.

31. Di Bennedetto M, Markey F: Electrodiagnostic localization of traumatic upper trunk brachial plexopathy. *Arch Phys Med Rehabil* 1984;65:15-17.

32. Markey KL, Di Benedetto M, Curl WW: Upper trunk brachial plexopathy: The stinger syndrome. *Am J Sports Med* 1993;21:650-655.

33. Meyer SA, Schulte KR, Callaghan JJ, et al: Cervical spinal stenosis and stingers in collegiate football players. *Am J Sports Med* 1994;22:158-166.

34. Levitz CL, Reilly PJ, Torg JS: The pathomechanics of chronic, recurrent cervical nerve root neurapraxia: The chronic burner syndrome. *Am J Sports Med* 1997;25: 73-76.

35. Wilbourn A, Bergfeld J: Value of EMG examination with sports related nerve injury. *Electroencephalogr Clin Neurophysiol* 1983;55:42P-54P.

5: Head and Neck

Tendinopathy

SECTION EDITOR:
KARIM KHAN, MD, PhD

Chapter 26

Tendon Overuse Pathology: Implications for Clinical Management

Alexander Scott, PhD   Karim Khan, MD, PhD

Introduction

Considerable progress has been made over the past several years with investigations into the nature of tendon overuse pathologies. Recent findings support classic descriptions in which the most commonly found pathology underlying overuse tendinopathies is tendinosis (the end result of a failed healing response) rather than tendinitis. Furthermore, key cellular events that may substantiate the chronicity of tendinosis pathology have been revealed.

Morphologically, five main features distinguish tendinosis tissue from a normal, healthy tendon: collagen disruption, increased proteoglycan, tenocyte abnormalities, altered cell populations, and increased presence of microvessels and nerves. The cellular processes that regulate these five features of tendinosis are starting to be understood, and these advances have paved the way for new treatments, allowing more realistic descriptions of the pathology and time frame of recovery.

Normal Tendon Structure and Function

Tendons are load-bearing structures that transmit the forces generated by muscles to their bony insertion (enthesis), thereby making joint movement possible. To meet the mechanical demand of transmitting high tensile loads, tendons are composed primarily of tightly packed, longitudinally oriented collagen fibrils. This collagen is predominantly type I, extensively cross-linked to provide stiffness, with small amounts of type III collagen. Normal tendons also contain small amounts of noncollagenous components, including glycosaminoglycans, both proteoglycan and hyaluronan, that help maintain a hydrated matrix, allow fibril sliding, and regulate collagen fibril assembly.[1] Tenocytes are surrounded by a pericellular sheath containing versican, fibrillin, and type VI collagen that may provide some protection from their mechanical environment.

Tenocytes, which form the primary cell population of tendons, are a poorly defined population of fibroblasts linked into longitudinal and lateral arrays by functional gap junctions. Tenocytes form load-responsive cell networks, and their ongoing metabolic and repair activity (collagen synthesis and breakdown) is regulated by the extent of loading to which they are exposed. Upon tenocytes' exposure to mechanical load, calcium-dependent signaling is activated, leading to the stimulation of extracellular matrix gene expression. Thus, ongoing loading is a required stimulus for tenocytes to maintain normal tendon structure.

Tendons are covered by epitenon, a loose, fibrous sheath containing the vascular, lymphatic, and nerve supply. The epitenon is continuous with the endotendon, which also houses the nerves and vessels and divides the tendon proper into fascicles. More superficially, the epitenon is surrounded by paratendon, a loose, fibrous, adipose tissue with an inner synovial lining containing type I and II synoviocytes.

The normal blood supply of tendons varies greatly depending on the anatomic location. In areas outside the tendon and in the epitendon, a range of vessels, including arteries, arterioles, and capillaries, predominate. In the endotendon, the blood supply consists of arterioles and capillaries. The density of vessels in a normal tendon is particularly poor at certain key regions, such as Codman's zone or the Achilles watershed zone.[2]

Tendon Response to Acute Injury

Tendon healing following acute insult occurs over a prolonged time course compared with more vascularized soft tissues such as muscle or skin. Approximately 10% of chronic tendinopathies are precipitated by an acute overload event that the patient can clearly recall. Following the initial inflammatory phase, repair and remodeling phases occur over several months. In the first 24 to 48 hours, monocytes and macrophages predominate, and phagocytosis of necrotic materials occurs. After a few days, vascular and fibroblastic cells proliferate

6: Tendinopathy

Table 1

Features of Tendinosis and Underlying Cellular Changes[*]

Feature	Morphologic Changes	Cellular Changes
Collagen	Separation Disorganization Fibril breaks/tears ↓ fibril diameter	↑ MMP activity ↑ Collagen synthesis Altered expression of collagen types (↑ type I, II, III)
Proteoglycan	Microvessel thickening Fibrocartilage metaplasia Scarring	↑ Versican ↑ Aggrecan ↑ Biglycan
Tenocytes	Abnormal distribution Mitotic figures Pyknotic nuclei	↑ Proliferation ↑ Apoptosis ↑ Migration
Abnormal cell populations	Mononuclear cells Granulocytes Mast cells Chondroid cells Fatty degeneration	↑ CD3 ↑ CD68 ↑ Mast cell tryptase
Vessels/nerves	Vascular hyperplasia Neural sprouting Edema Increased blood flow	↑ VEGF ↑ Substance P

[*]MMP = matrix metalloproteinase; VEGF = vascular endothelial growth factor; ↑= increasing; ↓ = decreasing

and secrete high amounts of reparative tissue rich in type III collagen and glycosaminoglycan. The remodeling stage lasts for months, and although cell populations and activities decline as collagen matures and strengthens, the tissue is left permanently in a hypercellular and hypervascular state. The stages of tendon healing are presented in detail in chapter 29.

Depending on anatomic configuration, some tendons are able to regenerate and reattach following injury, whereas others are incapable of regeneration and reattachment. Supraspinatus or biceps long head tendon ruptures do not heal, whereas Achilles tendons have healing ability, given successful apposition of the torn ends and adequate immobilization. However, the quality of self-repaired tendon is vastly inferior to the original tissue.[3] As an example, hamstring tendons, when removed for autografting, can completely regrow and reattach, but their structure is inferior, with thinner and less tightly packed collagen fibrils and greater cellularity.[4] Healed tendons also remain hypervascular for months or years.[3] The histology of healed tendons often demonstrates most of the major features of tendinosis.

The different regions of tendon (tendon proper, endotendon/paratendon, enthesis) appear to respond differently after injury. The endotendon and the paraten-

don appear to be more metabolically active, demonstrating aggressive proliferation and expansion, whereas the tendon proper is relatively quiescent but still capable of intrinsic repair mechanisms.[5] In addition to phenotypic differences between these cell types, proximity to blood vessels and invading inflammatory cell types and cytokines after injury may influence local injury responses. The expansion of the endotendon phenotype, rather than the tendon proper, may in part account for the abnormal histology of postinjury tendon.

Chronic Tendon Overuse Pathology and Histopathology

In contrast with acute tendon injuries, chronic tendon overuse pathology, by definition, fails to resolve. Tendon overuse pathology can occur in all elements of the tendon, including the enthesis (both bony and fibrocartilage elements), the paratendon or endotendon, and the tendon proper, either alone or together. Thus, all load-bearing elements of the tendon as well as its sheaths, linings, and adjacent structures are prone to injury.

Tendinosis Compared With Enthesopathies

Most tendon overuse injuries (with the exception of injuries to the Achilles, peroneal, and tibialis posterior tendons) occur adjacent to their bony attachment (the enthesis) and are sometimes referred to as enthesopathies. The prevalence of enthesopathies is not surprising when considering that the point of attachment of adult tendon is its weakest area biomechanically.[6] Distinctive pathologic changes occur at the enthesis itself, including irregularities in the tidemark, narrowing of cortical bone, bone marrow edema, and formation of bony spurs or fragments. However, despite the presence of abnormalities at the enthesis, the tendon itself usually appears to be the source of symptoms in overuse tendinopathies.

Tendinopathy Compared With Paratendinopathy

The five main histologic features of tendinosis (Table 1) can occur both in the vascular compartments of the tendon (endotendon and paratendon) and the tendon proper. Distinguishing between chronic tendinopathy and paratendinopathy can be challenging in some tendons. The histopathology of large tendons, such as the patellar or Achilles tendon, often shows a breakdown of boundaries between tissue compartments, with more vascularized tissue that is apparently continuous with the endotendon expanding and/or replacing regions normally occupied by tendon proper.[7] Thus, it is possible that tendinopathy results from pathologic changes both in the tendon and in the endotendon/paratendon, but this has been difficult to assess because of uncertainty about the tissue boundaries when obtaining surgical samples.

One notable difference between tendinopathy and paratendinopathy is that the paratendon appears to be more prone to cellular inflammation than the tendon proper. In a rat model of generalized lower limb inflammation, the paratendon became significantly inflamed, whereas the adjacent tendon proper maintained a normal appearance.[8] Conversely, injections of a proinflammatory substance (prostaglandin E$_1$) directly into the rat paratendon resulted in degenerative changes consistent with several features of tendinosis, including collagen disruption and tenocyte hypercellularity and hypocellularity in the underlying tendon proper. Thus, there appears to be significant overlap and interaction between tendinopathy and paratendinopathy.

Cellular Mechanisms Underlying Tendinosis

Collagen Degeneration

The collagen degeneration and disarray in tendinosis lesions probably represents a combination of accelerated breakdown (both mechanical and enzyme-mediated) and dysregulated fibril assembly.

In terms of collagen breakdown, it has been established that physiologic levels of loading lead to ongoing microtrauma within tendon. Thus, increased repetitive tendon loading can lead to a gradual loss of mechanical properties if there is insufficient time for adaptation and repair. Matrix metalloproteinase (MMP) activity also is induced by repetitive loading, and MMP activity (including collagen and gelatinase activity) is crucial both in physiologic remodeling in normal tendon, as well as in postinjury repair mechanisms.[9] In general, MMP activity is found to be higher in tendinosis tissue[10] despite some variability in the reported expression levels and activities of particular isoforms.[11,12] Increased MMP activity results in a high rate of collagen breakdown in tendinosis.

Collagen synthesis involves upregulation of type I and III collagens in tendinosis tissue, although type III collagen appears to predominate because of either scarring or expansion of the endotendon. Comparison of cross-linking profiles shows that the collagen in tendinosis is less mature than in normal, healthy tendon, and, therefore, tendinosis collagen is likely to be mechanically inferior. Studies have shown either reduced total collagen content or a trend toward suboptimal collagen content.[10]

The clinical implication of these advances in the understanding of collagen metabolism in tendinosis is that in theory, either blocking MMP activity or encouraging type I collagen synthesis may be beneficial. Aprotinin is a serine-proteinase inhibitor that acts as a nonspecific collagenase inhibitor. Pilot studies of aprotinin injections for Achilles and patellar tendinopathy have been promising. Data on the efficacy of these injections are being studied, with one recent randomized controlled trial reporting no significant benefit in Achilles tendinopathy.[13] Both nitric oxide therapy and controlled mechanical loading (therapeutic exercise) have been shown to stimulate collagen synthesis in tenocytes.[14,15] Nitric oxide therapy has randomized controlled trial support at the shoulder and elbow, although results at the Achilles tendon are controversial.[16-20] Substantial evidence exists to support exercise in patients with injury to the upper and lower extremity tendons; this information is discussed in chapter 27. It is likely that stimulating collagen synthesis is among the beneficial effects of therapeutic exercise.

Glycosaminoglycan

Tendinosis tendons contain more water than normal tendons (approximately 75% and 65%, respectively).[10] This high water content in tendinosis tendons is believed to be a result of increased levels of glycosaminoglycan, which is hydrophilic. Increased water content corresponds both to increased MRI signal and ultrasound hypoechogenicity and is a key feature contributing to a diagnosis of tendinosis (tendon pain with confirmed imaging changes).

Active vascular remodeling and associated cellular proliferation may be responsible for much of the proteoglycan produced in tendinosis tissue. Therefore, therapies that target the vessels, such as sclerosing or minimally invasive surgical procedures, may be capable of directly influencing the abnormal extracellular matrix. Perhaps a reduction in proteoglycan contributes to the trend toward "normal" tendon structure observed on ultrasound follow-up in some successfully treated tendons.

Tenocytes

Normal tenocytes are elongated, spindle-shaped cells with elaborate sheaths of cytoplasm branching among the collagen fibrils, continuously remodeling the tissue and responding to changes in loading. Tenocytes respond to the direction of tensile loading by depositing collagen fibrils along the line of tension. After collagen fibril ruptures (an expected consequence of mechanical loading), tenocytes either group together and express genes related to remodeling and repair or undergo apoptosis.[21,22]

In comparison with normal tendon, tendinosis tissue (including tenocytes and other cell types) generally demonstrates hypercellularity and increased proliferation. Hypocellular regions in areas with morphology typical of prior microtrauma (for example, fibrin deposition) also are seen, as is an increased rate of apoptosis.[23]

Reduction of one or more of the factors leading to vascular and cellular proliferation is an alternative clinical strategy that may be more in line with the hypercellular nature of tendinosis and could be beneficial in not only reducing the abnormal bulk of the tissue but also decreasing the metabolic demand in the tissue. For example, therapies that either promote tendon oxygenation or interfere with the ingrowing nerves could eliminate a substantial source of proliferative sub-

6: Tendinopathy

stances such as vascular endothelial growth factor (VEGF) or substance P.

Abnormal Cell Populations

Degeneration is a term used to describe a tissue that has changed in nature to a lower structural and functional state. Tendinosis frequently fits this description, with increased numbers of fat cells and mast cells. Perivascular inflammation is rarely seen, although one case series of acute Achilles paratendinopathy revealed the presence of inflammatory cells in most cases. At the chronic stage, these cells are usually absent, even in well-known paratendinopathies such as de Quervain tenosynovitis. In addition to fraying and disarray of collagen and synovium, a proliferation of synovial cells and chondroid metaplasia on the inner lining of the tendon sheath may be seen in patients with de Quervain tenosynovitis. Chondroid metaplasia also is observed in the tendon proper in patellar and Achilles tendinopathies and in ruptured supraspinatus tendons. Presumably, a loss of longitudinally oriented, collagen-producing tenocytes in exchange for other connective tissue cell types contributes to a loss of tendon biomechanical function, thus predisposing to further injury. Increased mast cell numbers also could contribute to a neurogenic component of the symptoms because of their close anatomic association with sensory nerves.[24,25]

The clinical implication is that in rare, acute cases of tendinopathy, anti-inflammatory strategies may initially be of benefit, but additional features of pathology may require treatment. Ongoing symptoms despite rest or anti-inflammatory drugs are a sure indication that other aspects of tendinosis pathology need to be considered. In patients with symptoms lasting longer than 3 months, anti-inflammatory drugs are unlikely to be beneficial.

Neurovascular Proliferation

Tendinosis is sometimes called angiofibroblastic tendinosis in reference to the most common biopsy finding: increased presence of vessels (and accompanying nerves). Immunohistochemistry reveals the presence of proliferating (Ki67+) endothelial and smooth muscle cells in tendinosis biopsies. The microvessel density may be increased by as much as 300%, with a predominance of capillaries and arterioles.[26]

Accompanying the abnormally increased microvasculature are nerves, including both autonomic and sensory fibers. These nerve fibers demonstrate positive labeling with common markers for sympathetic (tyrosine hydroxylase), parasympathetic (acetylcholine esterase), and sensory nerves (substance P).[27-31]

The causes of neurovascular proliferation have not yet been determined in tendinopathy, beyond the general recognition that earlier episodes of inflammation repair could lead to the release of a variety of angiogenic substances such as VEGF and nerve growth factor, both of which also cause axonal sprouting. In-

growth of both vessels and nerves is an important component of a healing response; however, the persistent presence of these elements in fibrotic or healed tissue is associated with chronic pain.

Angiogenesis involves an array of positive and negative regulators that could be implicated in the pathophysiology of tendinosis. Increased prominence of VEGF+ endothelial cells have been identified in patellar tendinosis. The clinical implications of neurovascular proliferation are detailed in chapter 30.

Summary

Tendinosis pathology demonstrates features of ongoing soft-tissue injury and repair, including disturbances in collagen and proteoglycan synthesis and breakdown, cell population abnormalities (proliferation, death, and metaplasia), and neurovascular proliferation. Inflammation is likely to play a role in the early stages of tendon overuse injury; however, the other (noninflammatory) pathologic features are probably responsible for the recalcitrant nature of many tendinopathies.

Annotated References

1. Vogel KG, Peters JA: Histochemistry defines a proteoglycan-rich layer in bovine flexor tendon subjected to bending. *J Musculoskelet Neuronal Interact* 2005;5:64-69.

   The authors suggest that the increased glycosaminoglycan present in tendon vessels at wraparound regions may represent an adaptive response to resist compression.

2. Pufe T, Petersen WJ, Mentlein R, Tillmann BN: The role of vasculature and angiogenesis for the pathogenesis of degenerative tendons disease. *Scand J Med Sci Sports* 2005;15:211-222.

   The hypothesis that invading or expanding vessels responding to angiogenic signals contribute to chronic tendinopathy is discussed.

3. Svensson M, Kartus J, Christensen LR, Movin T, Papadogiannakis N, Karlsson J: A long-term serial histological evaluation of the patellar tendon in humans after harvesting its central third. *Knee Surg Sports Traumatol Arthrosc* 2005;13:398-404.

   The authors discuss features of tendinosis in the healed patellar tendon that persist for at least 3 years after surgical transection.

4. Okahashi K, Sugimoto K, Iwai M, et al: Regeneration of the hamstring tendons after harvesting for arthroscopic anterior cruciate ligament reconstruction: A histological study in 11 patients. *Knee Surg Sports Traumatol Arthrosc* 2006;14:542-545.

   The authors discuss the inherent regenerative capacity of the human hamstrings tendons, which regrow and reattach after harvesting for anterior cruciate ligament repair but have an inferior matrix quality.

5. Dahlgren LA, Mohammed HO, Nixon AJ: Expression of insulin-like growth factor binding proteins in healing tendon lesions. *J Orthop Res* 2006;24:183-192.

    A prominent role for insulin-like growth factor-I is discussed along with its binding proteins in tendon healing. The expansion of the endotendon after injury is described.

6. Huang TF, Perry SM, Soslowsky LJ: The effect of overuse activity on Achilles tendon in an animal model: A biomechanical study. *Ann Biomed Eng* 2004;32:336-341.

    The authors show that tendon pathology does not result from treadmill running in rats.

7. Provenzano PP, Alejandro-Osorio AL, Valhmu WB, Jensen KT, Vanderby R Jr: Intrinsic fibroblast-mediated remodeling of damaged collagenous matrices in vivo. *Matrix Biol* 2005;23:543-555.

    The authors discuss the capacity of subfailure ligament injuries to mount an intrinsic repair response characterized by upregulation of genes involved in matrix repair and remodeling.

8. Bring DK, Heidgren ML, Kreicbergs A, Ackermann PW: Increase in sensory neuropeptides surrounding the Achilles tendon in rats with adjuvant arthritis. *J Orthop Res* 2005;23:294-301.

    Lower limb inflammation leads to nerve remodeling in the paratendon but not the tendon proper. This finding is in line with those of other studies that demonstrate a paucity of inflammation within the tendon proper. Many tendinopathies may result from changes in the paratendon and/or endotendon, which is more responsive to inflammatory mediators.

9. Dudhia J, Scott CM, Draper ER, Heinegard D, Pitsillides AA, Smith RK: Aging enhances a mechanically-induced reduction in tendon strength by an active process involving matrix metalloproteinase activity. *Aging Cell* 2007;6:547-556.

    This study conclusively shows that the accumulation of fatigue damage in tendons at physiologic levels of strain is cell mediated rather than a passive process of collagen fibril failure. The damage accumulates preferentially in aged tendons.

10. de Mos M, van El B, DeGroot J, et al: Achilles tendinosis: Changes in biochemical composition and collagen turnover rate. *Am J Sports Med* 2007;35:1549-1556.

    The authors discuss the increased rate of collagen synthesis and degradation (turnover) in Achilles tendinosis. Tendinosis involves an ongoing, cell-mediated matrix remodeling response.

11. Jones GC, Corps AN, Pennington CJ, et al: Expression profiling of metalloproteinases and tissue inhibitors of metalloproteinases in normal and degenerate human achilles tendon. *Arthritis Rheum* 2006;54:832-842.

    The authors report a distinctive expression profile of genes involved in matrix metabolism in chronically painful Achilles tendon. The histology and gene expression profiles of chronically painful tendon are distinct from acutely ruptured or normal tendons and involve the upregulation of MMP-23.

12. Riley G: The pathogenesis of tendinopathy: A molecular perspective. *Rheumatology (Oxford)* 2004;43:131-142.

    The current knowledge of matrix metabolism in human tendinopathies is summarized.

13. Orchard J, Massey A, Brown R, Cardon-Dunbar A, Hofmann J: Successful management of tendinopathy with injections of the MMP-inhibitor aprotinin. *Clin Orthop Relat Res* 2008;466:1625-1632.

    This study reports improved outcomes in Achilles tendinopathy patients receiving paratendinous aprotinin injections, compared with placebo. Level of evidence: IV.

14. Magnusson SP, Narici MV, Maganaris CN, Kjaer M: Human tendon behaviour and adaptation, in vivo. *J Physiol* 2008;586:71-81.

    The authors review recent work on human tendon physiology, with implications for injury prevention and rehabilitation.

15. Xia W, Szomor Z, Wang Y, Murrell GA: Nitric oxide enhances collagen synthesis in cultured human tendon cells. *J Orthop Res* 2006;24:159-172.

    The potential cellular basis for the reported beneficial effects of nitric oxide on tenocytes is discussed. Nitric oxide directly enhanced collagen synthesis in human tenocytes at clinical doses.

16. Kane TP, Ismail M, Calder JD: Topical glyceryl trinitrate and noninsertional Achilles tendinopathy: A clinical and cellular investigation. *Am J Sports Med* 2008; 36:1160-1163.

    No difference in clinical outcome or biopsy findings was reported in patients treated with nitric oxide or placebo. Level of evidence: I.

17. Murrell GA: Using nitric oxide to treat tendinopathy. *Br J Sports Med* 2007;41:227-231.

    This article summarizes recent randomized controlled trials and clinical experience using topical glyceryl trinitrate to treat a variety of tendinopathies.

18. Paoloni JA, Appleyard RC, Nelson J, Murrell GA: Topical glyceryl trinitrate treatment of chronic noninsertional achilles tendinopathy: A randomized, double-blind, placebo-controlled trial. *J Bone Joint Surg Am* 2004;86:916-922.

    The authors report a significant clinical benefit of topical glyceryl trinitrate in the treatment of Achilles tendinopathy. Level of evidence: I.

19. Paoloni JA, Appleyard RC, Nelson J, Murrell GA: Topical glyceryl trinitrate application in the treatment of chronic supraspinatus tendinopathy: A randomized, double-blinded, placebo-controlled clinical trial. *Am J Sports Med* 2005;33:806-813.

    The authors report a significant clinical benefit of topical glyceryl trinitrate in the treatment of chronic supraspinatus tendinopathy. Level of evidence: I.

6: Tendinopathy

20. Paoloni JA, Murrell GA: Three-year followup study of topical glyceryl trinitrate treatment of chronic noninsertional Achilles tendinopathy. *Foot Ankle Int* 2007;28:1064-1068.

    This study discusses persistent long-term benefits in response to topical glyceryl trinitrate treatment of Achilles tendinopathy. Level of evidence: I.

21. Arnoczky SP, Lavagnino M, Egerbacher M: The mechanobiological aetiopathogenesis of tendinopathy: Is it the over-stimulation or the under-stimulation of tendon cells? *Int J Exp Pathol* 2007;88:217-226.

    The authors present the hypothesis that tenocyte remodeling responses or apoptosis may be triggered by the rupture of adjacent collagen fibrils.

22. Scott A, Khan KM, Heer J, Cook JL, Lian O, Duronio V: High strain mechanical loading rapidly induces tendon apoptosis: An ex vivo rat tibialis anterior model. *Br J Sports Med* 2005;39:e25.

    This pilot study demonstrates that short-term supraphysiologic loading leads to apoptosis of tenocytes.

23. Lian O, Scott A, Engebretsen L, Bahr R, Duronio V, Khan K: Excessive apoptosis in patellar tendinopathy in athletes. *Am J Sports Med* 2007;35:605-611.

    An increased rate of apoptosis was shown in the patellar tendons of athletes with chronic patellar tendinopathy.

24. Hart D, Frank CB, Kydd A, Iveie T, Sciore P, Reno C: Neurogenic, mast cell and gender variables in tendon biology: Potential role in chronic tendinopathy, in Maffulli N, Renstrom P, Leadbetter W (eds): *Tendon Injuries: Basic Science and Clinical Medicine*. London, England, Springer, 2005, pp 1-48.

    Paratendon tissue responds to substance P by modulating extracellular matrix production, likely via a mast cell–mediated pathway.

25. Scott A, Lian O, Bahr R, Hart D, Duronio V, Khan KM: Increased mast cell numbers in human patellar tendinosis: Correlation with symptom duration and vascular hyperplasia. *Br J Sports Med* 2008;42:753-757.

    The increased mast cell density in tendinosis is demonstrated.

26. Scott A, Lian O, Roberts CR, et al: Increased versican content is associated with tendinosis pathology and vascular hyperplasia in the patellar tendon of athletes with jumper's knee. *Scand J Med Sci Sport* 2008;18:427-435.

    A large amount of abnormal glycosaminoglycan present in tendinopathy lesions consists of versican and is present in association with areas of vascular remodeling as well as regions of fibrocartilage metaplasia.

27. Andersson G, Danielson P, Alfredson H, Forsgren S: Nerve-related characteristics of ventral paratendinous tissue in chronic Achilles tendinosis. *Knee Surg Sports Traumatol Arthrosc* 2007;15:1272-1279.

    This article discusses the presence of perivascular sensory and autonomic nerves in the region anterior to the Achilles tendon, which is targeted by sclerosing injections or minimally invasive vessel-ablating procedures.

28. Danielson P, Alfredson H, Forsgren S: Distribution of general (PGP 9.5) and sensory (substance P/CGRP) innervations in the human patellar tendon. *Knee Surg Sports Traumatol Arthrosc* 2006;14:125-132.

    The authors demonstrate that many vessels in the tendinopathic tendon are mature vessels with an accompanying sensory innervation, which is implicated in chronic tendon pain.

29. Danielson P, Alfredson H, Forsgren S: In situ hybridization studies confirming recent findings of the existence of a local nonneuronal catecholamine production in human patellar tendinosis. *Microsc Res Tech* 2007;70:908-911.

    The upregulation of gene expression for sympathetic and parasympathetic mediators by tenocytes in the tendinopathic tendon is confirmed.

30. Danielson P, Alfredson H, Forsgren S: Studies on the importance of sympathetic innervation, adrenergic receptors, and a possible local catecholamine production in the development of patellar tendinopathy (tendinosis) in man. *Microsc Res Tech* 2007;70:310-324.

    The authors demonstrate the characteristics of nerves in tendinosis tissue and suggest that tenocyte-nerve interactions may be responsible for some aspects of tendon pathology.

31. Forsgren S, Danielson P, Alfredson H: Vascular NK-1 receptor occurrence in normal and chronic painful Achilles and patellar tendons: Studies on chemically unfixed as well as fixed specimens. *Regul Pept* 2005;126:173-181.

    The existence of substance P receptors in vessels of normal and pathologic tendon is discussed.

6: Tendinopathy

Chapter 27

Exercise for the Treatment of Tendinopathy

Jill L. Cook, PhD   Bill Vicenzino, BPhty, Grad Dip Sports Phty, MSc, PhD

Load Response of Tendons

Exercise has an important role in the management of tendinopathy because tendons can respond positively to appropriate loading. In normal tendons, blood flow, glucose, and oxygen uptake immediately increase twofold to fivefold during exercise. Exercise also improves protein production by tenocytes; type I collagen production increases after a single exercise session and after a period of exercise.[1,2] However, collagen production can take 3 days or longer to reach maximum levels.[1] Long-term effects of loading in normal adult tendons appear to be on the mechanical properties such as increased stiffness (decreased strain); few studies in adults have demonstrated an increase in cross-sectional area of the tendon after exercise.[3] Rest is catabolic for tendons because they require a load stimulus to maintain structure and function.[4]

Exercise has short-term effects in tendon of patients with tendinopathy that can be detected clinically. MRI studies have shown that one session of eccentric training resulted in a substantial increase in signal and volume in tendons with signs of abnormality.[5] Similar short-term changes in tendon vascularity have been reported, with a threefold increase in blood flow in abnormal tendons after exercise.[6]

Evidence for Exercise

The effects and outcomes of exercise are modulated by several parameters (for example, contraction type, load, repetitions, sets, and speed of contraction). Eccentric exercise has been the most commonly applied component of the nonsurgical treatment of tendinopathy since it was first proposed in 1984.[7] Concentric exercise does not appear to have the same effect, especially in the lower limb.[8]

Although the effects of eccentric exercise are clear, why it works is not understood. Several mechanical and structural hypotheses have been proposed but none have been substantiated. For example, most eccentric exercise involves a substantial amount of musculotendinous lengthening. In one study that compared stretch-ing to eccentric exercise in lateral elbow tendinopathy, outcomes were better in the eccentric exercise group, suggesting that muscle-tendon lengthening is not critical to outcome in tendinopathy.[9] This finding is supported by a study showing that ballistic stretching significantly decreased tendon stiffness more than static stretching.[10] Ballistic stretching is a fast eccentric contraction, again suggesting that muscle contraction in a lengthening muscle-tendon unit is a requirement for good outcomes.

Exercise in Specific Tendinopathies

Achilles Tendinopathy

Standard eccentric exercise has been shown in a range of studies to be effective in approximately 90% of those treated.[11] Studies on the effect of exercise on tendon pathology as assessed with imaging suggest that tendon structure improves and neovascularization decreases over the long term.[3,12]

Comparing exercise to more passive treatments has shown mixed results. In a recent study, therapeutic ultrasound was compared with eccentric exercise; no difference in outcomes was reported.[13] In another recent study, it was reported that exercise delivered better outcomes than passive therapies such as ultrasound and transverse friction massage.[14]

Patellar Tendinopathy

The decline squat (squat performed facing downhill on a 25° decline) was developed to increase loading on the patellar tendon. It has been demonstrated biomechanically that, compared with the normal squat, the decline squat increased the load on the patellar tendon, the magnitude of tendon strain, and the extent of quadriceps activation as measured with electromyography.[15] Clinically, an initial pilot study of the decline squat showed better outcomes in comparison with a standard squat, and further studies have shown that the decline squat is superior to other eccentric exercise programs and passive conservative management[16-18] (Figure 1). The addition of low-dose ultrasound to a decline squat exercise program for the patellar tendon does not

6: Tendinopathy

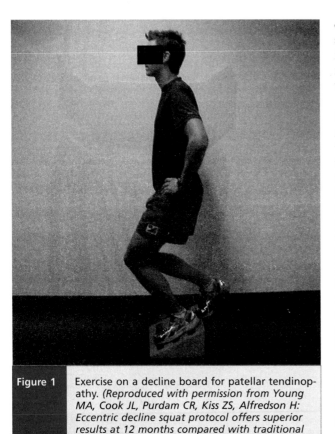

Figure 1 Exercise on a decline board for patellar tendinopathy. (Reproduced with permission from Young MA, Cook JL, Purdam CR, Kiss ZS, Alfredson H: Eccentric decline squat protocol offers superior results at 12 months compared with traditional eccentric protocol for patellar tendinopathy in volleyball players. Br J Sports Med 2005; 35:102-105.)

cent randomized clinical trial that showed improved satisfaction and lower recurrence rates following an isotonic exercise program (combined with elbow manipulation) when compared with corticosteroid injections at 12 months.[23]

Shoulder Tendinopathy

Although eccentric exercise as a treatment for shoulder tendinopathies has not been as extensively studied as in the lower limb, a recent pilot study of supraspinatus tendinopathy in impingement syndrome indicates that it is likely to be of some benefit.[24] Nine patients were evaluated who had an average 41 months of shoulder pain, a diagnosis of impingement, were on a surgery waiting list (on average for 14 months) and did not have acromioclavicular joint arthritis or calcification. Five patients were sufficiently satisfied to withdraw from the surgery waiting list at both the 12-week and 52-week follow-up. The similarity in outcome to that seen in lower limb tendons is perhaps not surprising considering that the underlying pathology appears similar.[25]

An isotonic exercise program (as opposed to solely eccentric exercise) for all the rotator cuff (shoulder joint stabilizers) as well as the periscapular muscles is also beneficial.[26] This form of exercise was as effective as arthroscopic decompression surgery in a randomized clinical trial of 90 patients with subacromial impingement.[27] In the upper limb, eccentric exercise may not be the sole exercise type to produce benefits.

enhance recovery.[19] Athletes who perform decline squats with eccentric exercise during a competitive season reported no improvement in outcome in comparison with a control group.[20]

Tennis Elbow

There is good evidence that exercise is beneficial in treating tennis elbow, but eccentric exercise is not necessarily better than concentric exercise. A recent systematic review reported that eccentric exercise of the forearm extensors is no better than concentric exercise or stretching in reducing pain or improving function and patient satisfaction/return to activity measures, but patient satisfaction 6 months after treatment was better with eccentric exercise than after ultrasound.[21]

According to one study, a combined isometric and isotonic exercise program for the forearm muscles appears to confer benefits such as less pain and shorter sick leave, as well as fewer physician consultations and operations, than a course of ultrasound.[22] This exercise program also improved forearm muscle strength, which has been implicated in protection against protracted symptoms and recurrence. Patients in this study had chronic pain that had previously failed to respond to a wide range of treatments including physiotherapy, corticosteroid injections, orthotics, and systematic and topical drugs. These findings are consistent with a re-

Variations of Standard Eccentric Exercise Programs

An important consideration in exercise programs is the amount and nature of other physical activity participation outside the exercise program during the rehabilitation period, especially with respect to pain provocation. One randomized controlled trial allowed half the participants in an Achilles tendon program to continue sports activities if their pain was ranked less than 5 on a scale of 1 to 10 during the participation of that sport as long as pain ranking had reverted to 0 by the next morning and that pain did not increase from week to week.[28] The control group participated in pain-free activity only during this early rehabilitation period. Allowing activity with pain did not affect outcome, suggesting that pain may be used to guide physical activity levels during rehabilitation.

The use or addition of braces and splints has been investigated in several studies. Patients with Achilles tendinopathy were assigned to one of three treatment groups: eccentric training, AirHeel brace (Aircast, Vista, CA), or a combination of eccentric training and AirHeel brace. At three time intervals (6, 12, and 54 weeks), there was no significant difference between groups and no synergistic effect when both treatment strategies were combined.[29] Another study used a similar protocol, examining the effect of a night splint in comparison with an eccentric exercise program. At 12 weeks, the eccentric exercise group reported significantly less pain than the splint-only group; more patients in the eccentric exercise group than in the splint group returned to sports activity after 12 weeks.[30] The addition of a night splint to an eccentric exercise program did not improve outcomes over eccentric exercise only in the Achilles tendon.[31]

The use of patches to deliver nitrous oxide has been investigated in three randomized controlled trials as an adjunct to a standard exercise program.[32-34] Overall, exercise improved in approximately 50% of the patients in both groups, and the addition of the patches resulted in improvement in approximately 75% of the patients. The effects of the patches were seen after 8 weeks of the exercise program.

Limitations of Prescription Eccentric Exercise Programs

Prescription exercise programs have been shown to be effective in specific groups, such as to treat an injured Achilles tendon in middle-aged recreational athletes or to treat an injured patellar tendon in athletes whose season has ended.[17] Changing the timing of exercise programs may alter outcomes because the same patellar tendon exercise program delivered in season showed no benefit.[20] Similarly, eccentric programs in different populations have a different effect; in a nonathletic group with Achilles tendinopathy, improvement was seen in only 56% of the participants; the rest required other interventions to improve pain.[35]

Eccentric exercise programs that use only one form of muscle contraction and movement are not likely to fully address all aspects of an athlete's sporting/participation requirements. A recent study showed that musculotendinous function does not recover after such a program;[36] therefore, it would seem reasonable to suggest that the lack of full functional recovery may predispose to further episodes of pain.[22]

Summary

Exercise clearly has a place in the treatment of tendinopathies and should be the first treatment option used. Care should be taken in choosing the type of muscle contraction to be exercised, the speed of movement, and the range through which the muscle-tendon unit is exercised as well as the staging of the exercises within the context of other activities that the patient is undertaking and that load the tendon. It would appear that tendinopathies of the lower limb are best treated with eccentric exercises, but this does not seem to be the case in the upper limb. Although these prescriptions focus in a limited exercise mode on the particular injured muscle-tendon unit, it is also important to use a diverse range of exercises to ensure that the patient is fully rehabilitated to his or her desired level of function.

Annotated References

1. Langberg H, Skovgaard D, Petersen LJ, Bulow J, Kjaer M: Type I collagen synthesis and degradation in peritendinous tissue after exercise determined by microdialysis in humans. *J Physiol* 1999;521:299-306.

2. Langberg H, Ellingsgaard H, Madsen T, et al: Eccentric rehabilitation exercise increases peritendinous type I collagen synthesis in humans with Achilles tendinosis. *Scand J Med Sci Sports* 2007;17:61-66.

   The authors investigated the local effect of a 12-week, heavy-resistance eccentric training regimen on 12 elite soccer players, 6 with chronic Achilles tendinopathy. Collagen synthesis was increased only in the injured tendons. The clinical effect of the eccentric training was a decrease in pain on loading in all of the chronically injured tendons.

3. Kongsgaard M, Aagaard P, Kjaer M, Magnusson SP: Structural Achilles tendon properties in athletes subjected to different exercise modes and in Achilles tendon rupture patients. *J Appl Physiol* 2005;99:1965-1971.

   The structural properties of the Achilles tendon in male elite athletes and in those with a ruptured Achilles tendon were studied using MRI, anthropometric measurements, and maximal isometric plantar flexion. No structural differences of the Achilles tendon were found between the groups; however, athletes who played volleyball had a larger normalized cross-sectional area than the control group.

4. Shalabi A, Kristoffersen-Wilberg M, Svensson L, Aspelin P, Movin T: Eccentric training of the gastrocnemius-soleus complex in chronic Achilles tendinopathy results in decreased tendon volume and intratendinous signal as evaluated by MRI. *Am J Sports Med* 2004;32:1286-1296.

   MRI scans of Achilles tendons were examined in 25 patients using five different MRI sequences. Tendon volume and mean intratendinous signal were calculated. Eccentric training resulted in decreased tendon volume and intratendinous signal and was correlated with an improved clinical outcome.

5. Ohno K, Yasuda K, Yamamoto N, Kaneda K, Hayashi K: Effects of complete stress-shielding on the mechanical properties and histology of in situ frozen patellar tendon. *J Orthop Res* 1993;11:592-602.

6. Cook J, Kiss ZS, Ptasznik R, Malliaras P: Is vascularity more evident after exercise? Implications for tendon imaging. *AJR Am J Roentgenol* 2005;185:1138-1140.

   This study investigated patellar tendon vascularity before and after exercise in volleyball players. Tendons that had demonstrable vessels at baseline on color Doppler imaging were reexamined within 30 minutes of completing a volleyball match. Standardized ultrasound settings were used, and the same examiner did baseline

6: Tendinopathy

and follow-up imaging. On average, the amount of vascularity increased threefold after exercise.

7. Curwin S, Stanish WD (eds): *Tendinitis: Its Etiology and Treatment.* Lexington, KY, Collamore Press, 1984, p 189.

8. Jonsson P, Alfredson H: Superior results with eccentric compared to concentric quadriceps training in patients with jumper's knee: A prospective randomised study. *Br J Sports Med* 2005;39:847-850.

   Painful eccentric quadriceps training on a decline board was superior to painful concentric exercises (3 sets of 15 repetitions, twice daily, 7 days a week for 12 weeks, with no other training for the first 6 weeks) in improving pain and function, as well as requiring less surgery at 32.6-month follow-up in patients with jumper's knee.

9. Martinez-Silvestrini JA, Newcomer KL, Gay RE, Schaefer MP, Kortebein P, Arendt KW: Chronic lateral epicondylitis: Comparative effectiveness of a home exercise program including stretching alone versus stretching supplemented with eccentric or concentric strengthening. *J Hand Ther* 2005;18:411.

   There was no difference in outcome in patients following a 6-week program of stretching, concentric strengthening with stretching, or eccentric strengthening with stretching on pain-free grip strength. Assessment of the three patient groups was with pain-free grip strength; the patient-rated Forearm Evaluation questionnaire; the Disabilities of the Arm, Shoulder and Hand questionnaire; the Medical Outcomes Study Short Form-36; and the visual analog pain scale.

10. Mahieu NN, McNair P, De Muynck M, et al: Effect of static and ballistic stretching on the muscle-tendon tissue properties. *Med Sci Sports Exerc* 2007;39:494-501.

    Static stretching and ballistic stretching of the calf muscles over 6 weeks was studied. Static stretching decreased passive resistive torque but not Achilles tendon stiffness. Ballistic stretching decreased tendon stiffness but not passive resistive torque. Dorsiflexion was increased in both groups.

11. Alfredson H, Lorentzon R: Chronic Achilles tendinosis: Recommendations for treatment and prevention. *Sports Med* 2000;29:135-146.

12. Ohberg L, Alfredson H: Effects on neovascularisation behind the good results with eccentric training in chronic mid-portion Achilles tendinosis? *Knee Surg Sports Traumatol Arthrosc* 2004;12:465-470.

    At a mean 28 months after eccentric exercise training, there was no tendon pain during activity in 36 of 41 tendons studied; 34 of these tendons were of normal structure, and 32 had no remaining neovascularization. Neovessels remained in all tendons with a poor clinical result.

13. Chester R, Costa ML, Shepstone L, Cooper A, Donell ST: Eccentric calf muscle training compared with therapeutic ultrasound for chronic Achilles tendon pain: Shepstone L, Cooper A, Donell ST: A pilot study. *Man Ther* 2008;13:484-491.

    In a pilot study, 16 recreational athletes with Achilles tendon pain of a minimum of 4 weeks duration were randomized to either eccentric loading or ultrasound over 6 weeks. There were no clear differences or trends on the visual analog scale, the fibromyalgia impact questionnaire, or the EuroQoL health status questionnaire over 2, 4, 6, and 12 weeks, which was not unexpected given the small sample size.

14. Herrington L, McCulloch R: The role of eccentric training in the management of Achilles tendinopathy: A pilot study. *Phys Ther Sport* 2007;8:191-196.

    The authors investigated the effect of adding eccentric exercise to conventional therapy of transverse friction massage and ultrasound in 25 subjects who were randomly allocated. Twelve-week follow-up showed that eccentric exercise improves the efficacy as measured on the Victorian Institute of Sports Assessment score.

15. Kongsgaard M, Aagaard P, Roikjaer S, et al: Decline eccentric squats increases patellar tendon loading compared to standard eccentric squats. *Clin Biomech (Bristol, Avon)* 2006;21:748-754.

    The use of a 25° decline board increases the load and the strain of the patellar tendon during unilateral eccentric squats as measured using electromyography and patellar tendon strain and joint angle kinematics in 13 subjects.

16. Purdam CR, Jonsson P, Alfredson H, Lorentzon R, Cook JL, Khan KM: A pilot study of the eccentric decline squat in the management of painful chronic patellar tendinopathy. *Br J Sports Med* 2004;38:395-397.

    This nonrandomized pilot study investigated the effect of eccentric quadriceps training on patients with painful chronic patellar tendinopathy. Two different eccentric exercise regimens were used: eccentric exercise with the ankle joint in a standard (foot flat) position or eccentric training standing on a 25° decline board, which was designed to increase load on the knee extensor mechanism. Good clinical results were obtained in the group who trained on the decline board; in comparison, results were poor in the standard squat group, with only one athlete returning to previous activity.

17. Young MA, Cook JL, Purdam CR, Kiss ZS, Alfredson H: Eccentric decline squat protocol offers superior results at 12 months compared with traditional eccentric protocol for patellar tendinopathy in volleyball players. *Br J Sports Med* 2005;39:102-105.

    In a prospective, randomized controlled trial, 17 elite volleyball players with patellar tendinopathy that was clinically diagnosed and confirmed by imaging were studied. The patients were randomly assigned to one of two treatment groups: a decline group and a step group. Both groups had improved significantly from baseline at 12 weeks and 12 months. Analysis of the likelihood of a 20-point improvement in the Victorian Institute of Sports Assessment score at 12 months revealed a greater likelihood of clinical improvements in the decline group than in the step group.

18. Stasinopoulos D, Stasinopoulos I: Comparison of effects of exercise programme, pulsed ultrasound and trans-

verse friction in the treatment of patellar tendinopathy. *Clin Rehabil* 2004;18:347-352.

Thirty subjects with chronic patellar tendinopathy were randomized into either exercise, pulsed ultrasound, or transverse friction over a 4-week period. The exercise program was the superior treatment at 4-, 8-, and 12-week follow-up.

19. Warden S, Metcalf BR, Kiss ZS, Cook JL, Purdam CR: Low-intensity pulsed ultrasound for chronic patellar tendinopathy: A randomised, double-blind, placebo-controlled trial. *Rheumatology* 2008;47:467-471.

The study investigated the efficacy of low-intensity pulsed ultrasound (LIPUS) in the management of patellar tendinopathy. Thirty-seven subjects were randomized to receive active LIPUS or a placebo. The results showed that LIPUS does not provide any additional benefit over placebo in the management of symptoms associated with patellar tendinopathy.

20. Visnes H, Hoksrud A, Cook J, Bahr R: No effect of eccentric training on jumper's knee in volleyball players during the competitive season: A randomized clinical trial. *Clin J Sport Med* 2005;15:227-234.

Fifty-one players with patellar tendinopathy were randomized to either a training group that performed squats on a 25° decline board as a home exercise program or a control group that trained as usual. There was no change in the Victorian Institute of Sports Assessment score during the intervention period in either group nor was there any change during the follow-up period at 6 weeks or 6 months.

21. Woodley BL, Newsham-West RJ, Baxter GD: Chronic tendinopathy: Effectiveness of eccentric exercise. *Br J Sports Med* 2007;41:188-198.

This systematic review identified 20 relevant studies of eccentric exercise in Achilles, patellar, and lateral elbow tendinopathy, 11 of which met the inclusion criteria. Limited levels of evidence exist in support of eccentric exercise on pain, function, and patient satisfaction/ return to work when compared with concentric exercise, stretching, splinting, friction, and ultrasound.

22. Pienimaki TT, Siira PT, Vanharanta H: Chronic medial and lateral epicondylitis: A comparison of pain, disability, and function. *Arch Phys Med Rehabil* 2002;83: 317-321.

23. Bisset L, Beller E, Jull G, Brooks P, Darnell R, Vicenzino B: Mobilisation with movement and exercise, corticosteroid injection, or wait and see for tennis elbow: Randomised trial. *BMJ* 2006;333:939-939.

Elbow manipulation and exercise is superior to a wait-and-see policy at 6 weeks and to corticosteroid injection afterward in patients with tennis elbow. The significant short-term benefits of corticosteroid injection are paradoxically reversed after 6 weeks, with high recurrence rates, implying that this treatment method should be used with caution.

24. Jonsson P, Wahlström P, Ohberg L, Alfredson H: Eccentric training in chronic painful impingement syndrome

of the shoulder: Results of a pilot study. *Knee Surg Sports Traumatol Arthrosc* 2006;14:76-81.

Nine patients with shoulder impingement (mean duration, 41 months) underwent 12-week painful eccentric exercises of the supraspinatus and deltoid. At 52 weeks, five patients were satisfied, had withdrawn from the surgery waiting list, and had mean visual analog scale and Constant scores of 31 and 81, respectively, from a baseline of 71 and 51, respectively.

25. Khan KM, Cook JL, Bonar F, Harcourt P, Astrom M: Histopathology of common tendinopathies: Update and implications for clinical management. *Sports Med* 1999; 27:393-408.

26. Desmeules F, Côté CH, Frémont P: Therapeutic exercise and orthopedic manual therapy for impingement syndrome: A systematic review. *Clin J Sport Med* 2003;13: 176-182.

Four of the seven studies that met inclusion criteria (randomized controlled trial, shoulder impingement syndrome, rotator cuff, bursitis, and treatment including therapeutic exercise or manual therapy), including the three trials with the best methodological score on the tool developed by the Cochrane Musculoskeletal Injuries Group, suggested some benefit of therapeutic exercise or manual therapy compared with other treatments such as acromioplasty, placebo, or no intervention.

27. Haahr JP, Østergaard S, Dalsgaard J, et al: Exercises versus arthroscopic decompression in patients with subacromial impingement: A randomised, controlled study in 90 cases with a one year follow up. *Ann Rheum Dis* 2005;64:760-764.

Randomly allocated arthroscopic subacromial decompression was not superior to graded physiotherapeutic training of the rotator cuff ($n = 90$) at 12-month follow-up. Mean Constant scores (baseline to 12 months) were 33.7 to 52.7 and 34.8 to 57.0 for surgery and physiotherapy, respectively.

28. Silbernagel KG, Thomee R, Eriksson BI, Karlsson J: Continued sports activity, using a pain-monitoring model, during rehabilitation in patients with Achilles tendinopathy: A randomized controlled study. *Am J Sports Med* 2007;35:897-906.

No negative effects could be demonstrated from continuing Achilles tendon-loading activity, such as running and jumping, with a pain-monitoring model during treatment.

29. Petersen W, Welp R, Rosenbaum D: Chronic Achilles tendinopathy: A prospective randomized study comparing the therapeutic effect of eccentric training, the AirHeel brace, and a combination of both. *Am J Sports Med* 2007;35:1659-1667.

One hundred patients were randomly assigned to eccentric training, AirHeel brace, and a combination of the two. All outcomes (ultrasonography, pain visual analog scale, American Orthopaedic Foot and Ankle Society, and Medical Outcomes Study Short Form-36) at 6, 12, and 54 weeks improved in all groups. Eccentric training and AirHeel brace are equally effective and not synergistic in the treatment of chronic Achilles tendinopathy.

6: Tendinopathy

30. Roos EM, Engstrom M, Lagerquist A, Soderberg B: Clinical improvement after 6 weeks of eccentric exercise in patients with mid-portion Achilles tendinopathy: A randomized trial with 1-year follow-up. *Scand J Med Sci Sports* 2004;14:286-295.

Forty-four patients with Achilles tendinopathy were randomized into three treatment groups for 12 weeks: the eccentric exercise group, the night splint group, or a combination of the two treatments. More patients in the exercise group returned to sports activity after 12 weeks and experienced less pain, emphasizing the need for eccentric exercise before surgery.

31. de Vos RJ, Weir A, Visser RJ, de Winter T, Tol JL: The additional value of a night splint to eccentric exercises in chronic midportion Achilles tendinopathy: A randomised controlled trial. *Br J Sports Med* 2007;41:e5.

In this single-blind, prospective, single-center, randomized controlled trial, 70 tendons were included and randomized into one of two treatment groups: eccentric exercises with a night splint or eccentric exercises only. Both groups completed a 12-week heavy-load eccentric training program. One group received a night splint in addition to eccentric exercises. After 12 weeks, patient satisfaction in the eccentric group was 63% compared with 48% in the night splint group. There was no significant difference between the two groups in the Victorian Institute of Sport Assessment-Achilles score ($P = 0.815$) and patient satisfaction.

32. Paoloni J, Appleyard R, Nelson J, Murrell GA: Topical nitric oxide application in the treatment of chronic extensor tendinosis at the elbow: A randomized, double-blinded, placebo-controlled clinical trial. *Am J Sports Med* 2003;31:915-920.

Eighty-six patients with extensor tendinosis underwent a standard tendon rehabilitation and were randomized into receiving an active glyceryl trinitrate transdermal patch or placebo. At 6 months, 81% of the treated patients were asymptomatic during activities of daily living, compared with 60% of the patients who had tendon rehabilitation and placebo patch.

33. Paoloni JA, Appleyard RC, Nelson J, Murrell GA: Topical glyceryl trinitrate treatment of chronic noninsertional achilles tendinopathy: A randomized, double-blind, placebo-controlled trial. *J Bone Joint Surg Am* 2004;86:916-922.

Sixty-five patients (84 Achilles tendons) all underwent exercises and were randomly assigned to either a topical glyceryl trinitrate patch or a placebo patch. Seventy-eight percent of 36 tendons in the active patch group were asymptomatic with activities of daily living at 6 months, compared with 49% of 41 tendons in the placebo group.

34. Paoloni JA, Appleyard RC, Nelson J, Murrell GA: Topical glyceryl trinitrate application in the treatment of chronic supraspinatus tendinopathy: A randomized, double-blinded, placebo-controlled clinical trial. *Am J Sports Med* 2005;33:806-813.

Topical glyceryl trinitrate therapy patch or placebo patch was randomly assigned to 57 shoulders with supraspinatus tendinopathy. Forty-six percent of patients on glyceryl trinitrate patches were asymptomatic with activities of daily living at 6 months compared with 24% of patients with tendon rehabilitation.

35. Sayana MK, Maffulli N: Eccentric calf muscle training in non-athletic patients with Achilles tendinopathy. *J Sci Med Sport* 2007;10:52-58.

Eccentric exercises were effective only in 56% of sedentary patients and likely are not as effective in this population as in athletes.

36. Silbernagel KG, Thomee R, Eriksson BI, Karlsson J: Full symptomatic recovery does not ensure full recovery of muscle-tendon function in patients with Achilles tendinopathy. *Br J Sports Med* 2007;41:276-280.

Only 25% of the patients who had full symptomatic recovery at 12 months had achieved full recovery of muscle-tendon function following a physical therapist-supervised rehabilitation program over 6 months. The program produced significant improvements in symptoms.

The Nonsurgical Treatment of Tendinopathy

Brett Andres, MD   *George A.C. Murrell, MD, DPhil

Introduction

Pain in and around tendons associated with activity is common and can be debilitating for the athletic population. These painful conditions have traditionally been termed tendinitis. This terminology implied that the pain associated with these conditions results from an inflammatory process. Thus, treatment modalities have mainly been aimed at controlling this inflammation. The mainstays of treatment have included rest, nonsteroidal anti-inflammatory drugs (NSAIDs), and periodic local corticosteroid injections; however, nonsurgical treatment has been problematic for two reasons. Several studies have demonstrated that little or no inflammation is actually present in tendons exposed to overuse.[1,2] Traditional treatment modalities aimed at modulating inflammation have had limited success in treating chronic, painful conditions arising from tendon overuse. More recently, the term tendinopathy has been used to describe the variety of painful conditions that develop in and around tendons in response to overuse. Histopathologic changes associated with tendinopathy include degeneration and disorganization of collagen fibers, increased cellularity, and minimal inflammation.[1,2] Macroscopic changes include tendon thickening, loss of mechanical properties, and pain. Recent work investigating the etiology of tendinopathy has shown several changes occur in response to overuse. Although many of these biochemical changes are pathologic and result in tendon degeneration, others appear to be beneficial or protective. Tendinopathy appears to result from an imbalance between the protective/regenerative changes and the pathologic responses that result from tendon overuse. The net result is tendon degeneration, weakness, tearing, and pain. As the basic science of tendin-

opathy has evolved, so have the treatment options for these conditions.

An extensive systematic review of the treatment options for tendinopathy has recently been published,[3] and this chapter draws on the findings of this review to discuss the multitude of options proposed for this condition.

Nonsteroidal Anti-inflammatory Drugs

Oral NSAIDs have been used extensively for decades for the treatment of tendon-mediated pain. Oral NSAIDs have been effective in the treatment of acute shoulder bursitis/tendinopathy, lateral epicondylitis, and Achilles tendinopathy.[4-6] NSAIDs clearly act rapidly and have been effective in providing pain relief in tendinopathy in the short term (2 weeks). NSAIDs do not appear to be as effective for patients with chronic tendinopathy with symptoms present for 6 to 12 months.[7,8] There is little evidence to support the use of oral NSAIDs over the long term. In addition, long-term NSAID use increases the risk of gastrointestinal, cardiovascular, and renal complications associated with these medications. Although cyclooxygenase-2 (COX-2)-specific medications limit gastrointestinal risks, cardiovascular risks still exist with the long-term use of these medications. Overall, a short course of NSAIDs appears to be a reasonable option for the treatment of acute tendon-mediated pain, particularly about the shoulder.

More recently, the local administration of NSAIDs via gels or patches has been an option. These medications have the advantage of targeting the painful area and limiting the systematic dose of the medication. This may limit some of the systemic complications seen with oral NSAIDs. Early results using these preparations appear quite promising in decreasing pain in the treatment of acute tendinopathies and lateral epicondylitis.[4,7,9]

Physical Therapy

Physical therapy has been commonly used for the treatment of tendinopathies. There is, however, mixed data

*George A.C. Murrell, MD, DPhil or the department with which he is affiliated has received research or institutional support from Cure Therapeutics and holds stock or stock options in Cure Therapeutics.

This chapter was adapted with permission from Andres BM, Murrell GA: Treatment of tendinopathy: What works, what does not, and what is on the horizon. Clin Orthop Relat Res 2008;466:1539-1554.

6: Tendinopathy

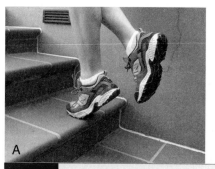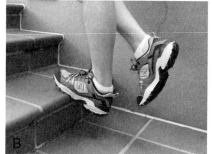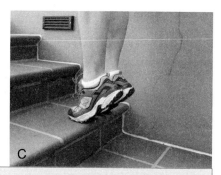

Figure 1 An eccentric training protocol for the treatment of Achilles tendinopathy is demonstrated. **A**, The patient starts in a single leg standing position with the weight on the forefoot and the ankle in full plantar flexion. **B**, The Achilles tendon is then eccentrically loaded by slowly lowering the heel to a dorsiflexed position. **C**, The patient then returns to the starting position using the arms or contralateral leg for assistance to avoid concentric loading of the involved Achilles tendon. (*Reproduced with permission from Andres BM, Murrell GA: Treatment of tendinopathy: What works, what does not, and what is on the horizon. Clin Orthop Relat Res 2008;466:1539-1554.*)

to support its use. The type of therapy used can be quite variable from one therapist to the next, and orthopaedic surgeons are often not involved in choosing the type of therapy. Stretching and strengthening programs are a common component of most therapy programs. Therapists also use other modalities, including ultrasound, iontophoresis, deep transverse friction massage, low-level laser therapy, and hyperthermia.

Stretching and Strengthening Programs

Eccentric strengthening programs have been advocated in the treatment of tendinopathy[10,11] (**Figure 1**). A 12-week course of eccentric strengthening exercises appears more effective than a traditional concentric strengthening program for treating Achilles and patellar tendinopathy in athletes.[11,12] Imaging of the Achilles tendon using ultrasound and MRI before and after a 12-week eccentric training protocol has shown thinning and normalization of the tendon structure.[13,14] Eccentric strengthening appears to be more effective in treating tendinopathy of the midsubstance of the Achilles compared with insertional tendinopathy.[15]

Eccentric strengthening protocols have also been successful in the treatment of lateral epicondylitis.[16] A 12-week course of eccentric strengthening can provide a considerable improvement in pain, strength, and function in these patients. A systematic review of the literature on eccentric strength training for the treatment of tendinopathy has been published.[17] Based on the variable results of the current studies, this review concluded there is only limited evidence to support the use of eccentric exercise over other treatments such as concentric exercise, stretching, splinting, massage, and ultrasound.

In addition to the data on eccentric strengthening, good results have been reported with a formal mobilization and strengthening program for rotator cuff tendinitis.[18-20] A formal supervised rotator cuff strengthening program has been shown to be as effective as acromioplasty for the treatment of shoulder impingement.[19] Based on this work, a course of physical therapy for mobilization and strengthening is recommended before proceeding with acromioplasty for the treatment of shoulder impingement.

Other Modalities

Because of the variety of modalities available to the physical therapist, it is difficult to predict which technique or group of techniques a given therapist will use. Although a typical orthopaedic surgeon is not involved in prescribing these treatments, it is worthwhile to have an understanding of what treatment options are available and their effectiveness. Ultrasound, iontophoresis, low-level lasers, and phonophoresis are Food and Drug Administration (FDA) approved; the 434-MHz hyperthermia device is not FDA approved for tendinopathy.

Low-level laser treatment (LLLT) has been studied extensively for the treatment of tendinopathy with mixed results. Although this treatment has been beneficial according to some controlled studies, most studies have shown little or no benefit in comparison with placebo.[21-25] Results from four systematic reviews on LLLT agree that the best current level of evidence does not support its use in the treatment of tendinopathy.[8,26-28]

The other physical therapy modalities have not been studied as extensively but have similar conflicting results in the literature. Iontophoresis and phonophoresis use ionizing current or ultrasound for local delivery of medications, along with corticosteroids and NSAIDs. Despite the widespread use of these modalities, there is conflicting evidence regarding their efficacy.[29-31]

Deep friction massage also has been described as a treatment modality for tendinopathy, but no studies have shown a benefit of deep friction massage over other physical therapy modalities.[32-34]

Therapeutic ultrasound has been fairly well evaluated and shows some benefit in the treatment of lateral epicondylitis and calcific tendinitis of the supraspinatus.[35,36] Pooled data from trials evaluating the treatment of lateral epicondylitis with ultrasound compared with controls showed the estimated difference in success rate to be 15%. Therapeutic ultrasound has not been effective in the treatment of noncalcific tendinopathy of the shoulder or Achilles tendinopathy.

Hyperthermia involves using deep-heating machines that combine a superficial cooling system with a microwave-powered heating system to increase the temperature of target tissues approximately 4°C without damaging the skin. Presumably this increase in temperature results in increased blood flow and subsequent healing to the damaged area. Two randomized clinical trials from a single institution evaluating hyperthermia and therapeutic ultrasound in the treatment of tendinopathy have been published.[37,38] These trials report improvements in pain and patient satisfaction in the hyperthermia group in comparison with the ultrasound group. No other clinical trials have evaluated hyperthermia in the treatment of tendinopathy.

Corticosteroids

Corticosteroid injections have been a mainstay in the treatment of tendinopathy. Despite their widespread use, there is some controversy as to their utility and safety. Several studies have shown good short-term pain control (in 6 weeks or less) with corticosteroid injections in patients with lateral epicondylitis and shoulder impingement.[39-41] The long-term efficacy of corticosteroid injections for tendinopathy has not been demonstrated. Corticosteroid injections for lateral epicondylitis have not shown a long-term benefit (6 to 12 months) compared with placebo, NSAIDs, or physical therapy in randomized controlled studies.[39-42] Mixed results have been published with regard to the long-term benefits of subacromial corticosteroid injections for rotator cuff tendinopathy. There are several well-controlled studies that show a small but significant level of improvement in the short term using corticosteroids in the treatment of shoulder impingement.[43,44] In contrast, several authors have reported no significant benefit with corticosteroid injections over control patients in the treatment of shoulder impingement.[25,45] A recent extensive systematic review to evaluate the efficacy of corticosteroid injections in the treatment of rotator cuff disease found little or no evidence to support the use of corticosteroid injections for these patients.[46]

In addition to uncertainty about the efficacy of corticosteroid injections in the medium-term treatment of tendinopathy, the safety of these medications has been questioned. Several cases of Achilles tendon rupture have been reported following corticosteroid injections to this region. More recently, the safe administration of corticosteroids to the Achilles region has been described.[47] This involves injecting the steroid under fluoroscopic guidance around the tendon but not within the substance of the tendon. Nevertheless, the efficacy of steroid injections for Achilles tendinopathy is questionable and is probably not worth the risk of tendon rupture.

Glyceryl Trinitrate Patches

Nitric oxide (NO) is a soluble molecule produced by a family of enzymes called nitric oxide synthases (NOS). In large doses, NO can be toxic, but in smaller, physiologic doses it acts as a cellular messenger and appears to play a role in blood pressure, memory, host defense, and tendon healing after injury. In a rat Achilles tendon healing model, inhibition of NOS resulted in decreased cross-sectional area and load to failure of the healing tendon.[48] The addition of NO in this model enhances tendon healing, suggesting that the addition of exogenous NO to an area of tendon damage may promote tendon healing.[49]

Based on this information, three randomized controlled double-blind clinical studies were designed to determine whether the topical administration of NO would enhance tendon healing in humans.[50-52] In these studies, NO was delivered transcutaneously to the area of painful tendinopathy using commercially available glyceryl trinitrate (GTN) patches (**Figure 2**). This series of trials studied the effectiveness of the GTN patch in the treatment of lateral epicondylitis, Achilles tendinopathy, and rotator cuff tendinopathy. In all three studies, 53 to 86 patients were randomly assigned to the treatment group or control group. The treatment group received GTN patches that delivered 1.25 mg of glyceryl trinitrate every 24 hours. The control group received a placebo patch. The patients and investigators were blinded to which patch was given to the patient. Both groups of patients were instructed to place the patch directly over the area of greatest tenderness or pain and to change the patch every 24 hours. The patches were worn until the symptoms subsided or the study ended (6 months).

All three studies showed statistically significant improvement in the treatment group compared with the control group. In addition to decreased pain, patients demonstrated increased power and improved function in the area of interest. Most impressive was the percentage of patients who were asymptomatic with activities of daily living in the treatment group compared to the control group. In the tennis elbow study, 81% of the treatment group was asymptomatic compared with 60% of the control group ($P = 0.005$).[50] The Achilles tendinopathy study showed 78% of the treatment group was asymptomatic with activities of daily living at 6 months compared with 49% of the control group ($P = 0.001$).[51] The supraspinatus tendinopathy data showed that 46% of patients were asymptomatic in the treatment group compared with 24% of the control group ($P = 0.007$).[52] As a whole, these studies provide convincing evidence that the administration of NO directly over an area of tendinopathy via a GTN patch enhances healing and recovery of the tendon.

6: Tendinopathy

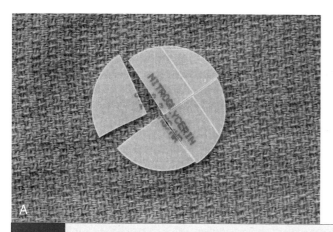
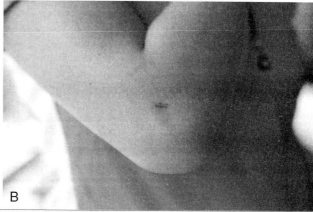

Figure 2 A 5-mg, 24-hour glyceryl trinitrate patch is cut into quarters (**A**) and placed over the area of maximal tenderness and pain in a patient with lateral epicondylitis (**B**). The patch is left in place for 24 hours and then replaced with a new quarter patch. *(Reproduced with permission from Andres BM, Murrell GA: Treatment of tendinopathy: What works, what does not, and what is on the horizon. Clin Orthop Relat Res 2008;466:1539-1554.)*

Extracorporeal Shock Wave Therapy

Extracorporeal shock wave therapy (ESWT) has been advocated for the treatment of a multitude of soft-tissue conditions including plantar fasciitis, lateral epicondylitis, calcific and noncalcific tendinitis of the supraspinatus, and tendinopathy of the Achilles tendon. ESWT delivers a series of low-energy shock waves directly over the painful area of the tendon. The mechanism by which ESWT would provide pain relief or enhance tendon healing is not clear. One theory is that ESWT causes nerve degeneration. There is also evidence that tenocytes release growth factors in response to ESWT that may promote tendon healing.

The ideal method for applying ESWT is also not clear. Published trials vary greatly with regard to the intensity and frequency of the shock waves, the duration of the treatment, the timing and number of repeat treatments given, and the use of local anesthetic. This variability makes it difficult to compare one study to the next.

The most significant question about ESWT is whether it is effective in treating tendinopathy. There is a great deal of variability in the data surrounding this treatment modality. The most convincing data are seen in the treatment of calcific tendinitis of the supraspinatus. Several large randomized controlled trials have shown excellent results using ESWT compared with placebo in the treatment of calcific tendinitis of the rotator cuff.[53-55] One advantage to treating calcific tendinitis with this method is the ability to see the area of pathology and target this area with the shock waves. The effectiveness of ESWT for treating noncalcific tendinitis of the rotator cuff has been less promising.[56,57] Variable results have been demonstrated with the use of ESWT in the treatment of lateral epicondylitis and Achilles tendinopathy. For every trial showing good results with ESWT compared to controls, there is another trial showing no significant difference. Several random-ized controlled clinical trials and systematic reviews have shown no significant benefit with ESWT compared with placebo for the treatment of noncalcific tendinopathy of the supraspinatus, lateral epicondylitis, and Achilles tendinopathy.[56-58]

Sclerotherapy

Sclerotherapy involves injecting a chemical into a blood vessel, which results in sclerosis of that vessel. The rationale behind using sclerotherapy in tendinopathy is based on the finding that there is a proliferation of small blood vessels in areas of tendinopahty. Nerve fibers appear to travel in close proximity to these areas of neovascularization.[59] It is possible that these nerve fibers are the pain generators in tendinopathy. In theory, injecting a sclerosing agent into the areas of neovascularization could not only sclerose the vessels but also may eradicate the pain-generating nerve fibers. These injections are performed under Doppler ultrasound guidance (**Figure 3**).

This theory has been tested in a series of clinical trials evaluating the treatment of tennis elbow, patellar tendinopathy, and Achilles tendinopathy with sclerotherapy.[60-62] High-resolution ultrasonography with color Doppler was done in all studies to locate areas of neovascularization and to guide injection of the sclerosing agent. Polidocanol was used as the sclerosing agent in all of the studies. Of note, polidocanol is not currently an FDA-approved sclerosing agent. This treatment method showed promising results treating Achilles tendinopathy with up to 2-year follow-up. Similar results have been seen in treating lateral epicondylitis and patellar tendinopathy with polidocanol injections.

Although polidocanol injections appear to provide pain relief, it is unclear what role they may play in tendon healing in tendinopathy. Intuitively, one would think that sclerosing the neovessels of a damaged ten-

6: Tendinopathy

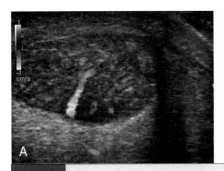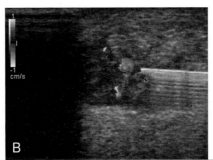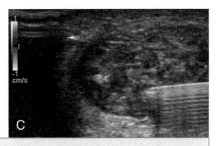

| Figure 3 | Injection of a sclerosing agent using Doppler ultrasound for guidance is shown. **A,** The presence of neovessels is detected in the Achilles tendon, using color Doppler ultrasound prior to injection. **B,** A 23-gauge needle is passed into the area of neovascularization under ultrasound guidance, and the sclerosant is injected. **C,** Ablation of blood flow within the neovessels is demonstrated after injection of the sclerosing agent. *(Reproduced with permission from Andres BM, Murrell GA: Treatment of tendinopathy: What works, what does not, and what is on the horizon. Clin Orthop Relat Res 2008;466:1539-1554.)* |

don would be detrimental to tendon healing and could possibly even cause more damage. Polidocanol injections do appear to be safe, however. Only two complications (one complete Achilles rupture and one partial rupture) possibly related to the treatment have been reported after injecting more than 400 Achilles lesions.[63]

Ablation of neovascularization with sclerosing agents is a promising option in the treatment of tendinopathy. Essentially all of the data published in this area to date have come from the group that originally described the technique. Additional data from other investigators or a multicenter study would be extremely valuable in validating the safety and efficacy of this technique.

Summary

Tendinopathy is a common and often debilitating condition that can be difficult to treat. Traditional first-line treatment methods include a short course of NSAIDs and physical therapy. Corticosteroids provide temporary pain relief but do not appear to have any longer term benefit. When these modalities fail, other options need to be considered. GTN patches are a good next step because they have been effective in well-controlled studies and cause minimal morbidity. ESWT is an excellent option for calcific tendinopathy of the shoulder, but more rigorous testing is required before it can be advocated to treat other types of tendinopathy. Sclerosing polidocanol injections appear to provide pain relief if the involved tendon has documented neovascularization seen on Doppler ultrasound. Further study is needed for optimal treatment of tendinopathy.

Annotated References

1. Soslowsky LJ, Thomopoulos S, Tun S, et al: Neer Award 1999: Overuse activity injures the supraspinatus tendon in an animal model. A histologic and biomechanical study. *J Shoulder Elbow Surg* 2000;9:79-84.

2. Khan KM, Cook JL, Bonar F, Harcourt P, Astrom M: Histopathology of common tendinopathies: Update and implications for clinical management. *Sports Med* 1999; 27:393-408.

3. Andres BM, Murrell GA: Treatment of tendinopathy: What works, what does not, and what is on the horizon. *Clin Orthop Relat Res* 2008;466:1539-1554.

   The authors present a systematic review of the literature investigating the options available for the treatment of tendinopathy. Level of evidence: II.

4. Mazières B, Rouanet S, Guillon Y, Scarsi C, Reiner V: Topical ketoprofen patch in the treatment of tendinitis: A randomized, double blind, placebo controlled study. *J Rheumatol* 2005;32:1563-1570.

   The efficacy of a topical ketoprofen patch in the treatment of tendinopathy was evaluated in this randomized, placebo-controlled study. The authors found that the ketoprofen patch provided significant pain relief after 1 week of treatment compared with a placebo patch. Level of evidence: I.

5. Mena HR, Lomen PL, Turner LF, Lamborn KR, Brinn EL: Treatment of acute shoulder syndrome with flurbiprofen. *Am J Med* 1986;80:141-144.

6. Petri M, Hufman SL, Waser G, et al: Celecoxib effectively treats patients with acute shoulder tendinitis/bursitis. *J Rheumatol* 2004;31:1614-1620.

   In this double-blind, placebo-controlled study, patients with acute bursitis were randomly assigned to one of three treatment groups: celecoxib, naprosyn, or placebo. The authors found that celecoxib and naprosyn were equally effective and superior to placebo in relieving pain at 7 and 14 days of treatment. Level of evidence: I.

7. Green S, Buchbinder R, Barnsley L, et al: Non-steroidal anti-inflammatory drugs (NSAIDs) for treating lateral elbow pain in adults. *Cochrane Database Syst Rev* 2002;2:CD003686.

8. McLauchlan GJ, Handoll HH: Interventions for treating

acute and chronic Achilles tendinitis. *Cochrane Database Syst Rev* 2001;2:CD000232.

9. Spacca G, Cacchio A, Forgács A, Moteforte P, Rovetta G: Analgesic efficacy of a lecithin-vehiculated diclofenac epolamine gel in shoulder periarthritis and lateral epicondylitis: A placebo-controlled, multicenter, randomized, double-blind clinical trial. *Drugs Exp Clin Res* 2005;31:147-154.

The authors of this study compared a topical diclofenac gel to a placebo gel in the treatment of lateral epicondylitis and shoulder periarthritis. The dicolfenac gel provided a statistically significant improvement in pain compared with placebo at 3- and 6-day intervals. Level of evidence: I.

10. Alfredson H, Pietilä T, Jonsson P, Lorentzon R: Heavy-load eccentric calf muscle training for the treatment of chronic Achilles tendinosis. *Am J Sports Med* 1998;26: 360-366.

11. Mafi N, Lorentzon R, Alfredson H: Superior short-term results with eccentric calf muscle training compared to concentric training in a randomized prospective multicenter study on patients with chronic Achilles tendinosis. *Knee Surg Sports Traumatol Arthrosc* 2001;9:42-47.

12. Jonsson P, Alfredson H: Superior results with eccentric compared to concentric quadriceps training in patients with jumper's knee: A prospective randomised study. *Br J Sports Med* 2005;39:847-850.

The authors of this small prospective, randomized study compared a 12-week course of eccentric quadriceps training to concentric training in the treatment of patellar tendinopathy. The authors reported significant improvement in pain and function with eccentric exercises. Level of evidence: II.

13. Ohberg L, Lorentzon R, Alfredson H: Eccentric training in patients with chronic Achilles tendinosis: Normalised tendon structure and decreased thickness at follow up. *Br J Sports Med* 2004;38:8-11.

Achilles tendon thickness and structure were evaluated via ultrasonography before and after a 12-week eccentric training program in patients with Achilles tendinopathy. The results showed a small but significant decrease in tendon thickness after treatment. Tendon structure was reported as abnormal in all tendons prior to the training program and normal in 19 of 26 tendons afterward. Level of evidence: II.

14. Shalabi A, Kristoffersen-Wilberg M, Svensson L, Aspelin P, Movin T: Eccentric training of the gastrocnemius-soleus complex in chronic Achilles tendinopathy results in decreased tendon volume and intratendinous signal as evaluated by MRI. *Am J Sports Med* 2004;32:1286-1296.

In this prospective cohort study, the authors demonstrated decreased Achilles tendon volume and intratendinous signal after a 3-month course of eccentric muscle training for the treatment of Achilldes tendinopathy. Level of evidence: II.

15. Fahlström M, Jonsson P, Lorentzon R, Alfredson H: Chronic Achilles tendon pain treated with eccentric calf-muscle training. *Knee Surg Sports Traumatol Arthrosc* 2003;11:327-333.

This prospective case series describes the results of eccentric calf muscle training in the treatment of Achilles tendinopathy. A satisfactory result was reported in 89% of patients with tendinopathy involving the midportion of the tendon compared with only 32% of those with insertional tendinopathy. The authors concluded that eccentric training is more effective in treating Achilles tendinopathy involving the midportion of the tendon than it is in treating insertional tendinopathy. Level of evidence: IV.

16. Croisier JL, Foidard-Dessalle M, Tinant F, Crielaard JM, Forthomme B: An isokinetic eccentric programme for the management of chronic lateral epicondylar tendinopathy. *Br J Sports Med* 2007;41: 269-275.

This randomized controlled study compared a physical therapy protocol without any strengthening to the same protocol with eccentric strengthening in the treatment of lateral epicondylitis. There was significant improvement in pain, strength, and function in the eccentrically trained group than in the control group. Level of evidence: I.

17. Woodley BL, Newsham-West RJ, Baxter GD: Chronic tendinopathy: Effectiveness of eccentric exercise. *Br J Sports Med* 2007;41:188-198.

Studies of eccentric strengthening programs in the treatment of tendinopathy were evaluated. The authors found very few high quality studies in this area. They concluded that there is only low level evidence currently available that supports the use of eccentric exercises for the treatment of tendinopathy.

18. Bang MD, Deyle GD: Comparison of supervised exercise with and without manual physical therapy for patients with shoulder impingement syndrome. *J Orthop Sports Phys Ther* 2000;30:126-137.

19. Brox JI, Staff PH, Ljunggren AE, Brevik JI: Arthroscopic surgery compared with supervised exercises in patients with rotator cuff disease (stage II impingement syndrome). *BMJ* 1993;307:899-903.

20. Conroy DE, Hayes KW: The effect of joint mobilization as a component of comprehensive treatment for primary shoulder impingement syndrome. *J Orthop Sports Phys Ther* 1998;28:3-14.

21. Basford JR, Sheffield CG, Cieslak KR: Laser therapy: A randomized, controlled trial of the effects of low intensity Nd:YAG laser irradiation on lateral epicondylitis. *Arch Phys Med Rehabil* 2000;81:1504-1510.

22. Bingöl U, Altan L, Yurtkuran M: Low-power laser treatment for shoulder pain. *Photomed Laser Surg* 2005;23:459-464.

The authors compared the effectiveness of low level laser treatment plus exercise with exercise alone for the treatment of shoulder pain. After 2 weeks of treatment, the laser treatment group reported decreased tenderness to palpation about the shoulder but showed no improvement in pain or active range of motion. Level of evidence: I.

23. Bjordal JM, Lopes-Martins RA, Iversen VV: A randomised, placebo controlled trial of low level laser therapy for activated Achilles tendinitis with microdialysis measurement of peritendinous prostaglandin E2 concentrations. *Br J Sports Med* 2006;40:76-80.

    Fourteen Achilles tendons with documented tendinopathy were randomly treated with a real or sham low level laser. Microdialysis was used to measure prostaglandin E2 concentrations in the tendons prior to treatment, after the real laser treatment, and after the sham treatment. Prostaglandin E2 levels were decreased after the real laser treatment. Level of evidence: I.

24. Stergioulas A, Stergioula M, Aarskog R, Lopes-Martins RA, Bjordal JM: Effects of low-level laser therapy and eccentric exercises in the treatment of recreational athletes with chronic achilles tendinopathy. *Am J Sports Med* 2008;36:881-887.

    The effectiveness of adding low-level laser treatment to an eccentric strengthening protocol in the treatment of Achilles tendinopathy was evaluated. The authors found that patients treated with laser therapy with eccentric exercise recovered significantly faster than those treated with exercise alone. Level of evidence: I.

25. Vecchio P, Cave M, King V, et al: A double-blind study of the effectiveness of low level laser treatment of rotator cuff tendinitis. *Br J Rheumatol* 1993;32:740-742.

26. Green S, Buchbinder R, Hetrick S: Physiotherapy interventions for shoulder pain. *Cochrane Database Syst Rev* 2003;2:CD004258.

    This systematic review found little evidence to guide the treatment of shoulder pain using physiotherapy modalities. The studies currently available lack the adequate design, quality, and power to draw useful conclusions. Level of evidence: I.

27. Stasinopoulos DI, Johnson MI: Effectiveness of low-level laser therapy for lateral elbow tendinopathy. *Photomed Laser Surg* 2005;23:425-430.

    This meta-analysis evaluated the results of low-level laser treatment for lateral epicondylitis. The authors found nine studies that met their search criteria. As a whole, these studies reported poor results with laser treatment for lateral epicondylitis. Level of evidence: I.

28. Trudel D, Duley J, Zastrow I, et al: Rehabilitation for patients with lateral epicondylitis: A systematic review. *J Hand Ther* 2004;17:243-266.

    Several rehabilitation modalities appear to be useful in the treatment of lateral epicondylitis, including acupuncture, exercise therapy, manipulations and mobilizations, ultrasound, phonophoresis, and ionization with diclofenac. Low level laser and pulsed electromagnetic field treatments appear ineffective. Level of evidence: I.

29. Klaiman MD, Shrader JA, Danoff JV, et al: Phonophoresis versus ultrasound in the treatment of common musculoskeletal conditions. *Med Sci Sports Exerc* 1998; 30:1349-1355.

30. Nirschl RP, Rodin DM, Ochiai DH, Maartmann-Moe C, DEX-AHE-01-99 Study Group: Iontophoretic administration of dexamethasone sodium phosphate for acute epicondylitis: A randomized, double-blinded, placebo-controlled study. *Am J Sports Med* 2003;31: 189-195.

    Iontophoresis with a dexamethasone cream was compared with placebo treatment for lateral epicondylitis. The dexamethasone treatment group reported significant improvement compared with placebo in the short term (2 days) but no significant improvement over the long term (1 month). Level of evidence: I.

31. Runeson L, Haker E: Iontophoresis with cortisone in the treatment of lateral epicondylalgia (tennis elbow)—a double-blind study. *Scand J Med Sci Sports* 2002;12: 136-142.

32. Brosseau L, Casimiro L, Milne S, et al: Deep transverse friction massage for treating tendinitis. *Cochrane Database Syst Rev* 2002;4:CD003528.

    This systematic review found that deep transverse friction massage was of no benefit in the treatment of lateral epicondylitis. Data available are insufficient to determine the efficacy of this modality in the treatment of other types of tendonitis. Level of evidence: I.

33. Ellis R, Hing W, Reid D: Iliotibial band friction syndrome: A systematic review. *Man Ther* 2007;12: 200-208.

    Little evidence was found in the current literature to support the use of NSAIDs, deep friction massage, phonophoresis, or corticosteroid injection in the treatment of iliotibial band syndrome. Additional research is needed in this field. Level of evidence: I.

34. Stasinopoulos D, Stasinopoulos I: Comparison of effects of exercise programme, pulsed ultrasound and transverse friction in the treatment of chronic patellar tendinopathy. *Clin Rehabil* 2004;18:347-352.

    This small randomized trial found that exercise was superior to ultrasound and transverse friction massage in the treatment of patellar tendinopathy. Level of evidence: II.

35. Robertson VJ, Baker KG: A review of therapeutic ultrasound: Effectiveness studies. *Phys Ther* 2001;81:1339-1350.

36. van der Windt DA, van der Heijden GJ, van den Berg SG, et al: Ultrasound therapy for musculoskeletal disorders: A systematic review. *Pain* 1999;81:257-271.

37. Giombini A, Di Cesare A, Casciello G, et al : Hyperthermia at 434 MHz in the treatment of overuse sport tendinopathies: A randomised controlled clinical trial. *Int J Sports Med* 2002;23:207-211.

6: Tendinopathy

38. Giombini A, Di Cesare A, Safran MR, Ciatti R, Maffulli N: Short-term effectiveness of hyperthermia for supraspinatus tendinopathy in athletes: A short-term randomized controlled study. *Am J Sports Med* 2006;34: 1247-1253.

Patients with supraspinatus tendinopathy were divided into three treatment groups: hyperthermia at 434 mHz, ultrasound at 1 MHz, or a stretching and strengthening program. The hyperthermia group reported significantly better pain relief than the other treatment groups at 6-week follow-up. Level of evidence: I.

39. Hay EM, Paterson SM, Lewis M, Hosie G, Croft P: Pragmatic randomised controlled trial of local corticosteroid injection and naproxen for treatment of lateral epicondylitis of elbow in primary care. *BMJ* 1999;319: 964-968.

40. Smidt N, van der Windt DA, Assendelft WJ, et al: Corticosteroid injections, physiotherapy, or a wait-and-see policy for lateral epicondylitis: A randomised controlled trial. *Lancet* 2002;359:657-662.

41. Verhaar JA, Walenkamp GH, van Mameren H, Kester AD, van der Linden AJ: Local corticosteroid injection versus Cyriax-type physiotherapy for tennis elbow. *J Bone Joint Surg Br* 1996;78:128-132.

42. Smidt N, Assendelft WJ, van der Windt DA, et al: Corticosteroid injections for lateral epicondylitis: A systematic review. *Pain* 2002;96:23-40.

43. Akgun K, Birtane M, Akarirmak U: Is local subacromial corticosteroid injection beneficial in subacromial impingement syndrome? *Clin Rheumatol* 2004;23: 496-500.

The short-term effects of subacromial injection of corticosteroid plus lidocaine compared with lidocaine alone in the treatment of subacromial impingment syndrome were evaluated in a randomized controlled study. All patients were given naproxen and did gentle stretching exercises. The corticosteroid injection group reported significantly less pain than the control group at 1 month after treatment, but no difference was noted at 3 months. Level of evidence: I.

44. Blair B, Rokito AS, Cuomo F, Jarolem K, Zuckerman JD: Efficacy of injections of corticosteroids for subacromial impingement syndrome. *J Bone Joint Surg Am* 1996;78:1685-1689.

45. Alvarez CM, Litchfield R, Jackowski D, Griffin S, Kirkley A: A prospective, double-blind, randomized clinical trial comparing subacromial injection of betamethasone and xylocaine to xylocaine alone in chronic rotator cuff tendinosis. *Am J Sports Med* 2005;33:255-262.

The authors reported that subacromial injection of betamethasone showed no benefit over xylocaine in improving quality of life or range of motion impingement signs in patients with rotator cuff disease. Level of evidence: I.

46. Koester MC, Dunn WR, Kuhn JE, Spindler KP: The efficacy of subacromial corticosteroid injection in the treatment of rotator cuff disease: A systematic review. *J Am Acad Orthop Surg* 2007;15:3-11.

The efficacy of corticosteroid injection in the treatment of rotator cuff disease was evaluated. There was little evidence to support the use of corticosteroid injection in the treatment of rotator cuff disease. Level of evidence: I.

47. Gill SS, Gelbke MK, Mattson SL, Anderson MW, Hurwitz SR: Fluoroscopically guided low-volume peritendinous corticosteroid injection for Achilles tendinopathy: A safety study. *J Bone Joint Surg Am* 2004;86-A: 802-806.

This retrospective review evaluated the safety of peritendinous corticosteroid injection in the treatment of Achilles tendinopathy. Of the 43 patients with 2-year follow-up who underwent this procedure, 40% described improvement, 53% had no change, and 7% thought their condition worsened. No tendon ruptures were reported. Level of evidence: IV.

48. Murrell GA, Szabo C, Hannafin JA, et al: Modulation of tendon healing by nitric oxide. *Inflamm Res* 1997; 46:19-27.

49. Yuan J, Murrell GA, Wei AQ, et al : Addition of nitric oxide via nitroflurbiprofen enhances the material properties of early healing of young rat Achilles tendons. *Inflamm Res* 2003;52:230-237.

Sixty-five rats with a transsected right Achilles tendon were randomly divided into three treatment groups: nitric oxide–flurbiprofen, flurbiprofen, or vehicle. Biomechanical and histologic testing showed better collagen organization and decreased cross-sectional are in both the nitric oxide–flurbiprogen and flurbiprofen groups but improved strength in the nitric oxide–flurbiprofen groups compared with the flurbiprofen group. Nitric oxide appears to have a beneficial effect on tendon healing.

50. Paoloni JA, Appleyard RC, Nelson J, Murrell GA: Topical nitric oxide application in the treatment of chronic extensor tendinosis at the elbow: A randomized, double-blinded, placebo-controlled clinical trial. *Am J Sports Med* 2003;31:915-920.

The efficacy of topical glyceryl trinitrate patches in the treatment of lateral epicondylitis was tested in comparison with that of control patches. The treatment group reported a significant improvement in pain and function compared with the control group. Level of evidence: I.

51. Paoloni JA, Appleyard RC, Nelson J, Murrell GA: Topical glyceryl trinitrate treatment of chronic noninsertional Achilles tendinopathy: A randomized, double-blind, placebo-controlled trial. *J Bone Joint Surg Am* 2004;86-A:916-922.

In this trial, topical glyceryl trinitrate patches proved better than control patches in the treatment of noninsertional Achilles tendinopathy. Level of evidence: I.

52. Paoloni JA, Appleyard RC, Nelson J, Murrell GA: Topical glyceryl trinitrate application in the treatment of

chronic supraspinatus tendinopathy: A randomized, double-blinded, placebo-controlled clinical trial. *Am J Sports Med* 2005;33:806-813.

In this trial, topical glyceryl trinitrate patches proved better than control patches in the treatment of supraspinatus tendinopathy. Level of evidence: I.

53. Cosentino R, De Stefano R, Selvi E, et al: Extracorporeal shock wave therapy for chronic calcific tendinitis of the shoulder: Single blind study. *Ann Rheum Dis* 2003; 62:248-250.

In this randomized controlled study, shock wave therapy proved superior to sham shock wave therapy in the treatment of calcific tendonitis. The treatment group had significant resorption of the calcium deposits and decreased pain in comparison with the control group. Level of evidence: I.

54. Loew M, Daecke W, Kusnierczak D, Rahmanzadeh M, Ewerbeck V: Shock-wave therapy is effective for chronic calcifying tendinitis of the shoulder. *J Bone Joint Surg Br* 1999;81:863-867.

55. Wang CJ, Yang KD, Wang FS, Chen HH, Wang JW: Shock wave therapy for calcific tendinitis of the shoulder: A prospective clinical study with two-year follow-up. *Am J Sports Med* 2003;31:425-430.

The efficacy of shock wave therapy in the treatment of calcific tendonitis of the rotator cuff was evaluated. The treatment group (39 shoulders) had 91% good to excellent results at 2 years. A small control group (6 shoulders) showed no good to excellent results. Level of evidence: II.

56. Schmitt J, Haake M, Tosch A, et al: Low-energy extracorporeal shock-wave treatment (ESWT) for tendinitis of the supraspinatus. A prospective, randomised study. *J Bone Joint Surg Br* 2001;83:873-876.

57. Speed CA, Richards C, Nichols D, et al : Extracorporeal shock-wave therapy for tendonitis of the rotator cuff: A double-blind, randomised, controlled trial. *J Bone Joint Surg Br* 2002;84:509-512.

58. Costa ML, Shepstone L, Donell ST, Thomas TL: Shock wave therapy for chronic Achilles tendon pain: A randomized placebo-controlled trial. *Clin Orthop Relat Res* 2005;440:199-204.

Shock wave therapy was compared with sham shock

wave therapy for the treatment of Achilles tendinopathy. The authors reported no significant difference between the treatment and control groups at 3 months. Level of evidence: I.

59. Bjur D, Alfredson H, Forsgren S: The innervation pattern of the human Achilles tendon: Studies of the normal and tendinosis tendon with markers for general and sensory innervation. *Cell Tissue Res* 2005;320:201-206.

Histologic samples of normal Achilles tendons and tendons with documented tendinopathy were stained with markers of nerve fibers. In both normal and tendinopathy samples, the nerves appeared in close proximity of the blood vessels in the specimens.

60. Hoksrud A, Ohberg L, Alfredson H, Bahr R: Ultrasound-guided sclerosis of neovessels in painful chronic patellar tendinopathy: A randomized controlled trial. *Am J Sports Med* 2006;34:1738-1746.

Polidocanol infections were compared with control injections with lidocaine for the treatment of patellar tendinopathy. Significant improvement was seen in the treatment group but not the control group at 4 months. The control group was crossed over to the treatment side at 8 months, and there was significant improvement after polidocanol injections. Level of evidence: II.

61. Ohberg L, Alfredson H: Ultrasound guided sclerosis of neovessels in painful chronic Achilles tendinosis: Pilot study of a new treatment. *Br J Sports Med* 2002;36: 173-175.

62. Zeisig E, Ohberg L, Alfredson H: Sclerosing polidocanol injections in chronic painful tennis elbow-promising results in a pilot study. *Knee Surg Sports Traumatol Arthrosc* 2006;14:1218-1224.

In this small pilot study, 13 patients were injected with a sclerosing agent for the treatment of lateral epicondylitis. A good clinical result was reported in 11 of the 13 patients at 8-month follow-up. Level of evidence: IV.

63. Alfredson H, Cook J: A treatment algorithm for managing Achilles tendinopathy: New treatment options. *Br J Sports Med* 2007;41:211-216.

The authors discuss the management of Achilles tendinopathy and report only two complications in their large series of polidocanol injections to the Achilles tendon. Level of evidence: V.

6: Tendinopathy

Chapter 29

Surgical Therapy for Tendinopathy

Nicola Maffulli, MD, PhD, FRCS(Orth)   Umile Giuseppe Longo, MD   Roald Bahr, MD, PhD

Primary Tendon Healing

As in other areas in the body, tendon healing occurs in three overlapping phases: inflammatory phase, reparative or collagen-producing phase, and organization or remodeling phase.[1] In the first 24 hours, monocytes and macrophages predominate, and phagocytosis of necrotic materials occurs.[1,2] Vasoactive and chemotactic factors are released, causing increased vascular permeability, initiation of angiogenesis, stimulation of tenocyte proliferation, and further recruitment of inflammatory cells. After a few days, the proliferative phase begins. Synthesis of type III collagen peaks during this stage, and lasts for a few weeks. Water content and glycosaminoglycan concentrations remain high during this stage. After approximately 6 weeks the remodeling phase commences, with decreasing cellularity and decreasing collagen and glycosaminoglycan synthesis. The remodeling phase can be divided into a consolidation stage and a maturation stage. The consolidation stage begins at about 6 weeks, and continues for up to 10 weeks. During this period, the repair tissue changes from cellular to fibrous. Tenocyte metabolism remains high during this period, and tenocytes and collagen fiber become more aligned in the direction of stress. A higher proportion of type I collagen is synthesized during this stage. After 10 weeks, the maturation stage occurs, with gradual change of the fibrous tissue to scar-like tendon tissue over the course of 1 year. During the latter half of this stage, tenocyte metabolism and tendon vascularity decline.[1]

Comparison of Intrinsic and Extrinsic Tendon Healing

Tendon healing can occur intrinsically, by proliferation of epitenon and endotenon tenocytes, or extrinsically, by invasion of cells from the surrounding sheath and synovium. Epitenon tenocytes typically initiate the repair process through proliferation and collagen production.[1] Healing of severed tendons can be achieved by cells from the epitenon and endotendon alone, without reliance on adhesions for vascularity or cellularity.[1] Initially, collagen is produced by epitenon cells, with endotenon cells synthesizing collagen later.[1,3] Internal tenocytes from the tendon proper also contribute to the intrinsic repair process and secrete larger and more mature collagen fibers than do epitenon or endotendon

tenocytes. The relative contribution of different cell types to tendon healing may be influenced by the type of trauma sustained, the anatomic location, the presence of a synovial sheath, and the amount of stress induced by motion after repair has taken place.[4]

Intrinsic healing results in better biomechanics and fewer complications; in particular, a normal gliding mechanism within the tendon sheath is preserved.[5] In extrinsic healing, scar tissue results in adhesion formation, which disrupts tendon gliding.[6] Different healing patterns may predominate in particular locations. For example, extrinsic healing tends to prevail in torn rotator cuffs.[6]

Limitations of Healing

Adhesion formation after intrasynovial tendon injury poses a major clinical problem.[7] Disruption of the synovial sheath at the time of the injury or surgery allows granulation tissue and tenocytes from surrounding tissue to invade the repair site. Exogenous cells predominate over endogenous tenocytes, allowing the surrounding tissue to attach to the repair site and resulting in adhesion formation. Despite remodeling, the biochemical and mechanical properties of healed tendon tissue never match those of intact tendon. In a study of transected sheep Achilles tendons that had spontaneously healed, the rupture force was only 56.7% of normal at 12 months.[8] One possible reason for this is the absence of mechanical loading during the period of immobilization.

Surgical Management of Tendinopathy

Surgery may be recommended for chronic overuse tendinopathy after unsuccessful nonsurgical treatment. Multiple surgical techniques have been reported, with the most common and consistent surgical intervention being the excision of the abnormal tissue in the tendinopathic lesion.[9-11]

The goal of surgical intervention is to excise the injured tissue and promote tendon repair to alleviate the pain associated with this chronic injury, and to promote wound repair induced by a modulation of the tendon cell-matrix environment.[12] Although surgeons agree on excising the injured lesion, there is much debate on exactly how to promote tendon repair.[10] Percutaneous needling of the tendon for such a purpose has been reported, even though no results have been published,[12] and open longitudinal tenotomy has been established.[13-15] In the absence of frank tears, the traditional operation involves a longitudinal skin incision over the tendon,[16] paratenon incision and stripping, multiple longitudinal tenotomies, and excision of the area of degeneration if present.[9] Even in very experienced surgeons the rate of complications can be high,[17] and success is not guaranteed.[18]

Minimally Invasive Stripping for Management of Achilles Tendinopathy

A new technique of minimally invasive stripping to treat Achilles tendinopathy appears to be safe and relatively inexpensive, with the potential to offer an alternative to open surgery.[19]

In Achilles tendinopathy accompanied by chronic painful tendinopathy (but not in normal pain-free tendons), there is neovascularization outside and inside the ventral part of the tendinopathic area.[20-24] The treatment technique involves stripping of neovessels from the Kager's triangle of the Achilles tendon to achieve safe and secure breaking of neovessels and the accompanying nerve supply.[19]

Percutaneous Longitudinal Tenotomies for Tendinopathy of the Main Body of the Achilles Tendon

Multiple percutaneous longitudinal tenotomies may be used when nonsurgical treatment has failed in patients with isolated tendinopathy who have no paratenon involvement and a well-defined nodular lesion less than 2.5 cm long.[25] If the multiple percutaneous tenotomies are performed in the absence of chronic paratendinopathy, the outcome is comparable to that of open procedures.

Percutaneous Longitudinal Tenotomy for Patellar Tendinopathy

A No. 11 surgical scalpel blade is inserted parallel to the long axis of the tendon fibers in the center of the area of tendinopathy, with the cutting edge pointing cranially and penetrating the entire thickness of the tendon. The blade is kept still and a full passive knee extension and flexion is produced. After reversing the blade, a full passive knee extension and flexion movement is produced.

Open Surgery for Patellar Tendinopathy

A variety of surgical methods for management of patellar tendinopathy have been described, including drilling of the inferior pole of the patella, realignment, excision of macroscopic tendinopathic areas, repair of macroscopic defects, longitudinal tenotomy, percutaneous needling, percutaneous longitudinal tenotomy, and arthroscopic débridement.[12,13,16,26-29]

A systematic review reported limited ability to make any substantial conclusions on the best surgical management of patellar tendinopathy.[10] The highest levels of evidence found on this topic were Level IV case series. The lack of a uniform assessment tool impairs the ability to compare results. The disparity of treatment options among the analyzed studies made it impossible to truly state that there is no difference between excising the inferior pole of the patella or leaving it alone, closing the paratenon or leaving it open, or immobilizing the postoperative patient instead of implementing early motion.

Drilling of the inferior pole of the patella was first described in 1962 with the idea that the blood would infuse the tendon and promote healing.[30] Some believe that a prominence of the inferior pole of the patella contributes to the tendinopathy process, and that excising the inferior pole helps alleviate the symptoms. Others believe that the drilling in the patella enhances healing of the excised tendon through the infusion of blood. A systematic review did not show any difference between those who did some surgical procedure on the inferior pole of the patella in comparison with those who did not.[10]

The need to address the paratenon during the excision of the tendinopathy lesion is another area for which surgeons hold disparate beliefs. Some maintain the paratenon holds many pain fibers and should be excised to control the pain, whereas others believe closing the paratenon could aid in the healing of the débrided tendon. Results from surgeons who closed the paratenon were not different from study results in which the paratenon was left open or treatment of the paratenon was not discussed.[10]

Open Procedure for Patellar Tendinopathy

The patellar tendon is exposed through a midline longitudinal incision. The paratenon is stripped and the tendon is palpated to locate the lesion, which is evident as a discrete area of intratendinous thickening just distal to the lower pole of the patella or proximal to the tibial tubercle. The lesion is exposed through a longitudinal tenotomy, the abnormal tissue is excised, and three to five longitudinal tenotomies are performed. The abnormal areas of the tendon are removed. The tendon and paratenon are not repaired.

Open Procedure for Achilles Tendinopathy

Surgical treatment of Achilles tendinopathy can be broadly grouped into four categories: (1) open tenotomy (**Figure 1**) with removal of abnormal tissue without stripping the paratenon; (2) open tenotomy with removal of abnormal tissue and stripping of the paratenon; (3) open tenotomy with longitudinal tenotomy and removal of abnormal tissue with or without paratenon stripping; and (4) percutaneous longitudinal tenotomy.[31-34]

The technical objective of surgery is to excise fibrotic adhesions, remove the areas of tendinopathy, and make multiple longitudinal incisions in the tendon to detect and excise intratendinous lesions. Reconstruction procedures may be required if large lesions are excised. Peroneus brevis tendon transfer may be used when the tendinopathic process has required debulking of at least 50% of the main body of the Achilles tendon.[35]

The biologic objective of surgery is to restore appropriate vascularity and possibly stimulate the remaining viable cells to initiate cell matrix response and healing.[32,36,37] The reasons why multiple longitudinal tenotomies work are still unclear. Studies have shown that the procedure triggers neoangiogenesis in the tendon, with increased blood flow.[38] This could result in improved nutrition and a more favorable environment for healing.

Open Procedure for Achilles Tendinopathy

Open surgery for tendinopathy of the main body of the Achilles tendon involves a longitudinal incision. Generally, the incision is made on the medial side of the tendon to avoid injury to the sural nerve and short saphenous vein. A straight posterior incision may also be more bothersome with the edge of the heel counter pressing directly on the incision. Preoperative imaging studies can guide the surgeon in the placement of the incision. The skin edge of the incision should be handled with extreme care throughout the procedure, because wound healing problems are possible and can be disastrous. The paratenon is identified and incised. In patients with evidence of coexisting paratendinopathy, the scarred and thickened tissue is generally excised. No studies have addressed the specific issue of the incidence of paratendinopathy. Care should be taken to minimize dissection and excision on the anterior side of the tendon. The anterior adipose tissue is thought to contain much of the vascular supply to the tendon. Based on preoperative imaging studies, the tendon is incised sharply in line with the tendon fiber bundles. The tendinopathic tissue can be identified, as it generally has lost its shiny appearance, and frequently contains disorganized fiber bundles that have more of a "crab-meat" appearance. This tissue is sharply excised. The remaining gap can be repaired using a side-to-side repair. If significant loss of tendon tissue occurs during the débridement, a tendon augmentation or transfer can be considered. A tendon turndown flap has been described for this purpose; one or two strips of tendon tissue from the gastrocnemius tendon are dissected out proximally while leaving the strip(s) attached to the main tendon distally. Each strip is then flipped 180° and sewn in to cover and bridge the weakened defect in the distal tendon. A plantaris weave has also been used. The plantaris tendon can be found on the medial edge of the Achilles tendon and traced proximally as far as possible and detached as close as possible to the muscle-tendon junction to gain as much length as possible. It can be left attached distally to the calcaneus, looped and weaved through the proximal Achilles tendon, and sewn back onto the distal part to the tendon.

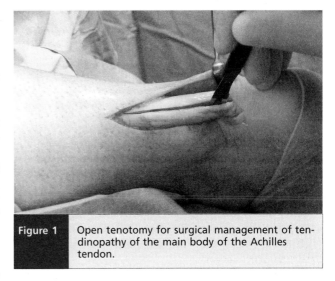

Figure 1 | Open tenotomy for surgical management of tendinopathy of the main body of the Achilles tendon.

Alternatively, the plantaris also can be detached distally and used as a free graft. Transfer and augmentation with the flexor hallucis longus tendon has been reported.[39]

Outcome of Surgery

The outcome of surgery for tendinopathy is entirely unpredictable. A review of 23 articles showed that the outcomes of surgery for patellar tendinopathy varied from 46% and 100%.[14] In the three studies in which more than 40 patients were studied, the authors reported combined excellent and good results of 91%, 82%, and 80% in series of 78, 80, and 138 patients, respectively. However, most authors report excellent or good results in up to 85% of patients with Achilles tendinopathy, and successful results in more than 70% of patients who had surgery.[40]

It was shown that the scientific methodology behind published articles on the outcome of tendinopathy after surgery is poor, and that the poorer the methodology the higher the success rate.[14] Therefore, the long-term outcome of surgical management is still not fully clarified.

Insertional Tendinopathy

Surgical management should be considered as a last resort and be limited to patients in whom 6 to 9 months of nonsurgical treatment has failed.[41] Goals of surgery include formation of scar tissue, removal of aberrant tissue, promotion of healing, relief of extrinsic pressure and tensile overload, repair of relevant tears, and replacement or augmentation of injured tendon structure.[12] These goals can be achieved by excising intratendinous or peritendinous abnormal tissue, decompression, bursectomy, synovectomy, longitudinal tenotomy and tendon repair or transfer.[42]

6: Tendinopathy

Achilles Insertional Tendinopathy

Achilles insertional tendinopathy is often associated with retrocalcaneal bursitis, which can be treated by bursectomy, excision of the diseased tendon, and resection of the calcific deposit.[43-45] If necessary, the Achilles tendon surrounding the area of calcific tendinopathy is detached by sharp dissection. The area of calcific tendinopathy is excised from the calcaneus. The area of hyaline cartilage at the posterosuperior corner of the calcaneus is excised using an osteotome, and, if needed, its base paired off with bone nibblers. The tendon is reinserted in the calcaneus using two to five bone anchors.

Soft-Tissue Arthroscopy, Tendoscopy, and Endoscopy

Arthroscopy is now in the armamentarium of orthopaedic surgeons for the routine treatment of rotator cuff disorders.[46] Tendoscopy has been used as a minimally invasive approach to several tendinopathic tendons, including the tibialis anterior; the Achilles tendon, where the surgical endoscopic technique includes peritenon release and débridement and longitudinal tenotomies; patellar tendon; peroneal tendons; tibialis posterior; and tennis elbow, with encouraging results.[47-53]

One study has compared arthroscopic techniques with classic open techniques.[13] Arthroscopic patellar tenotomy was as successful as the traditional open procedure, and both procedures provided virtually all subjects with symptomatic benefit. However, only about half the subjects who underwent either open or arthroscopic patellar tenotomy were competing at their former level of sports participation at follow-up.

More recently, endoscopic techniques have been used to manage tibialis posterior and peroneal tendinopathy showing that it is effective in controlling stage I tibialis posterior tendon dysfunction, with small scars, minimal wound pain, and a short hospital stay.[51,52]

Summary

Tendinopathy has been attributed to a variety of intrinsic and extrinsic factors. The source of pain in tendinopathy is still under investigation. Despite the morbidity associated with tendinopathy, management is far from scientifically based, and many of the therapeutic options described and in common use lack hard scientific background. There are few randomized prospective controlled trials using placebo to help select the best evidence-based management. Surgery should be reserved for patients in whom conservative treatment has been ineffective for at least 6 months; 24% to 45% of patients with tendinopathy fail to respond to nonsurgical treatment and eventually require surgery. Surgery is recommended for overuse tendon disorders, after nonsurgical treatment methods have been exhausted. The most common and consistent surgical intervention is

excision of the abnormal tissue in the tendinopathic lesion. Successful surgery for chronic overuse tendon conditions does not reconstitute a normal tendon; results are functionally satisfactory despite morphologic differences and biomechanical weakness in comparison with a normal tendon.

Annotated References

1. Sharma P, Maffulli N: Tendon injury and tendinopathy: Healing and repair. *J Bone Joint Surg Am* 2005;87:187-202.

   This article describes the function and structure of tendons and reviews the pathophysiology of tendon injury and the phases of tendon healing along with possible strategies for optimizing tendon healing and repair.

2. Murphy PG, Loitz BJ, Frank CB, Hart DA: Influence of exogenous growth factors on the synthesis and secretion of collagen types I and III by explants of normal and healing rabbit ligaments. *Biochem Cell Biol* 1994;72:403-409.

3. Becker H, Graham MF, Cohen IK, Diegelmann RF: Intrinsic tendon cell proliferation in tissue culture. *J Hand Surg [Am]* 1981;6:616-619.

4. Koob TJ: Biomimetic approaches to tendon repair. *Comp Biochem Physiol A Mol Integr Physiol* 2002;133:1171-1192.

5. Koob TJ, Summers AP: Tendon–bridging the gap. *Comp Biochem Physiol A Mol Integr Physiol* 2002;133:905-909.

6. Uhthoff HK, Sarkar K: Surgical repair of rotator cuff ruptures: The importance of the subacromial bursa. *J Bone Joint Surg Br* 1991;73:399-401.

7. Manske PR: History of flexor tendon repair. *Hand Clin* 2005;21:123-127.

   The authors discuss historical aspects of flexor tendon repair.

8. Bruns J, Kampen J, Kahrs J, Plitz W: Achilles tendon rupture: Experimental results on spontaneous repair in a sheep-model. *Knee Surg Sports Traumatol Arthrosc* 2000;8:364-369.

9. Khan KM, Maffulli N, Coleman BD, Cook JL, Taunton JE: Patellar tendinopathy: Some aspects of basic science and clinical management. *Br J Sports Med* 1998;32:346-355.

10. Kaeding CC, Pedroza AD, Powers BC: Surgical treatment of chronic patellar tendinosis: A systematic review. *Clin Orthop Relat Res* 2007;455:102-106.

    A systematic review was done to determine whether surgical débridement of abnormal tissue in proximal patellar tendinopathy is effective in relieving pain with activity, and to identify predictors of good surgical outcome for patellar tendinopathy. Level of evidence: I.

11. Khan KM, Visentini PJ, Kiss ZS, et al: Correlation of ultrasound and magnetic resonance imaging with clinical outcome after patellar tenotomy: Prospective and retrospective studies: Victorian Institute of Sport Tendon Study Group. *Clin J Sport Med* 1999;9:129-137.

12. Leadbetter WB: Cell-matrix response in tendon injury. *Clin Sports Med* 1992;11:533-578.

13. Coleman BD, Khan KM, Kiss ZS, Bartlett J, Young DA, Wark JD: Open and arthroscopic patellar tenotomy for chronic patellar tendinopathy: A retrospective outcome study: Victorian Institute of Sport Tendon Study Group. *Am J Sports Med* 2000;28:183-190.

14. Coleman BD, Khan KM, Maffulli N, Cook JL, Wark JD: Studies of surgical outcome after patellar tendinopathy: Clinical significance of methodological deficiencies and guidelines for future studies: Victorian Institute of Sport Tendon Study Group. *Scand J Med Sci Sports* 2000;10:2-11.

15. Orava S, Osterback L, Hurme M: Surgical treatment of patellar tendon pain in athletes. *Br J Sports Med* 1986; 20:167-169.

16. Martens M, Wouters P, Burssens A, Mulier JC: Patellar tendinitis: Pathology and results of treatment. *Acta Orthop Scand* 1982;53:445-450.

17. Paavola M, Orava S, Leppilahti J, Kannus P, Jarvinen M: Chronic Achilles tendon overuse injury: Complications after surgical treatment: An analysis of 432 consecutive patients. *Am J Sports Med* 2000;28:77-82.

18. Maffulli N, Binfield PM, Leach WJ, King JB: Surgical management of tendinopathy of the main body of the patellar tendon in athletes. *Clin J Sport Med* 1999;9:58-62.

19. Longo UG, Ramamurthy C, Denaro V, Maffulli N: Minimally invasive stripping for chronic Achilles tendinopathy [published online ahead of print]. *Disabil Rehabil* 2008; May 19:1-5.

A new minimally invasive technique for the management of chronic Achilles tendinopathy is discussed. This technique is advantageous because disruption of neovessels and the accompanying nerve supply is safe, secure, and minimally invasive.

20. Maffulli N, Testa V, Capasso G, et al: Similar histopathological picture in males with Achilles and patellar tendinopathy. *Med Sci Sports Exerc* 2004;36:1470-1475.

Biopsies from tendinopathic Achilles and patellar tendons were studied to determine possible differences in histopathologic appearance of tendinopathic Achilles and patellar tendons. The failed healing response pattern was common to both tendinopathic Achilles and patellar tendons.

21. Alfredson H, Ohberg L, Forsgren S: Is vasculo-neural ingrowth the cause of pain in chronic Achilles tendinosis? An investigation using ultrasonography and colour Doppler, immunohistochemistry, and diagnostic injections. *Knee Surg Sports Traumatol Arthrosc* 2003;11: 334-338.

Patients with the clinical diagnosis of painful chronic tendinopathy of the main body of the Achilles tendon were examined to investigate the origin of the pain. Findings support neovessels and accompanying nerves as the possible sources of pain.

22. Maffulli N, Sharma P, Luscombe KL: Achilles tendinopathy: Aetiology and management. *J R Soc Med* 2004; 97:472-476.

The current knowledge on etiology and management of Achilles tendinopathy is reviewed.

23. Maffulli N, Wong J, Almekinders LC: Types and epidemiology of tendinopathy. *Clin Sports Med* 2003;22: 675-692.

The current knowledge on types and epidemiology of tendinopathy is reviewed. Because of individual sport cultures and habits in different countries, national epidemiologic studies in each country are of importance.

24. Alfredson H, Ohberg L: Neovascularisation in chronic painful patellar tendinosis: Promising results after sclerosing neovessels outside the tendon challenge the need for surgery. *Knee Surg Sports Traumatol Arthrosc* 2005; 13:74-80.

Athletes with patellar tendinopathy were managed with ultrasound and color Doppler-guided injections of the sclerosing agent polidocanol, targeting the area with neovascularization.

25. Maffulli N, Testa V, Capasso G, Bifulco G, Binfield PM: Results of percutaneous longitudinal tenotomy for Achilles tendinopathy in middle- and long-distance runners. *Am J Sports Med* 1997;25:835-840.

26. Karlsson J, Lundin O, Lossing IW, Peterson L: Partial rupture of the patellar ligament: Results after operative treatment. *Am J Sports Med* 1991;19:403-408.

27. Raatikainen T, Karpakka J, Puranen J, Orava S: Operative treatment of partial rupture of the patellar ligament: A study of 138 cases. *Int J Sports Med* 1994;15: 46-49.

28. Puddu G, Cipolla M: Tendinitis, in Fox JM, Del Pizzo W (eds): *The Patellofemoral Joint*. New York, NY, McGraw-Hill, 1993.

29. Testa V, Capasso G, Maffulli N, Bifulco G: Ultrasound-guided percutaneous longitudinal tenotomy for the management of patellar tendinopathy. *Med Sci Sports Exerc* 1999;31:1509-1515.

30. Smillie I: *Injuries of the Knee Joint*. Edinburgh, Scotland, Churchill Livingstone, 1962, pp 264-267.

31. Testa V, Maffulli N, Capasso G, Bifulco G: Percutane-

6: Tendinopathy

ous longitudinal tenotomy in chronic Achilles tendonitis. *Bull Hosp Joint Dis* 1996;54:241-244.

32. Rolf C, Movin T: Etiology, histopathology, and outcome of surgery in achillodynia. *Foot Ankle Int* 1997; 18:565-569.

33. Nelen G, Martens M, Burssens A: Surgical treatment of chronic Achilles tendinitis. *Am J Sports Med* 1989;17: 754-759.

34. Leach RE, Schepsis AA, Takai H: Long-term results of surgical management of Achilles tendinitis in runners. *Clin Orthop Relat Res* 1992;282:208-212.

35. Pintore E, Barra V, Pintore R, Maffulli N: Peroneus brevis tendon transfer in neglected tears of the Achilles tendon. *J Trauma* 2001;50:71-78.

36. Astrom M, Rausing A: Chronic Achilles tendinopathy: A survey of surgical and histopathologic findings. *Clin Orthop Relat Res* 1995;316:151-164.

37. Benazzo F, Maffulli N: An operative approach to Achilles tendinopathy. *Sports Med Arthroscopy Review* 2000;8:96-101.

38. Friedrich T, Schmidt W, Jungmichel D, Horn LC, Josten C: Histopathology in rabbit Achilles tendon after operative tenolysis (longitudinal fiber incisions). *Scand J Med Sci Sports* 2001;11:4-8.

39. Wilcox DK, Bohay DR, Anderson JG: Treatment of chronic Achilles tendon disorders with flexor hallucis longus tendon transfer/augmentation. *Foot Ankle Int* 2000;21:1004-1010.

40. Tallon C, Coleman BD, Khan KM, Maffulli N: Outcome of surgery for chronic Achilles tendinopathy: A critical review. *Am J Sports Med* 2001;29:315-320.

41. Cook J, Khan K: The treatment of resistant, painful tendinopathies results in frustration for athletes and health professionals alike. *Am J Sports Med* 2003;31:327-328.

    Some tendinopathic tendons should undergo spontaneous resolution of the intratendinous changes on imaging. Changes resolved over 12 months in one third of elite athletes, despite continuation of elite sports activity.

42. Sandmeier R, Renstrom PA: Diagnosis and treatment of chronic tendon disorders in sports. *Scand J Med Sci Sports* 1997;7:96-106.

43. Yodlowski ML, Scheller AD Jr, Minos L: Surgical treatment of Achilles tendinitis by decompression of the retrocalcaneal bursa and the superior calcaneal tuberosity. *Am J Sports Med* 2002;30:318-321.

44. Baker BE: Current concepts in the diagnosis and treatment of musculotendinous injuries. *Med Sci Sports Exerc* 1984;16:323-327.

45. Kolodziej P, Glisson RR, Nunley JA: Risk of avulsion of the Achilles tendon after partial excision for treatment of insertional tendonitis and Haglund's deformity: A biomechanical study. *Foot Ankle Int* 1999;20:433-437.

46. Franceschi F, Ruzzini L, Longo UG, et al: Equivalent clinical results of arthroscopic single-row and double-row suture anchor repair for rotator cuff tears: A randomized controlled trial. *Am J Sports Med* 2007;35: 1254-1260.

    A comparison of single-row and double-row suture anchor repair for rotator cuff tears was performed in this randomized controlled study. Level of evidence: I.

47. Maquirriain J, Sammartino M, Ghisi JP, Mazzuco J: Tibialis anterior tenosynovitis: Avoiding extensor retinaculum damage during endoscopic debridement. *Arthroscopy* 2003;19:E9.

    The surgical technique of endoscopic débridement for the treatment of tibialis anterior tenosynovitis is discussed in this case report. Level of evidence: IV.

48. Maquirriain J, Ayerza M, Costa-Paz M, Muscolo DL: Endoscopic surgery in chronic achilles tendinopathies: A preliminary report. *Arthroscopy* 2002;18:298-303.

49. Maquirriain J: Endoscopic release of Achilles peritenon. *Arthroscopy* 1998;14:182-185.

50. Romeo AA, Larson RV: Arthroscopic treatment of infrapatellar tendonitis. *Arthroscopy* 1999;15:341-345.

51. van Dijk CN, Kort N: Tendoscopy of the peroneal tendons. *Arthroscopy* 1998;14:471-478.

52. van Dijk CN, Kort N, Scholten PE: Tendoscopy of the posterior tibial tendon. *Arthroscopy* 1997;13:692-698.

53. Grifka J, Boenke S, Kramer J: Endoscopic therapy in epicondylitis radialis humeri. *Arthroscopy* 1995;11:743-748.

Chapter 30

Sclerosing Polidocanol Injections for Chronic, Painful Tendinosis

Håkan Alfredson, MD, PhD   Eva Zeisig, MD

Introduction

Sclerosing polidocanol injection is a method of treatment of chronic (duration of symptoms more than 3 months) and painful tendinosis. Although not approved by the Food and Drug Administration for use in the United States, this treatment method has been evaluated in scientific studies of patients with chronic Achilles[1-4] and patellar tendinosis,[5,6] and also on patients with extensor carpi radialis brevis (ECRB) tendinosis (tennis elbow)[7] and chronic shoulder impingement syndrome (supraspinatus tendon).[8]

Color Doppler ultrasound with gray-scale ultrasonography revealed that all the painful tendons demonstrated high blood flow described as neovascularization in the regions with structural changes, whereas blood flow was normal in pain-free tendons[9] (**Figure 1**). Structural changes were located mainly in the ventral tendon, and the neovascularization was observed mainly in these same areas with structural changes as well as in the soft tissue just outside the ventral tendon. When color Doppler ultrasound was used to guide injections of small volumes of a local anesthetic, and by targeting only the areas with high blood flow on the ventral side of the tendon, patients were completely pain free after injection. Immunohistochemical analyses of tendon biopsies demonstrated the presence of nerves in close relation to vessels in tendinosis tendons.[10] This finding led to the hypothesis that blood vessels and nerves on the ventral side of the Achilles tendon were of significant importance for tendon pain. Polidocanol has been in use for many years to treat varicose veins and telangiectasis, with very few adverse effects.[11,12] The active substance is an aliphatic, nonionized, nitrogen-free surface anesthetic. Polidocanol has a sclerosing effect (primarily acting on the intimal layer in the vascular wall), and a local anesthetic effect.

It appears that the tendon with chronic, painful tendinosis is not a weak, but is instead a strong but painful tendon. Consequently, it is believed that these tendons can tolerate relatively early loading after treatment with sclerosing polidocanol injection. The current, routine rehabilitation protocol after polidocanol injection treatment consists of rest and very light Achilles tendon loading on the first day after treatment; range-of-motion exercises and short walks in slow tempo on days 2 through 7; longer walks and light bicycling on days 8 through 14; and gradual return to previous (pre-injury) Achilles tendon loading activity after 14 days.

Injection treatment should be instituted only in patients with both tendon pain and high blood flow on (outside and inside) the ventral side of the tendon. A maximum of five injection treatments, at intervals of 6 to 8 weeks, is recommended.

Clinical Studies

Achilles Midportion

The first pilot study of polidocanol included 10 patients (7 males and 3 females, mean age 55 years) with chronic painful midportion Achilles tendinosis.[1] Polidocanol (5 mg/mL) was injected in small fractions (0.1-0.2 mL per site; maximum of 2 mL) guided by color Doppler ultrasound to target the regions with high blood flow outside the ventral tendon (**Figure 2**). After a mean of two polidocanol injection treatments at intervals of 6 to 8 weeks, 8 of 10 patients were satisfied with the effect of the treatment and had resumed full Achilles tendon loading activity. At 6-month follow-up, the same eight patients were still satisfied, their mean visual analog scale score (Achilles tendon pain during loading) had decreased significantly from 73 before treatment to 8 after treatment, and there was no remaining high blood flow (neovascularization). The two patients who were not satisfied had ongoing pain and remaining high blood flow in the tendons.

The clinical results of this first study were encouraging, and a double-blind randomized controlled study was done on patients with chronic painful midportion Achilles tendinosis.[2] In this study, the effects of color Doppler ultrasound-guided polidocanol injections were compared with the effects of color Doppler ultrasound-guided lidocaine with adrenaline injections. The results showed that, despite a temporary reduction of pain, there was no clinical benefit of the lidocaine with adrenaline injections, whereas after a mean of two polidocanol (10mg/mL) injection treatments, 8 of 10 patients were satisfied and had resumed full Achilles tendon loading activity. According to this study, the

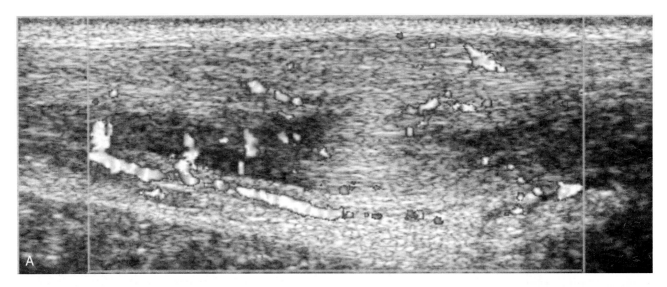

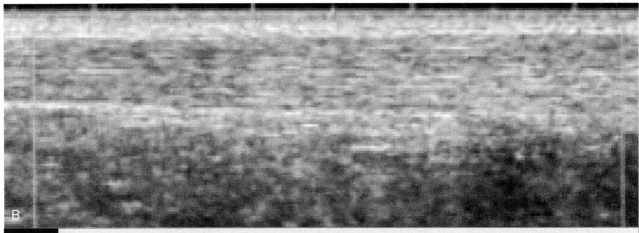

Figure 1   **A,** Chronic, painful midportion Achilles tendinosis. Gray-scale ultrasound (longitudinal view) shows thickened Achilles midportion, including structural changes and hypoechoic regions in a patient with chronic, painful midportion Achilles tendinosis. Color Doppler ultrasound shows high blood flow (neovascularization)—white/lighter structures—in regions with structural changes and hypoechoicity. **B,** Pain-free normal Achilles tendon. Gray-scale ultrasound (longitudinal view) shows normal thickness and normal structure in Achilles midportion. No color Doppler flow in the midportion.

clinical effects of polidocanol are superior to local anesthesia and adrenaline, and this may be because of the more destructive or irritating effects of polidocanol (which include fibrosis of blood vessels).

Because there were no observable short-term adverse side effects of polidocanol treatment, more patients were treated and longer follow-ups were conducted. In a 2-year clinical and color Doppler ultrasound follow-up study of 42 patients with Achilles tendinosis (23 men and 19 women, mean age 53 years), 38 patients remained satisfied with the results of the treatment; their visual analog scale during Achilles tendon loading activity had decreased from 75 before treatment to 7 at follow-up.[3] Ultrasound examination showed a significant reduction in the mean midportion tendon thickness (from 10 mm to 8 mm, $P < 0.05$) and a more "normal" structure (**Figure 3**). Color Doppler

ultrasound showed no, or a few, areas with remaining high blood flow (neovessels) in most of the successfully treated tendons, whereas there were multiple areas with high blood flow in the patients who were not satisfied. This follow-up study demonstrated that the initial, good clinical results observed in the pilot study were maintained in most patients at 2-year follow-up. Also, ultrasound showed that there was a decreased tendon thickness and improved structure 2 years after treatment, possibly indicating a remodeling potential.

Achilles Insertion
Patients with chronic pain from the Achilles tendon insertion often have pathology in the distal tendon (tendinosis), retrocalcaneal bursa, superficial bursa, and calcaneus (Haglund deformity, spurs, calcifications, fragments), either alone or in combination. Studies us-

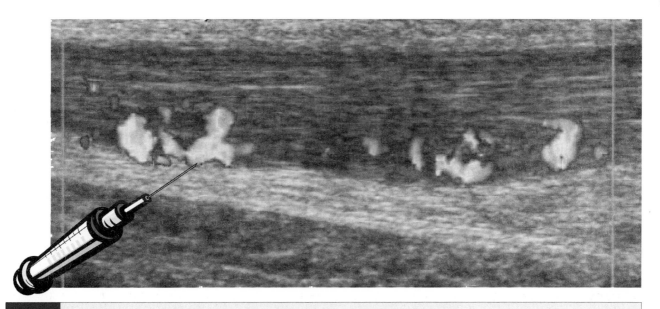

Figure 2 Gray-scale ultrasound (longitudinal view) shows thickening of Achilles midportion, including structural changes and hypoechoic regions in a patient with chronic painful midportion Achilles tendinosis undergoing sclerosing polidocanol injection treatment. Color Doppler shows high blood flow (neovascularization)—white/lighter structures—in regions with structural changes and hypoechoicity. The injection needle is placed just outside ventral tendon, in a region with high blood flow (neovascularization).

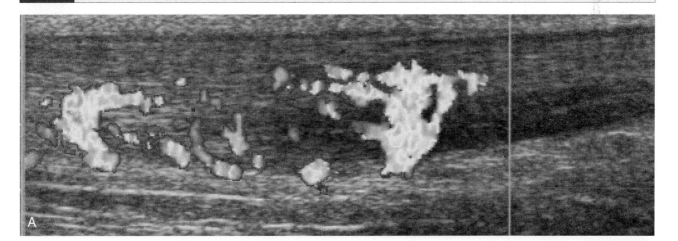

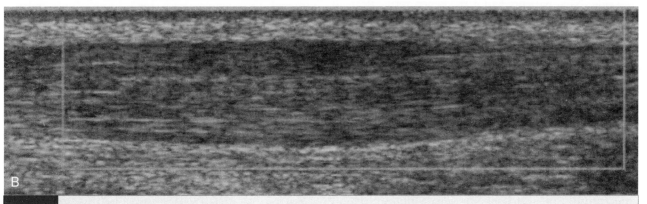

Figure 3 **A,** Ultrasound examination before sclerosing polidocanol injection treatment in a patient with chronic, painful midportion Achilles tendinosis. Gray-scale ultrasound (longitudinal view) shows thickening of Achilles midportion, including structural changes and hypoechoic regions. Color Doppler shows high blood flow (neovascularization)—white/lighter structures—in regions with structural changes and hypoechoicity. **B,** Two years after successful sclerosing polidocanol injection treatment. Gray-scale ultrasound (longitudinal view) shows thinner Achilles midportion, with more normal tendon structure. No color Doppler flow remains in the midportion.

6: Tendinopathy

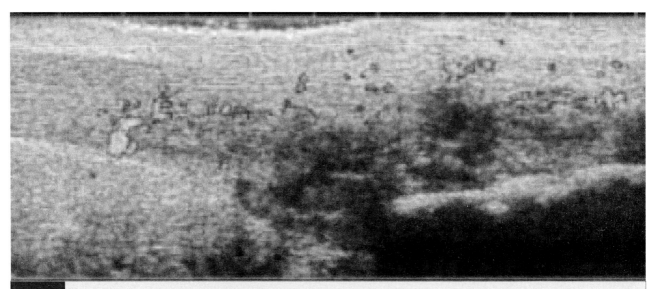

Figure 4 Gray-scale ultrasound (longitudinal view) shows thickening of the distal Achilles, thickened and enlarged retrocalcaneal bursae, Haglund deformity of the upper calcaneus, and thickening of the subcutaneous bursa in a patient with chronic pain in the Achilles insertion. Color Doppler shows high blood flow (neovascularization)—white/lighter structures—in the ventral Achilles tendon—(region with hypoechoicity) and dorsal to the enlarged retrocalcaneal bursa.

ing color Doppler ultrasound found that there were usually regions with high blood flow (neovascularization) in the ventral distal tendon, around the bursae, and in close relation to calcifications and bone spurs (**Figure 4**). With this information, a pilot study using color Doppler ultrasound-guided injections of polidocanol, targeting the regions with high blood flow, was performed.[4] The study included 11 patients (9 men and 2 women, mean age 44 years) with a long duration (mean 29 months) of chronic insertional Achilles tendon pain. All patients had structural changes in the distal tendon and regions with high blood flow (neovascularization) inside and outside the distal tendon on the injured/painful side, but not on the noninjured/pain-free side. Nine patients had a thickened retrocalcaneal bursae, and four patients showed bony pathology (calcification, spur, loose fragment) at the insertion; in these patients, high blood flow was observed in the bursae wall and/or in close relation to the bone changes. At follow-up (mean 8 months), sclerosing of the regions with high blood flow (neovessels) had stopped the pain in 8 of 11 patients, and in 7 of the 8 patients there was no remaining high blood flow. Pain during tendon-loading activity, recorded on a visual analog scale, decreased from 82 before treatment to 14 after treatment in the successfully treated patients. It can be concluded from this small pilot study that treatment focusing only on sclerosing the area with high blood flow (neovessels) seemed to have a potential to cure the pain despite the fact that tendon, bursae, and bone pathology were not directly treated. The findings support further use of this treatment method and continued scientific evaluation.

Patellar Tendinosis (Jumper's Knee)

Chronic, painful jumper's knee is a relatively common condition, especially among athletes involved in jumping and other high patellar tendon-loading activities.[13] The condition is known to be difficult to treat, and there is no gold standard for treatment. According to color Doppler ultrasound, there is an association between tendon pain and structural tendon changes combined with regions with high blood flow mainly located on the deep (dorsal) side of the tendon. However, patients also have a combination of high blood flow (neovascularization) located on both the deep and superficial sides of the tendon. A recent pilot study using color Doppler ultrasound-guided polidocanol injections targeted the regions with high blood flow outside the dorsal tendon. Fifteen elite or recreational athletes (12 men and 3 women) with a long duration of pain symptoms (mean 23 months) in 15 patellar tendons were studied.[5] In all patients, color Doppler ultrasound examination showed structural tendon changes with hypoechoic areas, and regions with high blood flow (neovascularization) corresponding to the painful area (**Figure 5**). At follow-up (mean, 6 months), after a mean of 3 treatments (with 6 weeks in between) there were good clinical results in 12 of 15 tendons. The patients returned to previous (preinjury) sport activity level, and the amount of pain had decreased significantly (visual analog scale from 81 to 12). The findings from this pilot study indicated that sclerosing polidocanol injections targeting the area with high blood flow outside the tendon may have the potential to cure the tendon pain and allow for a relatively fast return to full patellar tendon-loading activity. The findings from

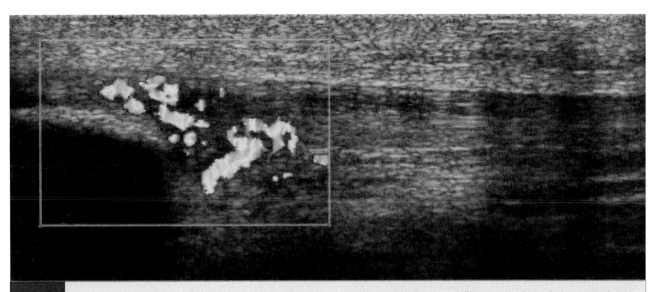

Figure 5 Patient with chronic painful proximal patellar tendinosis. Gray-scale ultrasound (longitudinal view) shows thickening of the proximal patellar tendon, including structural changes and hypoechoic regions, in a patient with chronic, painful proximal patellar tendinosis. Color Doppler shows high blood flow (neovascularization)—white/lighter structures—in regions with structural changes and hypoechoicity.

this study were of high interest, and led to an invitation to participate in a randomized, double-blind, placebo-controlled Norwegian study. The authors investigated and compared the effects of injections of the sclerosing substance polidocanol with the effects of injections of lidocaine with adrenaline on a group of elite athletes with chronic painful patellar tendinosis.[6] An initial 4-month double-blinded placebo-controlled treatment period (treatment period I) was followed by a second 4-month open treatment period, where the placebo group (lidocaine with adrenaline) crossed over to receive the active (polidocanol) treatment (treatment period II). Color Doppler ultrasound-guided injections targeting the regions with high blood flow (neovessels) on the dorsal side of the proximal patellar tendon were given to 33 patients (42 tendons) mainly from the Norwegian elite divisions in basketball, team handball, and volleyball. Pain and function were recorded using a Victorian Institute of Sport Assessment (VISA) score before the start of treatment, and 4 months (end of treatment period I), 8 months (end of treatment period II), and 12 months after the first injection (end of full competitive season). The results showed that in the treatment group there was a significant improvement in the VISA score from 52 (95% confidence interval: 45 to 57) to 62 (53 to 71) during the treatment period I ($P = .01$, paired Student's t test), whereas there was no change for the control group (55 [50 to 60] to 56 [48 to 62]) ($P = .86$, paired Student's t test) (group by time interaction; $F = 4.0$, $P = .052$, multivariate analysis of variance [MANOVA]). During treatment period II, when the placebo group also received active treatment with polidocanol, they had a greater improvement in VISA score from 4 to 8 months (58 [50 to 66] to 79 [71 to 87]) than the treatment group (54 [45 to 63] to 75 [66 to 84]) (group by time

interaction; $F = 5.76$, $P = .022$, MANOVA, time effect; $F = 24.9$, $P < .0001$). There was no further time or group effect in VISA score at the 12-month follow-up (treatment: 72 [62 to 82], placebo: 85 [79 to 91]). From this study it was concluded that treatment with sclerosing polidocanol injections resulted in a significant improvement in knee function and a reduction in pain in patients with chronic painful patellar tendinosis.

Extensor Carpi Radialis Brevis Tendinosis (Tennis Elbow)

The elbow common extensor origin, especially the ECRB tendon, is also known to be associated with chronic pain.[14,15] Histologically, the changes found in the ECRB tendon are similar to the findings in the Achilles, patellar, and supraspinatus tendons, and the challenges associated with treatment are similar.[16] Color Doppler ultrasound examinations showed high blood flow (neovascularization) in regions with structural tendon changes in patients with chronic painful tennis elbow, but not in pain-free elbows.[17] However, in contrast with the Achilles midportion and patellar tendon, in the extensor origin the high blood flow could be visualized only inside, and not outside, the tendon. These findings led to a pilot study using color Doppler ultrasound-guided injections of polidocanol targeting the region with structural changes and high blood flow inside the tendon insertion[7] (**Figure 6**). The study included 11 patients (4 men and 7 women, mean age 45 years) with the diagnosis of tennis elbow in 13 elbows. All patients had a long duration of pain symptoms (mean 24 months), and color Doppler ultrasound examination showed tendon changes corresponding to the painful area in the extensor origin. At follow-up 6

6: Tendinopathy

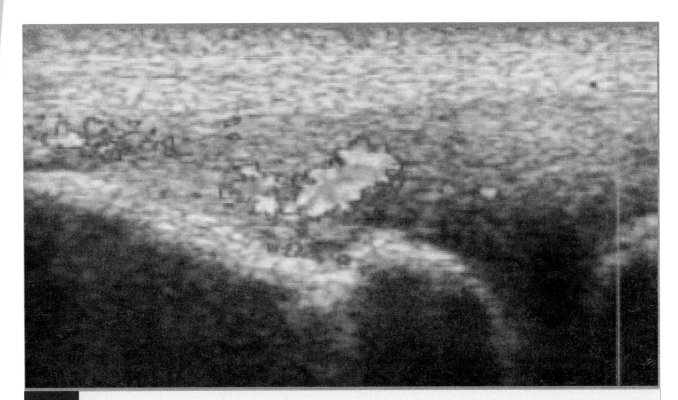

Figure 6 Gray-scale ultrasound (longitudinal view) shows thickening of the elbow extensor origin, including structural changes and hypoechoic regions, in a patient with chronic, painful ECRB tendinosis. Color Doppler shows high blood flow (neovascularization)—white/lighter structures—in regions with structural changes and hypoechoicity.

months after one injection treatment, there was a good clinical result in 11 of 13 elbows. Extensor origin pain during elbow loading activities was significantly reduced (mean visual analog scale from 75 to 34; $P < 0.003$), and maximal grip strength was significantly increased (from 29 to 40 kg; $P < 0.025$). The findings indicated that one treatment with sclerosing polidocanol injections targeting the area with high blood flow (neovascularization) inside the extensor origin may have the potential to reduce the tendon pain and increase grip strength in patients with chronic, painful tennis elbow. The results of this study led to a double-blind randomized study comparing the effects of color Doppler ultrasound-guided injections of polidocanol and lidocaine with adrenaline. Thirty-six patients with a long duration of elbow pain diagnosed as tennis elbow were included. The results of this study are currently under evaluation.

Chronic, Painful Shoulder Impingement Syndrome

The chronic, painful shoulder is another troublesome injury, for which the diagnosis is often difficult and the results of treatment are variable.[18] After excluding patients with pain from the glenohumeral and acromioclavicular joints and patients with mechanical impingement such as large calcifications, it was of interest to study the remaining group of patients diagnosed to have chronic painful subacromial impingement. In a

Swedish-Norwegian, collaborative, two-center pilot study, 15 patients (10 males and 5 females, mean age 46 years) with a long duration of shoulder pain (mean 28 months) with a diagnosis of chronic painful shoulder impingement syndrome were included.[8] All patients had tried rest, traditional rehabilitation exercises, and multiple subacromial corticosteroid injections without success. Using color Doppler ultrasound examination, regionally high blood flow (neovessels) was found in all chronically painful, but not in any pain-free, supraspinatus tendons. The clinical effects of color Doppler ultrasound-guided polidocanol injections were prospectively studied, targeting the area with high blood flow (neovascularization) in the supraspinatus tendon insertion. The patients evaluated the amount of shoulder pain during horizontal shoulder abduction on a visual analog scale, and treatment satisfaction. Two polidocanol injection treatments (median; range, 1 to 5) were given at 4- to 8-week intervals. At follow-up, 8 months after treatment (median; range, 4 to 17), 4 patients were satisfied with the result. Using the visual analog scale evaluation the pain dropped from 79 before treatment to 21 at follow-up ($P < 0.05$). It can be concluded that, in the short-term perspective, sclerosing polidocanol injections targeting the region with high blood flow in the supraspinatus tendon insertion seem to have the potential to reduce the pain during shoulder-loading activity. The findings support further use of this treatment method and scientific evaluations with larger patient groups.

Complications

Patients undergoing this treatment are followed closely, and many are involved in research projects with long follow-up periods. After completion of treatment, patients may return for follow-up care if they show any signs of complications in the treated tendon. Of more than 1,000 treated tendons at the Sports Medicine Unit in Umeå and the Capio Artro Clinic in Stockholm, there were 6 total and 2 partial Achilles tendon ruptures, and 1 partial patellar tendon rupture. Early full tendon loading was implemented, and there was no specific functional training program after treatment.

Summary

Ultrasound and Doppler-guided sclerosing polidocanol injections target the tendon region with high blood flow outside the tendon (with the exception of tennis elbow). Immediate weight-bearing activity (walking) is followed by a gradual return to full tendon loading activity 2 weeks after treatment. Regions with structural tendon changes and high blood flow in chronic painful Achilles, patellar, ECRB, and supraspinatus tendinosis tendons seem to be closely related to tendon pain during loading. Treatment with color Doppler ultrasound-guided injection of the sclerosing substance polidocanol targeting the area with neovascularization outside the tendon (or, in the case of the ECRB, inside the tendon) has been demonstrated to have a potential for reducing tendon pain. After treatment, a relatively fast return to tendon-loading activities without any specific functional training has been instituted. Few complications have been reported, possibly indicating that the tendinosis tendon is a strong tendon. Follow-up studies have shown a decrease in tendon thickness and a more normal structure in successfully treated tendons, suggesting a possible remodeling potential.

Annotated References

1. Öhberg L, Alfredson H: Ultrasound guided sclerosis of neovessels in painful chronic Achilles tendinosis: Pilot study of a new treatment. *Br J Sports Med* 2002;36: 173-177.

2. Alfredson H, Öhberg L: Sclerosing injections to areas of neovascularisation reduce pain in chronic Achilles tendinopathy: A double-blind randomized controlled trial. *Knee Surg Sports Traumatol Arthrosc* 2005;13:338-344.

   In a pilot study of 20 consecutive patients with chronic Achilles tendinopathy, local injections of polidocanol led to good clinical results, with the potential for reducing tendon pain during activity.

3. Lind B, Öhberg L, Alfredson H: Sclerosing polidocanol injections in mid-portion Achilles tendinosis: Remaining

good clinical results and decreased tendon thickness at 2-year follow-up. *Knee Surg Sports Traumatol Arthrosc* 2006;14:1327-1332.

   Long-term effects on tendon thickness, structure, and vascularity after sclerosing polidocanol injections were evaluated in 42 patients. At 2-year follow-up, 38 patients were satisfied with treatment results.

4. Öhberg L, Alfredson H: Sclerosing therapy in chronic Achilles tendon insertional pain-results of a pilot study. *Knee Surg Sports Traumatol Arthrosc* 2003;11:339-343.

   The authors present the clinical results of a pilot study using ultrasound with Doppler-guided sclerosing polidocanol injections to treat patients with chronic pain in the Achilles insertion. The group of patients had a mixture of tendon, bursae, and bone pathology.

5. Alfredson H, Öhberg L: Neovascularisation in chronic painful patellar tendinosis: Promising results after sclerosing neovessels outside the tendon challenges the need for surgery. *Knee Surg Sports Traumatol Arthrosc* 2005; 13:74-80.

   In 15 patients with patellar tendinosis/jumper's knee who were treated with ultrasound and color Doppler-guided injections of sclerosing polidocanol targeting neovascularization, clinical results were good in 12 of 15 patients.

6. Hoksrud A, Öhberg L, Alfredson H, Bahr R: Ultrasound-guided sclerosis of neovessels in painful chronic patellar tendinopathy: A randomized controlled trial. *Am J Sports Med* 2006;34:1738-1746.

   In a randomized controlled trial, 33 patients with patellar tendinopathy were divided into a treatment group (polidocanol injections in the area of neovascularization) and a control group (similar injections with lidocaine/epinephrine). The treatment group had improved VISA scores (improved knee function and reduced pain).

7. Zeisig E, Öhberg L, Alfredson H: Sclerosing polidocanol injections in chronic painful tennis elbow: Promising results in a pilot study. *Knee Surg Sports Traumatol Arthrosc* 2006;14:1218-1224.

   In 11 patients (13 elbows) with tennis elbow who were treated with sclerosing polidocanol injections, clinical results were good in 11 elbows, and extensor origin pain during wrist-loading activities was greatly reduced.

8. Alfredson H, Harstad H, Haugen S, Öhberg L: Sclerosing polidocanol injections to treat chronic painful shoulder impingement syndrome: Results of a two-center collaborative pilot study. *Knee Surg Sports Traumatol Arthrosc* 2006;14:1321-1326.

   In a study of 15 patients with long-term shoulder pain treated with ultrasound and color Doppler-guided polidocanol injections, 14 patients were satisfied with clinical results at 8-month follow-up.

9. Öhberg L, Lorentzon R, Alfredson H: Neovascularisation in Achilles tendons with painful tendinosis but not

6: Tendinopathy

in normal tendons: An ultrasonographic investigation. *Knee Surg Sports Traumatol Arthrosc* 2001;9:233-238.

10. Alfredson H, Öhberg L, Forsgren S: Is vasculo-neural ingrowth the cause of pain in chronic Achilles tendinosis? An investigation using ultrasonography and colour doppler, immunohistochemistry, and diagnostic injections. *Knee Surg Sports Traumatol Arthrosc* 2003;11: 334-338.

The authors present the results of using ultrasound with Doppler-guided injections of a local anesthetic, targeting the region where immunohistochemical analyses of paratendinous and tendinosis tissue have shown neovessels and nerves, to evaluate chronic Achilles tendon pain.

11. Conrad P, Malouf GM, Stacey MC: The Australian polidocanol (aethoxysklerol) study: Results at 2 years. *Dermatol Surg* 1995;21:334-336.

12. Guex JJ: Indications for the sclerosing agent polidocanol (aetoxisclerol dex, aethoxisklerol kreussler). *J Dermatol Surg Oncol* 1993;19:959-961.

13. Lian O, Refsnes PE, Engebretsen L, Bahr R: Performance characteristics of volleyball players with patellar tendinopathy. *Am J Sports Med* 2003;31:408-413.

The authors present information about volleyball and patellar tendinopathy, and show a relationship between jumping capacity and painful tendinopathy.

14. Nirschl RP: Elbow tendinosis/tennis elbow. *Clin Sports Med* 1992;11:851-870.

The condition from a histopathologic and clinical perspective is presented.

15. Ljung BO, Alfredson H, Forsgren S: Neurokinin 1-receptors and sensory neuropeptides in tendon insertions at the medial and lateral epicondyles of the humerus: Studies on tennis elbow and medial epicondylalgia. *J Orthop Res* 2004;22:321-327.

The authors studied muscle origin in patients with medial epicondylalgia and tennis elbow using immunohistochemistry, antibodies to substance P and calcitonin gene-related protein, and the general nerve marker protein gene product 9.5. Specific immunoreactions were seen, partly in association with blood vessels. Results indicate possible neurogenic involvement in the pathophysiology of tennis elbow and medial epicondylalgia.

16. Khan KM, Cook JL, Bonar F, Harcourt P, Åström M: Histopathology of common tendinopathies: Update and implications for clinical management. *Sports Med* 1999; 27:393-408.

17. Zeisig E, Öhberg L, Alfredson H: Extensor origin vascularity related to pain in patients with tennis elbow. *Knee Surg Sports Traumatol Arthrosc* 2006;14:659-663.

The common extensor origin was studied in 17 patients (22 elbows) with tennis elbow. After ultrasound and color Doppler-guided injection of a local anesthetic, patients had no pain during extensor loading activity.

18. Morrison D, Frogameni A, Woodworth P: Nonoperative treatment of subacromial impingement syndrome. *J Bone and Joint Surg Am* 1997;79:732-737.

Medical Issues

SECTION EDITOR:

MARGOT PUTUKIAN, MD, FACSM

Chapter 31

Sports Nutrition

Mandy Clark-Gruner, MS, RD, CSSD

Introduction

Team and individual nutrition strategies should strive to promote performance, health, and well-being. The goal of a performance eating plan is to achieve the appropriate nutrient timing and overall caloric intake to best support the daily metabolic, physical, and mental demands of an athlete's training and competition. In addition, body composition is often extremely important to an athlete, so practical and sound strategies for sustaining an optimal balance of fat-free mass and fat mass that best promotes a state of health and performance for the athlete are critical. It is important to emphasize that lifestyle habits off the field (for example, eating properly, adequate sleep) are just as influential to training as training itself.

Sports Nutrition Overview

The Physiology of Exercise

Adenosine triphosphate (ATP) is the high-energy compound derived from the oxidation of macronutrients (such as carbohydrates, protein, and fat) in food and allows cells to work. Because cells store a limited quantity of ATP, it must be continually synthesized. The amount of ATP that is synthesized depends on the intensity of the activity performed, thus determining which of the

three energy systems (Table 1) becomes the major contributing source of ATP for the working muscles.

Glucose and fatty acids are the primary sources of energy for skeletal muscle. Amino acids are not a preferred energy source for working muscles; they serve more regulatory, structural, and functional purposes. Muscle and liver glycogen are the storage reservoirs for dietary carbohydrates. Muscle glycogen levels can be further optimized through aerobic training and a diet high in carbohydrates. Adipose tissue and intramuscular triglycerides represent storage reservoirs for dietary fat. Endurance training increases the muscles' capacity to oxidize fat as a fuel source; thus, muscle glycogen is spared. The body's capacity to store fat far exceeds its capacity to store carbohydrates. However, at higher exercise intensities, fat cannot be oxidized as a fuel source; thus, the availability of muscle glycogen stores is crucial to exercise performance.

Nutrition Requirements for Athletes

Energy Intake

Balancing energy intake and expenditure represents a primary goal of physically active individuals who desire body mass maintenance and optimal adaptation to strenuous physical training. The reported energy intake of athletes is highly variable and depends on age, gender, and body size, as well as frequency, duration, and intensity of training. Male athletes may consume, on average, 4,000 to 6,000 kcal/day, whereas female ath-

---

Table 1

The Three Energy Systems

Energy is primarily transferred either anaerobically or aerobically, but no form of exercise is exclusively one or the other and may involve the following three energy systems:

The Immediate System: The ATP/phosphocreatine system fuels high-intensity or high-power bursts of activity lasting 5 to 6 s—for example, powerlifting, short all-out sprinting (50 to 100 m). Creatine is derived from animal food sources such as meat, fish, and poultry.

The Short-Term System: Human cells' capacity for glycolysis remains crucial during physical activities that require maximal effort for up to 90 s whenever adequate oxygen for aerobic activity is not available. Lactate accumulation results upon reaching a lactate threshold where work intensity will decrease because of increased muscle acidity and the inhibition of fatty acid breakdown. Carbohydrates are the only macronutrient that can act as a substrate to supply ATP anaerobically.

The Long-Term System: The aerobic energy system takes place in the mitochondria of cells and may use carbohydrates (glucose and glycogen), fats (fatty acids from adipose tissue and intramuscular triglyceride), or protein (amino acids) as substrates for ATP in the presence of oxygen. The two parts of this energy system include the Krebs cycle and the electron transport chain.

Table 2

Protein Recommendations for Athletes

Specific Athlete Group	Recommendation According to Body Weight (g/kg)
Endurance athletes	1.2-1.4
Strength athletes	1.6-1.8
Vegetarian athletes	1.3-1.8
Energy-restricted athletes	1.5-1.7

letes may consume between 1,600 and 3,000 kcal/day. However, a state of energy drain, a condition where energy demands far exceed energy intake, is commonly observed in female athletes.

Total daily energy expenditure (TDEE) determines an individual athlete's daily caloric needs. The amount of energy expended varies widely among individuals and even in the same individual on different days. The resting metabolic rate is the largest component of TDEE, accounting for 60% to 75%. The resting metabolic rate is largely determined by body size, specifically lean mass, including skeletal muscle and internal organs. Exercise thermogenesis is the second greatest contributor to TDEE (25% to 30%) and has two components: nonexercise activity thermogenesis, which includes energy expenditure from maintenance of posture, the activities of daily living, and even fidgeting; and physical activity energy expenditure, which includes energy expenditure from daily training and competition, in addition to recreational exercise. The thermic effect of food accounts for 5% to 10% and represents the increase in energy expenditure for digestion, absorption, and assimilation of macronutrients.

Carbohydrates

Dietary carbohydrates, which supply 4 kcal/g, are the preferred energy source for working muscles. Carbohydrates are the predominant fuel for exercise performed at intensities of 65% of maximal oxygen consumption (Vo_{2max}) or more, the level at which most athletes train and compete. Consumption of adequate daily carbohydrates by the athlete is imperative to maintain and replenish muscle and liver glycogen stores between bouts of training and competition. Nutrition recommendations for the general public are commonly expressed as a percentage of total energy intake, approximately 45% to 65%. For athletes, it is best to express recommendations in an absolute quantity or relative to body weight (that is, 5 to 10 g of carbohydrates per kilogram of body weight).[1]

Generally two thirds of an athlete's daily food intake should include foods that supply nutrient-dense, carbohydrate-rich foods (more whole foods versus processed foods). Many athletes derive most of their dietary carbohydrates from more convenience-type foods (for example, chips, crackers, candy bars, macaroni and cheese, and pizza) that are often higher in fat and lower in fiber, magnesium, selenium, and other micronutrients and health-benefiting phytochemicals.

A variety of fruits, vegetables, and whole grains is optimal at each of an athlete's primary daily meals. Because of the athlete's particularly high energy needs, foods containing simple sugars (honey, maple syrup, fruit preserves, juices, sport drinks) can easily fit into a sound training diet. Athletes who have difficulty eating enough food to satisfy the overall energy and carbohydrate requirements for daily training demands may consider incorporating commercially available nutritional supplementation that helps boost overall energy and carbohydrate intake. Overall, these products (for example, sport drinks, recovery beverages, nutrition shakes, sport bars) can be more practical and convenient before, during, and after training or competition, but they should be used only to supplement a well-balanced diet containing a wide variety of whole foods.

Protein

If carbohydrate and overall energy intake are adequate to support training, amino acids should account for less than 5% of the total energy expenditure. Unlike carbohydrates and fat, no "reservoir" for protein exists; protein contributes to tissue repair and acts as a component of metabolic, transport, and hormonal systems. Essential amino acids are the building blocks for synthesizing tissue. However, protein does supply 4 kcal/g and can become a significant energy source under certain circumstances, such as during a low carbohydrate condition or prolonged exercise.

In general, protein requirements for athletes are greater than those of their sedentary counterparts. Daily protein requirements are 1.6 to 1.8 g/kg for strength-trained athletes and 1.2 to 1.4 g/kg for endurance-trained athletes, with no benefit beyond 2.0 g/kg of body weight[1] (**Table 2**). Very few athletes are at risk of protein deficiency provided that energy intake is sufficient to maintain body weight and sound nutrition principles are followed. Athletes are encouraged to have a diet that includes a variety of plant and animal sources to obtain all of the essential amino acids along with essential vitamins, minerals, and antioxidants. Athletes are advised to choose leaner animal sources of protein, thus minimizing saturated fat intake. One third of an athlete's daily food intake should comprise protein-rich foods. There is no benefit to "bolusing" or eating large quantities of protein per meal; generally 20 to 40 g per meal spread over three meals and a couple of protein-containing snacks will easily satisfy an athlete's daily protein requirements.

The quality of vegetarian and vegan diets to meet an athlete's nutritional needs, specifically protein requirements, and support performance continues to be questioned. Although long-term studies are lacking, five observations can be made.[2] First, well-planned vegetarian diets can provide sufficient energy and an appropriate range of the macronutrients needed to support performance and health. Second, vegetarian athletes can satisfy protein requirements from plant sources, with both plant and animal protein sources appearing to provide equivalent support for athletic performance. Vegetarian athletes should aim toward the higher end of current recommendations because of the lower digestibility and essential amino acid profile of plant protein (Table 2). Third, female vegetarians are particularly at risk for nonanemic iron deficiency, given the lower bioavailability of iron from plant foods. Fourth, health professionals should be aware that disordered eating can be masked or perpetuated by adopting a vegetarian diet because it "legitimizes" restrictive eating. The athlete should be assessed for a potential eating disorder, especially if unwarranted weight loss occurs. Fifth, other nutrients of concern, depending on the degree of vegetarianism, may include zinc, vitamin B_{12}, vitamin D, and calcium.

There is no compelling scientific evidence to suggest that athletes need to supplement their habitual diets with protein powders or amino acid supplements. However, there is benefit to consuming a protein-containing snack or beverage after a muscle-damaging workout.[3] Because commercially available "protein shakes" are convenient, palatable, and portable, many athletes may prefer a drink immediately after a workout; in these circumstances, a drink that provides "supplemental protein" may be appropriate and beneficial. However, athletes should be advised of the proper amount of protein in a recovery beverage that is needed and beneficial versus excessive (Table 3).

Dietary Fat
Dietary fat plays several important physiologic roles, including protection of vital organs, thermal insulation, and acting as a vitamin carrier and hunger suppressor. Besides carbohydrates, fatty acids are an alternate energy source and reserve under lower intensity exercise. Free fatty acids, intramuscular triglycerides, and circulating plasma triglycerides can supply 30% to 80% of the energy for physical activity, depending on the training and nutritional status of the individual as well as the intensity and duration of exercise. Depletion of muscle glycogen stores will lower an individual's ability to exercise at higher intensities. As a result, the intensity of a training bout will be orchestrated to a lower intensity where the body can mobilize and oxidize fatty acids as fuel. Nonetheless, aerobic training enhances the ability of muscle mitochondria to oxidize fatty acids as fuel. In addition, the enhanced responsiveness of adipocytes to lipolysis allows endurance athletes to exercise at higher absolute submaximal exercise levels before experiencing the fatigue resulting from glycogen depletion.

According to the Dietary Guidelines for Americans, the recommendation for fat is in the range of 20% to 35% of total calorie intake. Recommendations should

Table 3	
Preworkout, During Workout, and Postworkout Carbohydrate, Protein, and Fluid Recommendations	
Preworkout	Carbohydrates: 1.0 g/kg—1 hour before; 2.0 g/kg—2 hours before; 3.0 g/kg—3 hours before; 4.0 g/kg—4 hours before Fluid: Drink 16-20 oz 2 hours before; additional 10 oz 20 minutes before
During Workout	Carbohydrates: 30-60 g/kg/hr Fluid: 4 oz per 15 minutes
Postworkout	Carbohydrates: 1.0-1.5 g/kg Protein: 0.1-0.2 g/kg Fluid: 24 oz per pound of body weight lost

be individualized based on an athlete's physical activity level, energy expenditure, growth stage, nutritional needs, and food preferences. Athletes should be encouraged to choose foods wisely to obtain "heart-healthy fats"—the essential fatty acids (omega-3 fatty acids) and unsaturated fats versus foods that are high in saturated and trans-fatty acids, which contribute to the onset of atherosclerosis and heart disease. However, very low-fat diets (< 15% of total caloric intake) may harm both performance and health and are highly discouraged.

Micronutrients
Micronutrients play a highly specific role in facilitating energy transfer and tissue synthesis. If an athlete adequately meets overall energy needs and incorporates a wide variety of nutrient-dense foods, vitamin and mineral recommendations can be met through the diet. Additionally, athletes tend to eat many highly fortified "sport" foods and drinks. However, athletes competing in lean sports (for example, distance running, gymnastics, diving) or weight-restricted sports (such as wrestling, lightweight rowing) are often at risk for low or marginal intakes of the micronutrients because of restrictions of overall food intake or certain food groups.

Iron
Iron functions as a component of hemoglobin, myoglobin, cytochromes of the electron transport chain, and in some iron-dependent enzymes; therefore, iron greatly influences oxygen transport and energy metabolism. Iron-deficiency anemia decreases the capacity of skeletal muscle to consume oxygen and produce ATP. Low iron stores are a frequent finding in elite endurance athletes. Endurance athletes and all female athletes should have serum ferritin, hemoglobin, and hematocrit levels monitored to treat both depletion and iron-deficiency anemia. Athletes should be informed about the types and sources of dietary iron to prevent or augment depletion or deficiency

(Table 4). The treatment for adults with known iron-deficiency anemia often involves consumption of 100 mg/day of elemental iron for 3 months or longer, taken on an empty stomach. The iron supplement formulation can be provided as ferrous gluconate or sulfate. In addition, supplementation also may be warranted for athletes with low serum ferritin levels.

Table 4

Common Food Sources of Iron

Food	Serving Size	Iron (mg)
Fortified ready-to-eat cereals	1 oz	23.8
Fortified instant cooked cereals	1 packet	4.9-8.1
Soybeans, mature, cooked	½ cup	4.4
Pumpkin and squash seed kernels, roasted	1 oz	4.2
Lentils, cooked	½ cup	3.3
Spinach, cooked from fresh	½ cup	3.2
Beef, cooked	3 oz	3.0
Kidney beans	½ cup	2.6
Chickpeas, cooked	½ cup	2.4
Lamb	3 oz	2.3
Prune juice	¾ cup	2.3
Refried Beans	½ cup	2.1

Source: Nutrient Values from Agricultural Research Service (ARS) Nutrient Database for Standard Reference, Release 17.

Calcium

Calcium deserves attention because of the incidence of amenorrhea in female athletes, the role of calcium in bone density, and the often low to marginal dietary intake of calcium in some athletes. These combined factors place athletes at risk for compromised bone health and/or increased risk for injury.

Female athletes should be asked about current and past intake of dairy products and calcium supplements, as well as menstrual history. Female athletes should be educated about the highly bioavailable dietary sources in addition to the role that menstrual function and overall diet adequacy has on bone health (Table 5). For athletes with known compromised bone density, 1,500 mg of calcium and 800 mg of vitamin D are recommended.[4] Calcium supplementation with calcium carbonate or citrate in doses of 500 mg or less taken between meals is recommended to optimize absorption.

Issues of Body Weight and Body Composition

Athletes who desire to lose weight commonly fall into three categories: the relatively lean, the excess body fat, and rapid weight loss groups. Athletes in the relatively lean group may desire weight loss for performance enhancement or appearance. If the athlete is female and amenorrheic, she may already be restricting food intake to a point beyond which further restriction is physiologically inappropriate. It is important to discuss with the athlete why chronically maintaining a lower than natural body weight is detrimental to both health and performance. Achieving energy balance and body fat that allow normal menstrual function is warranted. Body fat and lean body mass levels are largely determined by ge-

Table 5

Calcium Content of Dairy and Nondairy Food Sources

Dairy Food			Nondairy		
Sources	Serving Size	Calcium (mg)	Sources	Serving Size	Calcium (mg)
Plain yogurt	8 oz	452	Fortified cereals	1 oz	236-1043
Romano cheese	1.5 oz	452	Soy beverage	1 cup	368
Fruit yogurt	8 oz	345	Sardines	3 oz	325
Swiss cheese	1.5 oz	336	Tofu, firm	½ cup	253
Ricotta cheese, part skim	½ cup	335	Spinach	½ cup	146
American cheese, processed	2 oz	323	Soybeans, cooked	½ cup	130
Cheddar cheese	1.5 oz	307	Oatmeal, instant, fortified	1 packet	99-110
Skim milk	1 cup	306	Cowpeas	½ cup	106
2% reduced fat milk	1 cup	285	White beans, canned	½ cup	96
Chocolate milk	1 cup	280	Rainbow trout, cooked	3 oz	73

Source: Nutrient Values from Agricultural Research Service (ARS) Nutrient Database for Standard Reference, Release 17.

netics. An attempt to maintain a level of body fat that is lower than natural levels can harm both health and performance (recurrent injury or illness, amenorrhea, and diminished strength and endurance may occur). Clinicians should be aware of pathogenic weight control behaviors (for example, overexercise, purging, and the use of diuretics or laxatives) in which athletes may engage to achieve a lower weight or level of body fat. Athletes who carry excess body fat may need to lose weight for both health reasons and performance enhancement. If training is already maximal or further aerobic exercise would compromise strength or anaerobic training, a modest (300 to 500 kcal) daily calorie reduction may be warranted. Athletes in the rapid weight loss group have little or no excess body fat but wish to lose weight to compete in a weight-restricted sport (for example, lightweight rowing or wrestling). The process of rapid weight loss is usually called "cutting" and is typically accomplished by restricting food and fluids and increasing fluid loss (for example, via sweating or spitting) for 3 to 10 days before competition. Precompetition dieting and dehydration are followed by refeeding and rehydrating after weigh-in. This practice is repeated with each competition of the season. From a performance standpoint, even an acute negative energy balance and slight dehydration (1% to 2%) can negatively impact physiologic function and body composition, including decreased lean mass in addition to muscle and liver glycogen stores.

Guidelines for the Reduction of Excess Body Fat
Clinicians should review the following guidelines with the athlete who needs or desires to lose body fat: (1) basic bioenergetics (creation of an energy deficit); (2) timing (best accomplished in the off-season); (3) average rate of weight loss (for lean and normal weight athletes, 0.5-1.0 lb/week; for an athlete with excess body fat, up to 2 lb/week); (4) realistic schedule (based on average rates of weight loss; significant results take weeks to months); and (5) methods to achieve negative calorie balance (may include food choices and/or eating behaviors and exercise).[1]

Guidelines for Lean Tissue Gain
Progressive resistance training and adequate calories are critical for weight gain. However, genetic predisposition, somatotype, maturity level, and compliance determine progress. Initially increasing caloric intake by 500 to 700 kcal/day can facilitate success by considering meal and snack frequency, diet composition, and high-calorie supplements. Meal and snack frequency usually must increase to five to nine eating occasions per day. Continuous availability of food allows an athlete to eat whenever hunger occurs or on a predetermined schedule. If food volume is maximal, the next option is to concentrate calories without adding bulk. Strategies might include adding nut butters, nuts, dried fruit, chocolate milk, 100% fruit juices, cheese, and sport drinks. Athletes should still adhere to a high-carbohydrate, low-saturated fat diet. If an athlete is un-able to increase calories to the needed level with traditional foods alone, supplements are an option. High-calorie shakes, meal replacement beverages, smoothies, or bars are useful to increase frequency of eating as well as calories. The exact supplemental products can be individualized according to the athlete's personal preference.

Nutrient Timing
Precompetition or Workout Nutrition
Preexercise meals or snacks are geared to "top-off" muscle glycogen stores before activity, prevent the onset of hunger during exercise, and optimize hydration status. Because dehydration and energy depletion are a result of a cumulative effect of failing to properly recover from training, athletes should be conscious of optimal food and fluid choices each day, not only the few hours before a training session or competition. Athletes may choose to eat a larger meal 3 to 4 hours before activity because typically this allows adequate time for digestion. Some may "graze" throughout the time before activity, and some may fear eating altogether. Overall, carbohydrates and fluids are critical in the time before exercise (**Table 3**).

Both physiologic and practical considerations can greatly influence food and fluid choices before training and competition. Having an empty stomach before competition may be desirable for athletes in contact and high-intensity sports for fear of vomiting or discomfort. Athletes should know that the protein and fat content of a meal slows gastric emptying; therefore, higher carbohydrate foods at meals and snacks on the day of competition with more moderate amounts of fat and protein are warranted. Liquid meals can replace conventional foods for athletes who report problems with solid foods before training or competition. Athletes should be encouraged to try new or unfamiliar foods in a practice situation before eating such foods on a competition day. Personal preference and toleration needs to be considered; athletes should consume foods and fluids that are well liked, well tolerated, usually eaten, and believed to result in a winning performance.

Recovery Nutrition
Recovery from strenuous exercise or competition is optimal when athletes are following a diet high in carbohydrates because glycogen stores are maximized. Recovery of muscle glycogen can occur over a 24-hour period given that adequate dietary carbohydrates are consumed. Carbohydrates (1.0-1.5 g/kg) should be consumed immediately following activity and then an additional 1.0 to 1.5 g/kg every 2 hours thereafter (**Table 3**). For muscle-damaging workouts, the addition of protein to a recovery snack or beverage is beneficial in stimulating protein synthesis.[3,5]

Ingestion of carbohydrates and protein following intense exercise has been reported to increase insulin levels, optimize glycogen resynthesis, enhance protein synthesis, and lessen the immunosuppressive effects of intense exercise. There also has been interest in the different forms of carbohydrates (such as sucrose and maltodextrin) because the different forms of carbohydrates have varying glycemic effects. However, research suggests that each of these forms of carbohydrates serve as effective sources of carbohydrates to ingest with protein in an attempt to promote postexercise anabolic responses.[5] A combination of whey and casein protein, particularly in milk, may be an effective supplement that will provide both immediate and prolonged protein synthesis.[3] A whole protein and carbohydrate supplement should be consumed within 1 hour postworkout to allow for enhanced glycogen restoration, promote an anabolic hormonal environment, and facilitate protein synthesis and positive training adaptations.

Sport Supplements

More than 90% of collegiate athletes are currently using or have experimented with nutritional supplements.[6] "Supplements" is a very loose term for a wide range of products and ingredients, including vitamins, minerals, protein, and "ergogenic aids." Supplement recommendations should be highly individualized because vitamin and mineral supplements should only be recommended when a food-based solution is not possible; products such as sport drinks, energy bars, and carbohydrate-protein drinks may be beneficial and convenient in specific situations but should not be routinely used in place of regular meals and snacks.[7] Many athletes believe that a normal diet will not suffice for optimum performance and use supplements to gain a competitive edge. Because there are literally thousands of different products and supplements, every athlete should consult with a sports medicine professional before taking any nutritional supplements.

Eating Disorders

Eating disorders carry a high degree of medical and psychiatric morbidity, especially among female athletes who engage in competitive sports where appearance is important (such as gymnastics, distance running, dance, and figure skating). However, no sport is immune from association with these disorders; neither are males, who also commonly engage in pathogenic weight control behaviors that can develop into clinical eating disorders.[8]

Although there have been great advancements in the treatment of eating disorders in athletes over the past 20 years, the best form of treatment is prevention and early management by a multidisciplinary team of physicians, mental health–care professionals, and registered dietitians. The athletic trainer or medical clinician may be the first to detect signs and symptoms of an eating disorder that should prompt further screening. The SCOFF questionnaire is a brief and memorable tool designed to detect eating disorders and facilitate treatment. It has shown excellent validity in both a clinical population and a student population, where it detected all cases of anorexia nervosa and bulimia nervosa[9] (Table 6). If there is a high index of suspicion that the patient has an eating disorder or a positive response to any of these questions, the patient should be referred for mental health consultation.[10]

The Female Athlete Triad

Current understanding of the female athlete triad encompasses the spectrums of energy availability, menstrual dysfunction, and bone mineral density (Figure 1). The extremes of this spectrum pose significant health risks to physically active girls and women, including low energy availability (with or without eating disorders), amenorrhea, and osteoporosis, alone or in combination. Previously, the triad comprised disordered eating, amenorrhea, and osteoporosis, but researchers found that these criteria did not identify all physically active females who are at risk for developing components of the triad, suggesting the importance of traits such as osteopenia and exercise-related menstrual alterations as diagnostic criteria for early detection and treatment of the triad.[11]

In 2007, the American College of Sports Medicine pronounced and updated recommendations for screening, diagnosis, prevention, and treatment of the female athlete triad through the new Position Stand, which replaces the 1997 Position Stand.[4] The new model emphasizes how each component of the triad exists on its own independent spectrum, but the spectrums are interrelated and progression along each may occur at different rates. Many female athletes may display intermediate or "subclinical" presentations of one or more of the triad conditions, and the potentially irreversible consequences of the clinical conditions emphasize the need for prevention, early detection, and treatment. Treatment should model a team approach and include a physician or other health-care provider (physician's assistant or nurse practitioner), a registered dietitian, and, for athletes with an eating disorder or disordered eating, a mental-health practitioner.

Summary

Optimal diet composition, nutrient quality, and nutrient timing strategies can best help an athlete achieve peak performance goals. Athletes often need guidance based on sound and evidence-based information to attain the proper balance of macronutrients, micronutrients, and overall energy intake. Some sports place athletes at greater risk for nutritional issues because of the aesthetic or weight-restricted nature of that particular sport. These athletes may empirically benefit from sports nutrition strategies to meet protein, calcium, iron, and essential fatty acid requirements. Many athletes also seek nutritional supplements to achieve a competitive edge. Athletes taking supplements should be supervised by a sports medicine professional.

Table 6

The SCOFF Questionnaire

1. Do you ever make yourself **S**ick because you feel uncomfortably full?

2. Do you worry you have lost **C**ontrol over how much you eat?

3. Have you recently lost more than **O**ne stone in a 3-month period?

4. Do you believe yourself to be **F**at when others say you are too thin?

5. Would you say that **F**ood dominates your life?

A score of 2 indicates possible anorexia nervosa or bulimia nervosa. (The person taking this questionnaire should give themselves one point for each question answered affirmatively.)

(Reproduced with permission from Luck AJ, Morgan JF, Reid F, et al: The SCOFF questionnaire and clinical interview for eating disorders in general practice: Comparative study. BMJ 2002;325: 755-756.)

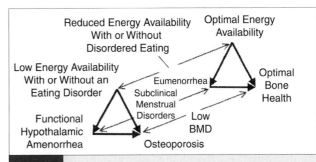

Figure 1   The female athlete triad: the spectrums of energy availability, menstrual function, and bone mineral density (BMD) along which female athletes are distributed (gray arrows). An athlete's condition moves along each spectrum at a different rate, in one direction or the other, according to her diet and exercise habits. Energy availability, defined as dietary energy intake minus exercise energy expenditure, affects bone mineral density both directly via metabolic hormones and indirectly via effects on menstrual function and thereby estrogen (black arrows). *(Reproduced with permission from Nattiv A, Loucks AB, Manore MM, et al: The Female Athlete Triad. Med Sci Sports Exerc 2007;29:1867-1882.)*

Annotated References

1. Position of Dietitians of Canada, the American Dietetic Association, and the American College of Sports Medicine: Nutrition and Athletic Performance. *Can J Diet Pract Res* 2000;61:176-192.

2. Barr SI, Rideout CA: Nutrition considerations for vegetarian athletes. *Nutrition* 2004;20:696-703.

   The quality of vegetarian diets to meet the nutritional needs and support peak performance among athletes is reviewed.

3. Elliot TA, Cree MG, Sanford AP, Wolfe RR, Tipton KD: Milk ingestion stimulates net muscle protein synthesis following resistance exercise. *Med Sci Sports Exerc* 2006;38:667-674.

   This randomized experimental study was designed to determine the response of net muscle protein balance following resistance exercise to ingestion of nutrients as components of milk. Findings included that milk ingestion stimulated net uptake of amino acids representing net muscle protein synthesis.

4. Nattiv A, Loucks AB, Manore MM, Sanborn CF, Sundgot-Borgen J, Warren MP: American College of Sports Medicine position stand: The female athlete triad. *Med Sci Sports Exerc* 2007;39:1867-1882.

   This update replaces the 1997 Female Athlete Position Stand, which updates understanding, and makes new recommendations for screening, diagnosis, prevention, and treatment of the female athlete triad.

5. Kreider RB, Earnest CP, Lundberg J, et al: Effects of ingesting protein with various forms of carbohydrate following resistance-exercise on substrate availability and markers of anabolism, catabolism, and immunity. *J Int Soc Sports Nutr* 2007;4:18.

   This randomized, double-blind study design investigated whether whey protein in combination with sucrose, maltodextrin, or honey influenced markers of anabolism and catabolism, finding that each of these forms of carbohydrate can serve as an effective source of carbohydrates to ingest with protein postexercise.

6. Froiland K, Koszewski W, Hingst J, Kopecky L: Nutritional supplement use among college athletes and their sources of information. *Int J Sport Nutr Exerc Metab* 2004;14:104-120.

   A survey was conducted to examine the source of information and usage of nutritional supplements in athletes at a Division I university. Eighty-nine percent of athletes were using supplements; in females, the use of supplements was for health reasons, whereas in men it was to improve agility, strength, or muscle/weight gain.

7. Maughan RJ, Depiesse F, Geyer H: The use of dietary supplements by athletes. *J Sports Sci* 2007;25(suppl 1): 103-113.

   This review examines the use of dietary supplements by athletes, including the risk of a positive doping result as a consequence of the presence of prohibited substances that are not declared on the label.

8. Baum A: Eating disorders in the male athlete. *Sports Med* 2006;36:1-6.

   This review examines the need for identifying and treating eating disorders in male athletes because they can be missed. Male athletes competing in weight-restricted and lean, aesthetic sports are especially at risk for eating disorders.

9. Luck AJ, Morgan JF, Reid F, et al: The SCOFF questionnaire and clinical interview for eating disorders in

general practice: Comparative study. *BMJ* 2002;325: 755-756.

10. Zerbe KJ: Eating disorders in the 21st century: Identification, management, and prevention in obstetrics and gynecology. *Best Pract Res Clin Obstet Gynaecol* 2007; 21:331-343.

This article on eating disorders discusses the benefits and limitations of contemporary treatment, special populations at risk (for example, athletes, patients with diabetes), and screening guidelines for an office practice.

11. Burrows M, Shepherd H, Bird S, MacLeod K, Ward B: The components of the female athlete triad do not identify all physically active females at risk. *J Sports Sci* 2007;25:1289-1297.

This cross-sectional investigation aimed to assess the effectiveness of the triad components (amenorrhoea, disordered eating, and osteoporosis) in identifying physically active women at risk of long-term health conditions.

Chapter 32

Sport Psychology and Mental Health Issues

David B. Coppel, PhD

7: Medical Issues

Introduction

Contemporary sport psychology has been defined as an area that explores the relationships among psychological factors and participation in sports and exercise/physical activity, and the impact of sports and exercise and physical activity on psychological development, health, and well-being over a person's life span. Sport psychologists help athletes and teams apply psychological principles to achieve improved or optimal sport performance and well-being.[1]

Efforts at sport psychology certification and proficiency have continued over several years, with the diversity of training backgrounds in sport psychology providing some controversy and conflict. The Association of Applied Sport Psychology, a multidisciplinary organization focusing on sport science, established the Certified Consultant status, which describes a consultant who provides information about the role of psychological factors in sports, exercise, and physical activity to individuals, groups, and organizations. These consultants can teach athletes specific mental, behavioral, psychosocial, and emotional skills for sports, exercise, and physical activity; consultants with clinical or counseling training also may be qualified to work with clinical disorders or issues relating to injury.

Over recent years, there has been an increase in the application of sport psychology at all levels of competition, for both performance-enhancement issues and mental health-related issues. Professional athletes have used sport psychologists over the years, and now many player associations, for example, the National Football League Players Assistance Program, have provided a variety of counseling and supportive services to athletes and their families. At the Olympic level, sport psychology has emerged as a crucial factor in athletic performance and is integrated with other sport sciences that help to prepare the athlete for Olympic competition.

Collegiate athletes and teams continue to use sport psychologists as consultants to teams, individuals, or athletic departments; clinical or counseling psychologists with specialty training and experience working with athletes also are available within university or college counseling centers. Collegiate athletes are vulnerable to the same adjustment/transition issues that all collegiate students face, and although some have built-in support systems within their team or athletic department programs, many athletes experience increasing emotional or behavioral symptoms related to pressures brought on by additional performance and athletic identity issues. High school athletes may receive some consultation or attend workshops on sport psychology. The role and value of the mental skills needed for peak athletic performance or general adjustment to competitive sports participation often are first introduced during the high school years. This information is increasingly important as athletes move upward competitively and can be applied in other life contexts; for example, skills in handling competition pressure and focus can be called upon when an athlete is experiencing test anxiety.

Sport Psychology Roles

Sport psychology also has experienced an expanding role within the field of sports medicine, as evidenced by the recent Team Physician Consensus Statement regarding the role of psychology in sports-related injuries.[2] Although psychology as a field has been linked with rehabilitation medicine (rehabilitation psychology) for decades, its potential role and contribution related specifically to sports injuries has primarily emerged as part of the multidisciplinary or interdisciplinary focus of sports medicine. The recognition that psychological factors contribute significantly to the general risk of injury, initial reactions to being injured, and attitudes and course of rehabilitation and recovery further substantiates the inclusion of the field of sport psychology with sports medicine. Furthermore, the secondary (or in some instances, primary) emotional reactions or clinical level symptoms that can emerge following injury or during recovery, such as depression, anger, anxiety, impatience, and frustration, may be best addressed by sport psychologists or licensed psychologists (or licensed mental health providers) with clinical/counseling experience/training in dealing with athletes and the athletic context/environment.

For example, physical injury can trigger depressive

reactions, and depressed athletes are likely to be at greater risk for injury. Athletic performance, at all levels, can be impacted by emotional or mental health factors and/or situational or adjustment factors. For athletes, having a greater understanding/awareness of the connections among the 3 M's (mind, mood, and movement) appears to make positive change or interventions more likely and effective. Psychologists may deal with negative or problematic cognitions with strategies for cognitive restructuring or challenging the negative thoughts; they may offer mood or affect management techniques to reduce anxiety or physiologic arousal; they may offer behavioral interventions to effect positive habit change or more adaptive behaviors. Sport psychiatry also may offer important interventions for clinical and mental health disorders in athletes.[3]

Sport Psychology and Developmental Issues in Youth Sports

Athletes in high school are as susceptible as nonathletes to a range of emotional or mental health issues. As suggested earlier, in certain instances the structure and demands of athletics may provide some protective or mediating role for certain clinical issues, such as depression, anxiety, substance abuse, or adjustment issues. However, athletic experience also may provide a context for the development of psychological difficulties. For adolescents (youth and high school sports participants), the impact of repeated failure/loss, criticism, negative peer interactions, maladaptive pressure to perform, and maladaptive parental or coach interactions may produce significant or problematic psychological consequences (for example, low self-esteem, mood lability, difficulty with impulse control and anger management, and anxiety/panic symptoms). Psychophysiological and/or somatoform effects (for example, exaggerated reports of pain or fatigue) also are noted, reflecting the manifestation of overtraining and stress.[4] In the absence of athlete-based data, the base rates for mental health issues in this high school age/developmental group must be seen as applicable for athletes and nonathletes, with the athlete's individual risk factors (negative) and mediating factors (positive) evaluated carefully. It is clear that in this age population, concerns over substance abuse, attention deficit disorder, impulse control, mood disorders, eating disorders, and anxiety must be evaluated carefully within a family and/or psychosocial context. For some athletes, sorting out the role of athletics in their lives, both the positive and the negative aspects, can provide insight about the adolescent's experiences and perceptions. It may be crucial for the sports medicine provider and/or sport psychologist to focus beyond mere return to play/performance levels and/or enhancing sport performance to the larger developmental, situational, or psychosocial issues faced by the adolescent athlete.

Of particular concern with adolescent athletes is the general trend of "professionalization" of youth sports, in which the focus of high athletic achievement becomes paramount and the environments (for example, family, training) adapt to this goal, making the enjoyment of athletics a secondary or absent goal. The role of parents and coaches in and contributions to these circumstances have been documented in newspapers and tabloids and in sport psychology literature. The pressures on high-achieving athletes are well documented and the concern over "distorted mentoring" effects is described as achievement by proxy distortion.[5] It is suggested that high-achieving youth athletes are at "risk for a broad range of neglect, boundary violation, and potential abuse in the push to achieve extraordinary success."[5] Sports medicine physicians may be positioned with athletes to recognize or evaluate if parents have distorted their role/ambition for the athletes' success.

The drive for high performance and success often has its origins in the youth sports experience. As expectations build over time, usually increasing quickly after successes, the athlete (and sometimes those associated with the athlete) may have a growing need to succeed.

Although this pressure situation can be stressful for athletes, the coping responses they choose to deal with this stress are of greater concern. In many instances, substance abuse, eating disorders, and steroid use in athletes can be seen as behavioral responses to perceived stress or pressure related to outcome focus. The focus on outcomes tends to increase as athletes move up the competitive scale (stakes or consequences are perceived as greater); in some instances, these behavioral responses continue or increase.

Sport Psychology and Collegiate Athletes

Collegiate student-athletes face the transitional adjustment issues that student nonathletes face, including adjustment to differences in living situations, academic demands or expectations, social and interpersonal situations, level of personal responsibility, and a potential shift in social supports. Incoming athletes often have to adjust to different coaching styles and interactions; some have to adjust to the new milieu where they are the proverbial small fish in a big pond. Although athletes have access to the same counseling and mental health support systems as nonathletes, athletic departments and the National Collegiate Athletic Association (NCAA) have developed several supportive programs specifically for athletes (Challenging Athletes' Minds for Personal Success, or CHAMPS); college counseling centers also may offer access to sport psychologists or other providers with experience in treating these adjustment and/or mental health issues. The NCAA's mental health handbook, *Managing Student-Athletes' Mental Health Issues*, discusses mood disorders, anxiety disorders, eating disorders, substance-related disorders, management and treatment issues, and resources.[6]

Sport Psychology and Injury

The psychological aspects of injury (including the experience of being injured and its consequences, the vulnerability, and the recovery or rehabilitation phase) are important areas in which a clinically trained sports psychologist can potentially make a valuable contribution. Sports medicine physicians and athletic trainers who recognize this contribution and make referrals for sport psychology consultation, when indicated, provide the athlete (and the team) a better chance at improved performance and overall adjustment. Referral for psychological consultation has been associated with enhanced physical recovery. The important and sometimes crucial role of psychology in treating sports-related injuries is described in the 2006 Team Physician consensus statement.[2] In the consensus statement, sports psychologists are described as being able to use training and experience to support the sports medicine team by addressing the factors (such as stress) that may influence the risk of injuries, as well as the emotional, cognitive, and behavioral factors related to feeling injured and handling recovery/rehabilitation. Some athletes with high levels of stress, low or ineffective coping skills, and inadequate social support may be at particular risk for injury and for a problematic injury response and recovery course.

Although there may be certain stages of physical recovery from a medical standpoint, the psychological efforts at coping with injury (and time frames for recovery) are more individualized and influenced by other factors, such as social support, impact on team or career, personality traits, and coping skills. The immediate postinjury phase can include shock and general emotional disorganization, with anxiety, apprehension, and uncertainty emerging during evaluation and treatment decision making. The recovery phase (or rehabilitation phase) may include impatience, anger, frustration, feelings of loss of control, and depressive symptoms; depending on team/coach policies and the circumstances, a sense of social isolation and loss of affiliation can occur. As an athlete gets closer to the return to play phase, fear of reinjury or not being at pre-injury levels of performance can emerge. This general self-doubt and rumination can undermine the athlete's confidence and focus. It is not abnormal for athletes to have emotional responses to being injured; however, if these symptoms worsen over time, such as progressing from disappointment and sadness to depression (with changes in sleep habits, appetite, and energy level), a referral to a licensed mental health provider with experience working with athletes is indicated.

Other signs of poor adjustment to injury can include exaggerated or generalized fear of reinjury, mood swings, irritability, withdrawal from significant others or social network, ruminative guilt for being injured or letting others down, increased somatic focus, general pessimism about a future in sports, or apathy. Because athletes often use their training/exercise as a coping mechanism and outlet for dealing with stress, the loss or reduction of access to this outlet because of injury can add to the emotional stress.

Sport Psychology and Clinical Disorders

Mental health issues or clinical level concerns in athletes can include varying levels of anxiety, depression, stress reactions, adjustment reactions, phobias, substance abuse, eating disorders, and burnout. All of these difficulties can be associated with sport performance decrements and often include some general decline or dysfunction in other areas of life functioning.[7]

Depression

Depressive symptoms can emerge in response to a specific event in one's life (situational), including a sense of loss, unmet expectation, worthlessness, or general disappointment; depression also can occur with no apparent precipitant and involve some predisposition to affective disorders or chemical or neurotransmitter imbalance (may be helped with antidepressant medication, but these medications can have adverse effects on athletic performance). Some athletes become depressed in response to their sport performance or situation; the sport performance level of other athletes is reduced because of depression and its consequences. A depressive condition in athletes can develop as a result of "overtraining" and often involves both the physical and psychological symptoms of depression. Athletes can become depressed in response to being injured, with the injury impacting their ability to participate or perform in their sport; for some this change in active involvement can produce significant negative self-worth or self-esteem and identity issues. Athletes' depression can be further compounded if the recovery or rehabilitation course does not go as planned or hoped, if the injury reduces the social support accessibility (out of sight, out of mind feeling), and if there is a lack of other stress reduction outlets now that sport training and participation have been reduced. Some depressive athletes (for example, those with dysthymia or low levels of depression over an extended period of time) may not report themselves as being depressed but will describe rumination, pessimism, and a reduction or loss of enjoyment in sports involvement. Bipolar disorder can involve both depressive episodes and manic or hypomanic episodes; it also may include a general dysregulation of affect. In athletes, bipolar disorder may present as extreme behavior change or self-destructive or violent behavior and may involve substance use/abuse; attention deficit disorder/attention deficit hyperactivity disorder and/or conduct disorders may be historic or concurrent. Psychological treatment by a licensed mental health professional and psychiatric consultation is often indicated.[7]

Anxiety

Feelings of anxiety in athletes can range from the continuum of "butterflies" to anxiety or panic disorders. Although most athletes report some precompetitive anxiety or apprehension, tension, nervousness, and physiologic changes, these symptoms may not meet the criteria of a diagnosable anxiety disorder. Anxiety disorders involve intense apprehension, fearfulness, the fear of losing control, physical symptoms such as palpitations, and avoidance efforts (avoidance of certain people, places, or things and mental avoidance in the form of worry). These avoidance efforts initially are made to reduce the anxiety but often create significant difficulties in life adjustment and reinforce the fear. Anxiety continuum disorders include panic disorder, generalized anxiety disorder, social anxiety disorder or social phobia, obsessive-compulsive disorder, posttraumatic stress disorder, or acute stress disorder.

Athletes with panic disorder (episodes of severe fear, fear of losing control, and physical symptoms that can result in suspected cardiac conditions or emergency department visits) often have difficulty maintaining focus or concentration, primarily because of their greater focus on anxiety or panic symptoms and sensations as they become worried about having a panic attack (anxious about being anxious); most individuals with panic disorder report a life stress event as a causative factor.

Generalized anxiety disorder involves long-standing anxiety symptoms, including rumination and worry in many (or all) spheres of life; hypervigilance to threats in the environment, in hopes of reducing bad things from happening, is a prominent symptom. Many athletes exhibit subclinical worry or perfectionism-related cognitions/behavior that can interfere with performance, but it is usually less severe and may not extend to other areas of functioning. Cognitive behavior interventions have been shown to be effective in helping athletes develop more adaptive cognitions and behaviors related to performance and other aspects of their life.

Social anxiety disorder involves the fear of evaluation in social situations; affected individuals are concerned about (or fear) poor or inadequate performance and negative evaluation. Many athletes describe competitive anxiety, but this does not usually rise to the threshold of social anxiety disorder. However, athletes with social anxiety disorder may have difficulty refocusing after distraction and have a greater negative reaction to real or perceived poor performance. In athletes with significant anxiety complaints and/or symptoms, a thorough assessment of the degree and pervasiveness of their symptoms and negative evaluation focus is strongly recommended; this assessment may involve a clinical interview and/or anxiety inventories or questionnaires. Medication may be indicated for certain patients, but psychological treatment aimed at the development of specific cognitive-behavioral coping skills should be the primary intervention.

Obsessive-compulsive disorder involves the intrusion of recurrent obsessions (thoughts, ideas, images, or impulses) and compulsions into daily functioning, creating significant difficulties. The compulsive (repetitive) behaviors serve to reduce the anxiety and distress so that the blockage of the behavior (or the thought of blockage) results in increased anxiety and decreased functioning. Athletes may have precompetitive routines or rituals, but these do not generally rise to the level of obsessive-compulsive disorder.

Posttraumatic stress disorder involves a group of symptoms emerging as an intense emotional response to an event that involved actual or possible death or injury (or as a witness to an event). Physiologic arousal symptoms include vigilance, extreme startle response, and decreased attention and concentration; individuals may reexperience symptoms from the event (flashbacks) and avoidance of all cues associated with trauma and emotional detachment. For some athletes a severe or career-ending injury may generate symptoms similar to posttraumatic stress disorder but would more likely meet criteria for acute stress disorder. Psychological or clinical sport psychological consultation/interventions are usually indicated.[8,9]

Eating Disorders/Disordered Eating

Athletic performance can be impacted by mental health conditions beyond the affective and anxiety continuum disorders. Disordered eating and/or eating disorders (such as anorexia nervosa or bulimia nervosa), while usually associated with some depressive or anxiety issues, can emerge in athletes who participate in sports that place significant focus or pressure on appearance or weight (such as figure skating, gymnastics, wrestling, and cross country running). Self-starvation or binge-purge behavior is common in athletes with these disorders, along with excessive or compulsive exercise; psychological consequences related to distortion of body image and perfectionism also can emerge. Physical effects from eating disorders include reduced physiologic functioning, lowered energy, fatigue, weakness, and dehydration. Psychological effects resulting from malnutrition can include decreased concentration, obsessional thinking, anxiety, and depression. Disordered eating can be one aspect of the female athlete triad, which also includes amenorrhea and osteoporosis; this triad requires evaluation and monitoring by sports medicine providers. Eating disorders may involve complex psychological and physiologic dynamics for individuals and respond best to a multidisciplinary sports medicine team approach.[10] Eating disorders also are discussed in chapter 31.

Substance-Related Disorders

Substance-related disorders can evolve from the use and abuse of legal, illegal, prescribed, or over-the-counter drugs. Steroid use/abuse is included in this category, with its primary objective being performance enhancement (or aiding rehabilitation or recovery from injury). Alcohol and other substances often are seen as part of the sports culture, and therefore the risk for related problems can be increased. Early educational and awareness programs may have a positive impact, but most athletes relate to the connection between their substance use and its negative impact on their sports participation or eligibility, for example, the result of a positive drug test.[11]

Attention Deficit Disorders

Attention deficit hyperactivity disorder involves symptoms related to inattention/disorganization and hyperactivity/impulsivity. Usually, symptoms emerge in childhood and may be comorbid with other adolescent disorders. Childhood symptoms can include difficulty concentrating, difficulty sitting still, excessive talking, impulsive behavior, and distractibility. Although symptoms decreases adulthood for some individuals, ongoing difficulty with focus, organization, concentration, and impulsivity can create problems in the workplace or in relationships. Athletes who have difficulty with attention, focus, or impulsivity may have difficulty with sports activities. However, the diagnosis of attention deficit hyperactivity disorder should not be made on inference, where poor performance or mistakes are attributed to inattention, or on the basis of self-reported difficulty with attention span. A thorough evaluation of history and other factors should be completed before the diagnosis is made; some schools have specific testing criteria and results they are required to qualify for accommodations related to attention deficit hyperactivity disorder (or learning disabilities). Primary treatment options for attention deficit hyperactivity disorder include behavioral interventions and medications.

Summary

Over recent years, the use of sport psychology at all levels of competition has increased in managing both performance enhancement and mental health issues. Mental health issues or clinical level concerns in athletes can include anxiety, depression, stress reactions, adjustment reactions, phobias, substance abuse, eating disorders, and burnout; these issues can be associated with sports performance decrements and decline and dysfunction in activities of daily living. Clinical sport psychologists can play an important role in supporting the team and sports medicine physician in dealing with sports-related injuries. Consultation with clinical sport psychologists can help athletes deal with subclinical and clinical issues and can potentially optimize the athletes' level of functioning in the sport and in life.

Annotated References

1. Murphy S (ed): *The Sport Psych Handbook.* Champaign, IL, Human Kinetics, 2005, pp xi-xv.

   This book contains descriptions of different roles that sport psychology can play, including dealing with injury and working with sports medicine. The increasing holistic approach to sports, in mind and body, is addressed.

2. American College of Sports Medicine, American Academy of Family Physicians, American Academy of Orthopaedic Surgeons, et al: Psychological issues related to injury in athletes and the team physician: A consensus statement. *Med Sci Sports Exerc* 2006;38:2030-2034.

   This article includes guidelines for team physicians regarding the importance and utilization of psychological issues in dealing with injury. Descriptions of the continuum of psychological responses/reactions to injury and possible interventions are offered.

3. Tofler IR, Morse ED: The interface between sport psychiatry and sports medicine. *Clin Sports Med* 2005;24:745-977.

   This article provides information from the sport psychiatry perspective and describes how psychiatry can play a role in sports medicine. Discussions of psychiatric diagnoses and the treatment of athletes, medication use, attention deficit hyperactivity disorder, suicide, aggression, and substance abuse are included.

4. Tofler IR, Butterbaugh GJ: Developmental overview of child and youth sports for the twenty-first century. *Clin Sports Med* 2005;24:783-804.

   This article describes the developmental issues that are often confronted in youth sports by children and adolescents and their parents. These issues are discussed within psychological, physical, social, and historic contexts.

5. Tofler IR, Knapp PK, Larden M: Achievement by proxy distortion in sports: A distorted mentoring of high-achieving youth. Historical perspectives and clinical intervention with children, adolescents, and their families. *Clin Sports Med* 2005;24:806-828.

   This article explores the pressure on high-achieving children in sports and the dynamics of parental roles and behavior in the pursuit of these sports goals. Vignettes and interventions are discussed.

6. Thompson R, Sherman R (eds): *Managing Student-Athletes' Mental Health Issues.* Indianapolis, IN, NCAA Publications, 2007.

   This book discusses factors related to sports participation and mental health.

7. Gardener FL, Moore ZE: *Clinical Sport Psychology.* Champaign, IL, Human Kinetics, 2006.

   This book provides an integration of clinical psychology and sport performance work and proposes a classification system for clinical sport psychologists to use in conceptualizing their work with athletes. It emphasizes the contributions of psychological perspectives in working with athletes.

8. Crossman J (ed): *Coping With Sports Injuries: Psychological Strategies for Rehabilitation.* New York, NY, Oxford University Press, 2001.

9. Brown C: Injuries: The psychology and recovery and rehab, in Murphy S (ed): *The Sport Psych Handbook*. Champaign, IL, Human Kinetics, 2005, pp 215-235.

This chapter provides an examination of the emotional and psychological aspects of athletic injury and recovery, including the impact of injury and coping strategies for recovery. The value of a treatment plan that focuses on the psychology of injury is discussed.

10. Cogan KD: Eating disorders: When rations become irrational, in Murphy S (ed): *The Sport Psych Handbook*. Champaign, IL, Human Kinetics, 2005, pp 237-253.

This chapter provides an overview of eating disorders in athletes, including their impact on the developing athlete, risk factors, etiology, identification/diagnoses, and treatment options.

11. Anshel MH: Substance use: Chemical roulette in sport, in Murphy S (ed): *The Sport Psych Handbook*. Champaign, IL, Human Kinetics, 2005, pp 255-276.

This chapter discusses the complex issues arising from the use or abuse of performance-enhancing drugs in sports, including the motives such as competitiveness, peer pressure, and self-esteem. The roles of sport psychologists, coaches, and sports organizations in controlling drug use are discussed.

Chapter 33
Cardiac Issues

David T. Bernhardt, MD

Introduction

Physical activity is promoted by health care providers because of its possible positive effects on health, including management of weight and blood pressure, insulin sensitivity, and overall well-being. However, in some individuals, vigorous physical activity increases the risk of sudden cardiac death. It is important to review preparticipation cardiac screening recommendations, common causes of sudden cardiac death, and the use of implantable cardioverter-defibrillators (ICDs) in the athlete.

Preparticipation Physical Examination and Cardiac Screening

More than 12 million athletes participate in competitive sports at the high school and collegiate levels, and these individuals often represent the pinnacle of health. Sudden cardiac death in an athlete has been defined as nontraumatic and unexpected sudden cardiac arrest that occurs within 6 hours of a previously normal state of health.[1] The dramatic, sudden, unexpected collapse and death of a young, otherwise healthy athlete is frightening to observe and is the cause of much consternation for the general public and health care providers. A stated purpose of the preparticipation physical examination (PPPE) is to detect life-threatening conditions. Recently, there has been significant debate about whether the traditional history and physical examination or the PPPE format is useful in meeting this goal.

The most recent screening guidelines are predicated on the premise that intense athletic participation may increase the risk of sudden cardiac death or disease progression in susceptible individuals.[2] The present screening guidelines rely heavily on the history provided by the patient. The 2007 American Heart Association preparticipation guidelines consist of eight personal and family history questions plus four items targeting the physical examination[2] (Table 1). Based on the experience of the health care provider and the reliability of the athlete, a positive response to one or more of the items may trigger a referral to a cardiologist for a more detailed assessment. The American Heart Association recommends repeat cardiovascular screening every 2 years with an abbreviated examination during the 2-year period. Routine diagnostic testing such as electrocardiogram (ECG), exercise testing, and echocardiograms were excluded from the American Heart Association's recommendations mainly because of cost and a lack of prospective evidence demonstrating a reduction in cardiovascular causes of sudden death. Controversy exists regarding the high rate of false positive test re-

Table 1

The 12-Element American Heart Association Recommendations for Preparticipation Cardiovascular Screening of Competitive Athletes

Medical History*

Personal History

1. Exertional chest pain/discomfort

2. Unexplained syncope/near-syncope†

3. Excessive exertional and unexplained dyspnea/fatigue, associated with exercise

4. Prior recognition of a heart murmur

5. Elevated systemic blood pressure

Family History

6. Premature death (sudden and unexpected, or otherwise) before age 50 years due to heart disease, in one or more relatives

7. Disability from heart disease in a close relative younger than 50 years of age

8. Specific knowledge of certain cardiac conditions in family members: hypertrophic or dilated cardiomyopathy, long-QT syndrome or other ion channelopathies, Marfan syndrome, or clinically important arrhythmias

Physical Examination

9. Heart murmur‡

10. Femoral pulses to exclude aortic coarctation

11. Physical stigmata of Marfan syndrome

12. Brachial artery blood pressure (sitting position)§

*Parental verification is recommended for high school and middle school athletes.
†Judged not to be neurocardiogenic (vasovagal); of particular concern when related to exertion.
‡Auscultation should be performed in both supine and standing positions (or with Valsalva maneuver), specifically to identify murmurs of dynamic left ventricular outflow tract obstruction.
§Preferably taken in both arms.

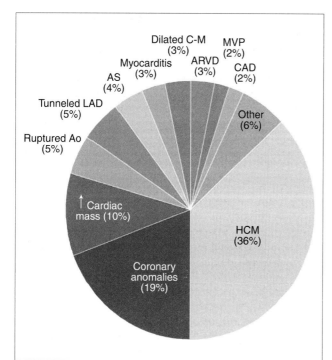

Figure 1 Causes of sudden cardiac death in young competitive athletes based on systematic tracking of 158 athletes in the United States. AO = aorta; LAD = left anterior descending coronary artery; AS = atherosclerosis; C-M = cardiomyopathy; ARVD = arrhythmogenic right ventricular dysplasia; MVP = mitral valve prolapse; CAD = coronary artery disease; HCM = hypertrophic cardiomyopathy *(Adapted with permission from Maron BJ, Shirani J, Poliac LC, Mathenge R, Roberts WC, Mueller FO: Sudden death in young competitive athletes: Clinical, demographic, and pathological profiles. JAMA 1996;276:199-204.)*

sults that such screening entails (estimated at 3% to 6% depending on the study). Given the high number of high school and college athletes in the United States, the consequences and implications of such screening must be considered.

In Italy, a legislative initiative led to a standardized screening procedure, including history, physical examination, and an ECG for all competitive athletes.[3] The screening program has been attributed as one of the reasons for the decrease in sudden cardiac death among Italian athletes. In addition, increasing numbers of athletes were identified as having cardiomyopathy.[4] The European Society for Cardiology and the International Olympic Committee recommend a 12-lead ECG for athletes younger than 35 years.[5]

Causes of Sudden Cardiac Death

Although much has been written about sudden cardiac death in athletes, the incidence of sudden death in all athletes is quite low. Most instances of sudden cardiac death in athletes younger than 35 years are related to

congenital cardiovascular diseases that result in either structural or conduction abnormalities. In the United States, the most frequent cause of death related to sports is hypertrophic cardiomyopathy; other causes include rupture of the aorta related to Marfan syndrome, aberrant coronary arteries, and myocarditis[6] (**Figure 1**). In athletes older than age 35 years, the most common etiology is coronary artery disease caused by atherosclerosis.

Athletic Heart Syndrome

Athletic heart syndrome is defined by a collection of normal structural and functional changes that occur in trained athletes. The condition is completely asymptomatic and is not associated with an increased risk for sudden cardiac death. The physiologic changes can lead to changes in diagnostic test results (for example, ECG, echocardiogram) that may indicate cardiac disease.

Repetitive exercise results in normal physiologic changes secondary to pressure and volume overload on the heart, which results in increased left ventricular muscle mass, wall thickness, and chamber size. These changes lead to increased stroke volume and cardiac output, which contribute to a lower heart rate. An alteration in autonomic feedback leads to increased vagal tone in the trained athlete that also contributes to a lower resting heart rate.

Electrocardiographic changes include sinus bradycardia and sinus dysrhythmias, including first-degree arteriovenous block. Other mild ECG changes may include ST-segment changes, T-wave changes, and increased QRS-voltage, including criteria for left and right ventricular hypertrophy.

Echocardiographic changes include increased left ventricular wall thickness with or without increased end-diastolic left ventricular volume depending on the type of dynamic versus static exercise. Left ventricular hypertrophy in the highly trained athlete usually results in concentric hypertrophy, with the left ventricular wall thickness measuring up to 13 to 16 mm. A wall thickness greater than 16 mm is suspicious for a pathologic process, including hypertrophic cardiomyopathy.

Hypertrophic Cardiomyopathy

Hypertrophic cardiomyopathy is the most common genetic cardiovascular malformation, with a prevalence of approximately 1 in 500 patients. Hypertrophic cardiomyopathy often presents as sudden cardiac death in previously asymptomatic individuals. Other symptoms that may precede sudden cardiac death include chest pain and/or dizziness with activity, or syncope. Diagnosis is based on characteristic findings seen with echocardiography, including asymmetric thickening of the left ventricular wall associated with a nondilated left ventricular cavity. Although most deaths related to hypertrophic cardiomyopathy occur while the patient is sedentary or during mild exertion, a significant percentage are associated with vigorous physical activity.[7] Athletes in whom hypertrophic cardiomyopathy is diagnosed are medically disqualified from participation in intense competitive sports with the exception of those with low static and dynamic demands, such as cricket, bowling, and golf.[2] Treatment of individuals with hypertrophic cardiomyopathy may include medications and/or placement of an ICD to reduce the risk of sudden death. Considerable controversy exists as to whether athletes with this device should be allowed to participate in competitive sports. The current Bethesda Guidelines conclude that an athlete with an ICD should not be allowed to participate in competitive sports.[8]

Aberrant Coronary Arteries

Malformation of the coronary arteries is another common cause of sudden cardiac death in the athlete. A variety of aberrant forms with a spectrum of clinical presentations, severity, and overall prognosis have been described. Most common is the anomalous origin of the right coronary artery from the left aortic sinus; anomalous origin of the left coronary artery from the right sinus occurs but is not as common. A recent study of sudden death in military recruits reported that 33% of sudden deaths related to a cardiac cause were the result of aberrant coronary arteries.[9] The mechanism related to sudden death in these scenarios is not fully understood but is at least partially related to coronary artery development, compression, or stenosis.[10] As in athletes with hypertrophic cardiomyopathy, sudden death is common in athletes with aberrant coronary arteries, although some may present with angina or syncope. Hypertrophic cardiomyopathy can be diagnosed using either transthoracic or transesophageal echocardiography, with the gold standard being traditional coronary artery angiography. The aberrant anatomy can be corrected surgically, and the athlete is allowed to return to play.

Arrhythmogenic Right Ventricular Dysplasia

Arrhythmogenic right ventricular dysplasia (ARVD) is another inheritable cardiomyopathy associated with ventricular arrhythmias and increased risk for sudden cardiac death. ARVD occurs as a result of fatty or fibrous replacement of diseased right ventricular myocardium involving either segments or diffuse portions of the right ventricle and less frequently the left ventricle. ARVD is the most common cause of sudden death among athletes in Italy and led to the mandatory screening of all athletes. Athletes may present with symptoms similar to those for hypertrophic cardiomyopathy (sudden death, syncope, or angina). MRI is the most sensitive and specific diagnostic test that may demonstrate abnormalities in right ventricle structure and function.[11] Treatment of ARVD may include medications and/or placement of an ICD. Activity restrictions are similar to those for hypertrophic cardiomyopathy.

Marfan Syndrome

Marfan syndrome is a genetic connective tissue disorder that affects many organ systems, including the cardiovascular system. Skeletal abnormalities typically include tall stature, arachnodactyly, pectus abnormalities, scoliosis, and pes planus. Other common abnormalities include myopia and mitral valve prolapse. Associated aortic root dilatation and risk of rupture increase the risk for sudden death in athletes with this condition. Athletes suspected of having Marfan syndrome should be referred for genetic and cardiology evaluation.

Myocarditis

Myocarditis is an inflammatory disease of the heart muscle characterized by inflammatory infiltrates associated with cell degeneration not related to ischemia. The most common infectious causes of myocarditis are viral and include coxsackievirus, adenovirus, and parvovirus. Noninfectious causes are usually related to medications or toxins, including lithium, doxorubicin, cocaine, alcohol, and carbon monoxide. Viral myocarditis usually resolves without complication, although progression to dilated cardiomyopathy may occur. Symptoms such as shortness of breath, chest pain, and fever may be preceded by a flulike illness. Endomyocardial biopsy is required to establish the diagnosis. The diagnostic accuracy of the biopsy is low, and immunologic evaluation may be necessary to establish the diagnosis. Athletes with a clinical diagnosis of myocarditis should be excluded from sports participation until symptoms completely resolve, at least 6 months after the onset of disease.[5,12] Final clearance for return to play should be determined by a cardiologist; some allow return to play sooner based on symptoms, normalization of laboratory tests, and diagnostic evaluation.

Wolff-Parkinson-White Syndrome

Wolff-Parkinson-White (WPW) syndrome involves pre-excitation of the ventricles caused by an accessory pathway that allows abnormal electrical communication between the atria and ventricles. Most patients with WPW syndrome will remain asymptomatic, and diagnosis will be made when a delta wave, a slurred upstroke in the QRS complex, is noted on a routine ECG. Treatment of WPW syndrome is based on risk stratification for possible tachyarrhythmias and risk of sudden cardiac death, which is quite low for most individuals with this condition. Risk stratification is usually determined by a cardiologist who has experience with electrophysiology. Individuals who demonstrate loss of the delta wave with high heart rates either associated with exercise or programmed electrical stimulation in the laboratory are believed to be at lower risk for sudden cardiac death. For patients who experience tachyarrhythmias, treatment with appropriate medication and definitive treatment with radiofrequency ablation of the electrical pathway usually is recommended.[13]

Commotio Cordis

Commotio cordis describes a condition where the heart rhythm is disturbed by sudden, low-impact, blunt trau-

7: Medical Issues

matic force in children age 13 to 16 years participating in sports. The trauma to the precordial area results in ventricular fibrillation with immediate death. Impact that occurs during a susceptible portion of the cardiac cycle just prior to the T wave peak creates the highest risk of causing the fibrillation.

Unlike with a myocardial contusion, there is very minimal damage to the heart tissue in commotio cordis. Most of the blunt trauma events are caused by baseballs, lacrosse balls, or hockey pucks. These injuries may occur even when the athlete is wearing a chest protector.

Treatment of commotio cordis is defibrillation, and the time to defibrillation has been shown to predict survival (as time to defibrillation increases, the likelihood of survival decreases). For sports with a high risk for commotio cordis, the emergency action plan should consider access to early defibrillation.

Prevention of commotio cordis has focused on safety baseballs, which are softer than regular baseballs and may reduce the risk of ventricular fibrillation in animal models.[14] In contrast, chest protectors currently used by baseball and lacrosse players have been shown to be ineffective protection against ventricular fibrillation in animal models.[15]

Implantable Cardiac Defibrillators

The ultimate cause of sudden cardiac death in many patients who experience commotio cordis and hypertrophic cardiomyopathy as well as arryhthmias is ventricular fibrillation. In some patients with a history of cardiac arrest or ventricular tachycardia, ICDs have been used to prevent recurrence. The use of these devices for the primary prevention of ventricular fibrillation in patients predisposed to this condition, such as those with genetic cardiovascular conditions, has been studied. ICDs should be considered for primary prevention when causes of ventricular fibrillation are not predictable or preventable with medication and when the risk of fibrillation is high.

The underlying condition that results in ICD placement usually requires sports restrictions in the athlete. ICD placement does not change this restriction because ventricular fibrillation is still considered a lethal rhythm that should be prevented rather than treated. The effectiveness of an ICD in treating fibrillation in the setting of intense exercise is unknown. The effect of brief impaired consciousness related to the arryhthmia is not considered desirable for sports participation and is not optimal for overall cardiac and central nervous system function.[16] Contact and collision sports are contraindicated in athletes with an ICD because of the risk of trauma to the device. Participation in sports where even a brief alteration in consciousness would be considered detrimental is also contraindicated.

Summary

Sudden cardiac death is a very rare event in athletes younger than 35 years. The inheritable conditions that cause most sudden deaths are difficult to detect through preseason screening because athletes are often asymptomatic, and physical examinations are normal. Guidelines from the European Society for Cardiology and the International Olympic Committee recommend using ECG to improve the sensitivity of screening. The application of this recommendation in the United States remains a topic of controversy. Prevention of sudden death in at-risk athletes may be possible through the use of an ICD, although continued athletic ability usually is not recommended. Emergency action planning is important in preparing for the treatment of sudden collapse associated with ventricular arrhythmias.

Annotated References

1. Maron BJ, Epstein SE, Roberts WC: Causes of sudden death in competitive athletes. *J Am Coll Cardiol* 1986; 7:204-214.

2. Maron BJ, Thompson PD, Ackerman MJ, et al: Recommendations and considerations related to preparticipation screening for cardiovascular abnormalities in competitive athletes: 2007 update. A scientific statement from the American Heart Association Council on Nutrition, Physical Activity and Metabolism: Endorsed by the American College of Cardiology Foundation. *Circulation* 2007;115:1643-1655.

   This consensus statement from the American Heart Association addresses the benefits and limitations of screening for the early detection of cardiovascular abnormalities in athletes and updates the 1996 consensus statement.

3. Pelliccia A, Maron BJ: Preparticipation cardiovascular evaluation of the competitive athlete: Perspectives from the 30-year Italian experience. *Am J Cardiol* 1995;75: 827-829.

4. Corrado D, Basso C, Rizzoli G, et al: Does sport activity increase the risk of sudden cardiac death in adolescents and young adults? *J Am Coll Cardiol* 2003;42:1959-1963.

   The authors report a 21-year prospective cohort study of all young people in the Veneto Region of Italy showing an incidence rate of cardiac death among athletes of 2.3 in 100,000 persons. Sports activity was associated with an increased risk of sudden death in those with underlying cardiovascular disease.

5. Corrado D, Pelliccia A, Bjornstad HH, et al: Cardiovascular pre-participation screening of young competitive athletes for prevention of sudden death: Proposal for a common European protocol. Consensus statement of the Study Group of Sport Cardiology of the Working Group of Cardiac Rehabilitation and Exercise Physiology and the Working Group of Myocardial and Pericar-

dial Diseases of the European Society of Cardiology. *Eur Heart J* 2005;26:516-524.

This consensus statement from the European Society of Cardiology takes into account the 25-year Italian experience on systematic preparticipation screening and highlights the key role of the ECG for identification of cardiovascular diseases that increase the risk of sudden death during sports participation.

6. Maron BJ, Shirani J, Poliac LC, et al: Sudden death in young competitive athletes: Clinical, demographic and pathologic profiles. *JAMA* 1996;276:199-204.

7. Maron BJ, Doerer JJ, Haas TS, et al: Profile and frequency of sudden death in 1,463 young competitive athletes: From a 25-year US national registry, 1980-2005. *Circulation* 2006;114(suppl II):830.

The authors of this research abstract reported epidemiology and etiology of sudden cardiac death in young athletes from the US National Registry.

8. Maron BJ, Zipes DP: 36th Bethesda Conference: Eligibility recommendations for competitive athletes with cardiovascular abnormalities. *J Am Coll Cardiol* 2005;48:1-64.

9. Eckart RE, Scoville SL, Campbell CL, et al: Sudden death in young adults: A 25-year review of autopsies in military recruits. *Ann Intern Med* 2004;141:829-834.

The authors reviewed causes of sudden death among military recruits from 1977 to 2001. Exercise was reported to be associated with sudden death in 86% (108 of 126 patients). The cause of sudden death was unexplainable in 35% (44 of 126 patients).

10. Angelini P: Coronary artery anomalies: An entity in search of an identity. *Circulation* 2007;115:1296-1305.

Presentation, pathophysiology, and possible treatment options for a diverse group of abnormal coronary artery anatomic variants were reviewed.

11. Tandri H, Macedo R, Calkins H, et al: Role of magnetic resonance imaging in arrhythmogenic right ventricular dysplasia: Insights from the North American arrhythmogenic right ventricular dysplasia (ARVD/C) study. *Am Heart J* 2008;155:147-153.

The authors reviewed the role of cardiovascular MRI in the diagnosis of ARVD.

12. Basso C, Carturan E, Corrado D, et al: Myocarditis and dilated cardiomyopathy in athletes: Diagnosis, management, and recommendations for sport activity. *Cardiol Clin* 2007;25:423-429.

The authors reviewed myocarditis and its etiology, diagnosis, and role in sudden death in young athletes and activity recommendations.

13. Tischenko A, Fox DJ, Yee R, et al: When should we recommend catheter ablation for patients with Wolff-Parkinson-White syndrome? *Curr Opin Cardiol* 2008;23:32-37.

The authors reviewed indications for catheter ablation in WPW syndrome.

14. Link MS, Maron BJ, Wang PJ, et al: Reduced risk of sudden death from chest wall blows (commotio cordis) with safety baseballs. *Pediatrics* 2002;109:873-877.

15. Weinstock J, Maron BJ, Song C, et al: Failure of commercially available chest wall protectors to prevent sudden cardiac death induced by chest wall blows in an experimental model of commotio cordis. *Pediatrics* 2006;117:e656-e662.

Ventricular fibrillation was induced in control subjects and chest-protected juvenile swine models subjected to a 40-mph baseball or lacrosse ball striking the chest during the vulnerable period of repolarization. There was no statistical difference in the rate of inducible ventricular fibrillation between the two groups.

16. Heidbuchel H: Implantable cardioverter defibrillator therapy in athletes. *Cardiol Clin* 2007;25:467-482.

ICD use among athletes as a primary and secondary prevention of sudden cardiac death was reviewed.

Chapter 34

Infectious Disease in Athletes

Karl B. Fields, MD, CAQSM   Mark Rowand, MD   Kristen Samuhel, MD

Introduction

Infectious disease is one of the most common reasons why athletes miss competition.[1] Although athletes are healthy in general, there are certain infectious diseases for which sports participation increases risk. It is important to review some of these specific diseases, their relationship to sports participation, the appropriate treatment of an athlete, and guidelines for return to sport.

Key factors that affect the likelihood of the development of a specific infection in an athlete include the physiologic stress of training for the event, mechanical irritations that occur during performance of a sport, exposure to environmental irritants, and crowding or skin contact with other athletes who are infected. Typical examples include the athlete who trains numerous hours but is unable to resist common infections because of inadequate rest; the contact or collision sport athlete with skin abrasions who is then exposed to another athlete with a bacterial viral or fungal infection; the swimmer or triathlete who ingests infectious agents or whose mucus membranes or skin is infected by contaminated water; the athlete with asthma who already has underlying respiratory tract inflammation and then runs distance races in air of poor quality, becoming susceptible to upper or lower respiratory infection; and the cyclist who has constant vibratory pressure from the bicycle seat and then develops a prostatitis, possibly triggered by tissue contusion.

Epidemiologic studies of marathon runners have been able to correlate clinical outcomes and infectious disease risk of upper respiratory infections with the phases of training and preparation for a marathon event. Similar data exist for other sports with stressful training programs, such as swimming. In addition to the epidemiologic data, studies of laboratory markers such as secretory antibody in saliva, natural killer cell activity, and the ability of white blood cells to respond to infectious threats in vitro have shown varying degrees of depressed immune responses in athletes who are at their most stressful phase of training.[2,3] Not all studies confirm this theory, and longitudinal follow-up of 20 elite distance runners in a study at the Australian Institute of Sport failed to show a correlation between training distance or intensity and incidence of respiratory infection.[4] In elite rowers, results failed to show a correlation of the immune parameters to upper respiratory infection outcomes.[2] These types of studies raise questions about the direct correlation between training stress, immunosuppression, and the occurrence of greater numbers of infections. One reason for this is that other confounding factors may also elevate infectious risk. For example, in marathon runners the risk of an upper respiratory infection for the first 2 weeks after a marathon increases twofold to fourfold. This increase could readily be ascribed to the immunosuppression that takes place from maximal effort. However, other studies of air quality also show a marked increase in upper respiratory infections after marathons that take place with poor air quality. During 1 hour of vigorous running, an elite marathon competitor will have a respiratory turnover equal to what a sedentary person would experience in 24 hours. The exposure to air pollutants, particulate matter, and pollens is dramatically increased during vigorous, prolonged distance running. This exposes the lungs to an extremely high risk of inflammatory changes. Similar concerns exist for swimmers who train in pools with excessive chlorination. Data have shown an increase in asthmatic events among swimmers in pools with high chlorine concentrations,[5] which also potentially increases the risk of upper respiratory infections. It is questioned whether the increased infection risk after a strenuous marathon is related to immunosuppression, lung inflammation, or a combination of these factors.

Another key concern is the risk of transmission of infectious disease in a particular sport. For example, wrestling has drawn the most attention to infectious disease of the skin. Numerous outbreaks of herpes gladiatorum have been documented in association with wrestling competitions, and have been severe enough to mandate temporary suspension of wrestling seasons. For this reason, guidelines that mandate the time of treatment and the type of occlusive dressing that a wrestler must use to return to competition are a standard for collegiate and high school wrestling in the United States. These guidelines for preventing skin transmission have generally been applied to other sports. However, wrestling continues to take the most aggressive approach to identifying and treating skin infections before competition.

Influenza outbreaks that spread among team members in sports such as basketball have led some schools to take an aggressive approach to vaccination before the influenza season. Similarly, the exclusion of athletes with untreated conjunctivitis, fever above 100.4°F, frequent coughing episodes, or an infectious rash are typical measures for preventing contagion in most sports. The key for most team physicians is early identification of a potentially contagious infection so that appropriate exclusion, treatment, or prophylaxis of uninfected teammates can take place.

When choosing a therapy, team physicians also should consider that adverse effects of particular medications could complicate performance. One example is doxycycline, which is effective for bacterial upper respiratory infections and community-acquired pneumonia but also is a sun sensitizer and may increase sunburn risk for skiers or other athletes competing in sunny conditions. In addition, recent case reports have led the Food and Drug Administration to require fluoroquinolone antibiotics to carry a black box warning for potential tendon rupture. Physicians should be cautious about the use of medications in athletes and should inform them of risks and adverse side effects of prescribed medications. Several medications such as amoxicillin-clavulanic acid combinations and clindamycin potentially cause diarrhea, which could increase risk of dehydration and impair an athlete's ability to participate.

The team physician should be confident that the risk to the individual teammates or competitors is minimal before deciding an athlete can return to play with an infectious condition. For the athlete given a specific treatment course, the physician's clinical judgment regarding the response to treatment guides the return-to-play decision unless there are specific written guidelines by the sport association. Rarely will an athlete be able to participate effectively if they have anything more than minimal temperature elevation. The athlete with cough, congestion, and impairment of respiratory function may not be at great risk but is also unlikely to perform at their best. The decision about which athletes participate is first about safety; the team physician should next offer advice about whether participation is practical.

Eye, Ear, Nose, and Throat Infections

Conjunctivitis

Conjunctivitis is the most common cause of red eye but traumatic irritation, keratitis, iritis, and glaucoma must be considered in atypical cases. Leading causes are allergic, chemical, and infectious agents. In young athletes, bacterial infections play a significant role. Bacterial infections affect both eyes in approximately 40% of patients and typically cause a purulent discharge that mats the eyelids and often makes them stick together in the morning. Profuse, purulent discharge should raise the suspicion of gonococcal conjunctivitis, a serious infection requiring aggressive therapy and consultation.[6]

In older athletes, viral infection is the most likely etiology of conjunctivitis. Viral conjunctivitis typically becomes bilateral in 24 to 48 hours. The discharge may be profuse but is more watery or lightly colored than that seen in bacterial infections. Both bacterial and viral conjunctivitis are highly infectious. Direct contact with an infected person, infected clothing, or sports equipment all potentially spread the pathogens. One viral type termed epidemic keratoconjunctivitis is particularly virulent, leading to foreign body sensation and a marked drop in visual acuity. Individuals with epidemic keratoconjunctivitis have an associated keratitis that potentially could damage vision. Severe symptoms that occur with a suspected viral infection become part of the differential and may warrant ophthalmologic consultation.

When the team physician determines that the infectious conditions are the result of viral or bacterial causes, the athlete should be held from competition in contact and collision sports until the team physician determines that they no longer pose a risk. Documented outbreaks of conjunctivitis from adenovirus have occurred in swimming pools and in freshwater lakes.[7] For this reason exclusion criteria also apply to swimmers and water sports athletes.

No specific treatment exists for most viral conjunctivitis (herpes gladiatorum is the exception), but fortunately the condition typically is self-limiting and lasts for 5 to 7 days. Bacterial infections can be treated with drops or ointments of standard antibiotic preparations. Allergic conjunctivitis does not require exclusion, but standard treatments with topical antihistamines, nonsteroidal anti-inflammatory drugs, and other allergy medications may allow the athlete to recover from symptoms.

Otitis Externa

Otitis externa, or swimmer's ear, occurs in water sports and has an increased frequency in sports in which mechanical trauma may occur, such as surfing, sailboarding, kayaking, and skiing. Polluted water can lead to infection in athletes participating in any water sport including swimming.[8] Water with high bacterial counts, particularly from typical waterborne pathogens such as *Pseudomonas*, gets into the ear canal and can lead to infection if there is any break in the skin barrier protection.

Treatment with drops that contain a combination of antibiotic and corticosteroid resolve most cases in 5 to 7 days. More resistant cases may be treated using cotton wicks usually soaked with a fluoroquinolone antibiotic drop. Once the acute infection clears, treatment with acidic agents or drying agents after water exposure may lessen the risk of recurrence. Heat from a hair dryer blown into the external ear canal facilitates drying and is an adjunct to treatment. Although exclusion from water sports is not required, refraining from water exposure for a few days may help speed resolution.

7. Medical Issues

Otitis Media

Upper respiratory infections often block normal eustachian tube functions, preventing the middle ear from ventilating, equalizing pressures, or clearing secretions. Bacterial overgrowth occurs on retained fluid or the virus itself may lead to excessive fluid retention. For this reason middle ear infections most commonly occur following viral upper respiratory infections. Athletes report ear pain and sometimes have fever, loss of equilibrium, or both. In children, treatment with antibiotics or with an antihistamine decongestant combination provide small treatment benefits according to the evidence-based analysis done for the Cochrane database.[9] Data do not support the use of antihistamines alone. There is not sufficient evidence to weigh the benefit of specific medications in the treatment of adolescents or older athletes.

The biggest risk to sports participation occurs in athletes who require good balance and have the symptom of disequilibrium. Equestrian sport, biking, gymnastics, and rock climbing are examples of activities in which altered balance from the infection would pose a risk. Treatment with an antihistamine that affected alertness or altered reaction time would also affect sports participation. Another specific risk is that for individuals with otitis media, diving even to levels as shallow as 6 feet increases the risk of tympanic membrane rupture. Otherwise, athletes without significant fever or intolerable treatment side effects can participate in other types of sport.

Group A Streptococcal Pharyngitis

Although most sore throats are caused by viral syndromes, team physicians particularly want to identify the athlete with streptococcal pharyngitis or mononucleosis.

The peak incidence of group A streptococcal (GAS) disease occurs in younger athletes age 5 to 15 years. Winter and spring are higher risk times. Particularly with indoor sports, spread by aerosolized droplets during close contact suggests that early identification and treatment can lessen the number of teammates likely to develop the infection. Unfortunately, clinical criteria based on physical examination alone have not helped identify GAS with accuracy. Clinical decision rules based on the Centor criteria coupled with rapid GAS antigen testing have proven the most useful strategy for identifying the likely GAS patient.[10,11] The Centor criteria are tender anterior cervical nodes, tonsillar exudates, fever by history, and absence of cough. When three or four of these criteria are negative, the predictive value approximates 80%. On the other hand, the positive predictive value is in the range of 50% even when three or four critieria are met. Thus the athlete with two, three, or four criteria can be considered for screening with a rapid GAS test. Those with positive tests would be treated with antibiotics because the sensitivity of rapid tests approaches 90% and the specificity is now 90% to 100%.

Treatment of GAS has remained the same for many years, with penicillins and oral cephalosporins the most effective antibiotic treatment. Oral penicillin is the drug of choice. Erythromycin is recommended for the patient who is allergic to penicillin. Amoxicillin has advantages over penicillin in that the taste is much more tolerable for younger athletes, a shorter course of 6 days is possible, and it penetrates the middle ear well for those who have concomitant otitis media.[12,13] In a large meta-analysis of adult patients, oral cephalosporins appear to slightly outperform penicillins in the treatment of GAS. The treatment failure rate was only 50% of that seen with penicillin.[14]

More common treatment mistakes include primary prescribing of macrolide drugs for treatment of GAS. Azithromycin has shown effectiveness for short course, 5-day treatment. However, resistance to macrolides in GAS has steadily increased and affects the entire class of drugs. The most appropriate use of this class would be in the patient allergic to penicillin or for the use of clindamycin in eradication of the carrier state. Tetracyclines, quinolones, and other oral antibiotics are not indicated for the treatment of GAS.

In the athlete with GAS, the most severe symptoms often resolve within 24 to 48 hours. Because this is typical of the clinical course, the team physician can often start antibiotic treatment and return the individual to practice and even competition sometimes as early as 24 to 48 hours. However, if symptoms and fever persist, return to activities should be delayed. A reasonable general guideline is to suggest 1 to 2 easy days of practice for every day the individual had significant fever.

Infectious Mononucleosis

Infectious mononucleosis is the other type of pharyngitis that most affects sports participation. Mononucleosis typically spreads through close contact and particularly salivary contact. Otherwise, the infection is not highly contagious; roommates of college students who have mononucleosis do not show an increased risk of contracting the disease. However, close contact such as sharing water bottles and participating in team sports do pose potential risks. The incidence in Caucasians age 15 to 24 years may be 30 times that of African Americans.

Clinical features of the disease include the triad of pharyngitis, posterior cervical adenopathy, and fever. More than 90% of affected athletes have this constellation of findings. The other key symptom that directly affects athletes is fatigue. In most cases the fatigue begins to resolve by 21 days. However, persistent fatigue that takes as long as 6 months to resolve develops in a small subset of individuals. Although this clinical picture affects most patients, a wide variety of clinical findings may arise with mononucleosis, including rash, splenomegaly, neurologic changes, hepatitis, and involvement of almost any organ system.

Screening testing for mononucleosis includes a complete blood count and differential. The key finding that suggests the presence of infection is an absolute lymphocytosis, in which lymphocytes and atypical lymphocytes constitute more than 50% of the cells in the differential.

A confirmatory test is the monospot or other rapid tests for heterophil antibodies. These tests have excellent sensitivity and specificity approaching 85% and 100%, respectively. This type of test also can be repeated after 1 week when the initial test is negative but the physician still has strong clinical suspicion of mononucleosis. Tests can be negative very early in the infectious process. When individuals with suspected mononucleosis and repeat negative monospot tests require diagnostic confirmation, clinicians can order additional Epstein-Barr virus-specific antibody tests. For example, immunoglobulins G and M antibodies for Epstein-Barr viral capsid antigen show a sensitivity and specificity of 94% and 97%, respectively.

Team physicians should be aware that several conditions can cause athletes to experience symptoms or syndromes similar to mononucleosis that are not distinguishable on clinical features. The most common of these is cytomegalovirus. Toxoplasmosis and human immunodeficiency virus (HIV) sometimes present with features suggestive of mononucleosis. In addition, monospot tests occasionally are positive in patients with lymphoma, leukemia, pancreatic cancer, systemic lupus erythematosus, rubella, and HIV. Infectious disease consultation may be useful in cases that simply do not fit the standard pattern or fail to resolve after a reasonable time frame.

After establishing that an athlete has mononucleosis, the team physicians should monitor the patient's clinical status to decide when return to sport is feasible. In general, athletes have significant fatigue during the first 2 weeks of the illness. Although normal activities and school attendance are still reasonable, even light training may slow recuperation. Most athletes with mononucleosis can begin light to moderate training and sports activity approximately 3 weeks after the onset of their symptoms. In general, physicians suggest a delay of return to contact sports for 4 weeks. This time frame is based on evidence that most splenic ruptures occur on days 4 to 21 of the illness. Only a very few cases have occurred later than 28 days. Persistent fatigue also should slow the return to sport. Other complications such as hemolytic anemia, thrombocytopenia, myocarditis, and neurologic symptoms delay return to activity. Individuals with mononucleosis-related hepatitis with elevated liver functions, right upper quadrant pain, or hepatomegaly also have a potential risk of organ damage; the safest approach is to wait for these symptoms to resolve before return to sport.

The risk of splenic rupture and mononucleosis in contact sports is based on numerous case reports in football, rugby, soccer, and other sports. Large case series nevertheless suggest that approximately 50% of splenic ruptures occur spontaneously and not because of contact. Physical examination unfortunately has not

been able to consistently detect enlarged spleens. The use of ultrasound to measure splenic size as a way to return an athlete to early contact is questionable at best. One study of 631 collegiate athletes showed that 7% had spleens longer than 13 cm. All of these individuals would meet the criteria for splenomegaly and disqualification from sports activity even though they were not ill or symptomatic. This study indicates the need to establish normal splenic size in athletes based on height, gender, and even race before ultrasound is used to guide clinical decision making.[15]

A final frustrating aspect in the treatment of mononucleosis is that no medications have been consistently beneficial. Corticosteroids are used to treat complications including airway obstruction, hemolytic anemias, myocarditis, and thrombocytopenia. However, neither corticosteroids nor the antiviral agent acyclovir have had results better than placebo in controlled clinical trials. Therefore, treatment focuses on symptomatic relief.[16] Key recommendations for mononucleosis are summarized in **Table 1**.

Pulmonary Infections

Bronchitis

Bronchitis in athletes typically results from a viral infection accompanied by a persistent cough and sometimes low-grade fever. The viruses most commonly implicated in outbreaks of bronchitis include respiratory syncytial virus, rhinovirus, influenza A and B, coronavirus, and other typical viruses affecting the upper respiratory system. Evidence for bacterial causes of acute bronchitis in adults without tracheal trauma is scant and not supported by the multiple epidemiologic studies of this disease. However, antibiotics are prescribed to 60% to 70% of individuals who seek medical care for acute bronchitis.

Viral bronchitis requires only symptomatic care, but influenza A, *Mycoplasma pneumoniae*, *Chlamydophila* (formerly *Chlamydia*) *pneumoniae* and *Bordetella pertussis* are some forms of acute bronchitis that are amenable to treatment. Probably the most important bronchial infection that affects sports participation is influenza A. Cough, high fever, purulent sputum, and systemic symptoms characterize the patient with influenza A. Rapid antigen tests now allow early identification of this infection; when treatment is instituted in the first 48 hours, the course of illness can be shortened by approximately 24 hours. The tests have reasonable sensitivity and specificity in the 70% to 90% range. The two agents approved for treating patients with positive test results are oseltamivir and zanamivir.

Although influenza vaccine remains the primary method of lowering the risk of influenza A, oseltamivir and zanamivir can be used for prophylaxis. Studies of efficacy show significant reduction of subsequent influenza infection in close contacts of the index case. The cost effectiveness of this approach has been questioned, but in the midst of a busy sports season the team physician can offer this option to unimmunized athletes exposed to influenza A.

How frequently should the physician consider treating the athlete with bronchitis for the atypical infections caused by *Mycoplasma, Chlamydophilia,* or pertussis? The most generous of epidemiologic estimates suggest that *Mycoplasma* and *Chlamydophilia* would not exceed 5% and less than 1% of the pathogens isolated in acute bronchitis and pertussis, respectively. These estimates are supported by meta-analysis of treatment trials in acute bronchitis that show minimal if any efficacy for the various antibiotics tested, including doxycycline, erythromycin, azithromycin, or trimethoprim-sulfamethoxazole. Any improvements noted (for example, shortening of cough by 0.6 days) have been negated by the frequency of adverse effects from the antibiotics.

Pneumonia

Pneumonia is a lower respiratory infection that has classic symptoms such as fever, tachypnea, and cough. Confirmation of pneumonia requires documentation with chest radiograph demonstrating interstitial or alveolar infiltrates. Physical examination often demonstrates an increase in respiratory rate, increased work of breathing, rales, rhonchi, or signs of consolidation on auscultation examination. In the younger athlete these findings strongly suggest pneumonia, although the differential diagnosis still must include pulmonary embolus, malignancy, collagen vascular disease, and atelectasis.

Pneumonia arises from viral, bacterial, and fungal pathogens. Although bacterial pneumonia may affect as many as 3% of adults who enter a primary care facility with respiratory disorders, the number of athletes developing a typical bacterial pneumonia is quite small. Atypical organisms such as *M pneumoniae* and *C pneumoniae* probably cause most significant pneumonias in younger athletes. The exception to this would be athletes with other chronic illness, particularly those who have moderate to severe asthma. These individuals would be more likely to have pneumonia caused by agents such as *Streptococcus pneumoniae, Haemophilus influenzae* and even *Staphylococcus*. Because of its relative resistance to most antibiotics, methicillin-resistant *Staphylococcus aureus* (MRSA) poses a risk for causing severe pneumonia even in otherwise healthy young athletes.[17]

Unless the athlete with pneumonia has typical generalized viral symptoms or rapid resolution of symptoms and a relatively mild clinical course, antibiotic treatment appropriate to cover the organisms seen in community-acquired pneumonia is warranted. Because most athletes are healthy hosts, oral antibiotic treatment usually leads to dramatic improvement in clinical symptoms within 72 hours. Acceptable choices for treatment of uncomplicated community-acquired pneumonia include azithromycin, clarithromycin or doxycy-

Table 1

Mononucleosis: Nine Key Recommendations*

Supportive care is standard treatment. (B)
Splenic rupture risk: 0.1% to 0.5% of cases (C)
Physical examination is a poor predictor of splenic size. (A)
One-time imaging of the spleen has limited utility. (B)
Ultrasound is the preferred modality for imaging to confirm splenic enlargement. CT examination is the preferred test for evaluating splenic rupture. (B)
Splenic imaging is not helpful in managing athletes with mononucleosis. (B)
Return to light activity generally can begin at 3 weeks after onset of symptoms but should be delayed for persistent symptoms or signs. (C)
Contact/collision sports: A minimum of 3 weeks delay following symptoms for return to play reduces risk of splenic rupture and longer time likely reduces risk. (C)
Premature return to activity may prolong symptoms and be associated with decreased performance. (C)

*Strength of recommendation shown in parentheses
(Reproduced with permission from Putukian M, O'Connor FG, Stricker P, McGrew C, Hosey RG, Gordon SM, et al: Mononucleosis and athletic participation: An evidence-based subject review. Clin J Sports Med 2008;18:309–315.)

cline. All of these cover the atypical pathogens well and have some activity against *Pneumococcus*, which is the next most common bacterial pathogen. Although quinolone antibiotics are generally effective against community-acquired pneumonia, emerging resistance to these antibiotics has led to recommendations against their routine use in treating pneumonia. Athletes too sick to be treated as outpatients are referred for standard inpatient therapies for adult pneumonia or pediatric pneumonia.

Return to play after pneumonia is significantly more delayed than for other respiratory infections. This relates to the fact that pneumonia causes tissue damage in the lung parenchyma and reflects a more significant level of end organ infection. Rarely will the individual recover sufficiently to effectively return to sport in less than 2 weeks.[18] More significant pneumonias, which cause greater lung damage, would further delay return to sport. The key to the decision of when the athlete can actually compete depends on functional testing to demonstrate that the athlete can tolerate the activity level required.

Blood-Borne Infections

Hepatitis B

Hepatitis B is a DNA virus that attacks the liver. The number of new infections per year has declined from 260,000 in the 1980s to 60,000 in 2004, presumably because of universal vaccination of children against hepatitis B. There are an estimated 1.25 million Americans with chronic hepatitis B infection; 30% of those

7: Medical Issues

infected have no symptoms. Symptoms of acute infection include jaundice, loss of appetite, abdominal pain, nausea and vomiting, and fatigue. Chronic infection develops in approximately 6% of persons infected after age 5 years, and of those patients 15% to 25% will die from chronic liver disease. Chronic liver disease can lead to cirrhosis of the liver, liver cancer, liver failure, and death.

Hepatitis B is primarily spread through the blood via parenteral exposure to blood and blood products, sexual contact, contamination of mucous membranes or open wounds with infected blood, as well as perinatally to a fetus or infant from an infected mother. The hepatitis B virus has a much higher concentration in the blood than HIV, and is also more stable in the environment. Estimates of infectivity from a needle stick range from 2% to 40%, depending on whether hepatitis E antigen is present. In comparison, the HIV rate of infectivity from a needle stick is 0.2% to 0.5%.[19] Hepatitis B is 50 to 100 times more infective than HIV.[20] The hepatitis B virus is resistant to alcohol and some detergents, and has been shown to persist on surfaces for more than 7 days.[21] As a result, sports participation may pose a risk for transmission of hepatitis B.

One study reported transmission in a high school sumo wrestling club in which hepatitis B developed in 5 of 10 members of the team in 1 year, with the source being one hepatitis E antigen asymptomatic carrier.[22] In another study of transmission in an American football team, there were 11 new cases of hepatitis B infection on the team during a 19-month period.[23] This represented 20% of the team, which was a significant difference in comparison with a group of nonfootball players (1.8%, $P < 0.001$) over the same period. An asymptomatic carrier of hepatitis B antigen on the team was considered the source. Both articles postulated that contamination was caused by exposure of open wounds and cuts. A recent study examined 70 male Olympic wrestlers.[24] None of the wrestlers were hepatitis B surface antigen positive, but 13% did have hepatitis B virus DNA detected via polymerase chain reaction in their blood. Furthermore, 11% of the wrestlers had hepatitis B virus DNA detected in their sweat via polymerase chain reaction, suggesting the possibility that hepatitis B can be transmitted via sweat.

Hepatitis B is best prevented by the hepatitis B vaccine. The vaccine is 95% effective in preventing chronic hepatitis in children and adults who do not have hepatitis B.[20] The American Academy of Pediatrics recommends that all athletes be vaccinated against hepatitis B if possible.[25] Sharing of razors, toothbrushes, or other personal care items that may have blood on them should be avoided. Intravenous drug use should be avoided, and recommended health practices should be followed during tattooing and body piercing to decrease the risk of transmission. The efficacy of latex condoms in preventing hepatitis B transmission is unknown, but they are still recommended because their use might reduce transmission.[26]

The treatment of acute hepatitis B is primarily supportive care because of the low risk of the development of chronic hepatitis B. Patients with chronic hepatitis B are treated with adefovir, dipivoxil, interferon alfa-2b, lamivudine, entecavir, telbivudine, or pegylated interferon alfa-2a.[26] These individuals usually have symptoms that limit activity levels.

Human Immunodeficiency Virus

HIV is a blood-borne pathogen that can be transmitted through contact with blood or blood products, sexual contact, or by contamination of a wound or mucous membrane with infected blood. The risk of transmission is much lower than in hepatitis and the risk of transmission through sports participation is extremely minimal (based on questionable case reports.) Some states require testing for some sports such as boxing. Prevention of transmission relies on universally accepted precautions and other measures such as those used to prevent the spread of hepatitis.[27,28] The joint statement of the American Medical Society for Sports Medicine (AMSSM) and the American Orthopaedic Society for Sports Medicine (AOSSM) provides additional information regarding HIV in sports.

Gastrointestinal Infections

Diarrhea

Infectious causes of acute diarrhea are very common and can spread quickly. Athletes with diarrhea must be monitored closely because dehydration is a common complication. Acute infectious diarrhea is most frequently transmitted through the fecal-oral route, and food and water sources contaminated with the infectious microorganisms can cause the rapid spread of illness. The major causes of acute infectious diarrhea are viruses, bacteria, and parasites. Acute, self-limiting diarrhea is most often caused by viral infections. The Centers for Disease Control and Prevention estimates that norovirus infection is the cause of 23 million cases of acute gastroenteritis in the United States annually.

The first steps in the evaluation of a patient with acute diarrhea are a history and physical examination to identify the possible causes, assess the severity of the illness, and determine the need for rehydration. Important information to gather in the history includes systemic symptoms such as fever, the presence of blood or pus in the diarrhea, recent travel, sick contacts, recent food and water sources, recent antibiotic use, and any chronic disease or immunocompromised state. The physical examination should primarily focus on determining the degree of dehydration and the need for rehydration. Examination of vital signs, orthostatic blood pressures and pulses, skin turgor, mucous membranes, and abdominal examination all are key components of the physical examination. Laboratory work is rarely needed and is guided by the history. Bloody stools warrant stool culture to look for *Shigella*, *Salmonella*, and

Table 2

Escherichia coli: Sources and Clinical Symptoms

Organism	Source	Clinical Symptoms
Enterotoxigenic *E coli*	Food products, water	Watery diarrhea
Enterohemorrhagic *E coli*	Undercooked beef	Hemorrhagic colitis Hemolytic uremic syndrome
Enteropathogenic *E coli*	Water	Diarrhea in infants/toddlers
Enteroinvasive *E coli*	Water, person to person	Fever Abdominal pain, diarrhea

Table 3

Treatment of Identified Intestinal Pathogens

Organism	Antibiotic Regimen
Campylobacter jejuni	Azithromycin 500 mg daily × 3 days or ciprofloxacin 500 mg bid × 3 days
Clostridium difficile	Metronidazole 500 mg tid × 10 to 14 days Alt: vancomycin 125 mg po qid × 10 to 14 days
Shigella	Ciprofloxacin 500 mg po bid × 3 days Alt: trimethoprim-sulfamethoxazole DS po bid × 3 days
Listeria	Ampicillin 50 mg/kg IV q 6 hours Alt: trimethoprim-sulfamethoxazole 20 mg/kg/day
Giardia lamblia	Tinidazole 2 g po × 1 or nitazoxanide 500 po bid × 3 days Alt: metronidazole 250 mg po tid x 5 days
Cryptosporidium	Nitazoxanide 500 mg po bid × 3 days

bid = twice daily; tid = three times daily; po = by mouth; qid = four times daily; IV = intravenous

Campylobacter. Recent antibiotic use should prompt investigation for *Clostridium difficile*. A patient who recently consumed untreated water should have the stool checked for parasites such as *Giardia* and *Cryptosporidium*.[29]

Treatment is based on the specific diagnosis. Antibiotics are usually not indicated because they do not change the clinical course and may increase symptoms in patients with *Escherichia coli* and *Salmonella*. The initial treatment of acute diarrhea is primarily supportive care. Oral rehydration is most important. Adults should drink plenty of fluids (preferably a glucose-based electrolyte solution) and consume salt such as in soups and crackers. Loperamide is an antimotility agent that also has antisecretory properties. In general, loperamide should be avoided in patients with bloody diarrhea because of its association with prolonged fever in cases of shigella, toxic megacolon in patients with *C difficile*, and hemolytic-uremic syndrome in cases of *Shigella* toxin-producing *E coli* (**Table 2**). Other over-the-counter antidiarrheal remedies include bismuth subsalicylate and kaolin.[29] Athletes must be clinically improving before resuming training or competition. Specifically, they must be afebrile and have normal orthostatic vital signs. Athletes should be able to toler-

ate fluids and have a regular diet prior to return, and weight should be within 2% to 3% of preillness weight. Functional testing is recommended to ensure that there is no fatigue or difficulty with training or competition. Athletes taking antibiotics must be assessed for common adverse effects of the medications, such as nausea or vomiting. For some bacterial and parasitic causes of diarrhea, antimicrobial treatment may be warranted[30] (**Table 3**).

Viruses

Norwalk virus is spread via food, water, and from person to person. The virus is very contagious; 10 viral particles are believed to be sufficient to cause infection. In 1998, acute gastroenteritis developed in 43 University of North Carolina football players who ate a contaminated boxed lunch the day before a game. The illness developed in 11 other North Carolina players who did not eat the lunch, and in 11 players from the opposing team following the game.[31] Viral shedding begins with symptoms and may continue 2 weeks after recovery.

The normal incubation period is 24 to 48 hours. Symptoms include acute onset of vomiting, nonbloody diarrhea, and occasionally low-grade fever. The dura-

7: Medical Issues

tion of illness is 24 to 60 hours. Treatment is primarily supportive care.

Parasites

Giardia intestinalis

Giardia is spread via fecal-oral transfer of cysts. The cysts are excreted by infected animals such as dogs, cats, beavers, and humans and can contaminate water supplies. Symptoms range from mild diarrhea to protracted illness with foul-smelling stools and abdominal distension. Diagnosis is via stool examination. Treatment is with tinidazole, nitazoxanide, or metronidazole.

Cryptosporidium

Cryptosporidium is transmitted via oocysts that are excreted in feces of infected animals. There have been extensive waterborne outbreaks. Symptoms include benign, self-limited diarrhea. However, severe, chronic diarrhea that can result in death may develop in immunocompromised patients (particularly those with HIV). Diagnosis is via stool examination. Treatment usually consists of supportive care.

Bacterial Infections of the Skin

Impetigo

Impetigo, one of the most common skin infections, is a contagious superficial infection caused by staphylococcal species and beta-hemolytic streptococcus. The infection usually consists of "honey-crusted" pustules on an erythematous base. Impetigo spreads quickly to other places on the body, but usually not to the palms or soles.

Options for treatment include both topical and systemic antibiotics. Topical treatment should be used if there are a limited number of lesions without bullae. Mupirocin, three times daily for 10 days, is the agent of choice (> 90% effective). Efforts should also be made to remove crusts with warm water soaks for 10 to 15 minutes before application of topical antibiotic for treatment to be effective. An alternative topical therapy is hydrogen peroxide cream, which is 70% to 80% effective.[32]

Systemic therapy may be warranted in more extensive cases. Appropriate agents include dicloxacillin, cephalexin, or clindamycin. Clindamycin should be used if MRSA is suspected. Penicillin is no longer recommended because of the significant role of *S aureus*.

National Collegiate Athletic Association wrestlers are required to have no new lesions for 48 hours, to complete 72 hours of oral antibiotic therapy, and to have no moist or exudative lesions. In addition, all lesions must be covered for competition. There are no formal guidelines for other sports, but contact sports, swimming, and gymnastics should follow guidelines similar to those set forth for wrestlers to prevent spread.[33,34]

Furuncles/Carbuncles

Furuncles are infections extending from hair follicles. Carbuncles are groups of several inflamed follicles. Early lesions may appear as cellulitis. They develop in individuals who are skin or nasal carriers of *S aureus*, which is the most common pathogen. Other pathogens include gram-negative bacteria and anaerobes, especially in the perioral, perirectal, and vulvovaginal areas. Close contact with affected individuals or poor hygiene can predispose to these infections.

Treatment can include antibiotics and warm compresses alone; however, definitive treatment usually requires incision and drainage. Material should be sent for cultures and susceptibilities. The evidence for addition of systemic antibiotics is unclear. Situations in which antibiotic therapy may be warranted are multiple abscesses, extensive surrounding cellulitis, immunosuppression, and systemic illness. Empiric antibiotic therapy for skin abscesses, furuncles, and carbuncles should include activity against MRSA in areas of high MRSA prevalence. Appropriate antibiotics include trimethoprim-sulfamethoxazole, doxycycline, and clindamycin. The parenteral agent of choice is vancomycin. The duration of treatment should be tailored to clinical improvement. Return-to-play guidelines are the same as those for impetigo.[35]

MRSA Infections of the Skin

Over the past 10 years there has been a dramatic increase in infections caused by MRSA in the community. These bacteria have the potential to cause disfiguration and life-threatening infections if not recognized and treated promptly. Prevalence of community-acquired MRSA varies by geographic location and population. It usually affects young healthy people. Sports teams are believed to have higher rates of carriage and infection than the general population. Approximately 30% of the population are asymptomatic carriers.[36]

Risk factors for transmission of MRSA include sharing equipment, contact with contaminated surfaces, skin-to-skin contact with others who are carriers or infected, skin abrasions, or cuts. Risk rises substantially with poor personal hygiene.

Incision and drainage along with systemic antibiotics are generally recommended. It is important to obtain cultures to guide treatment and provide epidemiologic data. Antibiotic regimens include trimethoprim-sulfamethoxazole (double strength, twice daily for 10 to 14 days) and doxycycline (100 mg twice daily for 10 to 14 days). Second-line agents are clindamycin (300 mg four times daily for 10 to 14 days) and linezolid (600 mg twice daily for 10 to 14 days). There are conflicting reports on decontamination for MRSA carriers.

Frequent hand washing is the best way to prevent MRSA. Athletic staff also should focus on cleaning frequently touched surfaces (using Environmental Protection Agency-approved disinfectant), covering infections, and cleaning and drying shared equipment after each use. Athletes should be instructed on proper hand hygiene (including the use of alcohol-based rubs on the field); showering immediately after practice and before using whirlpools; not sharing personal items (such as towels, razors, and ointments); and reporting possible infections immediately to coaches, athletic trainers, or parents. Some teams have adopted waterless cleansers and paper towels for sideline use with great success.

If sport-specific rules do not exist, in general, athletes should be excluded if wounds cannot be properly covered during participation in sports. Athletes with MRSA infections should not use whirlpools or swimming pools until wounds have healed (**Figure 1**).

Ecthyma
Ecthyma is an ulcerative form of impetigo with lesions that extend deep into the dermis. The painful lesions appear as punched-out ulcers with yellow crust and surrounding violaceous margins and are usually in the lower extremities. There may be associated regional lymphadenopathy. The lesions usually heal with scarring. Predisposing factors include high temperature and humidity, crowded conditions, and poor hygiene. Treatment follows the same recommendations discussed for impetigo.

Folliculitis
Folliculitis is inflammation of the superficial portion of hair follicles. The outbreak typically consists of clusters of pustules and papules on an erythematous base. The most common types of folliculitis include staphylococcal folliculitis and hot tub folliculitis. More common locations are areas traumatized by maceration (for example, under thigh pads or sweaty garments, or on the trunk, legs, and arms of wrestlers). Deep folliculitis can produce furuncles and boils. Systemic symptoms of fever, chills, and malaise can occur with widespread infections. Hot tub folliculitis, caused by *Pseudomonas aeruginosa*, is produced on areas of skin that come in contact with contaminated water. This infection is usually self-limited once water exposure ends and resolves in 7 to 10 days without specific treatment. Because lesions usually respond spontaneously, initial treatment involves keeping the area clean and dry and using antibacterial soap. For persistent lesions, topical mupirocin, 10% benzoyl peroxide can be used. Cephalexin (500 mg four times daily for 7 days), erythromycin (500 mg four times daily for 7 days), and azithromycin (500 mg on day 1, then 250 mg daily for 4 days) may be used unless MRSA is suspected. Those at high risk for MRSA require doxycycline or trimethoprim-sulfamethoxazole.

Cellulitis
Cellulitis occurs as an area of skin erythema, edema, and warmth involving the deeper dermis and subcutaneous fat. The infection may occur with or without underlying skin trauma. The infection most frequently oc-

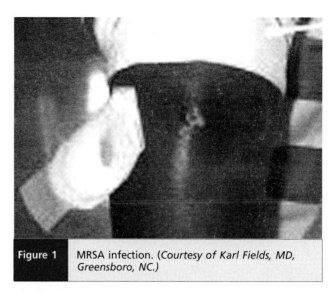

Figure 1   MRSA infection. (*Courtesy of Karl Fields, MD, Greensboro, NC.*)

curs in the lower extremities. In athletes, group A streptococcus and staphylococcus are the most common pathogens. Gram-negative bacteria sometimes are involved. The diagnosis is typically made clinically, without the aid of cultures.

Initial management involves elevation of the affected extremity and treatment of underlying conditions. The skin also should be hydrated to avoid cracking. A patient with signs of systemic toxicity or rapidly progressing erythema should be treated with parenteral antibiotics. Small peripheral infections can be treated with cephalexin (500 mg four times daily for 7 to 10 days) or erythromycin (500 mg four times daily for 7 to 10 days). The patient should be closely monitored and switched to MRSA-covering antibiotics if the infection extends. Appropriate regimens include doxycycline (100 mg by mouth twice daily for 10 to 14 days) and trimethoprim-sulfamethoxazole (double strength, twice daily for 10 to 14 days). Joints underlying infected areas should be monitored for synovitis and septic arthritis, although these complications are rare.

Patients should not play until they are afebrile and without systemic symptoms. Again, for most sports, with the exception of wrestling, there are no established guidelines. For wrestling, athletes must be free of new lesions for 2 days, have completed 3 days of oral antibiotics, and have no draining lesions.

Erythrasma
Erythrasma is a chronic bacterial infection involving intertriginous areas and interdigital areas. The causative agent is *Corynebacterium minutissimum* and the clinical picture mimics a topical fungal infection (**Figure 1**). The rash consists of reddish-brown patches. Diagnosis is made by the presence of coral-red fluorescence on Woods light examination and the absence of fungal elements on potassium hydroxide preparation.

Treatment includes topical 2% erythromycin or 1% clindamycin four times a day for 14 days. More severe cases usually require the addition of oral erythromycin

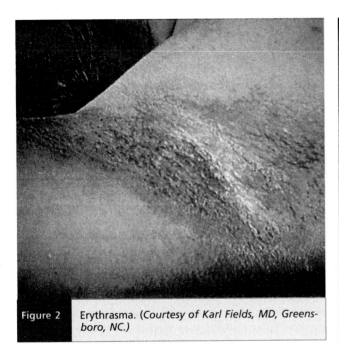

Figure 2   Erythrasma. (*Courtesy of Karl Fields, MD, Greensboro, NC.*)

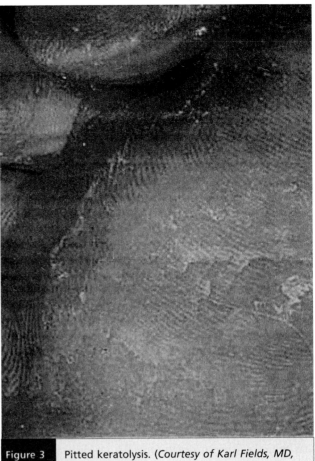

Figure 3   Pitted keratolysis. (*Courtesy of Karl Fields, MD, Greensboro, NC.*)

or tetracycline 250 mg four times daily for 5 to 14 days. An easier alternative is a single 1-g dose of clarithromycin, which is equally effective.

This infection is contagious but does not cause serious problems. As such there are no return-to-play guidelines. Affected areas should be covered during practice and competition, but participation should not be restricted (**Figure 2**).

Pitted Keratolysis
Pitted keratolysis, also called stinky foot and sweaty sock syndrome, is a bacterial condition of the foot that is often confused with tinea pedis. The lesion appears as multiple pits 1 to 3 mm in diameter overlying a plaque usually on the heel or toes (weight-bearing areas). The infection has a pungent odor and the involved skin is typically slimy with hyperhidrosis. Causative organisms include *Corynebacterium*, *Dermatophilus*, and *Micrococcus*.

Because the condition is associated with moist environments, treatment includes moisture-wicking socks, frequent changing of socks, shoes, and insoles, and use of drying agents (20% aluminum chloride foot powder and 5% benzoyl peroxide soap). Topical antibiotics can usually cure the infection if applied for 2 to 4 weeks. Effective agents include 5% erythromycin cream. There is no return-to-play restriction on athletes with this condition[1] (**Figure 3**).

Viral Infections of Skin

Herpes Simplex
Herpes simplex virus (HSV-1) can cause primary and recurrent infections in athletes. It is transmitted through direct contact with breaks in the skin. Because

of its prevalence in rugby and football it is also known as herpes gladiatorum and herpes rugbiformus or scrumpox.

The lesions appear as a cluster of painful vesicles on an erythematous base. The infection may be heralded by prodromal symptoms of fever, sore throat, headache, and painful adenopathy. These symptoms do not usually occur with reactivation infection. Outbreaks can be triggered by emotional or physical stress (illness, sun, cold, wind). The incubation period in a primary outbreak is 2 to 20 days. Most individuals do not recollect their initial infection because 90% occur in early childhood. After initial infection, the virus enters a dormant phase and resides in neural ganglion.

The diagnosis is usually made based on clinical presentation. A Tzanck test can be done on fluid from an unroofed vesicle. Viral titers, immunologic tests, monoclonal antibody tests, and cultures also can be done.

Treatment of HSV-1 is mostly based on studies of HSV-2 treatment. However, some studies have shown that treatment with acyclovir decreased the duration of active disease and viral shedding by 50%. Antiviral agents should be administered as soon as prodromal symptoms (pain and tingling) begin. The agent of choice is acyclovir, which can be dosed in several different ways: 200 mg five times a day for 5 days, 400 mg three times a day for 5 days, or 800 mg twice a day for 5 days. Valacyclovir (500 mg twice a day for 5 days) and famcyclovir (125 mg twice daily for 5 days) may also be used. For symptomatic relief from neuralgia, capsaicin cream, viscous lidocaine, and nonsteroidal anti-inflammatory drugs have been used.

Suppressive therapy can be considered in athletes with frequent recurrences. Commonly used regimens include acyclovir (400 mg twice daily), valacyclovir (500 to 1,000 mg once daily), and famcyclovir (250 mg twice daily). These can be used throughout the year or only during periods of stress. When two or more athletes on a team have active lesions, prophylactic treatment of the entire team may be appropriate.

Rules regarding return to play for wrestlers mandate a minimum 120 hours of oral antiviral agents, no new lesions over the previous 72 hours, and no moist lesions. All lesions must have a firm adherent crust, and individuals with primary infections must be free of systemic symptoms for 72 hours[1] (**Figure 4**).

Herpes Zoster

Following primary infection with varicella zoster virus, the virus may later be reactivated from its dormant state in dorsal root ganglia and cause herpes zoster. It is contagious to those who have not had varicella or the vaccine. The rash usually occurs in one dermatome and does not cross midline. It is characterized by an erythematous base with multiple overlying macropapular lesions that become vesicles. The rash may be preceded by prodromal symptoms or burning, itching, pain, and hypersensitivity in the affected dermatome along with fever, malaise, and headache.

Treatment options include acyclovir 800 mg five times a day for 7 days, famciclovir 500 mg three times daily for 7 days, or valacyclovir 1,000 mg three times daily for 7 days. These medications promote healing of lesions, reduce severity and duration of pain, and reduce the incidence of postherpetic neuralgia. Prednisone may be used as an adjunct in severe cases. Zoster may be prevented in individuals who have not had primary infection with the administration of the varicella zoster vaccine.

Athletic participation requires lesions to be surrounded by a firm adherent crust and have no evidence of secondary bacterial infection.[36]

Molluscum Contagiosum

Molluscum contagiosum arises from the pox virus. Characteristically the lesions form a pearly nodule with an umbilication in the center. The lesions are single or clustered and usually only 1 to 2 mm in diameter. These are not invasive deeper than superficial layers of the skin and the nodules represent viral inclusion bodies. Spread occurs from close contact and has been documented in sports teams.

Treatment options including unroofing, desiccation, freezing, application of chemicals, curetting, or any strategy that destroys the integrity of the nodule usually

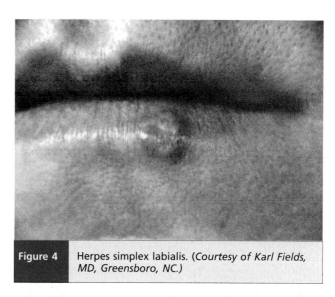

Figure 4 Herpes simplex labialis. (*Courtesy of Karl Fields, MD, Greensboro, NC.*)

results in death of the virus. Curettage results in destruction of the lesions with the least number of office visits.[37]

In wrestlers, NCAA guidelines call for lesions to be curetted or removed before the meet or tournament. Solitary or localized, clustered lesions can be covered with a gas permeable membrane such as OpSite or Bioclusive (OpSite: Smith & Nephew, Memphis, TN; Bioclusive: Johnson & Johnson, Cincinnati, OH), followed by an inherent wrap or tape.[35]

Verruca Vulgaris

Warts arise from infections with human papilloma virus. Classic appearance of rough, hyperkeratotic papules that interrupt skin lines make warts relatively easy to identify. Plantar warts are often more difficult and calluses on the feet can be mistakenly identified as warts. Scraping off the surface of the wart reveals seedlike material comprising thrombosed capillaries. This diagnostic test helps distinguish them from thickened calluses or other skin lesions. The human papilloma virus has approximately 150 subtypes and the particular subtype influences both the location where the wart occurs and the appearance.

Various methods of destruction are effective for resolving warts. Among these are application of liquid nitrogen, other forms of cryotherapy, topical application of salicylic and other acids, application of cantharidin, topical immunomodulators such as imiquimod or intralesional immunotherapy, and a variety of novel therapies such as oral cimetidine or occlusion with duct tape.[38] Therapies frequently take time to achieve full success.

According to NCAA guidelines, wrestlers with multiple digitate verrucae of the face are disqualified if the infected areas cannot be covered with a mask. Solitary or scattered lesions can be curetted away before the meet or tournament. Wrestlers with multiple verrucae plana or verrucae vulgaris must have the lesions adequately covered.[1]

Surgical excision might be desirable for athletes with an isolated lesion on the face that could not be covered well. An athlete with a plantar wart who participates in a jumping or running sport usually would not choose surgery or an aggressive destructive technique because the ability to compete may be limited.

Fungal Infections of the Skin

Tinea Pedis, Cruris, and Corporis

Hygiene standards have fortunately lessened the frequency of tinea pedis infections so that athlete's foot is no longer a right of passage for participation in sport. Wet floors, unclean locker room surfaces, and shared towels and clothing in past years helped spread this infection. Currently, most locker rooms have daily cleaning, foot baths with antifungal disinfectants, and policies that discourage sharing towels and clothing. All these measures have dramatically reduced the frequency of tinea pedis.

However, foot trauma and moisture from sweating and participation in wet shoes continue to provide an environment in which tinea pedis thrives. As a result, this infection will always be relatively common in sports. Current topical treatments offer slightly faster resolution of symptoms and higher cure rates than older therapies. Terbinafine and naftifine have shown excellent efficacy. Limited infections may be treated in time courses as short as 1 week, with more extensive ones requiring up to 4 weeks of topical therapy. Treatment failures may indicate a misdiagnosis so that the patient actually has eczema or contact dermatitis. Potassium hydroxide scraping for diagnosis helps confirm the infection and should be used whenever doubt exists.

Tinea cruris often worsens because of maceration or dampness. Clean clothing changes and garments that cause less sweating or chafing can help lessen risk. The rash that starts along the upper thigh and may extend throughout the groin should have an elevated border. If not, the possibility of erythrasma or a monilial infection should be considered. Again, potassium hydroxide testing and even cultures can confirm difficult diagnostic cases. Antifungal powders and drying agents can play adjunctive roles in eliminating this infection.

Tinea corporis refers to a superficial infection of nonhairy portions of the skin. Isolated lesions may expand in size leaving a clearing central area and an elevated border. These lesions can remain local or multiple lesions may develop. Topical application of antifungals resolves most isolated lesions. Tinea gladiatorum refers to the widespread outbreaks of tinea corporis that have occurred in wrestlers in past years. These led to specific restrictions and studies of the most effective way to make this infection less contagious. Both topical and oral treatment resolved the infection but oral fluconazole 200 mg weekly for 3 weeks showed culture-negative lesions in 11 days. Topical clotrimazole showed similar efficacy at 3 weeks but cultures did not become negative until 23 days.[39,40]

For patients with tinea pedis, cruris or corporis, NCAA wrestling guidelines stipulate that a minimum of 72 hours of topical therapy is required for skin lesions. The cidal topic antifungals terbinafine or naftifine are suggested for treatment. A minimum of 2 weeks of systemic antifungal therapy is required for scalp lesions. Wrestlers with extensive and active lesions will be disqualified. Activity of treated lesions can be judged either by use of potassium hydroxide preparation or a review of therapeutic regimen. Wrestlers with solitary, or closely clustered, localized lesions will be disqualified if lesions are in a body location that cannot be adequately covered. Covering routine should include selenium sulfide washing of lesion or ketoconazole shampoo, followed by application of naftifine gel or cream or terbinafine cream, then gas-permeable dressing such as OpSite or Bioclusive, followed by an inherent wrap or tape. Dressing changes should be done after each match so that the lesion can air dry. The disposition of tinea cases will be decided on an individual basis as determined by the examining physician and/or certified athletic trainer.[1]

Summary

Infectious disease causes considerable time loss from sport. Excessive training, skin injuries, exposures to environmental toxins, and the crowding and close contact that are integral parts of sport all contribute to the risk of specific infections. A principal concern of the team physicians is to ensure the safety of the competitor, team members, and opponents, as well as helping the individual athlete return successfully to their sport. Team physicians should choose treatments and return-to-play strategies based on knowledge of the specific demands of the individual sport and the best evidence established from medical studies.

Annotated References

1. NCAA Wrestling Committee: *NCAA Wrestling: 2008 Men's Rules and Interpretations*. Indianapolis, IN, 2007, pp 1-182.

   Wrestling has established guidelines for participation with skin disease. Treatment recommendations as well as types of dressings that would allow an athlete to continue sports participation are discussed.

2. Nieman D, Nehlsen-Canarella S, Fagoaga OR, et al: Immune function in female elite rowers and non-athletes. *Br J Sports Med* 2000;34:181-187.

3. Gleeson M, McDonald WA, Pyne DB, et al: Salivary IgA levels and infection risk in elite swimmers. *Med Sci Sports Exerc* 1999;31:67-73.

4. Fricker P, Pyne D, Saunders PU, et al: Influence of training loads on patterns of illness in elite distance runners. *Clin J Sport Med* 2005;15:246-252.

   Longitudinal follow-up of elite distance runners did not demonstrate a correlation between respiratory infection and the training intensity or load. This calls into question the relationship of immune function and training suppression.

5. Drobnic F, Freixa A, Casan P, Sanchis J, Guardino X: Assessment of chlorine exposure in swimmers during training. *Med Sci Sports Exerc* 1996;28:271-274.

6. Jacobs D: Conjunctivitis. UpToDate Website. Available at www.uptodate.com. Accessed May 2008.

   This review text provides an overview of the types of conjunctivitis and its treatment.

7. Weinberg SK: Medical aspects of synchronized swimming. *Clin J Sport Med* 1986;5:159-167.

8. Turbeville S, Cowan L, Greenfeld R: Infectious disease outbreaks in competitive sports: A review of the literature. *Am J Sports Med* 2006;34:1860-1865.

   This review documents 59 outbreaks of infectious disease in sport and indicates activities with high risks.

9. Glasziou PP, Del Mar CB, Sanders SL, Hayem M. Antibiotics for acute otitis media in children. *Cochrane Database Syst Rev* 2004;CD000219.

   The authors concluded that antibiotic treatment for acute otitis media is beneficial and may play a role in reducing the risk of mastoiditis.

10. Cooper RJ, Hoffman JR, Bartlett JG, et al: Principles of appropriate antibiotic use for acute pharyngitis in adults: Background. *Ann Emerg Med* 2001;37:711-719.

11. Centor RM, Witherspoon JM, Dalton HP, Brody CE, Link K: The diagnosis of strep throat in adults in the emergency room. *Med Decis Making* 1981;1:239-246.

12. Cohen R, Levy C, Doit C, et al: Six-day amoxicillin vs. ten-day penicillin V therapy for group A streptococcal tonsillopharyngitis. *Pediatr Infect Dis J* 1996;15:678-682.

13. Peyramond D, Portier H, Geslin P, Cohen R: 6-day amoxicillin versus 10-day penicillin V for group A beta-haemolytic streptococcal acute tonsillitis in adults: A French multicentre, open-label, randomized study. The French Study Group Clamorange. *Scand J Infect Dis* 1996;28:497-501.

14. Casey JR, Pichichero ME: Meta-analysis of cephalosporins versus penicillin for treatment of group A streptococcal tonsillopharyngitis in adults. *Clin Infect Dis* 2004;38:1526-1534.

   Treatment failure rates appear lower in patients with GAS infections treated with cephalosporin instead of penicillin antibiotics.

15. Hosey RG, Mattacola CG, Kriss V, et al: Ultrasound assessment of spleen size in collegiate athletes. *Br J Sports Med* 2006;40:251-254.

   This study sought to determine normal spleen dimensions in a healthy athletic population. A single ultrasound was of limited value in determining splenomegaly. Wide variation in splenic size was found in athletes such that normative data need to be established.

16. Doolittle R: Pharyngitis and infectious mononucleosis, in Fields K, Fricker P (eds): *Medical Problems in Athletes*. Cambridge, MA, Blackwell Science, 1997, pp 11-20.

17. File T: Treatment of community-acquired pneumonia in adults in the outpatient setting UpToDate Website. Available at http://www.uptodate.com. Accessed January 7, 2008.

18. Fields KB: Bronchitis and pneumonia, in: Fields K, Fricker P (eds): *Medical Problems in Athletes*. Cambridge, MA, Blackwell Science, 1997, pp 26-33.

19. Gerberding JL: Management of occupational exposures to blood-borne viruses. *N Engl J Med* 1995;332:444-451.

20. World Health Organization Website. Hepatitis B fact sheet. Available at http://www.who.int/mediacentre/factsheets/fs204/en/index.html. Accessed June 21, 2008.

21. Beltrami EM, Williams IT, Shapiro CN, et al: Risk and management of bloodborne infections in healthcare workers. *Clin Microbiol Rev* 2000;12:385-407.

22. Kashiwagi S, Hayashi J, Ikematsu H, et al: An outbreak of hepatitis B in members of a high school sumo wrestling club. *JAMA* 1982;248:213-214.

23. Tobe K, Matsuura K, Ogura T, et al: Horizontal transmission of hepatitis B virus among players of an American football team. *Arch Intern Med* 2000;160:2541-2545.

24. Bereket-Yücel S: Risk of hepatitis B infections in Olympic wrestling. *Br J Sports Med* 2007;41:306-310.

   Seventy Olympic wrestlers had their blood and sweat examined for the presence of HBV DNA. There was a statistically significant correlation between HBV DNA in the blood and sweat of the wrestlers, suggesting that hepatitis B may be transmitted via sweat.

25. Human immunodeficiency virus and other blood-borne viral pathogens in the athletic setting: Pediatrics Committee on Sports Medicine and Fitness: American Academy of Pediatrics. *Pediatrics* 1999;104:1400-1403.

26. Centers for Disease Control and Prevention Website. Hepatitis B fact sheet. Available at http://www.cdc.gov/ncidod/diseases/hepatitis/b/fact.htm. July 27, 2007. Accessed June 21, 2008.

27. Centers for Disease Control and Prevention Website. *CDC HIV/AIDS Facts* Available at http://www.cdc.gov/hiv/resources/factsheets/us.htm. Accessed June 21, 2008.

7: Medical Issues

The CDC offers information about HIV and acquired immunodeficiency virus.

28. Clem KL, Borchers JR: HIV and the athlete. *Clin J Sports Med* 2007;26:413-424.

This review article presents a discussion on the diagnosis and treatment of HIV, benefits of athletic participation and exercise in patients with HIV, and participation safety.

29. Thielman N, Guerrant RL: Clinical practice: Acute infectious diarrhea. *N Engl J Med* 2004;350:38-47.

This review article discusses the epidemiology, cause, and treatment of acute, infectious diarrhea.

30. DuPont HL: Therapy for and prevention of traveler's diarrhea. *Clin Infect Dis* 2007;45:S78-S84.

This review article discusses prevention and treatment of traveler's diarrhea.

31. Becker KM, Moe CL, Southwick KL, MacCormack JN: Transmission of Norwalk virus during a football game. *N Engl J Med* 2000;343:1223-1229.

32. Sedgwick PE, Dexter WW, Smith CT: Bacterial dermatoses in sports. *Clin Sports Med* 2007;26:383-396.

This review article summarizes the common skin problems encountered during sports that are related to bacterial infection.

33. Batts KB: Dermatology, in O'Connor FG, Sallis RE, Wilder RP, St. Pierre P (eds): *Sports Medicine: Just the Facts*. New York, NY, McGraw-Hill, 2005, pp 149-157.

This chapter provides concise information about several sports-related dermatologic issues, including impetigo.

34. Baddour LA: Impetigo. UpToDate Website. Available at http://www.uptodate.com. January 2008. Accessed December 2008.

35. Lillegard WA, Butcher JD, Fields, KB: Dermatologic problems in athletes, in Fields KB, Fricker PA (eds): *Medical Problems in Athletes*. Cambridge, MA, Blackwell Science, 1997, pp 234-246.

36. Centers for Disease Control and Prevention Website: *Epidemiology and Management of MRSA in the Community*. October 2007. Available at http://www.cdc.gov/ncidod/dhqp/MRSA-inthe-community.html. Accessed June 2008.

The CDC continues to track the outbreaks of MRSA and also offers information about susceptibility to treatment. Guidelines for prevention of spread and educational materials are included at their Website.

37. Isaacs S: *Molluscum Contagiosum*. UpToDate Website. Available at http://www.uptodate.com. 2007. Accessed December 2008.

38. Goldstein B, Goldstein A: *Cutaneous Warts*. 2003. UpToDate Webiste. Available at http://www.uptodate.com. Accessed December 2008.

39. Goldstein B, Goldstein A: Dermatophyte (Tinea) Infections. 2008. UpToDate Website. Available at http://www.uptodate.com. Accessed December 2008.

40. Kohl TD, Martin DC, Berger MS: Comparison of topical and oral treatments for tinea gladiatorum. *Clin J Sport Med* 1999;9:161-166.

7: Medical Issues

Chapter 35

Heat and Hydration

Susan M. Joy, MD

Introduction

Heat production by the human body during exercise is 15 to 20 times greater than it is at rest.[1] Heat illness in its various forms is encountered frequently in athletes, particularly when exercising in warmer environments. Heat illness represents a spectrum of disease, the most serious of which may be life threatening. Heat illness is preventable with proper interventions and education to address training parameters and hydration. Sports medicine personnel must be familiar with the signs and symptoms of heat illness so prompt treatment can be initiated. Appropriate hydration strategies have the potential to mitigate the negative performance effects of dehydration as well as minimize the risk of both heat illness and overhydration with resultant dilutional hyponatremia. This chapter summarizes various clinical entities within the spectrum of heat illness; provides an overview of issues related to heat, hydration, and performance; outlines current considerations related to exercise-associated hyponatremia; and highlights current recommendations for treatment and prevention.

Epidemiology

The exact incidence of heat illness in athletes is not known and likely is underestimated. The National Collegiate Athletic Association (NCAA) Football Study Oversight Committee evaluated "time loss heat illness" (TLHI) in collegiate football players using NCAA Injury Surveillance System data for the 2001 and 2002 football seasons.[2] Of five fall sports monitored (football, men's soccer, women's soccer, field hockey, women's volleyball), football accounted for 80% of the reported TLHI, with 95% of cases reported during preseason football. Players who wore at least helmets and shoulder pads or participated in multiple sessions in a single day accounted for more than 80% of TLHI cases. Thus, football players seem to be at increased risk for heat illness, although it is important to recognize the potential for heat illness in all athletes depending on the scenario.

Pathophysiology of Heat Illness

Exercising muscles generate metabolic heat that must be dissipated to maintain balance and allow for the continuation of exercise. To maintain a body temperature of 37°C, thermoregulatory processes are initiated by peripheral and hypothalamic heat receptors when the temperature of the blood rises just 1°C.[3] Cardiac output is increased, and blood is shunted to the peripheral circulation to facilitate cooling via four basic mechanisms: conduction, convection, radiation, and evaporation. At lower ambient temperatures, convection and conduction play larger roles in dissipating heat. In warmer, more humid environments, evaporation of sweat is the primary means by which heat is dissipated.[4] Anything that limits this evaporative response will impair the body's ability to maintain a normal core temperature while exercising in the heat, thereby increasing the potential for heat illness.

Dehydration can result in a decrease in circulating blood volume and stroke volume and thus hamper the delivery of blood to the skin's surface for the dissipation of heat.[1] Without adequate compensation, sustained heat stress can lead to cardiorespiratory collapse and direct injury to tissue. Respiratory alkalosis, lactic acidosis, coagulation disorders, and endothelial cell injury also have occurred during heat stroke.[3] At the cellular level, multiple factors have been implicated in heat stress, including interleukin-1, interleukin-6, tumor necrosis factor-alpha, cytokines, and heat-shock proteins, all responding through pathways similar to those observed during sepsis.[3] These pathways increase the risk for progression to multiorgan system dysfunction and ultimate failure.

The ability to withstand the effects of exercise in extreme heat varies among individuals. This likely stems from a complex interplay of multiple issues, including genetic alterations in circulating neuroendocrine factors, training and acclimatization variables, and differences in sweat composition and sweat rate.[5]

Heavy, tight-fitting clothing and layers of protective equipment, such as football equipment, have been shown to impede sweat evaporation and may decrease athletes' tolerance of exercise in the heat. American football players have been estimated to have at least twice the daily sweat loss of cross-country runners training in the same environment.[4]

Children are more susceptible to heat illness. Because smaller children generally have greater surface area to body mass ratios, they will gain more heat from the environment when exercising on a hot day.[6] Compared with dehydrated adults in the same environment, chil-

Table 1

Risk of Heat Illness

Risk	WBGT (°C)
Very high risk	> 28
High risk	23-28
Moderate risk	18-23
Low risk	< 18

Table 2

Recommendations for Children Exercising in the Heat

Recommendation	WBGT (°C)
Cancel all activities	> 29
Stop activity in at-risk children, limit in others	26-29
Longer rest periods in shade; fluids every 15 min	24-26
No limitations	< 24

(Data from American Academy of Pediatrics: Climactic heat stress and the exercising child and adolescent: American Academy of Pediatrics committee on sports medicine and fitness. Pediatrics 2000;106:158-159.)

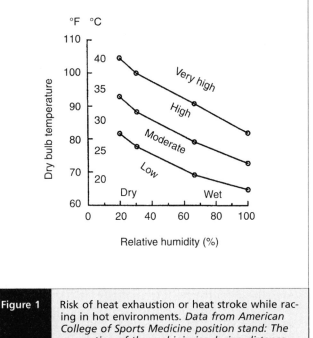

| Figure 1 | Risk of heat exhaustion or heat stroke while racing in hot environments. *Data from American College of Sports Medicine position stand: The prevention of thermal injuries during distance running.* Med Sci Sports Exerc 1987;19:529-533. |

dren also have a lower sweat rate, cannot dissipate heat as efficiently via sweat evaporation, and can become hyperthermic faster.[5] Heat illness in young athletes is discussed in detail in chapter 39.

Classification of Heat Illness

Heat illness represents a spectrum of disorders ranging in severity from mild to severe. Milder forms of heat illness include heat fatigue, heat syncope, and heat cramps. Heat fatigue may manifest as general fatigue, headache, and weakness. When blood pools in the peripheral venous circulation with cessation of exercise in the heat, heat syncope can occur, most often in unacclimatized individuals. The etiology of heat cramps is not well understood. They appear to be associated with dehydration, electrolyte disturbances, or sodium deficits and muscle fatigue[4] and are more common in individuals not acclimated to the heat and in those who sweat profusely, resulting in large sodium losses during exercise.[4] When severe, heat cramps can represent a sign of impeding heat exhaustion.[1]

Heat exhaustion is a more severe condition. In response to high workload, high ambient temperature, and dehydration, the cardiovascular system may fail to meet the demands placed on it; as a result, the athlete is unable to continue exercising in the heat. Symptoms include headache, weakness, nausea, vomiting, and mild confusion. Clinical findings may include increased

sweating, increased heart rate, and hypotension. Mild elevations in core temperature may be seen but usually will remain below 40.5°C.[1]

The most serious form of heat illness is heat stroke, a medical emergency with potentially fatal consequences. Core temperature elevations greater than 40.5°C, central nervous system involvement, and decreased or complete cessation of sweating distinguish heat stroke from milder forms of heat illness.[1] The degree of organ damage and mortality rate have been shown to be proportional to the length of time elapsed between core temperature elevation and initiation of cooling therapy.[7]

Measurement of Environmental Heat Stress

To reliably assess the risk of heat illness in athletes, some measure of environmental heat stress must be made before practice or competition commences. The wet bulb globe temperature (WBGT), which represents a standardized index of environmental heat stress from air temperature, amount of radiant heat, and percent humidity, is the temperature at which no more evaporation can occur.[1] It is measured using a commercially available psychrometer. The greatest risk for heat stroke has been described when the WBGT exceeds 28°C (**Table 1**). The American Academy of Pediatrics has presented recommendations for activity modification in children based on WBGT to minimize the risk of heat illness[6] (**Table 2**).

If WBGT is not available, climacteric heat stress can be estimated by charting the relative humidity versus the dry bulb temperature[7] (**Figure 1**). The temperature and humidity either can be recorded locally or gathered from local weather sources.

Risk Factors for Heat Illness

Multiple risk factors have been identified that increase an individual's susceptibility to ill effects while exercising in the heat[1,5,8] (Table 3). Athletes should be carefully screened before participation, and educational efforts should be targeted toward risk reduction strategies whenever possible.

Heat, Hydration, and Performance

There is strong evidence that dehydration adversely affects performance and decreases the time to exhaustion in athletes,[9] particularly when body fluid losses exceed 2% of baseline body weight.[5] Cardiac output and oxygen delivery during exercise can be impaired by both hypohydration and environmental heat stress independently, with the combination reducing exercise capacity and performance to a greater degree than either factor alone.[3] Dehydrated athletes are at increased risk of developing heat illness.[10]

Hydration status can be assessed several ways. Tracking daily weight is the easiest, most accessible way for athletes to monitor acute hydration status. The level of dehydration is best expressed as a percentage of baseline body mass (average of three consecutive weights taken while nude first thing in the morning), and postpractice or daily fluctuations correlate with acute water loss from exercise. A loss of 1 mL of sweat represents a 1-g loss of body weight (specific gravity of sweat estimated to be 1.0 g/mL); losses exceeding 1% have been shown to correlate with dehydration.[4] The total volume of fluid needed to replenish this deficit is 125% to 150% of lost body mass to offset the obligatory increased urinary loss that accompanies rehydration. Replenishment of fluid is more effective when consumed in 500-mL increments every 20 to 30 minutes.[5]

Another method to measure hydration status is to assess urine color and specific gravity. Euhydrated athletes generally have pale, yellow urine with a specific gravity less than 1.020 and a measured urine osmolality of less than 700 mOsm/kg.[4]

Sports performance is negatively affected by fluid losses of at least 2% dehydration or more,[11] and the greater the level of dehydration, the greater the level of systemic strain.[12] Dehydration exceeding 2% impairs cardiac output and aerobic performance in the heat, but it has less effect in colder environments and results in little change in muscular strength or anaerobic performance.[4] There is strong evidence that 2% to 3% dehydration increases the perception of exercise difficulty and additional evidence that mental function, memory, processing, and mood also can be impaired.[5]

Athletes should consume fluids well in advance of exercise to prehydrate and allow urine output to normalize before sports participation. The recommended fluid intake of 5 to 7 mL/kg body weight 4 hours before the sports activity should allow the athlete to begin

Table 3

Risk Factors for Heat Illness

Prepubescent or advanced age

Body mass index (obesity)

Dehydration

Prior history of heat illness

Lack of acclimatization

Poor fitness

Medications (antidepressants, diuretics, antihypertensives, antihistamines)

Stimulant use (amphetamines, certain supplements, pseudoephedrine)

Sunburn

Acute illness

Tight-fitting, dark, nonbreathable clothing and equipment layers

in a euhydrated state.[4] Athletes should consume enough fluid during sports activity to prevent the performance impairment and potential heat illness associated with dehydration of 2%. Fluid intake should never exceed sweat loss. It has been suggested that the athlete monitor daily weight, sweat rate, and weather conditions and individualize their fluid intake accordingly.[4] Carbohydrate-electrolyte beverages improve athletic performance more than plain water during vigorous exercise longer than 45 minutes, are more palatable and therefore result in greater voluntary intake than water, and, when 30 to 60 g of carbohydrates per hour are replenished, delay mental performance decline and increase perceived exertion better than plain water.[5] Carbohydrate concentration should not exceed 8% because it will result in delayed gastric emptying and increased gastrointestinal discomfort.[4]

After exercise, athletes should strive to replace 1.5 L of fluid for each kilogram of body weight lost during exercise in smaller boluses to limit urinary losses.[4] Sodium and glycogen generally can be replenished via normal meals, although athletes may need to resume vigorous activity before their next meal and correct fluid and electrolyte imbalances accordingly.[12]

Hyponatremia

Hyponatremia is defined as a serum sodium level below 135 mEq/L and refers to a clinical syndrome resulting from rapid lowering of sodium levels, usually to 130 mEq/L or lower. It has been increasingly seen in endurance athletes, such as those participating in ultramarathon, triathlon, or marathon events, particularly in warmer weather.[13]

Hyponatremia is believed to occur when consumption of water or low-sodium fluid exceeds sweat losses with or without large sodium losses via sweating that also dilute extracellular sodium.[5] Neuroendocrine responses to changes in body fluid homeostasis with prolonged exercise also may affect secretion of antidiuretic hormone and arginine vasopressin and may contribute to increased risk of exercise-associated hyponatremia in certain patients.

Risk factors for hyponatremia include extremes of body mass index and substantial weight gain (1 kg or more) during a race.[14] One large retrospective study described a linear relationship between serum sodium and percentage weight change during endurance racing, with greater weight gain corresponding to lower postrace sodium levels.[10] Slower marathon race times of greater than 4 hours also have been shown to correlate with risk for hyponatremia, presumably because of increased fluid intake during the lengthier race time.[13] Women in whom hyponatremia develops may be more at risk for cerebral edema as a result of estrogen and progesterone inhibition of Na^+-K^+-adenosine triphosphatase (ATPase).[15] Inexperienced marathon runners also appear to be at increased risk of hyponatremia. Despite a relatively high incidence of heat illness and increased sweating in collegiate football players, there is no documented risk of hyponatremia.[2,16]

When sodium loss and water excess lead to a decreased sodium concentration in extracellular fluid, water is forced into the intracellular milieu, resulting in clinical symptoms such as pulmonary and cerebral edema, seizure, coma, and cardiorespiratory arrest.[5] Early symptoms are similar to those seen with dehydration and include confusion, disorientation, headache, nausea, vomiting, aphasia, impaired coordination, muscle cramps, and weakness.[5] The severity of symptoms is not necessarily correlated with the absolute decrease in serum sodium level but rather the rate and extent of decreased extracellular tonicity.[12]

When recognized, exertional hyponatremia is generally treatable and does not result in any significant long-term sequelae. It is important to assess the fluid and sodium status of symptomatic athletes during any endurance event. Athletes with mildly depressed postevent sodium levels who have recently ingested a large amount of water also may be at risk for worsening hyponatremia and should be carefully monitored.[12]

Participants in endurance events should be educated about the risk of hyponatremia associated with excessive fluid intake during a race. When combined with efforts to space water stops at intervals to limit consumption, such educational efforts have shown a decreased incidence of symptomatic hyponatremia without an increase in other untoward effects.[16] Fluid intake should never exceed sweat loss, and body weight measures should be used to estimate fluid losses.[5] Athletes should learn to estimate their individual sweat losses and appropriately tailor personal hydration strategies.[16] Race personnel should be aware of the risk of hyponatremia, recognize symptoms and signs, and be prepared for rapid hospital transfer. There is no convincing evidence

or existing consensus at this time as to whether on-site electrolyte measurements should be performed and 3% NaCl intravenous fluid administered before hospital arrival.[16]

Management of Heat Illness in Athletes

Assessment of the acutely ill athlete should begin with an assessment of airway, breathing, and circulation and focus on notable signs and symptoms of heat illness. An athlete experiencing heat cramps should be removed from competition. Prolonged stretching may help lengthen affected muscle groups, and oral rehydration should be instituted with sports beverages or salt and water.[9] Intravenous fluid administration may be recommended by the treating physician, particularly if the athlete has difficulty tolerating oral fluid intake or is orthostatic.[17]

Any athlete experiencing more severe symptoms, such as fatigue, syncope, exhaustion, or confusion, should be removed from competition to a cool environment and carefully evaluated. Assessment of airway, breathing, circulation, and mental status should be done. It is vital to determine a core temperature via a rectal thermometer because oral, tympanic, and axillary temperature measurements are falsely lowered by environmental factors and thus are not accurate.[9] Elevations in body temperature above 40°C indicate heat stroke and are a medical emergency. Rapid whole-body cooling should be instituted immediately using ice water immersion, although application of ice packs to the neck, axillae, and groin with water-soaked towels on the head, trunk, and extremities also has been used when immersion is unavailable.[9] It is important to recognize the potential need for basic and advanced cardiac life support when the patient collapses as a result of heat stroke and that immersion therapy may complicate the delivery of resuscitative efforts.[1] To date, no pharmacologic cooling methods have been shown to be effective in treating heat stroke.[3]

Mental status and core temperature should be serially reassessed during treatment in the field. Persistent core temperature elevation despite aggressive cooling is associated with a poor outcome and should prompt emergent hospital referral from the field. A return of normal mental status and central nervous system function is a favorable prognostic sign.[3] Intravascular volume may be maintained during cooling through the administration of intravenous normal saline and help maintain tissue perfusion, thereby decreasing the risk of rhabdomyolysis.[9]

Moderate symptoms of heat illness can be managed by removing the athlete from competition and carefully assessing and monitoring fluid status and core temperature. Heat exhaustion by definition is not associated with significant hyperthermia, although cooling measures should be instituted if mild or moderate elevations in core temperature are observed. Intravenous flu-

Table 4

WGBT Levels for Modification or Cancellation of Workouts or Athletic Competition for Healthy Adults

WBGT °F	°C	Continuous Activity and Competition	Training and Noncontinuous Activity Nonacclimatized, Unfit, High-Risk Individuals *	Acclimatized, Fit, Low-Risk Individuals *†
≤ 50.0	≤ 10.0	Generally safe; exertional heat stroke can occur associated with individual factors	Normal activity	Normal activity
50.1-65.0	10.1-18.3	Generally safe; exertional heat stroke can occur	Normal activity	Normal activity
65.1-72.0	18.4-22.2	Risk of exertional heat stroke and other heat illness begins to rise; high-risk individuals should be monitored or not compete	Increase the rest:work ratio; monitor fluid intake	Normal activity
72.1-78.0	22.3-25.6	Risk for all competitors is increased	Increase the rest:work ratio and decrease total duration of activity	Normal activity; monitor fluid intake
78.1-82.0	25.7-27.8	Risk for unfit, nonacclimatized individuals is high	Increase the rest:work ratio; decrease intensity and total duration of activity	Normal activity; monitor fluid intake
82.1-86.0	27.9-30.2	Cancel level for exertional heat stroke risk	Increase the rest:work ratio to 1:1, decrease intensity and total duration of activity; limit intense exercise; watch at-risk individuals carefully	Plan intense or prolonged exercise with discretion §; watch at-risk individuals carefully
86.1-90.0	30.1-32.2		Cancel or stop practice and competition	Limit intense exercise§ and total daily exposure to heat and humidity; watch for early signs and symptoms
≥ 90.1	> 32.3		Cancel exercise	Cancel exercise, uncompensable heat stress‡ exists for all athletes§

(Data from Casa DJ, Armstrong LE: Exertional heat stroke: A medical emergency, in Armstrong LE (ed): Exertional Heat Illness. Champaign, IL, Human Kinetics, 2005, pp 26-56.)
*While wearing shorts, T-shirt, socks, and sneakers
†Acclimatized to training in the heat at least 3 weeks
‡Internal heat production exceeds heat loss, and core body temperature rises continuously, without a plateau
§Differences of local climate and individual heat acclimatization status may allow activity at higher levels than outlined in the table, but athletes and coaches should consult with sports medicine staff and should be cautious when exceeding these limits

ids have been shown to restore plasma volume more quickly and thus may help with acute symptoms, although heat tolerance with subsequent exercise may not be superior to that achieved through rehydration with oral fluids.[9,18] Most athletes with heat exhaustion will recover with on-site management and can be released when clinically stable under the auspices of a relative or friend for rest and rehydration at home.[9]

Return to play depends not only on the resolution of any symptoms of heat illness but also the correction of dehydration and electrolyte imbalances. It is recommended that athletes be cleared for sports participation by a physician after experiencing heat exhaustion, heat stroke, or exertional hyponatremia[17] and that they be closely monitored when training resumes. Additionally, the NCAA recommends that athletes experiencing

acute loss of 5% or more body weight as a result of dehydration be restricted from activity, medically evaluated, and cleared for sports participation only when they are euhydrated.[19]

Prevention Strategies

Death from heat illness is preventable. All athletes should be screened for risk factors for heat illness before sports participation (Table 3). A prior history of heat illness also should be documented; at-risk athletes should be educated about hydration, sodium balance, acclimatization, and recovery; and any deficits should be rectified before clearance.[9]

A systematic review of existing heat illness prevention guidelines reported five common themes: fluid intake, heat limits, clothing, acclimatization, and precautionary interventions.[20] Acclimatization via a gradual increase in duration and intensity of exercise over a 10- to 14-day period appears to be the best means of protecting athletes from heat exhaustion and heat stroke.[9] It has been suggested that 75% of the acclimatization occurs in the first 5 days, but it may be a full 2 weeks or longer before full acclimatization occurs.[20] In children, the process is slower and should progress in a more conservative fashion with approximately 8 to 10 exposures of 30 to 45 minutes each before levels of activity in the heat are increased.[6]

Personnel involved with teams practicing in the heat should be vigilant with the assessment of climacteric stress, whether by WBGT or heat stress index, and should be prepared to impose practice limitations when unsafe conditions are present[9] (Table 4). Even at lower heat stress indices, a risk of heat illness exists in certain individuals; therefore, a high index of suspicion should remain when evaluating symptomatic athletes.

Based on findings from the NCAA Football Study Oversight Committee of significant TLHI in collegiate football players during the preseason, strategies designed to reduce the risk of heat illness in preseason football were implemented in 2003 and included the following recommendations: 5-day acclimatization period of time-limited, single practice sessions; gradual addition of protective equipment during the acclimatization period; no consecutive multipractice days; and limited practice times outside the acclimatization period.[2] Data on the incidence of heat illness occurring after the institution of these guidelines have not yet been formally reported.

Prior to engaging in any organized practices or competitions, careful forethought should be given to all levels of the response to a downed or ill athlete. First responders should be identified and trained in emergency response protocols. They also should be educated on the constellation of symptoms associated with heat illness and recognize the warning signs of heat stroke. Athletes exercising in the heat should have ready access to water and carbohydrate-electrolyte beverages to maintain fluid-electrolyte balance and performance.[4] Rectal thermometers and methods to institute rapid cooling should be available. In certain situations, it is appropriate to have additional supplies such as intravenous fluid therapy, an ice bath, and fans or air conditioning. In all instances, an emergency response protocol should be available with access to emergency medical and local hospital services.

Summary

More epidemiologic studies on the incidence of heat illness in different athletic populations are warranted. Further study of individual risk factors and genetic susceptibility also will help to identify at-risk athletes and

allow appropriate screening and prevention strategies. The use of ingestible sensors hopefully will facilitate the transition of the study of body temperature, fluid status, and physiologic responses to exercise from the laboratory to the playing field. Further exploration of biologic effects of sports beverages has the potential to determine which fluids are most appropriate for which individuals. The contribution of precooling techniques to the prevention of heat stress and heat illness also warrants further investigation. Continued efforts to educate athletes, coaches, and parents about heat illness are vital. Furthermore, local and national sports governing bodies should emphasize safe practice recommendations borne from thoughtful scientific discussion and systematic investigation.

Annotated References

1. Coris EE, Ramirez AM, Van Durme DJ: Heat illness in athletes: The dangerous combination of heat, humidity and exercise. *Sports Med* 2004;34:9-16.

   This review article discusses heat illness, including pathophysiologic mechanisms, clinical syndromes and classification, effects of hydration status, assessment of environmental heat stress, and risk reduction strategies.

2. Dick RW, Schmalz R, Diehl N, Newlin C, Summers E, Klossner D: Process and rationale behind safety modifications to 2003 NCAA preseason football practice. *Med Sci Sport Exerc* 2004;36(Suppl 5):S324.

   Data from the NCAA Injury Surveillance System collected on TLHI in preseason football are presented. Level of evidence: II.

3. Bouchama A, Knochel JP: Heat stroke. *N Engl J Med* 2002;346:1978-1988.

4. American College of Sports Medicine, Sawka MN, Burke LM, et al: American College of Sports Medicine position stand: Exercise and fluid replacement. *Med Sci Sports Exerc* 2007;39:377-390.

   This consensus statement from the American College of Sports Medicine addresses specific issues related to hydration assessment and fluid replacement in athletes based on an in-depth review of the literature and including strength of evidence statements.

5. Casa DJ, Clarkson PM, Roberts WO: American College of Sports Medicine roundtable on hydration and physical activity: Consensus statements. *Curr Sports Med Rep* 2005;4:115-127.

   This document represents an outline of statements and recommendations weighted by strength of evidence regarding heat illness in athletes as derived from a consensus panel.

6. American Academy of Pediatrics: Climatic heat stress and the exercising child and adolescent: American Academy of Pediatrics committee on sports medicine and fitness. *Pediatrics* 2000;106:158-159.

7. Armstrong LE, Epstein Y, Greenleaf JE, et al: American College of Sports Medicine position stand: Heat and cold illnesses during distance running. *Med Sci Sports Exerc* 1996;28:i-x.

8. Selected issues in injury and illness prevention and the team physician: A consensus statement. *Med Sci Sports Exerc* 2007;39:2058-2068.

   Representatives from major medical organizations convened for this consensus statement to discuss existing evidence pertaining to injury and illness, including the prevention of heat illness in athletes. This statement of expert opinion was presented.

9. American College of Sports Medicine, Armstrong LE, Casa DJ, et al: American College of Sports Medicine position stand: Exertional heat illness during training and competition. *Med Sci Sports Exerc* 2007;39:556-572.

   This expert panel presents an up-to-date review of existing evidence including strength of evidence statements pertaining to dehydration, exertional heat illness, and athletic activity recommendations during times of heat stress.

10. Noakes TD, Sharwood K, Speedy D, et al: Three independent biological mechanisms cause exercise-associated hyponatremia: Evidence from 2,135 weighed competitive athletic performances. *Proc Natl Acad Sci USA* 2005;102:18550-18555.

    This retrospective study of pooled data on cases of exercise-associated hyponatremia addresses the concept of fluid overload in pathogenesis. Level of evidence: III.

11. Hew-Butler T, Verbalis JG, Noakes TD, International Marathon Medical Directors Association: Updated fluid recommendation: Position statement from the International Marathon Medical Directors Association (IMMDA). *Clin J Sport Med* 2006;16:283-292.

    These authors present six physiologic considerations of fluid balance, review current evidence, and provide six practical recommendations applicable to athletes participating in marathon running for maintaining proper hydration status.

12. Casa DJ, Armstrong LE, Hillman SK, et al: National Athletic Trainers' Association position statement: Fluid replacement for athletes. *J Athl Train* 2000;35:212-224.

13. Rosner MH, Kirven J: Exercise-associated hyponatremia. *Clin J Am Soc Nephrol* 2007;2:151-161.

    The authors present an in-depth review of the pathogenesis of exercise-associated hyponatremia through a discussion of hormonal, cellular, and renal pathophysiology.

14. Almond CS, Shin AY, Fortescue EB, et al: Hyponatremia among runners in the Boston Marathon. *N Engl J Med* 2005;352:1550-1556.

    This article describes the findings of a prospective study of subjects at the 2002 Boston Marathon in terms of the incidence of and risk factors for hyponatremia for existing recommendations. Level of evidence: II.

15. Hew-Butler T, Almond C, Ayus JC, et al: Consensus statement of the 1st international exercise-associated hyponatremia consensus development conference, Cape Town, South Africa 2005. *Clin J Sport Med* 2005;15:208-213.

    An expert panel presents their consensus statements on evidence pertaining to current beliefs on the pathophysiology of hyponatremia, risk factors, prevention strategies, and future study design.

16. Cooper ER, Ferrara MS, Broglio SP: Exertional heat illness and environmental conditions during a single football season in the southeast. *J Athl Train* 2006;41:332-336.

    An observational study of the rate of heat illness and WBGT readings over a 3-month period in the southern United States was undertaken to monitor the rate of heat illness and environmental stress. Level of evidence: II.

17. Binkley HM, Beckett J, Casa D, Kleiner DM, Plummer PE: National Athletic Trainers' Association position statement: Exertional heat illnesses. *J Athl Train* 2002;37:329-343.

18. Kenefick RW, O'Moore KM, Mahood NV, Castellani JW: Rapid IV versus oral rehydration: Responses to subsequent exercise heat stress. *Med Sci Sports Exerc* 2006;38:2125-2131.

    A small study of nonheat-acclimated males was performed using three experimental designs in a randomized order to determine the effect of oral versus intravenous fluid administration on recovery and performance in the heat. Level of evidence: I.

19. *National Collegiate Athletic Association 2007-2008 Sports Medicine Handbook*, ed 18. Indianapolis, IN, NCAA, July 2007.

    Guidelines are put forth by the NCAA regarding the prevention of heat illness, outlining screening, risk factors, the measurement of heat stress, general hydration strategies, and initial treatment for heat illness. Level of evidence: V.

20. Larsen T, Kumar S, Grimmer K, Potter A, Farquharson T, Sharpe P: A systematic review of guidelines for the prevention of heat illness in community-based sports participants and officials. *J Sci Med Sport* 2007;10:11-26.

    This paper provides a systematic review of heat illness prevention strategies formulated with particular attention to a critical appraisal of study design behind current recommendations and weighting based on the quality of guidelines.

The Youth Athlete

SECTION EDITOR:

ANDREW GREGORY, MD, FAAP, FACSM

Chapter 36

Osteochondroses and the Young Athlete

John P. Batson, MD, FAAP   Brian L. Bixler, MD

Introduction

The family of conditions known as osteochondroses affects skeletally immature children and adolescents. Impaired blood supply to the various bones is believed to be a result of repetitive microtrauma in many instances. Because of this observation, sports activity is often associated with the development of osteochondroses. These disorders most commonly affect the elbow, hip, foot, and wrist.

Panner Disease

Overview

Panner disease is a type of osteochondrosis that affects the capitellum of the humerus. The etiology of the disorder is not fully understood; as with other osteochondroses, impaired blood supply to the immature capitellum is believed to be responsible. Repetitive microtrauma, such as valgus stress during overhead throwing or axial compression to the elbow during gymnastics, has been associated with the condition.[1] Children younger than age 10 years are most often affected.[2] It is unknown if the condition is a milder version of an osteochondritis dissecans (OCD) lesion of the capitellum or if the two are separate entities.[1] Adolescents older than age 10 years with more mature bony anatomy are more likely to be affected with OCD lesions than Panner disease. A comparison of Panner disease and OCD is presented in **Table 1**.

Clinical Presentation

The child will usually present with pain localized to the elbow that worsens with physical activity. Young athletes may report impaired performance because of pain and limited motion. Physical examination reveals tenderness over the lateral elbow. Range of motion, both the extremes of extension and flexion and all pronation/supination motions, may be limited, and strength may be reduced because of pain. An effusion may be present. Mechanical symptoms are more common with OCD than Panner disease. Valgus laxity is rare in patients with Panner disease. In most instances, the nondominant arm can serve as a normal comparison to the affected arm.

Diagnostic Imaging

AP, lateral, and oblique radiographic views are typically obtained with comparison views of the unaffected elbow to demonstrate more subtle findings. In patients with Panner disease, the entire capitellum is often affected, with irregularity of the bony contours, fissuring, and fragmentation[1] (**Figures 1** and **2**). If the diagnosis is in question or a more detailed image is necessary, MRI helps show bony edema, an effusion, or cartilage irregularity with the disease.

Treatment and Prognosis

The management of Panner disease is directed at symptomatic care. Rest from any aggravating sport or activity is important and should be emphasized. A brief period of immobilization may be necessary to control the symptoms. Ice and anti-inflammatory drugs can help in the acute phase. Physical therapy may resolve any strength deficits or poor flexibility in the upper extremity. The prognosis for a child with Panner disease is excellent, with symptom resolution, remodeling potential, and little to no residual deformity.[1,2]

Legg-Calvé-Perthes Disease

Overview

Despite the tremendous work performed since the early 19th century in understanding and treating Legg-Calvé-Perthes disease, many questions remain regarding the disease etiology, best treatment, and ultimate prognosis.[3]

Etiology

Legg-Calvé-Perthes disease is an osteochondrosis affecting the capital femoral epiphysis in the growing child. The exact pathogenesis of the condition remains unknown. As with the other osteochondroses, interruption of the blood supply to the femoral head appears to be a universal event that leads to the typical changes seen on physical examination and imaging.

8: The Youth Athlete

Table 1

Comparison of Panner Disease and Osteochondritis Dissecans (OCD)

	Panner Disease	OCD Lesion
Age affected	Younger than 10 years	Older than 10 years
Size of lesion	Entire capitellum	Focal area in capitellum
Presence of loose bodies	No	Possible
Treatment	Symptomatic care	Variable
Prognosis	Excellent	Variable

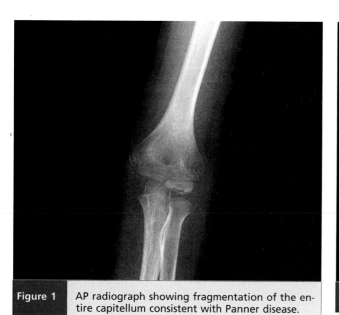

Figure 1 | AP radiograph showing fragmentation of the entire capitellum consistent with Panner disease.

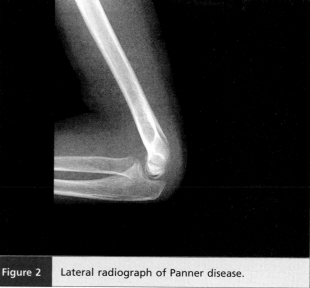

Figure 2 | Lateral radiograph of Panner disease.

Some have suggested Legg-Calvé-Perthes disease in certain children is the hip's manifestation of a systemic bony dysplasia.[3] Short stature, delayed bone age relative to chronologic age, and bilateral hip involvement are associations that lend some evidence to a possible underlying systemic bony abnormality.[3,4] Endocrine abnormalities have been implicated in some studies.[5] Associations with hyperactivity and preceding trauma have led some to think that repetitive microtrauma or an isolated traumatic event may impair the femoral head's vascular supply and trigger the disease process.

The association of thrombophilia and Legg-Calvé-Perthes disease has been studied.[6-9] Many prothrombotic factors have been implicated, including protein C or S deficiency, antithrombin III deficiency, factor V Leiden mutation, MTHFR C677T mutation, and the prothrombin gene G20210A polymorphism. Some studies show associations between Legg-Calvé-Perthes disease and thrombus risk factors, whereas others do not.

Environmental factors also have been implicated with Legg-Calvé-Perthes disease, including passive smoke exposure, nutritional deficiencies, and lower socioeconomic class.[3,10,11] Initially, it was believed that some cases of transient (toxic) synovitis developed into Legg-Calvé-Perthes disease. It is now believed that synovitis is one of the early manifestations of Legg-Calvé-Perthes diseases and few, if any, cases of Legg-Calvé-Perthes disease are causally related to transient synovitis.

Clinical Features and Differential Diagnosis

Children with Legg-Calvé-Perthes disease frequently present with the insidious onset of unilateral hip pain or a limp. The pain and limp are more noticeable after sports activities and will improve with rest and anti-inflammatory drugs. The condition affects males more frequently than females at a ratio of approximately 3-4:1.[3] It is seen in children age 6 to 8 years with an age range of 2 to 12 years.[3] The prevalence of bilateral involvement is reportedly 8% to 24%.[12] In most children with bilateral disease, the hips are in different stages of disease, but up to one third have been shown to be in the same stage of disease.[12] An antalgic gait may be present in the acute phase secondary to related synovitis and muscle spasm. Later in the disease process, the limp may be related to disuse muscle atrophy or a limb-length discrepancy. On physical examination, the child with Legg-Calvé-Perthes disease in the acute phase will have limited and painful range of motion in the affected hip, with loss of internal rotation a particularly sensitive indicator of intra-articular pathology. As the disease progresses, range of motion is often limited to varying degrees by the altered bony femoral head and acetabular relationship.

The clinician should always be alert for hip pathology referring pain to the ipsilateral knee. In this scenario, the child will present with vague knee pain and a normal knee examination. In addition, it is important to determine if a patient has a history of trauma, unexplained fever, weight loss, other joint symptoms or systemic issues (for example, rashes, ophthalmologic or gastrointestinal symptoms). The differential diagnosis of a child with an irritable hip includes occult fracture or injury, infection, transient synovitis, or rheumatologic disease. Childhood skeletal dysplasia, such as multiple epiphyseal dysplasia and spondyloepiphyseal dysplasia, also may present with hip pathology. A family history of bony abnormalities, a child with short stature, or a child with bilateral hip involvement should trigger a thorough evaluation. Slipped capital femoral epiphysis is another common hip disorder in childhood, but this typically affects older, overweight adolescents. Previously unrecognized cases of developmental dysplasia of the hip also may become apparent, with children having hip pain as they grow and become more active with sports. Vascular congestion with subsequent femoral head osteonecrosis also can occur in hematologic disorders such as sickle cell disease, thalassemia, and childhood cancers.[3]

Diagnostic Imaging

The initial evaluation of a child with suspected Legg-Calvé-Perthes disease includes AP and frog-leg pelvic radiographs. The condition is unilateral in most children, and radiographs of the pelvis allow comparison between the affected and asymptomatic (presumably normal) side. Initial radiographs may appear normal. Associated synovitis may be visible with widening of the joint space. Other findings early in the disease process include a smaller femoral ossific nucleus and lateralization of the femoral head.[3] A subchondral fracture of the femoral head may be present in the initial disease stage. As the disease progresses, radiographic changes become more pronounced. Findings in the femoral head include increased density, irregularity, fragmentation, sclerosis, and collapse. Plain radiographs also may demonstrate radiolucent cystic changes in the metaphyseal region[3,13] (**Figure 3**).

If the initial plain radiographs are normal in appearance, the child may be managed conservatively for 1 to 2 weeks; the physical examination and radiographs are then repeated. Further evaluation (laboratory and diagnostic imaging) is warranted in a child with continued symptoms and normal plain radiographs. An ultrasound may be obtained to document the presence of effusion, especially if an aspiration is planned. MRI is helpful to demonstrate subtle early findings related to Legg-Calvé-Perthes disease. MRI provides a more de-

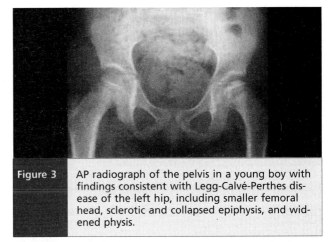

Figure 3 AP radiograph of the pelvis in a young boy with findings consistent with Legg-Calvé-Perthes disease of the left hip, including smaller femoral head, sclerotic and collapsed epiphysis, and widened physis.

tailed and functional study by allowing visualization of the femoral head in multiple planes.[14] A bone scan can detect early impaired blood flow to the femoral epiphysis before findings on plain films;[3] however, its lack of specificity limits its clinical utility.

Staging and Classification of Disease

The disease process is staged based on radiographic evaluation.[3] The classification has been modified and condensed into four stages: initial, fragmentation, healing, and residual.[3] The initial stage of the disease (6 months average duration; range 1 to 14 months) may show a smaller, denser ossific nucleus. During the fragmentation phase (8 months average duration; range 2 to 35 months), collapse of the femoral head becomes more pronounced. Lateral migration of the femoral head becomes more apparent. Reossification with new bone formation occurs as hips enter the healing phase (51 months average duration; range 2 to 122 months). The residual phase is generally regarded as the conclusion of the disease process when little growth or remodeling remains.

Much work has been performed to determine a classification scheme for Legg-Calvé-Perthes disease that would allow consistent disease description, physician communication, and treatment planning. A problem with past disease classifications (for example, Catterall and Salter-Thompson) has been poor interobserver and intraobserver agreement and reliability.[15,16] The lateral pillar classification has shown improved interobserver agreement.[3,15,17] The lateral pillar classification is determined on an AP radiograph of the pelvis early in the fragmentation stage, typically 6 months after symptom onset.[15] The lateral pillar is distinguished from the center of the femoral head by a radiolucent line of fragmentation.[15] Changes seen on plain radiographs, including radiolucency and collapse of bony height, determine the classification severity (**Table 2**).[15,17] In recent years, this classification has been refined to include an intermediate group and was again found to have good to excellent interobserver and intraobserver reliability.[15,18]

Table 2

Modified Lateral Pillar Classification of Legg-Calvé-Perthes Disease

Group	Radiographic Findings
A	No significant lucency or collapse noted on plain radiographs
B	Radiolucency present, less than 50% original height lost
B/C	A narrow lateral pillar more than 50% original height, or a lateral pillar with little ossification, but at least 50% original height, or a lateral pillar with exactly 50% original pillar height
C	More lucency, lateral pillar collapse with more than 50% original height lost

Table 3

Suggested Treatment and Prognosis Based on the Lateral Pillar Group (LPG) and the Presenting Age

LPG/Presenting Age	Proposed Treatment	Prognosis
Group A, any age	No treatment necessary	Excellent
Group B, younger than 8 years	Symptomatic treatment	Good
Group B, older than 8 years	Surgery recommended	Fair
Group B/C, younger than 8 years	+/- Benefit with surgery	Fair
Group B/C, older than 8 years	Surgery recommended	Fair-Poor
Group C, any age	Surgery no benefit	Poor

Treatment

Given the complexities of staging, classification, and treatment options, management of the child with Legg-Calvé-Perthes disease by a physician specializing in the disorder is optimal. Initially, if the hip is extremely painful, a period of rest from activity, crutch use to minimize weight bearing, and a course of an anti-inflammatory drugs is helpful. When tolerable, physical therapy often is initiated to maintain motion, flexibility, and strength in the hip and muscles of the leg. Radiographs are taken, and the child is observed to determine the severity of the disease. Prolonged periods of traction, bracing, and casting have fallen out of favor in recent years. A limb-length discrepancy of clinical significance must be treated.

A key concept that has emerged in recent years is containment of the femoral head within the acetabulum. Surgical strategies such as femoral varus osteotomy, Salter innominate osteotomy, and shelf arthroplasty are reserved for femoral heads at risk of deformity and poor acetabular coverage. An adductor tenotomy may accompany the surgical procedure to assist with motion and limit distracting forces in the hip. Emerging surgical techniques include distraction of the femoral head with an external fixator secured in the femur and pelvis. Core decompression of the femoral head to promote vascular ingrowth is another newer concept. Timing of containment surgery is important and typically recommended early in the course of disease before advanced fragmentation, when radiographs show increased density or collapse of the femoral head.[19] Once a significant deformity is present, the role of surgery is deemphasized in the young patient. Surgical techniques often are chosen based on the surgeon's preference and experience. Adolescents with a history of Legg-Calvé-Perthes disease and new-onset hip pain with activity should be evaluated for conditions such as femoroacetabular impingement or an osteochondritis dissecans lesions, which are known to occur in the hip after Legg-Calvé-Perthes disease.[20,21]

Overall Prognosis in Legg-Calvé-Perthes Disease

The ultimate prognosis of Legg-Calvé-Perthes disease is related to the shape of the femoral head at the conclusion of the active disease process. Although many children have significant abnormality during the disease, most have a good prognosis into adulthood.[3] According to results from a large multicenter trial, the strongest predictor in disease outcome was the revised lateral pillar classification system.[22] As the radiographic changes advance from group A to C, the prognosis changes from good to poor. This study also reinforced the belief that younger children in whom the disease develops fare better than those who are older at presentation. Remodeling potential is likely limited in older children and, in a similar fashion, girls who reach skeletal maturity earlier than boys. The study allows for some helpful treatment recommendations and gives some prognostic value based on the disease stage and the presenting age (Table 3). It will be years before physicians can determine how newer treatment concepts and modalities have affected the disease process.[23]

Osteochondroses of the Foot

Overview

The two most common osteochondroses of the foot are Köhler disease, which affects the tarsal navicular bone, and Freiberg disease, which affects the metatarsal heads. Both conditions are believed to be the result of interrupted blood supply to the affected bone secondary to repetitive microtrauma.

Köhler Disease

Köhler disease affects children age 4 to 8 years. It is up to four times more common in boys than girls.[23] Hyperactivity is a frequent association in patients with Köhler disease. Patients present with the insidious onset of midfoot pain or a limp. On physical examination, the patient may have an antalgic gait, walking on the lateral side of the foot. Point tenderness is present over the navicular bone. Subtle erythema and soft-tissue swelling may be present. The differential diagnosis includes posterior tibialis tendinitis, navicular stress fracture, and a symptomatic accessory navicular bone. All of these conditions are much more common in older patients. AP, lateral, and oblique radiographic views of the foot will show the typical radiographic changes (Figure 4). The navicular bone is sclerotic, fragmented, and smaller than normal. Accessory bones and multiple centers of ossification are common radiographic normal variants, and clinical correlation is required. Additional imaging studies such as a bone scan or MRI generally are not necessary.

Treatment of Köhler disease is with symptomatic care. A short leg cast or walking boot may be used for 4 to 12 weeks. Weight bearing is allowed as tolerated. An ankle support orthotic device and footwear with a supportive arch may be helpful as the symptoms subside. The prognosis for patients with Köhler disease is excellent, with no residual deformity or persistent conditions at the conclusion of the disease process.[2,23,24] The radiographic changes may take up to 1 year or longer to normalize; however, if the pain is resolved, there is no need for activity limitation.

Freiberg Disease

Freiberg disease tends to affect adolescent females between ages 10 and 15 years. These patients may be involved in activities such as dance, ballet, or sports involving running. Patients typically present with the gradual onset of vague forefoot pain. The second and third metatarsal heads are most frequently affected. On clinical examination, tenderness is isolated to the metatarsal head. An effusion and painful range of motion at the adjacent metatarsophalangeal (MTP) joint may be present. The remainder of the physical examination is often unre-

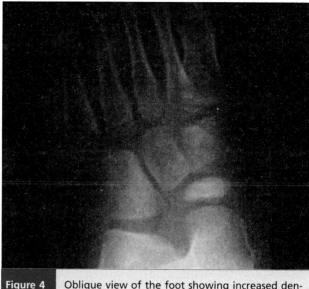

Figure 4 Oblique view of the foot showing increased density of the navicular bone consistent with Köhler disease.

markable. The differential diagnosis includes a metatarsal stress fracture, metatarsalgia, interdigital neuroma, and a MTP joint sprain. Radiographs will show a flattened metatarsal head with sclerotic margins. Advanced disease may show cystic changes, irregular margins, and loose bodies within the MTP joint. Additional imaging studies (bone scans, MRI, and CT) may be needed for surgical planning but often are not necessary.

Prompt diagnosis and treatment is important for patients with Freiberg disease. The foot should be immobilized with either a walking boot or short leg cast with toe extension so motion at the MTP joint is limited. Ice and anti-inflammatory drugs help reduce inflammation and pain. The patient should be completely asymptomatic before transitioning back to athletics. An orthotic device with a stiff last may be helpful when the patient is ready for shoe wear. Although most patients do not have significant long-term disability, arthritis of the affected MTP joint can occur. Patients with persistent pain and disability may require surgery, such as débridement, bone grafting, metatarsal head resection, or joint arthroplasty.[23,24]

Osteochondrosis of the Wrist: Kienbock Disease

Osteochondrosis of the carpal lunate bone is known as Kienbock disease. The disorder is less common in younger athletes, but it is an important condition to consider in the differential diagnosis of any individual with wrist pain unresponsive to conservative measures. The athlete typically presents with vague pain in the dominant wrist. Common sports involved include tennis and weight lifting. As with other disorders in the osteochondrosis family, an impaired blood supply to the lunate has been implicated as an initial insulting event.

As such, repetitive microtrauma or an acute traumatic injury to the affected wrist may be recalled by the athlete. The physical examination is significant for limited range of motion in the wrist, decreased strength about the wrist and hand, and point tenderness over the dorsal lunate. Radiographs will show typical findings, including sclerosis, fragmentation, and adjacent arthritis. Early in the disease process, MRI is a more sensitive modality to demonstrate bony pathology. Grading systems have been proposed based on the radiographic findings, which can assist with formulating a treatment plan.[25] Given the complexities of the disease and frequent need for advanced surgical management, referral of these patients to an upper extremity orthopaedic specialist should be strongly considered.

Summary

The osteochondroses are a group of conditions affecting children of all ages. The disease process can occur in any bone in the body, but it is more common in the elbow, wrist, hip, and foot. Affected children often are involved in sports and fitness endeavors. Athletic trainers, therapists, and educated coaches and other members of the athletic care network should be familiar with the common osteochondroses and can assist with recognition, therapeutic modalities, and transitioning back to sport. Physicians involved in the care of these athletes, in particular children with Legg-Calvé-Perthes disease, should recognize the complexities involved in these disease processes and have experience in their management. Many of these conditions respond to simple conservative measures, including rest, ice, and anti-inflammatory drugs.

Annotated References

1. Kobayashi K, Burton KJ, Rodner C, Smith B, Caputo AE: Lateral compression injuries in the pediatric elbow: Panner's disease and osteochondritis dissecans of the capitellum. *J Am Acad Orthop Surg* 2004;12:246-254.

   In this review of the literature, the authors compare and contrast lateral compression injuries in the pediatric elbow, including Panner disease and OCD. Etiology, the clinical presentation, the physical examination, radiographic findings, and treatment options are discussed.

2. Tachdjian MO: *Clinical Pediatric Orthopedics: Art of Diagnosis.* Stamford, CT, Appleton and Lange, 1997, pp 67-70, 304, 322, 333.

3. Herring JA: *Legg-Calvé-Perthes Disease.* Rosemont, IL, American Academy of Orthopaedic Surgeons, 1996.

4. Lee ST, Vaidya SV, Song HR, Lee SH, Suh SW, Telang SS: Bone age delay patterns in Legg-Calve-Perthes disease: An analysis using the Tanner and Whitehouse 3 method. *J Pediatr Orthop* 2007;27:198-203.

The authors assessed the bone age delay patterns seen in different stages of Legg-Calvé-Perthes disease using both the Tanner and Whitehouse 3 and the Greulich and Pyle systems. The bone age in the 83 patients was found to lag behind the mean chronologic age in various stages of the disease. Bone age delay was most evident in the early stages of the disease. Decreases in the bone age delay as the disease progresses were observed and are thought to be a result of skeletal maturation acceleration. No significant differences were seen between male and female children with Legg-Calvé-Perthes disease in terms of the age of onset of the disease, the severity of the disease, or bone age delay patterns.

5. Kealey WD, Lappin KJ, Leslie H, Sheridan B, Cosgrove AP: Endocrine profile and physical stature of children with Perthes disease. *J Pediatr Orthop* 2004;24:161-166.

The authors compared 139 children with Legg-Calvé-Perthes disease with 40 healthy matched control subjects and assessed the endocrine profile and body habitus. They found no significant differences that would be suggestive of an endocrine abnormality associated with children with Legg-Calvé-Perthes disease.

6. Balasa VV, Gruppo RA, Glueck CJ, et al: Legg-Calvé-Perthes disease and thrombophilia. *J Bone Joint Surg Am* 2004;86:2642-2647.

In this retrospective study, the blood from 72 patients with Legg-Calvé-Perthes disease was compared with that of a control group of 172 healthy children and analyzed for various coagulation abnormalities. The G1691A Leiden mutation in the factor V gene was more common in patients with Legg-Calvé-Perthes disease (11%) than control subjects (4%). In addition, anticardiolipin antibody levels were higher in patients with Legg-Calvé-Perthes disease than in control subjects. No other case-control differences were noted, including protein C or S deficiencies, antithrombin III deficiencies, homocystine levels, and plasminogen activator inhibitor-1 activity.

7. Hresko MT, McDougall PA, Gorlin JB, Vamvakas EC, Kasser JR, Neufeld EJ: Prospective reevaluation of the association between thrombotic diathesis and Legg-Perthes disease. *J Bone Joint Surg* 2002;84:1613-1618.

8. Lopez-Franco M, Gonzalez-Moran G, De Lucas JC Jr, et al: Legg-Perthes disease and heritable thrombophilia. *J Pediatr Orthop* 2005;25:456-459.

The authors studied 90 children with Legg-Calvé-Perthes disease who were analyzed for any association with inheritable thrombophilic disorders, including the G20210A prothrombin gene, factor V Leiden, and MTHFR C677 mutation. No relationship was found with these markers, and thus the authors did not recommend screening for these disorders in patients with Legg-Calvé-Perthes disease.

9. Mehta JS, Conybeare ME, Hinves BL, Winter JB: Protein C levels in patients with Legg-Calve-Perthes disease: Is it a true deficiency? *J Pediatr Orthop* 2006;26:200-203.

The authors of this observational study found lower end

normal protein C levels but no true deficiency in 51 patients with Legg-Calvé-Perthes disease. However, 74.5% of patients with Legg-Calvé-Perthes disease had a history of secondhand smoke exposure.

10. Gordon JE, Schoenecker PL, Osland JD, Dobbs MB, Szymanski DA, Luhmann SJ: Smoking and socioeconomic status in the etiology and severity of Legg-Calvé-Perthes disease. *J Pediatr Orthop B* 2004;13: 367-370.

   In this prospective study, the authors found 63.3% of children with Legg-Calvé-Perthes disease were exposed to at least one smoker in the house. They suggest secondhand smoke is a significant risk factor for the development of Legg-Calvé-Perthes disease.

11. Garcia Mata S, Ardanaz Aicua E, Hidalgo Ovejero A, Martinez Grande M: Legg-Calve-Perthes disease and passive smoking. *J Pediatr Orthop* 2000;20:326-330.

12. Guille JT, Lipton GE, Tsirikos AI, Bowen JR: Bilateral Legg-Calve-Perthes disease: Presentation and outcome. *J Pediatr Orthop* 2002;22:458-463.

13. Kim HK, Skelton DN, Quigley EJ: Pathogenesis of metaphyseal radiolucent changes following ischemic necrosis of the capital femoral epiphysis in immature pigs: A preliminary report. *J Bone Joint Surg Am* 2004;86: 129-135.

   The prevalence of metaphyseal radiographic changes and histologic changes seen in the metaphyseal region of patients with Legg-Calvé-Perthes disease was studied in piglet models of ischemic necrosis of the femoral head. Ischemic changes were induced in the femoral head of 53 piglets via ligature of the femoral neck. Metaphyseal radiolucent changes, ranging from cystic lesions to diffuse radiolucency around the proximal physis, were seen in 13 piglets. Histologic changes observed included focal physeal thickening, fibrovascular tissue replacement of trabecular bone, and physeal cartilage resorption. The femoral necks with metaphyseal lesions were significantly shorter than those of control subjects and diseased hips without metaphyseal changes. The presence of these metaphyseal radiolucent changes is associated with a poor prognosis in Legg-Calvé-Perthes disease.

14. Cho TJ, Lee SH, Choi IH, Chung CY, Yoo WJ, Kim SJ: Femoral head deformity in Catterall groups III and IV Legg-Calve-Perthes disease: Magnetic resonance image analysis in coronal and sagittal planes. *J Pediatr Orthop* 2002;22:601-606.

15. Herring JA, Kim HT, Browne R: Legg-Calvé-Perthes disease: Part I: Classification of radiographs with use of the modified lateral pillar and Stulberg classifications. *J Bone Joint Surg Am* 2004;86:2103-2120.

   As part of a multicenter prospective study, the authors performed interobserver and intraobserver trials of the lateral pillar and Stulberg classifications in 345 hips with Legg-Calvé-Perthes disease. Important classification schemes for Legg-Calvé-Perthes disease also are reviewed. A new intermediate B/C border group was added to the lateral pillar classification in an effort to refine the original classification system. The lateral pil-

lar classification showed good to excellent interobserver and intraobserver reliability. Stulberg classifications showed excellent interobserver and intraobserver reliability between six orthopaedic examiners. A new technique for measuring femoral head sphericity applicable to the Stulberg classification is also suggested.

16. Kalenderer O, Agus H, Ozcalabi IT, Ozluk S: The importance of surgeons' experience on intraobserver and interobserver reliability of classifications used for Perthes disease. *J Pediatr Orthop* 2005;25:460-464.

   In this study, 18 reviewers evaluated 10 radiographs of patients with Legg-Calvé-Perthes disease. They found physicians with more experience in pediatric orthopaedics had improved intraobserver and interobserver reliability for the Catterall, Salter-Thompson, Herrin, and Stulberg classifications. However, overall error rates were high for all examiners, including resident, senior, and orthopaedic surgeons.

17. Herring JA, Neustadt JB, Williams JJ, Early JS, Browne RH: The lateral pillar classification of Legg-Calvé-Perthes disease. *J Pediatr Orthop* 1992;12: 143-150.

18. Akgun R, Yazici M, Aksoy MC, Cil A, Alpaslan AM, Tumer Y: The accuracy and reliability of estimation of lateral pillar height in determining the herring grade in Legg-Calve-Perthes Disease. *J Pediatr Orthop* 2004;24: 651-653.

   The authors sought to determine if the amount of preserved lateral pillar height had an effect on interobserver agreement when assigning Herring grades for Legg-Calvé-Perthes disease. They found good interobserver agreement in 29 of the 50 cases but poor interobserver reliability in the rest, which were borderline cases between groups A, B, and C. The authors suggested measurements of the lateral pillar height should be used rather than estimates, particularly with these borderline cases. This is important if the Herring classification is to be used to determine prognosis and treatment options.

19. Joseph B, Nair NS, Narasimha Rao KL, Mulpuri K, Varghese G: Optimal timing for containment surgery for Perthes disease. *J Pediatr Orthop* 2003;23:601-606.

   In an effort to identify the optimal timing for containment surgery, the authors studied 97 children following femoral osteotomy for Legg-Calvé-Perthes disease. The results of surgery were not as successful to prevent femoral head deformation if the surgery was performed after the fragmentation stage of the disease.

20. Rowe SM, Chung JY, Moon ES, Yoon TR, Jung ST, Lee KB: Computed tomographic findings of osteochondritis dissecans following Legg-Calve-Perthes Disease. *J Pediatr Orthop* 2003;23:356-362.

   CT revealed osteochondritis dissecans in 13 hips with Legg-Calvé-Perthes disease. Three-dimensional reconstruction helped determine the extent of the lesions and the presence of loose bodies and to follow the healing process.

21. Parvizi J, Leunig M, Ganz R: Femoroacetabular impingement. *J Am Acad Orthop Surg* 2007;15:561-570.

Femoroacetabular impingement is reviewed, including mechanisms of the disease, the types of impingement, clinical and radiographic features related to the disorder, and treatment options. Legg-Calvé-Perthes disease is discussed as a potential preceding disorder.

22. Herring JA, Kim HT, Browne R: Legg-Calvé-Perthes disease: Part II. Prospective multicenter study of the effect of treatment on outcome. *J Bone Joint Surg Am* 2004;86:2121-2134.

The effect of various treatment options on outcome of the disease was studied in a multicenter, prospective cohort trial comprising 438 patients with 451 affected hips with Legg-Calvé-Perthes disease. Three hundred forty-five hips in 337 patients were available for follow-up. The lateral pillar classification and age at onset of the disease correlated most with disease outcome. Patients older than age 8 years at disease onset and who had a lateral pillar B or B/C intermediate group faired better with surgical intervention. Patients younger than age 8 years with lateral pillar B hips at disease onset had good outcomes unrelated to the treatment provided. Patients with lateral pillar C hips had poor outcomes unrelated to the treatment.

23. Olney BW: Conditions of the foot, in Abel MF (ed): *Orthopaedic Knowledge Update: Pediatrics 3*. Rosemont, IL, American Academy of Orthopaedic Surgeons, 2006, pp 236-240.

The author lists possible surgical options for Freiberg disease and reminds the reader that Köhler disease is a self-limiting process with little or no residual problems in the foot, regardless of the treatment.

24. DiGiovanni CW, Patel A, Calfee R, Nickisch F: Osteonecrosis in the foot. *J Am Acad Orthop Surg* 2007; 15:208-217.

Osteonecrosis in the foot, including Köhler disease and Freiberg disease, is discussed; these conditions are reviewed in terms of etiology, treatment recommendations, and prognosis.

25. Allan CH, Joshi A, Lichtman DM: Kienböck's disease: Diagnosis and treatment. *J Am Acad Orthop Surg* 2001;9:128-136.

Chapter 37

Pediatric Anterior Cruciate Ligament Injuries

William Hennrikus, MD

Introduction

Tears of the anterior cruciate ligament (ACL) in skeletally immature athletes are occurring more frequently because of the increased number of children participating in organized year-round sports and are being diagnosed because of a greater awareness of the injury and improved diagnostic tests.[1] In children, athletic injuries cause 70% of acute knee hemarthroses, and approximately two thirds of acute knee hemarthroses occur in conjunction with an ACL tear.[2-4] ACL tears are more common in the female child athlete than the male child athlete.[5]

Natural History and Mechanism of Injury

Pediatric patients with an ACL tear have a natural history similar to that of adults with the same injury. Pediatric patients who are unable to modify their activities are at risk of recurrent instability, swelling, pain, meniscal tears, chondral injury, and arthritis.[6-15]

ACL tears in the pediatric athlete are caused by noncontact and contact mechanisms of injury. Often a "pop" is heard at the time of injury. The patient with an acute ACL tear typically presents with pain, a knee effusion, a reduction in knee motion, and difficulty bearing weight. The patient with a chronic ACL tear typically presents with recurrent effusions and instability.

Physical Examination

In the child, palpating the area of the physes is important to rule out physeal injury. When indicated, varus or valgus stress testing with fluoroscopy also helps rule out physeal injury. In the child with an acute ACL tear, the Lachman and anterior drawer tests typically demonstrate excess anterior translation of the knee with a soft end point. The pivot-shift test often is difficult to perform in the child with an acute knee injury because of pain and guarding.

Imaging

Plain radiographs should be obtained to rule out fracture, dislocation, osteochondral injury, or physeal injury. In addition, the amount of physeal closure can be estimated with plain radiographs. In patients with tenderness over the physis and valgus or varus laxity on physical examination, stress radiographs may be needed to differentiate between physeal and collateral ligament injury. The accuracy of MRI for diagnosing meniscal and ACL tears in children with acute knee injuries has been questioned.[16-19] However, MRI is a valuable ancillary tool to determine ligamentous, meniscal, and chondral injuries in the child whose physical examination is difficult to perform because of pain, swelling, and lack of cooperation[20] (**Figure 1**).

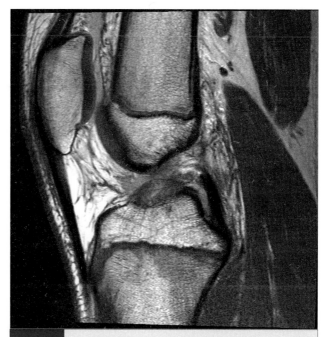

Figure 1   Sagittal MRI scan showing an ACL tear in a skeletally immature athlete with open physes.

Determination of Skeletal Maturity

Tanner staging has been suggested as a basis for determining the treatment of ACL tears in children.[1,9,21] Physical examination of the genital area and the breasts is done during Tanner staging. For example, Tanner stage II indicates the first signs of genital development and secondary sexual characteristics. Tanner stage V indicates maturity as the child proceeds to a physiologic epiphysiodesis. The accuracy of Tanner staging by orthopaedic surgeons has not been reported.

A more practical and more accurate method to determine skeletal maturity is to obtain the skeletal age of the patient, which can be obtained by comparing an AP radiograph of the athlete's left hand and wrist to the radiographs in the Greulich and Pyle atlas.[22] Most skeletal growth has been achieved in males with a bone age of 16 years and in females with a bone age of 14 years. A bone age of 16 years in a male and 14 years in a female corresponds to a radiograph of the hand and wrist showing that all growth plates have closed except for those of the distal radius and ulnar styloid.

In female patients, menarche history is a helpful physiologic indicator of diminished skeletal growth. The peak height velocity occurs before menarche. In most females, the physes will completely close 2 years following menarche. An equivalent physiologic indicator of diminished skeletal growth does not exist in males.

Treatment Approach

An ACL tear in a pediatric athlete is not a surgical emergency. Discussions with the parents and the child about the appropriate management options and understanding their goals and expectations are key.[1] The level of commitment to therapy by the child and the parents also should be determined, along with the full extent of the knee injury. MRI can help to assess whether additional physeal, ligamentous, meniscal, or chondral injury has occurred.[20] An accurate understanding of skeletal maturation using the patient's skeletal age is important.

Nonsurgical Treatment

Nonsurgical treatment such as activity modification, rehabilitation, and functional bracing avoids the risk of physeal injury and angular or longitudinal growth disturbance;[8] however, repeat instability episodes and additional meniscal or articular cartilage injury may occur.[6-13,15,23-25] In a small percentage of pediatric athletes, nonsurgical treatment can be definitive in those willing to limit their activity, such as cessation of sports involving cutting, pivoting, acceleration, and deceleration motions. Sports such as swimming, biking, and golf may be played by most athletes with an ACL-deficient knee. Nonsurgical treatment also can be used temporarily in some pediatric athletes with the goal of

protecting the menisci and articular surfaces until skeletal maturity has been achieved. At skeletal maturity, a definitive transphyseal ACL reconstruction may be successful in patients with low physical demands.[14,26] In pediatric athletes who perform activities that involve forceful deceleration and cutting movements, nonsurgical treatment of the ACL tear often is unsuccessful, leading to secondary injury and subsequent meniscal tears and knee arthritis.[6,10,11,14] In pediatric athletes who participate in sports such as soccer, basketball, gymnastics, wrestling, and football, nonsurgical treatment is likely to fail. It may be unrealistic to commit pediatric athletes involved in high-demand sports to years of activity modification and bracing.

Surgical Treatment

Current data are insufficient to provide absolute guidelines for the treatment of ACL tears in children.[27] The safest and most effective techniques continue to evolve.[8] However, as a result of reviewing the evidence-based literature, the following management recommendations are suggested. Patients with open physes and a skeletal age less than 14 years in females and less than 16 years in males should be counseled about activity modification, bracing, rehabilitation, and careful follow-up. Surgery can be performed at a later date when skeletal maturity has been achieved. Early surgery is indicated for those pediatric athletes (and parents) who are unable to comply with nonsurgical treatment or in whom nonsurgical treatment fails. Patients and parents who request surgery before maturation of the growth plates should be counseled about the small but real risk of angular or longitudinal growth injury and the possible need for additional surgery.[13,28-30] In addition, one case of overgrowth following transphyseal reconstruction with a hamstring graft has been reported.[31] Extraphyseal, transepiphyseal, partial transphyseal, and transphyseal ACL reconstruction methods have been used. Surgical treatment of the torn ACL also may be indicated in patients of any age with additional knee injuries, such as a meniscal tear that is amenable to repair.

Extraphyseal Surgery

In the skeletally immature athlete (skeletal age less than 11 years in females and less than 13 years in males), extraphyseal surgery can provide physiologic stabilization until full skeletal maturity occurs. The physes are avoided to prevent the risk of growth disturbance. Two types of extraphyseal procedures have been popularized. A hamstring graft can be routed through a groove in the anterior tibia through the notch and over the top of the lateral femoral condyle.[32-36] Alternatively, a strip of iliotibial band can be placed around the outside of the lateral femoral condyle through the notch and then sutured to the periosteum of the proximal tibia.[21,37,38] Patients and parents should be counseled that these surgical procedures are nonanatomic. Patients may have continued instability requiring activity modification. In addition, an anatomic reconstruction may be needed when the child reaches skeletal maturity.

Transepiphyseal Surgery

In the skeletally immature athlete and in the older child (skeletal age 11 to 14 years in females and 13 to 16 years in males), transepiphyseal surgery reportedly helps prevent iatrogenic growth disturbance. Using arthroscopy and fluoroscopy for precise tunnel placement, a hamstring graft is placed through the proximal tibia and distal femoral epiphyses.[34,39] Graft fixation is performed away from the physes. This procedure is more technically demanding than extraphyseal surgery, with the smallest margin of error that could result in physeal injury.

Partial Transphyseal Surgery

In the older child, a hamstring graft can be placed through a small 6- to 7-mm centrally placed, vertical, tibial drill hole and via the over-the-top position at the femur.[34,40,41] A soft-tissue allograft also has been used for this method.[23] Physeal injury can be avoided by using a small drill hole, using soft-tissue grafts only, avoiding injury to the physis at the over-the-top position,[42] and placing the fixation away from the physes. Patients and parents should be counseled that there is a small risk for physeal injury, along with the possibility of additional surgery for angular or longitudinal growth disturbance.

Complete Transphyseal Surgery

In the older child, a hamstring graft can be placed through a small 6- to 7-mm centrally placed tibial drill hole and via an equally small femoral drill hole.[28,31,43-45] As with partial transphyseal surgery, physeal injury can be avoided by using a small drill hole, using soft-tissue grafts only, avoiding injury to the tibial tubercle, and placing the fixation away from the physes. Patients and parents should be counseled that physeal injury may still occur, and additional surgery for angular or longitudinal growth disturbance may be necessary.

Adolescents who are approaching skeletal maturity (skeletal age of 14 years for females and 16 years for males) can undergo anatomic ACL surgery with tibial and femoral drill holes and the surgeon's graft of choice with minimal risk of physeal injury.[6,25,46-50]

Rehabilitation

Rehabilitation in children can be more difficult than in adults with respect to compliance with therapy and activity restrictions. Rehabilitation may need to be modified for the individual patient and for the particular surgical procedure performed. In general, a graduated rehabilitation program emphasizing full extension, active range of motion, strength (quadriceps, hamstring, hip, and core), and endurance training can be started in the first few days after surgery. Progressive rehabilita-

tion during the first 3 months after surgery includes range-of-motion exercises, patellar mobilization, proprioceptive exercises, and closed chain strengthening exercises. Straight line jogging, plyometric exercises, and sport-specific exercises are added after 3 to 6 months. Return to play typically occurs 6 to 9 months following surgery.

Summary

The rate of ACL tears in pediatric athletes is increasing. Treatment should be based on skeletal maturity and activity level. Patients in whom nonsurgical management has failed or those who wish to return to high-risk athletic activity without a trial of nonsurgical management can be treated with surgery. The surgical technique selected is influenced by skeletal age. For children with large growth potential, nonanatomic, extraphyseal reconstruction is recommended. For young adolescents with decreasing growth potential, partial transphyseal reconstruction is recommended. For older adolescents near skeletal maturity, anatomic transphyseal reconstruction is recommended. Unfortunately, the study designs in the current literature—small case series—are inadequate to completely answer the question of whether early or delayed ACL reconstruction results in the best possible outcome in skeletally immature individuals. Future prospective studies are needed with larger patient series.

Annotated References

1. Stanitski CL: Anterior cruciate ligament injury in the skeletally immature patient: Diagnosis and treatment. *J Am Acad Orthop Surg* 1995;3:146-158.

2. Kocher MS, Di Canzio J, Zurakowski D, et al: Diagnostic performance of clinical examination and selective magnetic resonance imaging in the evaluation of intraarticular knee disorders in children and adolescents. *Am J Sports Med* 2001;29:292-295.

3. Luhmann SJ: Acute traumatic knee effusions in children and adolescents. *J Pediatr Orthop* 2003;23:199-202.

   The etiology of traumatic knee effusions is described in 44 patients younger than 18 years. Of 55 total diagnoses, 16 (29%) were ACL injuries, 16 (29%) were meniscal tears, 14 (25%) were patellofemoral subluxations or dislocations, 3 (5%) were medial collateral ligament sprains, 2 (4%) were patellar osteochondral fractures, 2 (4%) were retinacular injuries, 1 (2%) was a posterior cruciate ligament rupture, and 1 (2%) was a tibial eminence fracture. Level of evidence: IV.

4. Stanitski CL, Harvell JC, Fu F: Observations on acute knee hemarthrosis in children and adolescents. *J Pediatr Orthop* 1993;13:506-510.

5. Shea KG, Pfeiffer R, Wang JH, Curtin M, Apel PJ: Anterior cruciate ligament injury in pediatric and adolescent soccer players: An analysis of insurance data. *J Pediatr Orthop* 2004;24:623-628.

   Injury claims from an insurance company specializing in soccer coverage are studied. Like adult females, skeletally immature females demonstrated a higher rate of ACL injury in comparison with male counterparts. A significant increase in ACL injuries occurred in the 11- to 12-year-old age group. Level of evidence: IV.

6. Aichroth PM, Patel DV, Zorrilla P: The natural history and treatment of rupture of the anterior cruciate ligament in children and adolescents: A prospective review. *J Bone Joint Surg Br* 2002;84:38-41.

7. Angel KR, Hall DJ: Anterior cruciate ligament injury in children and adolescents. *Arthroscopy* 1989;5:197-200.

8. Beasley LS, Chudik SC: Anterior cruciate ligament injury in children: Update of current treatment options. *Curr Opin Pediatr* 2003;15:45-52.

   The safest and most effective treatment method for ACL injuries in children is still evolving. Level of evidence: V.

9. Dorizas JA, Stanitski CL: Anterior cruciate ligament injury in the skeletally immature. *Orthop Clin North Am* 2003;34:355-363.

   The natural history of ACL tears in children mirrors the natural history in adults. Pediatric patients who are unable to modify their activities risk recurrent instability, swelling, pain, meniscal tears, chondral injury, and arthritis. Level of evidence: V.

10. Graf BK, Lange RH, Fujisaki CK, et al: Anterior cruciate ligament tears in skeletally immature patients: Meniscal pathology after attempted conservative treatment. *Arthroscopy* 1992;8:229-233.

11. Janarv PM, Nyström A, Werner S, Hirsch G: Anterior cruciate ligament injuries in skeletally immature patients. *J Pediatr Orthop* 1996;16:673-677.

12. Kannus P, Jarvinen M: Knee ligament injuries in adolescents: Eight year follow up of conservative management. *J Bone Joint Surg Br* 1988;70:772-776.

13. McCarroll JR, Rettig AC, Shelbourne KD: Anterior cruciate ligament injuries in the young athlete with open physes. *Am J Sports Med* 1988;16:44-47.

14. Mizuta H, Kubota K, Shiraishih M, Otsuka Y, Nagamoto N, Takagi K: The conservative treatment of complete tears of the anterior cruciate ligament in skeletally immature patients. *J Bone Joint Surg Br* 1995;77:890-894.

15. Pressman AE, Letts RM, Jarvis JG: Anterior cruciate ligament tears in children: An analysis of operative versus non-operative treatment. *J Pediatr Orthop* 1997;17:505-511.

16. King SJ, Carty HM, Brady O: Magnetic resonance imaging of knee injuries in children. *Pediatr Radiol* 1996;26:287-290.

17. McDermott MJ, Bathgate B, Gillingham BL, Hennrikus WL: Correlation of MRI and arthroscopic diagnosis of knee pathology in children and adolescents. *J Pediatr Orthop* 1998;18:675-678.

18. Stanitski CL: Correlation of arthroscopic and clinical examinations with magnetic resonance imaging findings in the injured knee in children and adolescents. *Am J Sports Med* 1998;26:2-6.

19. Williams JS, Abate JA, Fadale PD, Tung GA: Meniscal and nonosseous ACL injuries in children and adolescents. *Am J Knee Surg* 1996;9:22-26.

20. Lee K, Siegel MJ, Lau DM, Hildebolt CF, Matava MJ: Anterior cruciate ligament tears: MR imaging-based diagnosis in a pediatric population. *Radiology* 1999;213:679-704.

21. Kocher MS, Sumeet G, Micheli LJ: Physeal sparing reconstruction of the anterior cruciate ligament in skeletally immature prepubescent children and adolescents. *J Bone Joint Surg Am* 2005;87:2371-2379.

   The authors of this study performed physeal sparing reconstruction using an iliotibial band graft placed around the outside of the lateral femoral condyle through the notch and then sutured to the periosteum of the proximal tibial in 44 children. Drill holes were not used. Growth disturbance did not occur during an average follow-up period of 5.3 years. Only two patients needed a revision ACL procedure because of graft failure. Level of evidence: IV.

22. Greulich WW, Pyle SI: *Radiographic Atlas of Skeletal Development of the Hand and Wrist*, ed 2. Stanford, CA, Stanford University Press, 1959.

23. Andrews M, Noyes FR, Barber-Westin SD: Anterior cruciate ligament allograft reconstruction in the skeletally immature athlete. *Am J Sports Med* 1994;22:48-54.

24. Koman JD, Sanders JO: Valgus deformity after reconstruction of the anterior cruciate ligament in a skeletally immature patient: A case report. *J Bone Joint Surg Am* 1999;81:711-715.

25. McCarroll JR, Shelbourne KD, Porter DA, Rettig AC, Murray S: Patellar tendon graft reconstruction for midsubstance anterior cruciate ligament rupture in junior high school athletes: An algorithm for management. *Am J Sports Med* 1994;22:478-484.

26. Woods GW, O'Connor DP: Delayed anterior cruciate ligament reconstruction in the adolescent with open physes. *Am J Sports Med* 2004;32:201-210.

   The outcomes of a period of conservative treatment to allow skeletal maturity before performing ACL reconstruction in 13 patients are reported in this study. There was no evidence that intentionally delayed ACL reconstruction increased the rate of additional knee injuries. Delayed reconstruction is a valid treatment option for adolescents with open physes at injury. Absolute activity restriction is key to decreasing the risk of additional knee injuries. Level of evidence: IV.

27. Mohtadi N, Grant J: Managing ACL deficiency in the skeletally immature individual: A systematic review of the literature. *Clin J Sport Med* 2006;16:457-464.

A comprehensive meta-analysis review of more than 600 articles about ACL injuries in children was done to determine if early ACL reconstruction resulted in improved outcomes compared with nonsurgical treatment or delayed surgical treatment until skeletal maturity was achieved. Only seven studies had acceptable study design. The question could not be answered based on current literature. Future prospective studies are needed. Level of evidence: III.

28. Kocher MS, Saxon JS, Hovis WD, et al: Management and complications of anterior cruciate ligament injuries in skeletally immature patients: Survey of the Herodicus Society and the ACL study group. *J Pediatr Orthop* 2002;22:452-457.

29. Koman JD, Sanders JO: Valgus deformity after reconstruction of the anterior cruciate ligament in a skeletally immature patient. A case report. *J Bone Joint Surg Am* 1999;81:711-715.

30. Lipscomb AB, Anderson AF: Tears of the anterior cruciate ligament in adolescents. *J Bone Joint Surg Am* 1986; 68:19-28.

31. McIntosh AL, Dahm DL, Stuart MJ: Anterior cruciate ligament reconstruction in the skeletally immature patient. *Arthroscopy* 2006;22:1325-1330.

In this study, 16 skeletally immature patients were treated with a transphyseal hamstring graft. Seven patients required a reoperation, two had a traumatic graft tear, and symptomatic overgrowth developed in one patient. Level of evidence: IV.

32. Brief LP: Anterior cruciate ligament reconstruction without drill holes. *Arthroscopy* 1991;7:350-357.

33. DeLee JC, Curtis R: Anterior cruciate ligament insufficiency in children. *Clin Orthop Relat Res* 1983;172: 112-118.

34. Guzzanti V, Falciglia F, Stanitski CL: Physeal sparing intra-articular anterior cruciate ligament reconstruction in preadolescents. *Am J Sports Med* 2003;31:949-953.

The use of a soft-tissue graft placed via a groove in the proximal tibia and in the over the top position in the femur is described in eight patients. No growth disturbances were reported with an average follow-up period of 4.5 years. Level of evidence: IV.

35. Kim SH, Ha KI, Ahn JH, et al: Anterior cruciate ligament reconstruction in the young patient without violation of the epiphyseal plate. *Arthroscopy* 1999;15: 792-795.

36. Parker AW, Drez D Jr, Cooper JL: Anterior cruciate ligament injury in patients with open physes. *Am J Sports Med* 1994;22:44-47.

37. Micheli LJ, Rask B, Gerberg L: Anterior cruciate ligament reconstruction in patients who are prepubescent. *Clin Orthop Relat Res* 1999;364:40-47.

38. Nakhostine M, Bollen SR, Cross MJ: Reconstruction of the mid-substance anterior cruciate ruptures in adolescents with open physes. *J Pediatr Orthop* 1995;15: 286-287.

39. Anderson AF: Transepiphyseal replacement of the anterior cruciate ligament in skeletally immature patients. *J Bone Joint Surg Am* 2003;85:1255-1263.

Twelve children underwent ACL reconstruction using a hamstring graft placed through drill holes in the distal femoral and proximal tibial epiphysis. Fluoroscopic imaging was used for precise tunnel placement. No growth disturbance occurred during an average follow-up period of 4.1 years. Level of evidence: IV.

40. Bisson LJ, Wickiewicz T, Levinson M, Warren R: ACL reconstruction in children with open physes. *Orthopedics* 1998;21:659-663.

41. Lo IK, Kirley A, Fowler PJ, Miniaci A: The outcome of operatively treated anterior cruciate ligament disruptions in the skeletally immature child. *Arthroscopy* 1997;13:627-634.

42. Behr CT, Potter HG, Paletta GA: The relationship of the femoral origin of the anterior cruciate ligament and the distal femoral physeal plate in the skeletally immature knee: An anatomic study. *Am J Sports Med* 2001; 29:781-787.

43. Aronowitz ER, Ganley TJ, Goode JR, et al: Anterior cruciate ligament reconstruction in adolescents with open physes. *Am J Sports Med* 2000;28:168-175.

44. Simonian PT, Metcalf MH, Larson RV: Anterior cruciate ligament injuries in the skeletally immature patient. *Am J Orthop* 1999;28:624-628.

45. Volpi P, Galli M, Bait C, et al: Surgical treatment of anterior cruciate ligament injuries in adolescents using double-looped semitendinosis and gracilis tendons: Supraepiphyseal femoral and tibial fixation. *Arthroscopy* 2004;20:447-449.

The authors discuss a hamstring graft fixed with two transverse femoral and tibial bioabsorbable cross pins without interfering with the growth cartilage. Level of evidence: IV.

46. Fuchs R, Wheatly W, Uribe JW, Hechtman KS, Zvijac JE, Schurhoff MR: Intra-articular anterior cruciate ligament reconstruction using patellar tendon allograft in the skeletally immature patient. *Arthroscopy* 2002;18: 824-828.

47. Gaulrapp HM, Haus J: Intraarticular stabilization after

8: The Youth Athlete

anterior cruciate ligament tear in children and adolescents: Results 6 years after surgery. *Knee Surg Sports Traumatol Arthrosc* 2006;14:417-424.

A transphyseal graft was placed in 29 skeletally immature patients. A hamstring graft was used in 15 patients, and a patella tendon graft was used in 14 patients. Follow-up averaged 6 years. No growth disturbance was reported. Level of evidence: IV.

48. Matava MJ, Seigel MG: Arthroscopic reconstruction of the ACL with semitendinosis-gracilis autograft in skeletally immature adolescent patients. *Am J Knee Surg* 1997;10:60-69.

49. Shelbourne KD, Gray T, Wiley BV: Results of transphy-

seal anterior cruciate ligament reconstruction using patellar tendon autograft in Tanner stage 3 or 4 adolescents with clearly open growth plates. *Am J Sports Med* 2004;32:1218-1222.

This article describes ACL reconstruction in adolescent patients using drill holes and a patella tendon autograft. Bone plugs were placed proximal to the physes, and the graft was not overtensioned. No growth disturbance was reported in 16 patients with an average follow-up of 3.4 years. Level of evidence: IV.

50. Schachter AK, Rokito AS: ACL injuries in the skeletally immature patient. *Orthopedics* 2007;30:365-370.

This review article discusses the diagnosis and management of ACL tears in children. Level of evidence: V.

Chapter 38

Spondylolysis

Akin Cil, MD   Lyle J. Micheli, MD

Introduction

Spondylolysis is the most common stress injury involving the lumbar spine of adolescent athletes. Injuries to the back in child and adolescent athletes are being seen more frequently in recent years because of greater participation in organized sports, increased training time and competition in this age group, and increased awareness of athletic injuries by physicians and trainers.[1]

Sports injuries of the back are caused by acute macrotrauma or repetitive microtrauma. As a result, low back pain has a broad differential diagnosis. Although uncommon in most athletes, acute lumbar spine fractures may occur in athletes who participate in contact sports or who fall during participation in equestrian sports, trampolining, skiing, snowboarding, hockey, and football. Macrotrauma also can result in apophyseal avulsion in skeletally immature athletes. Herniation of the nucleus pulposus can be seen with lumbar flexion, axial compression, or rotation, which occurs during weightlifting, rowing, collision sports, and bowling. During the adolescent growth spurt, the thoracolumbar fascia and peripelvic tendons cannot grow at the same pace with the spine, resulting in traction injury to the spinous process and facet joints or pain at the site of pseudarthrosis of transitional vertebrae.[2] Athletes participating in sports that require repeated hyperextension and flexion are at particularly high risk for back injury.[2-4]

Stress fractures in the adolescent spine occur because of risk factors that make it susceptible to injury.[1] The growth plates and ossification centers of the adolescent spine are the weakest links in the transfer of torsional, compressive, and distractive forces through the spine.[2] Consequently, abutment of the inferior articular facet of the L4 vertebra subjects the incompletely ossified arch of the L5 vertebra to repetitive loading and stress that may lead to a stress fracture.[2] Additionally, morphometric studies have shown that the isthmic and lateral buttress portions of the pars interarticularis are thinnest in the lower lumbar spine.[5,6] Cadaver biomechanical studies have demonstrated that the greatest flexion-extension loads occur at the L5-S1 segments, with high tensile and shear stresses predominantly concentrated at the pars interarticularis region.[7]

Spondylolysis is a stress fracture of the pars interarticularis and is by far the most common site of stress injury in the lumbar spine. Stress fractures also can involve the pedicles[8,9] and sacrum,[10,11] but these are rare[12] when compared with stress fractures in the pars interarticularis, which reportedly are present in 47% of adolescent athletes with significant back pain.[13]

Etiology

Spondylolysis was once believed to be congenital (present at birth or detected within 1 year of birth). The belief that spondylolysis has a congenital etiology has been discounted because in multiple cases early radiographs of the spine were normal.[14] Additionally, spondylolytic defects have not been reported in newborns or patients who have not assumed an upright posture and are absent in other primates.[15] These findings suggest the hypothesis of an acquired etiology of a mechanically vulnerable pars interarticularis at the lower lumbar spine.[5-7]

A genetic predisposition for spondylolytic defects has been documented.[16] Anatomic variations such as transitional vertebrae, spina bifida occulta, and an elongated pars interarticularis may predispose to spondylolysis.[3] Unilateral spondylolysis can lead to a stress fracture or sclerosis on the contralateral side because of increased stresses in the region.[17] Recently, it has been demonstrated that an insufficient increase in interfacet distance results in the inferior articular processes of L4 and the superior articular processes of S1 contacting the same cross-section of the intervening pars interarticularis (L5). This increases the likelihood of spondylolytic fracture, resorption, and separation of the pars interarticularis. The development of spondylolysis is more likely in individuals with less than normal mediolateral separation of facets from L4-L5 to L5-S1 than in their counterparts with normal spines.[18]

Thus, spondylolysis appears to be an acquired stress fracture of the lumbar spine, although there may be a genetic risk for sustaining this injury.

Epidemiology

The prevalence of spondylolysis in the general population is 4% to 6%. It most commonly involves L5 (85% to 95% of cases) and L4 (5% to 15% of cases).[19] Although the prevalence is as high as 26% in certain

8: The Youth Athlete

ethnic groups such as Alaskan Native Americans,[20] spondylolysis generally affects 6.4% of white males, with the least affected group being black females (1.1%). Spondylolysis in adulthood is uncommon.

The prevalence of spondylolysis in athletes is variable. In general, the prevalence is not higher than in the general population.[21] However, athletes who participate in sports that require repetitive hyperextension, extension, and rotational movements of the back have an increased incidence of spondylolysis. Among 3,132 competitive athletes, the rate of spondylolysis was reported to be 43% in divers, 30% in wrestlers, and 23% in weight-lifters.[22] Similarly, among these same 3,132 athletes, the prevalence of spondylolysis was 27% in throwing athletes, 17% in gymnasts, and 17% in rowers.[21]

In contrast to the general population in which males are twice as likely to develop spondylolysis, recent studies suggest that young female athletes may be at an increased risk.[23] The number of young females participating in high school sports such as gymnastics, rowing, and throwing has increased nearly tenfold, and these activities are associated with a higher incidence of spondylolysis. The female athlete triad also places these athletes at an increased risk of stress fracture because of lower bone density in this group.[1,24,25]

Clinical Presentation

Most children with spondylolysis remain asymptomatic. However, spondylolysis in the athletic population is commonly symptomatic.[4,21] The mean age of athletes with clinically significant low back pain is 15 to 16 years. Pain is usually insidious in onset, and the patient may or may not recall a recent injury. Sometimes pain can radiate to the buttocks or the back of the thigh with associated hamstring tightness. Radicular pain, weakness, and bowel or bladder dysfunction are rare in patients with spondylolysis. Initially, the pain is elicited by strenuous activity; however, the pain often becomes progressively more severe and is associated with activities of daily living. Rest may relieve the symptoms temporarily, and persistent night pain is uncommon.

On physical examination, paraspinal tenderness, spasm, and point tenderness to palpation at the affected level may be detected. Range of motion may be limited or painful in flexion and extension but is more compromised in extension. During the stork test, single leg lumbar hyperextension will often produce pain on the affected side, with less pain during testing on the contralateral leg. The stork test may be positive in many posterior element derangements and should not be relied on to confirm the diagnosis.[26] Eighty percent of patients have tight hamstrings on physical examination.[27]

Diagnostic Imaging

In the patient with extension-based pain, plain radiographs of the lumbar spine should be obtained. The AP view may demonstrate evidence of scoliosis, spina bifida occulta, or other sources of pain. On the lateral view, a spondylolytic defect can be seen as a lucent gap in the area of the pars interarticularis. Oblique views may provide evidence of more subtle unilateral spondylolysis. However, only chronic spondylolytic fractures usually can be demonstrated on these views. Additionally, iliac wings tend to obscure the images in the lower lumbar spine. Consequently, using only AP and lateral views to rule out other pathologic conditions or spondylolisthesis has been advocated.

When plain radiographs of a patient with symptoms suggesting spondylolysis are nondiagnostic, bone scan, single photon-emission computed tomography (SPECT), CT, or MRI all have been advocated. The imaging study that provides the most accurate evaluation, particularly for posterior element stress injury, is a topic of debate.

A bone scan can sometimes detect stress reactions in the pars interarticularis before a complete stress fracture develops. Additionally, a bone scan helps to differentiate acute painful (biologically active) pars interarticularis lesions from chronic asymptomatic nonunion lesions seen on plain radiographs.[28] SPECT has the same advantages as a bone scan; in addition, it improves diagnostic localization by permitting spatial separation of bony structures that overlap on the standard planar images of a bone scan[29,30] (Figure 1). Several studies have shown that SPECT is more sensitive and specific than a bone scan.[30,31]

CT offers detailed visualization of bony morphology and therefore is superior to plain radiography in the detection and characterization (early, progressive, or terminal) of pars interarticularis defects[32,33] (Figure 2). However, CT exposes a patient to approximately 50 times the radiation dose of plain radiographs.[34] To decrease radiation exposure, CT can be localized (when SPECT shows a lesion) to the level of increased bone scan activity.[3] CT also has significant limitations as a primary diagnostic tool in patients with an early stress reaction in the pars interarticularis without overt fracture.[35]

A lack of ionizing radiation, the ability to image disk abnormalities and other pathologies, and the ability to demonstrate bony anatomy and bony edema in a single test as opposed to obtaining both CT and SPECT imaging are properties that theoretically make MRI the gold standard of imaging in spondylolysis. However, there is a dearth of literature on the specificity and sensitivity of MRI in the diagnosis of spondylolysis[36,37] when compared with SPECT and/or CT, especially in the absence of overt fracture.[26,37] Recently, high signal changes of the pedicles on axial T2-weighted MRI were compared with the CT-based stages of spondylolysis in children and adolescents. High signal changes of the pedicle were found to be an indicator for early spondylolysis.[38]

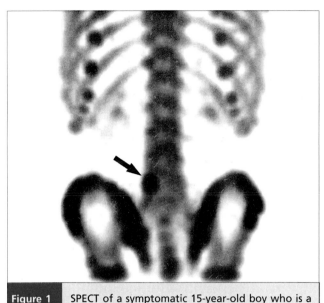

Figure 1   SPECT of a symptomatic 15-year-old boy who is a football player. Localized uptake at the L5 left-sided pars interarticularis (*arrow*) is indicative of spondylolysis.

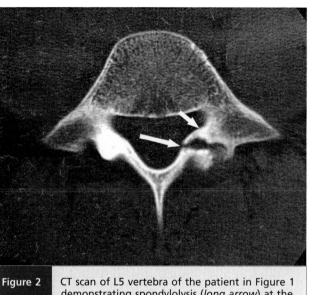

Figure 2   CT scan of L5 vertebra of the patient in Figure 1 demonstrating spondylolysis (*long arrow*) at the left-sided pars interarticularis. Sclerosis at the right-sided pars interarticularis (*short arrow*) also can be seen.

In the future, MRI also may prove useful for follow-up studies of these fractures.

Positron emission tomography-CT (PET-CT) has recently been used to evaluate low back pain in adolescents and detected spinal lesions with a high diagnostic accuracy. However, because of its associated costs and radiation exposure, PET-CT currently should be used only in patients with long-standing and disabling back pain for which other imaging modalities are inconclusive.[39] SPECT presently remains the first-line imaging modality for active athletes with suspected spondylolysis, followed by limited CT if SPECT is positive.[26]

Treatment

Ideally, the goal of spondylolysis treatment should be painless participation in athletic activity and prevention of the formation and progression of spondylolisthesis. Because spondylolysis is a stress fracture of the pars interarticularis, the logical goal of treatment of young athletes with this type of injury is osseous union.

Nonsurgical Treatment

There is a lack of consensus on the type of nonsurgical treatment for spondylolysis. Rest and avoiding aggravating activities have been proposed as a way to symptomatically manage spondylolysis. Physical therapy alone or in combination with other modalities also has been proposed to have a beneficial effect on symptomatic management.[40] Rehabilitation in patients with spondylolysis should consist of deep abdominal muscle strengthening, hamstring stretching, and pelvic tilt exercises.[41] However, few studies in the literature report on the use of activity modification or physical therapy alone.[40]

Although many authors advocate the routine use of a lumbosacral orthosis in the treatment of spondylolysis, there is still no consensus on the type of brace (soft or rigid, lordotic or antilordotic), duration of brace use, and return to sports criteria.[3,42-45] Wiltse and associates[46] were the first to demonstrate that healing of the spondylolytic lesion can occur with a cast, corset, brace, or no immobilization. Subsequently, Steiner and Micheli[45] introduced the concept of antilordotic brace treatment of spondylolisthesis. The primary goal of antilordotic bracing was to decrease lumbar lordosis, rendering the sagittal alignment of the pars interarticularis more vertical, thus reducing shear forces. A recent update reported effective utilization of the antilordotic rigid overlapping brace in 73 adolescent athletes with symptomatic spondylolysis or low-grade spondylolisthesis.[3] The brace was worn for 23 hours per day for 6 months; the period of weaning from the brace was several months. In addition, a physical therapy regimen that initiated both peripelvic flexibility and antilordotic strengthening was prescribed. Athletes having no pain on lumbar extension after 6 weeks were allowed to return to sports activity with the brace if they remained pain free. With this treatment, a favorable outcome allowing pain-free sports participation was achieved in 80% of the patients, similar to the results from the Steiner and Micheli study[45] (**Figure 3**). In a 1993 study, 82 athletes with lumbar spondylolysis or spondylolisthesis were treated with bracing and activity restriction for 2 to 6 months.[47] However, these patients used a lumbosacral brace that maintained lumbar lordosis. No sports or exercise was permitted during the entire treatment period. Pain-free return to sports was attained in 92% of the patients.

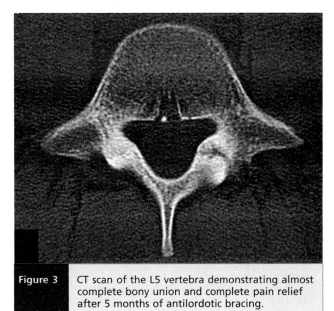

| Figure 3 | CT scan of the L5 vertebra demonstrating almost complete bony union and complete pain relief after 5 months of antilordotic bracing. |

A 2007 study reported on a large series involving conservative treatment of symptomatic patients ($n = 436$) treated with a custom-fit thoracolumbar orthosis and activity cessation for 3 months followed by an organized physical therapy program.[48] The authors reported that 95% of the patients had excellent results; 5% had good results, but anti-inflammatory drugs occasionally were needed to relieve pain, and none of the patients required surgery.

Several recent studies that include patients treated with and without bracing found that bracing had no effect on bony union or clinical outcome.[44,49] One study suggested that patients with a rigid lumbosacral brace may actually experience an increase in intervertebral motion without any stabilizing effect of the brace.[50] Bracing may aid in restricting activity and limiting painful extension while decreasing lumbar lordosis, thus rendering the sagittal alignment of the pars interarticularis more vertical and reducing shear.[3,45]

The success of nonsurgical treatment may depend on the type of sport, with participation in high-risk sports (gymnastics, football, dance, soccer) five times more likely to lead to an unfavorable clinical outcome than participation in low-risk sports (basketball, track, swimming, baseball). Acute onset of pain and hamstring tightness also was found to be associated with a less favorable outcome.[3] Delay in brace treatment was reported to result in persistent symptoms in comparison with prompt treatment.[30,45,51]

Healing of the pars interarticularis defect may not be necessary for a favorable outcome, at least in the short term.[52] The most important factors to affect bony healing were the presence of a unilateral lesion as opposed to a bilateral lesion,[42,51,53] and early detection (stress reaction stage).[35,42,53] Apart from these prognostic factors for bony union, a recent study found that an L4 defect heals better than an L5 defect, a lower lumbar lordosis

increases the chance of bony union, and a defect closer to the vertebral body heals better than a defect that is not close to the vertebral body.[42] It is generally agreed that attaining osseous union is the ideal goal of treatment; however, pain-free function with fibrous union is acceptable.

Electrical stimulation has been used to successfully treat established lower extremity stress fractures or spinal fusions.[52,54] It is believed that electrical stimulation results in a sustained increase of multiple osteogenic genes, suggesting that the biologic mechanism for the increased bone formation in the electrical field observed clinically may be mediated by the upregulation of these osteoinductive factors.[55] Several case series have reported its successful use in spondylolysis, but results of prospective studies are needed before the use of electrical stimulator can be advocated.[56] Electrical stimulation presently is used in selected patients when other conservative measures have been unsuccessful.

Surgical Treatment

Most children and adolescent athletes respond to nonsurgical treatment of spondylolisthesis.[57] A 45-year follow-up study of 500 first-grade children showed that unilateral defects never experienced slippage over the course of the study. In addition, subjects with a pars interarticularis defect had a similar clinical course in terms of low back pain and Medical Outcomes Study 36-Item Short Form scores compared with that of the general population.[58] Consequently, surgical intervention usually is not necessary.

Patients who have persistent pain with activities of daily living after an appropriate nonsurgical treatment regimen for 6 months or who have neurologic dysfunction or progression of their spondylolisthesis may require surgery. Surgical treatment involves either fusion of the motion segment or direct repair of the pars interarticularis defect.

Posterolateral in situ fusion of L5-S1 is usually performed for L5 spondylolysis and accepted as the standard treatment for children and adolescents.[59] Arthrodesis clinical outcomes generally are good, with relatively low rates of complications.[60] However, there is presently no report on athletes treated with posterolateral fusion detailing return to play and levels of subsequent participation. After posterolateral in situ fusion, the spine is immobilized with a spica cast or a brace. The timing of return to sports participation after fusion remains unanswered in the literature. Bono[4] reported that the athlete should be pain free and have nearly normal function (strength, flexibility, and endurance), along with the added requirement of a solid fusion by CT. Decompression in conjunction with fusion is reserved for a clear neurologic deficit and a readily discernible lesion such as the hypertrophied fibrocartilaginous mass at the level of the pars interarticularis defect, irritating the L5 root.

For spondylolysis of L4 or above, direct repair of the pars interarticularis defect with débridement of the painful fibrous nonunion can maintain the motion segment. This is especially important for spondylolysis involving multiple levels.[61,62] Individuals with single-level defects, minimal slippage, a normal intervening disk, and no radicular symptoms are candidates for pars interarticularis repair.[63] Various fixation methods have been described, including direct fixation of the pars interarticularis defects with screws[57,64,65] and indirect compression of the pars interarticularis defect with wiring technique[62,66] or a pedicle screw-rod-hook construct.[67] In a study comparing direct repair versus uninstrumented in situ posterolateral fusion in symptomatic spondylolysis and low-grade spondylolisthesis, with a mean follow-up of approximately 15 years, a significant clinical or radiologic difference between the two could not be demonstrated, but the reoperation rate was higher in the direct repair group.[68]

Summary

Most instances of spondylolysis occur in early childhood and are asymptomatic. Adolescent athletes, especially those participating in sports that require repetitive extension or rotation of the low back, are at risk for the development of symptomatic spondylolysis; therefore, the physician should suspect the presence of spondylolysis in an active adolescent. Spondylolysis was once believed to be a contraindication to high-level sports participation and, in particular, contact sports. It has been shown that most young athletes can safely return to sports participation, without pain, after nonsurgical treatment. Although attaining bony union of a spondylolytic stress fracture still remains the ideal outcome of treatment, this can actually be achieved in only approximately 50% of the treated patients, yet most of the remaining athletes can return to sports participation without pain.

Annotated References

1. Loud KJ, Gordon CM, Micheli LJ, Field AE: Correlates of stress fractures among preadolescent and adolescent girls. *Pediatrics* 2005;115:e399-e406.

   The authors present a cross-sectional analysis of females younger than age 17 years to determine the risk factors of stress fracture development in a population-based national cohort.

2. d'Hemecourt PA, Gerbino PG II, Micheli LJ: Back injuries in the young athlete. *Clin Sports Med* 2000;19:663-679.

3. d'Hemecourt PA, Zurakowski D, Kriemler S, Micheli LJ: Spondylolysis: Returning the athlete to sports participation without brace treatment. *Orthopedics* 2002;25:653-657.

4. Bono CM: Low-back pain in athletes. *J Bone Joint Surg Am* 2004;86:382-396.

   The author presents a review of differential diagnosis, evaluation, and management of low back pain in the athletic population.

5. Ebraheim NA, Lu J, Hao Y, Biyani A, Yeasting RA: Anatomic considerations of the lumbar isthmus. *Spine* 1997;22:941-945.

6. Weiner BK, Walker M, Wiley W, McCulloch JA: The lateral buttress: An anatomic feature of the lumbar pars interarticularis. *Spine* 2002;27:E385-E387.

7. Dietrich M, Kurowski P: The importance of mechanical factors in the etiology of spondylolysis: A model analysis of loads and stresses in human lumbar spine. *Spine* 1985;10:532-542.

8. Crim JR: Winter sports injuries: The 2002 Winter Olympics experience and a review of the literature. *Magn Reson Imaging Clin N Am* 2003;11:311-321.

   The author describes injury patterns and types of the joints involved from a radiological perspective at the 2002 Winter Olympics, including the underreported injuries.

9. Parvataneni HK, Nicholas SJ, McCance SE: Bilateral pedicle stress fractures in a female athlete: Case report and review of the literature. *Spine* 2004;29:E19-E21.

   The authors present a clinical case report of bilateral stress fractures of the pedicle in a female athlete with back pain who was treated surgically with circumferential fusion.

10. Shah MK, Stewart GW: Sacral stress fractures: An unusual cause of low back pain in an athlete. *Spine* 2002;27:E104-E108.

11. Johnson AW, Weiss CB Jr, Stento K, Wheeler DL: Stress fractures of the sacrum: An atypical cause of low back pain in the female athlete. *Am J Sports Med* 2001;29:498-508.

12. Micheli LJ, Curtis C: Stress fractures in the spine and sacrum. *Clin Sports Med* 2006;25:75-88.

   The authors review the current literature on stress fractures of the spine and sacrum for etiology, diagnosis, and management of the problem and include insights from their clinical experience.

13. Micheli LJ, Wood R: Back pain in young athletes: Significant differences from adults in causes and patterns. *Arch Pediatr Adolesc Med* 1995;149:15-18.

14. Reitman CA, Gertzbein SD, Francis WR Jr: Lumbar isthmic defects in teenagers resulting from stress fractures. *Spine J* 2002;2:303-306.

15. Rosenberg NJ, Bargar WL, Friedman B: The incidence of spondylolysis and spondylolisthesis in nonambulatory patients. *Spine* 1981;6:35-38.

8: The Youth Athlete

16. Wynne-Davies R, Scott JH: Inheritance and spondylolisthesis: A radiographic family survey. *J Bone Joint Surg Br* 1979;61:301-305.

17. Sairyo K, Katoh S, Sasa T, et al: Athletes with unilateral spondylolysis are at risk of stress fracture at the contralateral pedicle and pars interarticularis: A clinical and biomechanical study. *Am J Sports Med* 2005;33:583-590.

    The authors present a case series in addition to a descriptive laboratory study to draw attention to increased stresses at the contralateral side of a unilateral spondylolysis that may cause persistent low back pain.

18. Ward CV, Latimer B, Alander DH, et al: Radiographic assessment of lumbar facet distance spacing and spondylolysis. *Spine* 2007;32:E85-E88.

    The authors evaluated articular facet spacing on clinical radiographs of normal and spondylolytic patients to identify anatomic differences predisposing to spondylolysis.

19. Standaert CJ, Herring SA, Halpern B, King O: Spondylolysis. *Phys Med Rehabil Clin N Am* 2000;11:785-803.

20. Stewart TD: The age incidence of neural-arch defects in Alaskan natives, considered from the standpoint of etiology. *J Bone Joint Surg Am* 1953;35:937-950.

21. Soler T, Calderon C: The prevalence of spondylolysis in the Spanish elite athlete. *Am J Sports Med* 2000;28:57-62.

22. Rossi F, Dragoni S: Lumbar spondylolysis: Occurrence in competitive athletes. Updated achievements in a series of 390 cases. *J Sports Med Phys Fitness* 1990;30:450-452.

23. Takemitsu M, El Rassi G, Woratanarat P, Shah SA: Low back pain in pediatric athletes with unilateral tracer uptake at the pars interarticularis on single photon emission computed tomography. *Spine* 2006;31:909-914.

    The authors report on the clinical characteristics and outcome of pediatric athletes with low back pain and unilateral tracer uptake on SPECT at the pars interarticularis with normal radiographs.

24. Loud KJ, Micheli LJ: Common athletic injuries in adolescent girls. *Curr Opin Pediatr* 2001;13:317-322.

25. Donaldson ML: The female athlete triad: A growing health concern. *Orthop Nurs* 2003;22:322-324.

    The author explains the female triad components in depth to increase awareness.

26. Masci L, Pike J, Malara F, Phillips B, Bennell K, Brukner P: Use of the one-legged hyperextension test and magnetic resonance imaging in the diagnosis of active spondylolysis. *Br J Sports Med* 2006;40:940-946.

    The authors report on the clinical role of the one-legged hyperextension test in the clinical detection of active spondylolysis and compare MRI with SPECT and CT in the visualization of active spondylolysis in a prospective cohort.

27. Phalen GS, Dickson JA: Spondylolysis and tight hamstrings. *J Bone Joint Surg Am* 1961;43:505-512.

28. Lowe J, Schahner E, Hirschberg E, Shapiro Y, Libson B: Significance of bone scintigraphy in symptomatic spondylolysis. *Spine* 1984;9:653-655.

29. Bellah RD, Summerville DA, Treves ST, Micheli LJ: Low-back pain in adolescent athletes: Detection of stress injury to the pars interarticularis with SPECT. *Radiology* 1991;180:509-512.

30. Anderson K, Sarwark J, Conway JJ, Logue ES, Schafer MF: Quantitative assessment with SPECT imaging of stress injuries of the pars interarticularis and response to bracing. *J Pediatr Orthop* 2000;20:28-33.

31. Bodner RJ, Heyman S, Drummond DS, Gregg JR: The use of single photon emission computed tomography (SPECT) in the diagnosis of low back pain in young patients. *Spine* 1988;13:1155-1160.

32. Harvey CJ, Richenberg JL, Saifuddin A, Wolman RL: The radiological investigation of lumber spondylolysis. *Clin Radiol* 1998;53:723-728.

33. Morita T, Ikata T, Katoh S, Miyake R: Lumbar spondylolysis in children and adolescents. *J Bone Joint Surg Br* 1995;77:620-625.

34. Brenner DJ, Hall EJ: Computed tomography: An increasing source of radiation exposure. *N Engl J Med* 2007;357:2277-2284.

    This review outlines the radiation doses of different CT studies and biologic effects, including the risk of cancer formation.

35. Standaert CJ, Herring SA: Expert opinion and controversies in sports and musculoskeletal medicine: The diagnosis and treatment of spondylolysis in adolescent athletes. *Arch Phys Med Rehabil* 2007;88:537-540.

    The authors reflect on the current controversies in diagnosis, treatment, and follow-up of spondylolysis in adolescent athletes and include insights from their clinical practice and literature support.

36. Udeshi UL, Reeves D: Routine thin slice MRI effectively demonstrates the lumbar pars interarticularis. *Clin Radiol* 1999;54:615-619.

37. Campbell RS, Grainger AJ, Hide IG, Papastefanou S, Greenough CG: Juvenile spondylolysis: A comparative analysis of CT, SPECT and MRI. *Skeletal Radiol* 2005;34:63-73.

    The authors evaluate the correlation of MRI with CT and SPECT imaging for the diagnosis of juvenile spondylolysis with its strength and weaknesses, especially on early lesions.

38. Sairyo K, Katoh S, Takata Y, et al: MRI signal changes of the pedicle as an indicator for early diagnosis of spondylolysis in children and adolescents: A clinical and biomechanical study. *Spine* 2006;31:206-211.

The authors evaluated the signal changes of the pedicles on MRI and compared this with CT-based stages of the defect. Also by using finite-element analysis, the authors investigated the pathomechanism of the signal changes based on stresses in the pedicles.

39. Ovadia D, Metser U, Lievshitz G, Yaniv M, Wientroub S, Even-Sapir E: Back pain in adolescents: Assessment with integrated 18F-fluoride positron-emission tomography-computed tomography. *J Pediatr Orthop* 2007;27:90-93.

The authors reported on their experience with PET-CT in adolescents with back pain.

40. McNeely ML, Torrance G, Magee DJ: A systematic review of physiotherapy for spondylolysis and spondylolisthesis. *Man Ther* 2003;8:80-91.

The authors systematically reviewed the literature and found very few prospective studies that examined the efficacy of physiotherapy on spondylolysis and spondylolisthesis.

41. O'Sullivan PB, Phyty GDM, Twomey LT, Allison GT: Evaluation of specific stabilizing exercise in the treatment of chronic low back pain with radiographic diagnosis of spondylolysis or spondylolisthesis. *Spine* 1997; 22:2959-2967.

42. Fujii K, Katoh S, Sairyo K, Ikata T, Yasui N: Union of defects in the pars interarticularis of the lumbar spine in children and adolescents: The radiologic outcome after conservative treatment. *J Bone Joint Surg Br* 2004;86: 225-231.

The authors retrospectively analyzed and outlined the prognostic factors that have an effect on union of pars interarticularis defects in patients younger than 18 years. Level of evidence: IV.

43. Standaert CJ, Herring SA: Spondylolysis: A critical review. *Br J Sports Med* 2000;34:415-422.

44. Ruiz-Cotorro A, Balius-Matas R, Estruch-Massana AE, Vilaro Angulo J: Spondylolysis in young tennis players. *Br J Sports Med* 2006;40:441-446.

The authors reported retrospectively on their results in the diagnosis, classification, treatment, and outcomes of spondylolysis with or without spondylolisthesis in young tennis players.

45. Steiner ME, Micheli LJ: Treatment of symptomatic spondylolysis and spondylolisthesis with the modified Boston brace. *Spine* 1985;10:937-943.

46. Wiltse LL, Widell EH Jr, Jackson DW: Fatigue fracture: The basic lesion is isthmic spondylolisthesis. *J Bone Joint Surg Am* 1975;57:17-22.

47. Blanda J, Bethem D, Moats W, Lew M: Defects of the pars interarticularis in athletes: A protocol for nonoperative treatment. *J Spinal Disord* 1993;6:406-411.

48. Kurd MF, Patel D, Norton R, Picetti G, Friel B, Vaccaro AR: Nonoperative treatment of symptomatic spondylolysis. *J Spinal Disord Tech* 2007;20:560-564.

The authors retrospectively reviewed the clinical outcomes of 436 juvenile and adolescent patients with symptomatic spondylolysis who were treated with bracing and activity cessation.

49. El Rassi G, Takemitsu M, Woratanarat P, Shah SA: Lumbar spondylolysis in pediatric and adolescent soccer players. *Am J Sports Med* 2005;33:1688-1693.

The authors reviewed the results of different nonsurgical treatment modalities of lumbar spondylolysis in young soccer players and recommend stopping sports for at least 3 months to allow return to their previous level of play without back pain. Level of evidence: IV.

50. Axelsson P, Johnsson R, Stromqvist B: Effect of lumbar orthosis on intervertebral mobility: A roentgen stereophotogrammetric analysis. *Spine* 1992;17:678-681.

51. Sys J, Michielsen J, Bracke P, Martens M, Verstreken J: Non-operative treatment of active spondylolysis in elite athletes with normal X-ray findings: Literature review and results of conservative treatment. *Eur Spine J* 2001; 10:498-504.

52. Mooney V: A randomized double-blind prospective study of the efficacy of pulsed electromagnetic fields for interbody lumbar fusions. *Spine* 1990;15:708-712.

53. Miller SF, Congeni J, Swanson K: Long term functional and anatomical follow-up of early detected spondylolysis in the young athlete. *Am J Sports Med* 2004;32: 928-933.

The authors report a longitudinal follow-up of 32 athletes with early detected spondylolysis in terms of radiographic union and functional outcome using the low back outcome score. Level of evidence: II.

54. Benazzo F, Mosconi M, Beccarisi G, Galli U: Use of capacitive coupled electric fields in stress fractures in athletes. *Clin Orthop Relat Res* 1995;310:145-149.

55. Fredericks DC, Smucker J, Petersen EB, et al: Effects of direct current electrical stimulation on gene expression of osteopromotive factors in a posterolateral spinal fusion model. *Spine* 2007;32:174-181.

The authors report on an in vivo model that was used to determine levels of messenger RNA expression in response to direct current electrical stimulation in a rabbit posterolateral fusion model to test whether electrical stimulation at the surgery site can increase expression of genes related to bone formation.

56. Fellander-Tsai L, Micheli LJ: Treatment of spondylolysis with external electrical stimulation and bracing in adolescent athletes: A report of two cases. *Clin J Sport Med* 1998;8:232-234.

8: The Youth Athlete

57. Debnath UK, Freeman BJ, Grevitt MP, Sithole J, Scammell BE, Webb JK: Clinical outcome of symptomatic unilateral stress injuries of the lumbar pars interarticularis. *Spine* 2007;32:995-1000.

The authors evaluated the results of nonsurgical and surgical (modified Buck's technique) treatment of symptomatic unilateral lumbar spondylolysis in a prospective cohort of 42 patients.

58. Beutler WJ, Fredrickson BE, Murtland A, Sweeney CA, Grant WD, Baker D: The natural history of spondylolysis and spondylolisthesis: 45-year follow up evaluation. *Spine* 2003;28:1027-1035.

The authors report the results of a prospective radiographic and clinical study of spondylolysis and spondylolisthesis, initiated in 1955 on 500 first-grade children to determine the natural history of spondylolysis and spondylolisthesis.

59. Lim MR, Yoon SC, Green DW: Symptomatic spondylolysis: Diagnosis and treatment. *Curr Opin Pediatr* 2004; 16:37-48.

The authors present a review of evaluation and current management of spondylolysis.

60. Frennered AK, Danielson BI, Nachemson AL, Nordwall AB: Midterm follow-up of young patients fused in situ for spondylolysis. *Spine* 1991;16:409-416.

61. Chung CH, Chiu HM, Wang SJ, Hsu SY, Wei YS: Direct repair of multiple levels lumbar spondylolysis by pedicle screw laminar hook and bone grafting: Clinical, CT and MRI-assessed study. *J Spinal Disord Tech* 2007; 20:399-402.

The authors present a prospective analysis of six patients with multiple-level spondylolysis treated by direct repair with pedicle screw laminar hook. The rate of union was 87%.

62. Ogawa H, Nishimoto H, Hosoe H, Suzuki N, Kanamori Y, Shimizu K: Clinical outcome after segmental wire fixation and bone grafting for repair of the defects in multiple level lumbar spondylolysis. *J Spinal Disord Tech* 2007;20:521-525.

The authors present a retrospective analysis of seven patients with multiple-level spondylolysis treated with segmental wire fixation and bone grafting. These patients had radiographic healing in 70% of lesions.

63. Bradford DS, Iza J: Repair of the defect in spondylolysis or minimal degrees of spondylolisthesis by segmental wire fixation and bone grafting. *Spine* 1985;10: 673-679.

64. Buck JE: Direct repair of the defect in spondylolisthesis: Preliminary report. *J Bone Joint Surg Br* 1970;52: 432-437.

65. Debnath UK, Freeman BJ, Gregory P, de la Harpe D, Kerslake RW, Webb JK: Clinical outcome and return to sport after the surgical treatment of spondylolysis in young athletes. *J Bone Joint Surg Br* 2003;85:244-249.

The authors reported on 22 young athletes who had undergone surgical treatment (Buck's or Scott's fusion) and were followed prospectively; 82% of patients returned to previous levels of sports participation.

66. Nozawa S, Shimizu K, Miyamoto K, Tanaka M: Repair of pars interarticularis defect by segmental wire fixation in young athletes with spondylolysis. *Am J Sports Med* 2003;31:359-364.

The authors present a retrospective study evaluating the outcome of surgical repair of pars interarticularis defects by segmental wire fixation in young athletes with lumbar spondylolysis in terms of radiographic results, the Japanese Orthopaedic Association score, preoperative and postoperative sports activity levels and intensities, and the presence of complications.

67. Kakiuchi M: Repair of the defect in spondylolysis: Durable fixation with pedicle screws and laminar hooks. *J Bone Joint Surg Am* 1997;79:818-825.

68. Schlenzka D, Remes V, Helenius I, et al: Direct repair for treatment of symptomatic spondylolysis and low-grade isthmic spondylolisthesis in young patients: No benefit in comparison to segmental fusion after a mean follow-up of 14.8 years. *Eur Spine J* 2006;15:1437-1447.

The authors compare the long-term clinical, functional, and radiographic outcome of direct repair of spondylolysis using cerclage wire fixation according to Scott in young patients with symptomatic spondylolysis or low-grade isthmic spondylolisthesis with the outcome after uninstrumented posterolateral in situ fusion.

Chapter 39

Exertional Heat Illness in Youth Sports

*Michael F. Bergeron, PhD, FACSM   Ronald A. Feinstein, MD

Introduction

More emphasis is being placed on the specific physiologic responses and tolerance of young athletes during sport and exercise in the heat and some of the challenges they face that can increase the risk for and contribute to the development of exertional heat illness. Certain controversies and perspectives that, in many instances, were based on limited laboratory studies or only anecdotal field evidence, have been clarified.

Thermoregulation and Exercise-Heat Tolerance

Previous studies suggested that children respond differently to thermal stress and are less effective than adults in regulating body temperature during exercise in the heat. Reasons for these reported differences included higher metabolic heat production, lower reliance on and capacity for evaporative cooling (thus a greater reliance on dry heat exchange), delayed and inadequate sweat production, a greater rate of increase in core body temperature for a given workload or fluid deficit, greater cardiovascular strain and instability, and less effective heat acclimatization in children than adults.[1-6]

More recent research provides a different perspective when children and adults are compared in response to equal relative physiologic and thermal stresses. Similar rectal temperatures, mean skin temperatures, and heart rate responses during 85 minutes of exercise in the heat (41°C) were found in physically active, heat nonacclimatized prepubertal boys (age 9.4 ± 0.6 years) compared with young men (age 22.7 ± 0.8 years) with similar aerobic fitness and heat acclimation state.[7] This was attributed to more efficient sweating and more effective thermoregulation in the younger group, which offset the age-related differences in relative metabolic heat production, sweating, and environmental heat

gain. Morever, it appears that elevated core body temperature and perceptual strain (central fatigue), not circulatory insufficiency, were the more likely determinants in limiting exercise endurance in a slightly older group of heat nonacclimatized prepubertal boys (age 11.7 ± 0.4 years) during exercise in the heat (31°C) when the incurred fluid deficit was minimal (< 0.5% of initial body mass).[8] Premenarcheal heat-acclimatized girls (age 11.3 ± 0.3 years) responded similarly to comparably fit and acclimatized women (age 26.8 ± 1.9 years) with respect to thermoregulatory and cardiovascular responses and exercise tolerance time, during exercise at the same relative intensity and in the same hot (33.7°C) and humid conditions when sufficient hydration was maintained.[9] These new findings do not support previous claims of less effective thermoregulation and tolerance during exercise in the heat in children (9 to 12 years of age) compared with adults and underscore the importance of making comparisons by age group only when environmental and exercise conditions and other modulating factors contributing to thermal and cardiovascular strain are the same. Notably, some young athletes (age 12.6 ± 0.5 and 16.5 ± 0.5 years) have been shown to experience greater thermal and cardiovascular strain and perceived effort during a second bout of exercise in the heat when the recovery period between bouts is short (1 hour), even when hydration is maintained.[10]

Sweat Fluid and Electrolyte Losses

As with adults, young athletes rely on evaporative cooling and have a high relative capacity for sweating during exercise in the heat. Hourly sweat losses can readily range from 300 to 700 mL per hour in 9- to 12-year-old boys and girls[7-10] and much higher (for example, 1 to 2 L or more per hour) as children mature and develop through their adolescent years.[10-13] As a young athlete's sweat rate increases through adolescence, the concomitant increased loss of sweat electrolytes (particularly sodium) can increase the risk for exertional heat cramps when sweat-induced fluid and electrolyte deficits are not sufficiently offset by water and salt intake during and after each training session or

*Michael F. Bergeron, PhD, FACSM or the department with which he is affiliated has received research or institutional support and miscellaneous nonincome support, commercially derived honoraria, or other nonresearch-related funding from the Gatorade Sports Science Institute.

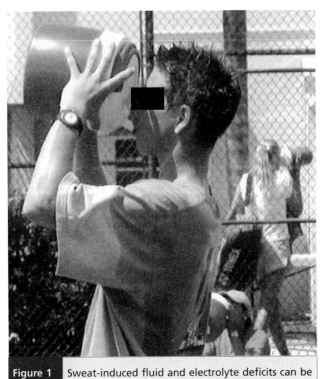

Figure 1 Sweat-induced fluid and electrolyte deficits can be extensive when not sufficiently offset by water and salt intake during and after each training session or competition in the heat. Such deficits can readily reduce performance and increase exertional heat illness risk.

competition.[14] Exertional heat cramps, which should be distinguished from those muscle cramps prompted by overload and fatigue, can be treated and averted by an appropriate amount of sodium and fluid ingestion or by intravenous rehydration as warranted by the severity of cramping or other related clinical conditions.[15]

Hydration

The effects of heat stress on a young athlete's well-being and safety are well recognized.[4,16-19] Moreover, cardiovascular and thermal strain and heat tolerance during exercise and sports activity are directly influenced by hydration status.[1,20-24] Considering the sweat loss potential, a young athlete can incur significant fluid deficits during training and competition in the heat (**Figure 1**). Accordingly, effective strategies to encourage sufficient fluid intake and optimize hydration can play an important role in maintaining performance and reducing exertional heat illness risk.

Despite a small difference in voluntary fluid intake, unflavored water was equally effective as a carbohydrate-electrolyte sports drink in maintaining no (or a minimal) change in body weight in physically active, heat nonacclimatized young girls (age 10.6 ± 0.9 years) during intermittent exercise in the heat (35°C).[25] There also was no statistical difference between beverages in cardiovascular or thermal strain. These results are somewhat in contrast to previous studies showing a stronger preference for and effectiveness of the same sports drink in preventing voluntary dehydration in young boys in hot and humid climates.[26,27] Such distinctions related to fluid intake and preference may be related to sex, fitness, or athletic level.[12] Effective rehydration during and after physical activity and extensive sweating involves more than ample fluid intake. As sodium replenishment more closely matches individual sweat sodium losses, the appropriate amount of ingested fluid is better retained and distributed to all fluid compartments.[28-31] The result is more complete rehydration, which underscores a key advantage of using higher sodium-containing sports drinks and other rehydration beverages over water alone.

American Football

New guidelines from the American College of Sports Medicine (ACSM) highlight the challenges facing high school and youth league American football players on the field, specific to hydration, heat strain, and related clinical risk during preseason practice and conditioning in the heat.[32] The expert panel notes that, although minimizing fluid deficits is integral to football safety, adequate hydration alone cannot guarantee safety in the heat and the prevention of exertional heatstroke. Progressive acclimatization is critical. Players must be given the opportunity to gradually and safely adapt to the climate, training intensity and volume, and the insulating effects of the football uniform.[33] The ACSM consensus statement outlines specific recommendations for preseason acclimatization, practice modification, the identification of risk factors, proper hydration and recovery strategies, and monitoring the athletes on the field that are intended to reduce the incidence of exertional heatstroke and other heat-related injuries during the time of greatest heat injury risk.[32] The panel also emphasizes the importance of prompt recognition of developing heat illness and rapid cooling to avert death in heatstroke incidents.

The need for increased awareness, education, and implementation of effective heat injury risk-reduction strategies in high school football is underscored by a recent survey of 540 high school football programs across the United States.[34] Although the reporting schools have a preseason period sufficiently long to achieve progressive, safe, and effective acclimatization to the environment, workload, and full uniform and protective equipment configuration, while still meeting individual and team training objectives, many programs need to more appropriately introduce and adjust uniform configurations, the duration and intensity of training, and demanding scheduling in the early preseason and in response to heat and humidity. Moreover, inadequate hydration strategies, environment and player monitoring tools (wet-bulb globe temperature monitors and rectal thermometers, respectively), education, and preparation for heat-related medical emergencies are among the other identified widespread shortcomings in preseason high school football that also contribute to avoidable heat-related injury and death.

Tennis

A carbohydrate-electrolyte sports drink may be more effective than water alone in maintaining hydration status and minimizing thermal strain during intense tennis training in the heat for fit adolescent players (age 15.1 ± 1.4 years).[12] However, core body temperature was not statistically related to prepractice hydration status (which was apparently quite poor for a number of players) or fluid intake or percentage change in body weight during the training sessions. The thermal challenges during junior tennis tournaments in the heat and the greater impact of precompetition hydration status in contributing to core body temperature during competitive play were emphasized in a study of elite young boys (age 13.9 ± 0.9 years) during the first round of play in a national championship event.[11] This study showed that preplay urine specific gravity (indicating hydration status) had a progressively stronger positive association, as the matches advanced, with core body temperature during singles matches, even though all of these matches were fairly short, were conducted mostly in the morning, and resulted in a minimal fluid deficit incurred during play. In contrast with recent statements,[35-37] it appears that hydration status does impact core body temperature in field situations, when intensity is maintained at a high level—that is, greater fluid deficits are associated with increased thermal strain. Notably, in examining the effect of previous play in the heat on performance, previous same-day, on-court, degree-minutes exposure was the most significant determinant (after controlling for seeding) of a second singles match outcome in a national junior competition.[38]

Basketball

Even though basketball is generally played indoors and the risk for excessive heat strain is usually not very high, sweat losses can be extensive, and the negative clinical (heat cramps and exhaustion) and performance effects of significant fluid and electrolyte deficits can be readily realized, especially in a repeated-bout tournament scenario where complete rehydration between games is often not achieved. The effects of prior exercise- and heat-induced 2% dehydration and hydration maintenance with either a commercial carbohydrate-electrolyte solution (sports drink) or flavored water on basketball skill drills and thermal and cardiovascular strain during a subsequent (following a

1-hour recovery period) simulated basketball game were examined in 12- to 15-year-old boys.[13] A 2% fluid deficit impaired shooting percentage and sprint and lateral movement speed. Moreover, at the end of the simulated game, heart rate and core body temperature were statistically higher in the 2% fluid deficit trial. Notably, many of the assessed basketball skill measures were enhanced further when hydration was maintained with the carbohydrate-containing sports drink (in comparison with flavored water). Similarly, a progressive decrease in movement and shooting performance paralleled progressive levels of prior exercise-induced dehydration in the heat.[39] However, the high school boys and collegiate players studied were able to tolerate (with no statistical difference in performance) a slight fluid deficit (1%), and carbohydrate intake during the euhydration trials did not provide a performance advantage.

Exertional Heatstroke: Treatment and Prevention

Exertional heatstroke (core body temperature greater than 40°C, thermoregulatory failure, and usually central nervous system dysfunction) can occur in a variety of weather conditions and is an acute medical emergency associated with a significant mortality rate if diagnosis is delayed and appropriate medical management is not promptly initiated.[40-43] Prognosis is predictably based on the degree and duration of excessive core body temperature. The term golden hour denotes the importance of initiating effective cooling as soon as possible, preferably at the site of the activity or event.[44] Myriad cooling methods have been used and are supposedly effective in treating exertional hyperthermia.[45] However, ice- or cold-water immersion arguably remains the gold standard and most effective mode of treating exertional heatstroke and rapidly lowering core body temperature, but other proven methods should be promptly initiated if immersion is unavailable or inappropriate.[46-48] Concerns about peripheral vasoconstriction and shivering impeding heat loss and prompting greater heat storage are not warranted, as the thermal gradients between the core and periphery and the periphery and surrounding water allow rapid heat transfer and dissipation, whereas shivering and reduced peripheral blood flow are either absent or only minor contributors to an increase in heat production and reduced rate of core temperature decrease.[49] It is critical, however, to monitor core body temperature throughout this process, so that the victim can be removed from the water well before becoming hypothermic.

Not all young athletes who stop or collapse during or after training or competition have excessive core body temperatures. Other primary underlying factors can include energy depletion, fatigue, dehydration, postexercise hypotension, or sudden cardiac arrest.[50,51]

8: The Youth Athlete

However, especially in hot weather and if the athlete is wearing a uniform and protective equipment that promote heat storage, rectal temperature should be checked. Central nervous system dysfunction, confusion, erratic behavior, nausea, and headache also could be related to hyponatremia and not excessive heat strain; young athletes exhibiting these signs and symptoms should have their blood sodium level assessed and be treated accordingly.[52]

Several new proposed options for predicting (and thus preventing) exertional heat illness should also be considered by health care professionals. Current and previous-day wet-bulb globe temperature can be assessed to better anticipate exertional heat illness risk and adjust training accordingly.[53] The Heat Illness Symptom Index can help health care staff identify milder forms of heat illness in athletes (while also focusing on contributing factors such as body weight change and player position), prompting earlier intervention, and adjusting the activity and/or schedule before more serious symptoms and clinical conditions evolve.[54] Another option is the heat tolerance test, which can be used as a screening tool to identify those who are particularly susceptible to the heat and are at greater risk for an earlier and more rapid than expected rise in core body temperature during physical activity in hot conditions.[55] The heat tolerance test also may be used following an episode of heat exhaustion or exertional heatstroke to determine if there is any residual compromise of the affected athlete's thermoregulation under similar conditions.

Summary

Young athletes do not seem to have less effective thermoregulatory and insufficient cardiovascular capacities compared with adults during exercise in the heat, if adequate hydration is maintained. The demands of inappropriate training and competition intensity, duration, uniform configurations, and scheduling are likely the primary determinants for excessive thermal strain and heat injury risk in youth sports versus any maturation-associated heat tolerance insufficiencies. Progressive acclimatization to the environment, uniform and protective equipment, and intensity and duration of activity is critical in helping young athletes to adapt safely and effectively to the heat.

Young athletes often begin training and competition measurably dehydrated, which can also increase cardiovascular and thermal strain, as well as the risk for exertional heat illness. Accordingly, especially in the heat, sufficient fluid and electrolytes (with a particular emphasis on sodium) should be consumed to offset sweat losses from previous exercise bouts and to prepare for upcoming training sessions or competition.

Young athletes may be able to cope with poorer hydration during practice, when they have the opportunity to reduce exercise intensity and effort. However,

during a meaningful competition or when a coach pushes athletes to maintain intensity during practice, the negative effects of insufficient hydration on cardiovascular and thermal strain, perceived effort, performance, and heat injury risk will likely be more readily apparent.

Multiple matches, games, or training sessions on the same day may pose a particular heat injury risk to young athletes because of insufficient recovery time and rehydration, as well as potential physiologic carryover effects from the previous bout(s). Practicing and competing in unsafe conditions and an insufficient recovery time between sessions can place a young athlete at great risk, even if he or she is fit and well hydrated. A well-prepared and properly hydrated player is no match for uncompensable heat stress or a coach or tournament director who does not appropriately adjust the workout, uniform configuration, or schedule to accommodate for the heat and emphasize player safety. Early recognition, immediate activation of the emergency response system, and prompt on-site whole-body cooling are critical in effectively treating exertional heatstroke and reducing morbidity and mortality.

Annotated References

1. Bar-Or O, Dotan R, Inbar O, Rotshtein A, Zonder H: Voluntary hypohydration in 10- to 12-year-old boys. *J Appl Physiol* 1980;48:104-108.

2. Drinkwater BL, Kupprat IC, Denton JE, Crist JL, Horvath SM: Response of prepubertal girls and college women to work in the heat. *J Appl Physiol* 1977;43:1046-1053.

3. Falk B: Effects of thermal stress during rest and exercise in the paediatric population. *Sports Med* 1998;25:221-240.

4. Falk B, Bar-Or O, MacDougall JD: Thermoregulatory responses of pre-, mid-, and late-pubertal boys to exercise in dry heat. *Med Sci Sports Exerc* 1992;24:688-694.

5. Haymes EM, Buskirk ER, Hodgson JL, Lundergren HM, Nicholas WC: Heat tolerance of exercising lean and heavy prepubertal girls. *J Appl Physiol* 1974;36:566-571.

6. Wagner JA, Robinson S, Tzankoff SP, Marino RP: Heat tolerance and acclimatization to work in the heat in relation to age. *J Appl Physiol* 1972;33:616-622.

7. Inbar O, Morris N, Epstein Y, Gass G: Comparison of thermoregulatory responses to exercise in dry heat among prepubertal boys, young adults and older males. *Exp Physiol* 2004;89:691-700.

Using an 85-minute intermittent exercise-in-heat protocol with eight subjects in each age group, these authors found that prepubertal boys were the most efficient thermoregulators, even with greater relative metabolic heat production and less relative sweating than the older subjects.

8. Rowland T, Garrison A, Pober D: Determinants of endurance exercise capacity in the heat in prepubertal boys. *Int J Sports Med* 2007;28:26-32.

Using a steady load cycling protocol to exhaustion, these authors found that elevated thermal and perceptual strain, instead of circulatory insufficiency, were the likely limiting factors for eight nonacclimatized, highly physically active, prepubertal boys during exercise in the heat.

9. Rivera-Brown AM, Rowland TW, Ramirez-Marrero FA, Santacana G, Vann A: Exercise tolerance in a hot and humid climate in heat-acclimatized girls and women. *Int J Sports Med* 2006;27:943-950.

Using a cycling protocol to fatigue, the authors showed that nine young girls responded similarly (with respect to thermoregulatory and cardiovascular responses) to nine young women with similar fitness and heat acclimatization states during exercise in hot and humid outdoor conditions, when sufficient hydration was maintained.

10. Laird MD, Bergeron MF, Marinik EL, Brenner JS, Lou M, Waller JL: Physiological strain and perceptual differences during repeated-bout exercise in the heat. *Med Sci Sports Exerc* 2007;39:S309.

With 24 fit boys and girls completing an experimental protocol consisting of two 80-minute intermittent exercise bouts, 1 hour of rest, cool-down, and rehydration between bouts was not sufficient recovery time to avert greater perceptual effort and, for some, greater physiologic strain during the second exercise session.

11. Bergeron MF, McLeod KS, Coyle JF: Core body temperature during competition in the heat: National Boys' 14's Junior Tennis Championships. *Br J Sports Med* 2007;41:779-783.

In an observational study conducted at a national championship event, the authors found that preplay hydration status had a progressively stronger association with core temperature during singles play in the heat.

12. Bergeron MF, Waller JL, Marinik EL: Voluntary fluid intake and core temperature responses in adolescent tennis players: Sports beverage versus water. *Br J Sports Med* 2006;40:406-410.

By comparing the on-court physiologic responses of 14 healthy, fit, young tennis players during two 2-hour tennis training sessions in the heat, these authors found that the consumption of a carbohydrate-electrolyte drink may be more effective than water in minimizing thermal strain.

13. Dougherty KA, Baker LB, Chow M, Kenney WL: Two percent dehydration impairs and six percent carbohydrate drink improves boys basketball skills. *Med Sci Sports Exerc* 2006;38:1650-1658.

Using a double-blind, randomized order protocol with 15 young boys, these authors found that basketball performance was impaired and cardiovascular and thermal strains were higher with a 2% fluid deficit.

14. Bergeron MF: Heat cramps: Fluid and electrolyte challenges during tennis in the heat. *J Sci Med Sport* 2003;6:19-27.

In this review, field observations of fluid-electrolyte losses in players with a cramping history are described, and the etiology and strategy to avert such muscle cramping are highlighted.

15. Bergeron MF: Exertional heat cramps: Recovery and return to play. *J Sport Rehabil* 2007;16:190-196.

This article outlines the specific etiology and treatment and prevention strategies for muscle cramps during exercise that are associated with extensive sweating and a sodium deficit.

16. American Academy of Pediatrics Committee on Sports Medicine and Fitness: Climatic heat stress and the exercising child and adolescent. *Pediatrics* 2000;106:158-159.

17. Gutierrez G: Solar injury and heat illness: Treatment and prevention in children. *Physician Sportsmed* 1995;23:43-48.

18. Hoffman JL: Heat-related illness in children. *Clin Pediatr Emerg Med* 2001;2:203-210.

19. Martin TJ, Martin JS: Special issues and concerns for the high school- and college-aged athletes. *Pediatr Clin North Am* 2002;49:533-552.

20. González-Alonso J: Separate and combined influences of dehydration and hyperthermia on cardiovascular responses to exercise. *Int J Sports Med* 1998;19:S111-S114.

21. González-Alonso J, Mora-Rodríguez R, Below PR, Coyle EF: Dehydration markedly impairs cardiovascular function in hyperthermic endurance athletes during exercise. *J Appl Physiol* 1997;82:1229-1236.

22. Nadel ER, Fortney SM, Wenger CB: Effect of hydration state on circulatory and thermal regulations. *J Appl Physiol* 1980;49:715-721.

23. Sawka MN, Latzka WA, Matott RP, Montain SJ: Hydration effects on temperature regulation. *Int J Sports Med* 1998;19:S108-S110.

24. Sawka MN: Physiological consequences of hypohydration: Exercise performance and thermoregulation. *Med Sci Sports Exerc* 1992;24:657-670.

25. Wilk B, Rivera-Brown AM, Bar-Or O: Voluntary drinking and hydration in non-acclimatized girls exercising in the heat. *Eur J Appl Physiol* 2007;101:727-734.

In this experimental study of 12 physically active girls during 3 hours of intermittent exercise in the heat, these authors found that unflavored water was equally effec-

8: The Youth Athlete

tive as a carbohydrate-electrolyte sports drink in maintaining hydration and with respect to thermal and cardiovascular strain.

26. Rivera-Brown AM, Gutiérrez R, Gutiérrez JC, Frontera WR, Bar-Or O: Drink composition, voluntary drinking, and fluid balance in exercising, trained, heat-acclimatized boys. *J Appl Physiol* 1999;86:78-84.

27. Wilk B, Bar-Or O: Effect of drink flavor and NaCl on voluntary drinking and hydration in boys exercising in the heat. *J Appl Physiol* 1996;80:1112-1117.

28. Mitchell JB, Phillips MD, Mercer SP, Baylies HL, Pizza FX: Postexercise rehydration: Effect of Na+ and volume on restoration of fluid spaces and cardiovascular function. *J Appl Physiol* 2000;89:1302-1309.

29. Sanders B, Noakes TD, Dennis SC: Sodium replacement and fluid shifts during prolonged exercise in humans. *Eur J Appl Physiol* 2001;84:419-425.

30. Sanders B, Noakes TD, Dennis SC: Water and electrolyte shifts with partial fluid replacement during exercise. *Eur J Appl Physiol Occup Physiol* 1999;80:318-323.

31. Shirreffs SM, Maughan RJ: Volume repletion after exercise-induced volume depletion in humans: Replacement of water and sodium losses. *Am J Physiol* 1998;274:F868-F875.

32. Bergeron MF, McKeag DB, Casa DJ, et al: Youth football: Heat stress and injury risk. *Med Sci Sports Exerc* 2005;37:1421-1430.

    These new evidence-based and panel consensus guidelines from the ACSM highlight strategies for acclimatization, practice modification, hydration, and monitoring athletes on the field to reduce the incidence of exertional heatstroke during preseason.

33. Yeargin SW, Casa DJ, Armstrong LE, et al: Heat acclimatization and hydration status of American football players during initial summer workouts. *J Strength Cond Res* 2006;20:463-470.

    By observing 11 collegiate football players during the first 8 days of preseason practices, gradual heat acclimatization and enhanced heat tolerance were noted.

34. Luke AC, Bergeron MF, Roberts WO: Heat injury prevention practices in high school football. *Clin J Sport Med* 2007;17:488-493.

    The results of a Web-based survey of 540 high school football programs from 26 states highlight the need for increased awareness, education, and implementation of effective heat injury risk-reduction strategies during the preseason.

35. Godek SF, Bartolozzi AR, Burkholder R, Sugarman E, Dorshimer G: Core temperature and percentage of dehydration in professional football linemen and backs during preseason practices. *J Athl Train* 2006;41:8-14.

    By measuring core body temperature and sweat loss in

14 professional football players during preseason two-a-day practices, these authors found that maximal thermal strain was not statistically associated with selected hydration measures.

36. Laursen PB, Suriano R, Quod MJ, et al: Core temperature and hydration status during an Ironman triathlon. *Br J Sports Med* 2006;40:320-325.

    By measuring core body temperature in 10 triathletes during a 226-km Ironman triathlon, these authors found that a body mass loss of up to 3% was well tolerated in warm conditions.

37. Noakes TD: Hydration in the marathon: Using thirst to gauge safe fluid replacement. *Sports Med* 2007;37:463-466.

    This article contrasts two models of fatigue with a proposed mechanism that allows athletes to anticipate exercise demands and modify their exercise response to prevent biological harm.

38. Coyle J: Cumulative heat stress appears to affect match outcome in a junior tennis championship. *Med Sci Sports Exerc* 2006;38:S110.

    For a period of 7 years, 370 singles matches at a national junior tennis championship event in the heat were analyzed. Degree-minutes of heat stress acquired during a previous same-day morning match could predict the winner of an afternoon match.

39. Baker LB, Dougherty KA, Chow M, Kenney WL: Progressive dehydration causes a progressive decline in basketball skill performance. *Med Sci Sports Exerc* 2007;39:1114-1123.

    By observing 17 male basketball players during 6 randomized trials each consisting of an 80-minute simulated game following 3 hours of interval treadmill walking with or without fluid replacement, these authors found that the athletes experienced a progressive decrease in performance that paralleled progressive dehydration levels.

40. Howe AS, Boden BP: Heat-related illness in athletes. *Am J Sports Med* 2007;35:1384-1395.

    This article highlights the causes and risk factors, distinguishing features, and recommended strategies for treatment and prevention of heat-related illness in athletes.

41. Roberts WO: Exertional heat stroke during a cool weather marathon: A case study. *Med Sci Sports Exerc* 2006;38:1197-1203.

    This case study of a well-trained male runner in his late 30s highlights how exertional heatstroke can occur in cool conditions and that rectal temperature should be checked in all collapsed runners who do not progress with prompt recovery.

42. Roberts WO: Exertional heat stroke in the marathon. *Sports Med* 2007;37:440-443.

    This article highlights the importance of rapid recognition and treatment of exertional heatstroke and provides strategies for effective field treatment.

43. Roberts WO: Heat and cold: What does the environment do to marathon injury? *Sports Med* 2007;37: 400-403.

The author examined course dropouts and finish-line medical encounter rates, as related to environmental conditions, from two well-known marathons in the United States.

44. Heled Y, Rav-Acha M, Shani Y, Epstein Y, Moran DS: The "golden hour" for heatstroke treatment. *Mil Med* 2004;169:184-186.

These authors use case reports to emphasize the importance of initiating prompt cooling and how exertional heatstroke prognosis is predictably based on the degree and duration of excessive core body temperature.

45. Hadad E, Rav-Acha M, Heled Y, Epstein Y, Moran DS: Heat stroke: A review of cooling methods. *Sports Med* 2004;34:501-511.

The authors highlight the importance of rapid cooling in treating heatstroke and describe various cooling techniques.

46. Casa DJ, McDermott BP, Lee EC, Yeargin SW, Armstrong LE, Maresh CM: Cold water immersion: The gold standard for exertional heatstroke treatment. *Exerc Sport Sci Rev* 2007;35:141-149.

This review emphasizes with conclusive evidence how ice- or cold-water immersion is the most effective way to treat exertional heatstroke.

47. Smith JE: Cooling methods used in the treatment of exertional heat illness. *Br J Sports Med* 2005;39:503-507.

This article discusses various methods of reducing core body temperature associated with exertional heatstroke. Seventeen papers from a literature review were analyzed to determine the most effective methods of treatment.

48. Hadad E, Moran DS, Epstein Y: Cooling heat stroke patients by available field measures. *Intensive Care Med* 2004;30:338.

The authors describe alternate methods of cooling heatstroke victims, when ice water immersion is not available, based on military field evidence.

49. Proulx CI, Ducharme MB, Kenny GP: Effect of water temperature on cooling efficiency during hyperthermia in humans. *J Appl Physiol* 2003;94:1317-1323.

Seven subjects were evaluated for cooling rate, after exercise-induced hyperthermia in the heat, using various water immersion techniques.

50. Blue JG, Pecci MA: The collapsed athlete. *Orthop Clin North Am* 2002;33:471-478.

51. Drezner JA, Courson RW, Roberts WO, Mosesso VN, Link MS, Maron BJ: Inter-association Task Force recommendations on emergency preparedness and management of sudden cardiac arrest in high school and college athletic programs: A consensus statement. *J Athl Train* 2007;42:143-158.

The authors present a consensus statement that summarizes the current understanding of sudden cardiac arrest and highlights emergency planning and treatment protocols for high school and collegiate athletic programs.

52. Hew-Butler T, Almond C, Ayus JC, et al: Consensus statement of the 1st International Exercise-Associated Hyponatremia Consensus Development Conference, Cape Town, South Africa 2005. *Clin J Sport Med* 2005; 15:208-213.

This consensus statement was developed from a comprehensive review of existing data on exercise-associated hyponatremia that helped formulate an evidence-based understanding and recommendations for treatment and prevention.

53. Wallace RF, Kriebel D, Punnett L, et al: The effects of continuous hot weather training on risk of exertional heat illness. *Med Sci Sports Exerc* 2005;37:84-90.

Based on a case-crossover study with Marine Corps recruits in basic training and weather measurements for 2,069 patients with exertional heat illness, the authors recommend assessing current and previous-day heat stress to better anticipate exertional heat illness.

54. Coris EE, Walz SM, Duncanson R, Ramirez AM, Roetzheim RG: Heat illness symptom index (HISI): A novel instrument for the assessment of heat illness in athletes. *South Med J* 2006;99:340-345.

The authors conducted a prospective observational pilot study on Division I football players during practice in the heat to initially validate a new Heat Illness Symptom Index scale for identifying milder forms of heat illness in an athletic population.

55. Moran DS, Erlich T, Epstein Y: The heat tolerance test: An efficient screening tool for evaluating susceptibility to heat. *J Sport Rehabil* 2007;16:215-221.

The authors describe how a controlled exposure to an exercise-heat stress can be applicable in identifying individuals' tolerance or intolerance to the heat.

8: The Youth Athlete

Chapter 40
Strength Training in Youth

Teri M. McCambridge, MD

Introduction

Society often rewards athletic prowess with elusive college scholarships, lucrative professional contracts, and celebrity status. Consequently, children are beginning year-round, sports-specific training at younger ages[1] and sometimes rely on alternative methods such as performance-enhancing substances, strength training, hypnosis or imagery, and speed or plyometric training to enhance sports performance. The reported rate of anabolic steroid use in adolescents is from 1.5% to 7%.[2,3] Orthopaedic surgeons and primary care providers need to discuss the risks and benefits of strength training in youth (those who have not reached skeletal maturity) and also counsel parents on how to implement an effective and proper strength training program.

This chapter discusses common strength training definitions, current safety data, and the current data on efficacy. The published data on injury prevention and effects on sports performance with strength training in youth will be reviewed. Special patient populations that might particularly benefit or suffer harm from participation in strength training are discussed.

Definition of Strength Training

Resistance training or strength training is defined as a specialized form of conditioning used to increase the ability to exert or resist force. In contrast, Olympic weight lifting, power lifting, or bodybuilding are competitive events that require maximal lifts, specific ballistic maneuvers, and/or judging of the aesthetic appearance and muscle definition. Historically, strength training was discouraged in preadolescents because of its presumed ineffectiveness, the potential risk of injury to growth plates, and impairment of flexibility.[4] However, recent research in well-designed studies has demonstrated reproducible strength gains in youth without adverse effects on growth, flexibility, or significant injuries. Youth strength training now is almost universally accepted among the leading sports medicine organizations. Guidelines have been established for youth strength training by the American Academy of Pediatrics (AAP) Council on Sports Medicine and Fitness, the National Strength and Conditioning Association, the American College of Sports Medicine (ACSM), and the American Orthopaedic Society for Sports Medicine.

Strength Training Safety

Strength training can be achieved with the use of free weights, therabands, kettle balls, the athlete's own body weight, or machines. In children, the use of free weights and weight machines poses unique challenges. Proper form, technique, weight, and adequately trained spotters are critical when free weights are in use. Balance and coordination in the preadolescent are underdeveloped, increasing the susceptibility of injury in those who use free weights. The main advantage of free weights is the ability to increase resistance in small increments. Weight machines, in contrast, require large weight increases (5- or 10-lb weight plates), which may be inappropriate for the smaller athlete. Additionally, the lever arms on weight machines may be inappropriately sized for smaller children. The main advantage of weight machines is that they do not require balance or spotters.

The original concerns regarding weight training safety in youth arose from data reported from the US Consumer Product Safety Commission's National Electronic Injury Surveillance System. According to 2007 data, there were 23,332 estimated injuries attributed to weightlifting or weight equipment in individuals between 8 and 19 years of age.[5] These data are difficult to use in assessing injury rates because proper supervision, proper use of weight equipment, and type of training are not taken into account.

Most injuries reported in the National Electronic Injury Surveillance System are sprains or strains, most commonly involving the low back. Retrospective studies have reported more serious injuries, including intervertebral disk herniation, epiphyseal plate fracture, spondylolysis, dislocations, meniscal tears, and even death.[6-9] According to a 2000 study, most injuries resulted from unsafe behavior, equipment malfunction, poor supervision, and inattention. Most of the serious injuries occurred while using free weights.[7]

In a recent evidence-based review that evaluated 10 prospective weight training studies during which good supervision and proper technique were practiced, injuries were reported for only 3 of these studies.[10] The injuries sustained were two shoulder strains and one

8: The Youth Athlete

thigh contusion, with injury rates estimated at 0.176, 0.053, and 0.055 per 100 participant hours, respectively.[11-13]

Adverse effects on growth have not been demonstrated in children as young as 6 years or in preadolescents participating in strength training in programs up to 20 weeks in duration.[14-16] Research has been variable in its effects on flexibility, as determined by sit and reach testing. Flexibility has been improved in some training programs[11,17] and unchanged in others.[18-20] Only one study has demonstrated decreased flexibility (8%), but that included incorporation of soccer agility training with resistance training in adolescents.[21]

Although youth strength testing is now considered almost universally safe and effective, there is still debate about the safety of 1 repetition maximum (1-RM; the maximum amount of weight an individual can displace at one time) for training or to assess strength gains. A recent study demonstrated no injuries with 1-RM strength testing in healthy children, with proper supervision on a child-sized weight training machine.[22] The AAP Council on Sports Medicine and Fitness does not endorse the use of 1-RM until skeletal maturity is attained.[23]

Olympic weight lifting is a competitive sport evaluating maximum lifting ability during the snatch (a lift during which a barbell is raised from the floor to above the head in one continuous movement) and clean and jerk (a lift during which a barbell is lifted to shoulder height and then jerked overhead so that the arms are completely extended, with the thrust overhead generally accompanied by a lunge of the legs) maneuvers. The AAP has cautioned against participation in Olympic weight lifting until skeletal maturity because of concerns about the risk of injury to the growing skeleton and to the epiphyseal plates and spine in an unsupervised setting, using improper techniques.[23] Studies performed at the USA Weightlifting Development Center reported significant strength gains in children studied over a 22-month period.[12-15] The Center provided a highly supervised setting, emphasizing proper form and gradual weight progression. There were no reported injuries.[6] The applicability of the safety of Olympic weight lifting to a poorly supervised setting or to a setting without proper weight progression and technique is difficult to guarantee.

Strength Gains

Strength training initially was not recommended in prepubescent patients because it was believed that muscular hypertrophy and strength gains were impossible without adequate circulating androgen levels. It is now known that even with low levels of circulating androgens, strength gains are possible. Research suggests that the strength gains are attributable to enhanced motor unit activation, alterations in patterns of motor unit recruitment, improved motor unit coordination, and in-

creased neuromuscular firing as demonstrated on electromyographic testing[24] rather than muscular hypertrophy.[14] Some recent studies suggest early physical training, rather than strength training, in gymnasts, figure skaters, and dancers resulted in an increased cross-sectional area of the erector spinae, multifidus, and psoas musculature on axial MRI studies in comparison with age-matched, nonathletic control patients. The cross-sectional area, after adjustment for body mass, was directly correlated with trunk flexion and extension strength. This study presents evidence to suggest that long-term sports involvement, rather than strength training, may result in more significant muscular hypertrophy and strength gains in the adolescent.[25]

Early studies in the literature that used inadequate control groups, low volume training, and short duration studies failed to demonstrate significant strength gains in the preadolescent.[16] However, more recent strength training studies in children and preadolescents using training programs of adequate intensity, frequency (two to three times per week) and duration (8 to 20 weeks) generally demonstrated strength gains from 30% to 50% of those expected from natural growth and maturation.[17-20,26] Maximal strength gains of up to 74.3% have been reported. Training modalities to achieve these strength gains have been accomplished with pediatric and adult weight machines, pneumatic and hydraulic machines, free weights, and isometric contractions. Studies specifically evaluating once versus twice weekly strength training in males and females between 7 and 12 years of age revealed significant gains (above age-matched control patients) in the effectiveness of the chest press only with twice weekly training.[19] There are few studies in children and adolescents evaluating strength changes after withdrawal of the training program (detraining). Evaluation of strength maintenance in children is further complicated by natural gains in strength with growth and development. Studies suggest that withdrawal of a strength training program, despite continued participation in sports, results in a regression of strength gains to pretraining levels.[18] In the aforementioned study, the magnitude of strength loss during detraining averaged 3.0% a week. There is currently no evidence-based research in children determining the amount or frequency of training required to maintain strength gains. Prepubescent athletes need to lift weights approximately twice a week to maintain strength.[27]

Injury Prevention

Preventive exercise (prehabilitation) refers to strength training programs that address areas commonly subjected to overuse in specific sports. Rotator cuff and scapular stabilization exercises are used to reduce overuse injuries of the shoulder in overhead sports. Quadriceps and hamstring exercises are used to reduce lower extremity injuries in football. There has been limited evidence to suggest that prehabilitation may help decrease injuries in adolescent swimmers and high school football players, but it is unclear whether it has the same benefit in preadolescent athletes.[28,29]

It is well known that the rate of noncontact ACL injuries is greater in females than in males. Considerable research has been done in the past decade to identify and modify neuromuscular and biomechanical factors that make the female athlete more susceptible to ACL injuries. A recent research study of adolescent females (age 14.5 years ± 1.3 years) has suggested that a simple resistance training program alone may improve neuromuscular and biomechanical factors to decrease the athlete's risk of ACL injury.[30] However, further research is needed. Prospective studies using an appropriate age-matched control group are needed to evaluate whether the basic strength training program and improved neuromuscular and biomechanical factors actually reduce ACL injuries. Another research study suggested a reduction in sports-related ACL injuries in adolescent girls when strength training was combined with specific plyometric exercises.[31] Some research has demonstrated a decreased risk of ankle injuries in collegiate soccer players who perform resistance training.[32] There is no evidence that strength training will reduce the incidence of catastrophic sports-related injuries in youth.

Sports Performance

A major goal of strength training is to improve sports performance. Many studies have demonstrated improvement in specific measurable motor skills in sports such as the long jump,[11,26] the vertical jump,[17] the 30-m dash,[11,21] the squat jump,[21] and agility runs.[11,21] A few studies have failed to demonstrate improvements in vertical jump,[17,18] 40-yd sprint speed,[33] and flexibility.[19,34] In studies demonstrating increased lower extremity muscle strength and improved sprint speeds, the actual transfer of strength gains to increased speed is minimal. For example, one study demonstrated a 52% increase in leg strength, but only a 2.5% increase in 30-m speed.[21] Strength training has not been shown to be effective in increasing anaerobic capacity as measured with repeated jumps or Wingate testing.[21,33]

In addition to improvement in motor skills, sports-specific improvements with resistance or strength training have been documented in several studies. In studies of handball players, there has been a direct improvement in handball throwing velocity in adolescents after strength training.[35] According to results from two other studies, one of age-group swimmers and the other of competitive gymnasts, there were improvements in swim times and gymnastic event-specific performance following a resistance training program.[36,37] Results from studies of soccer players have failed to show improvement in 10-m sprint speed or soccer technique tests (dribbling between cones) after twice-weekly participation in a 16-week strength training program. At

Table 1
Medical Conditions Exacerbated by Strength Training
Late cardiac dysfunction and acute cardiomyopathy in patients treated for childhood cancer with anthracyclines
Aortic dissection in the absence of hypertension or dilated aortic root in patients with Marfan syndrome
Uncontrolled hypertension
Systemic pulmonary hypertension
Complex congenital heart disease
Cardiomyopathy

this time it is difficult to conclude that strength training during preadolescence and adolescence directly affects sports performance. Practicing sports-specific exercises may be as effective or more effective in enhancing sports performance then resistance training per se.

Preparticipation Clearance

In the context of proper supervision and program progression, strength training is relatively safe. However, some medical conditions can be acutely exacerbated by strength training.[38-40] Several medical conditions should be considered before strength training is recommended (Table 1).

Medical Conditions That Benefit From Strength Training

Youths who are either at risk of being overweight (body mass index (BMI) from 85% to 95%) or obese (BMI > 95%) may find strength training to be the ideal form of exercise. Agility and aerobic conditioning are not required for participation, and the effects of strength training can be seen 2 to 3 weeks after program initiation. Additionally, because these patients are larger than their peers, they also are relatively stronger; their ability to lift heavier weights provides them with a psychological advantage.[1] Although resistance training programs have failed to increase basal metabolic rate or reduce body weight, numerous health benefits have been demonstrated.[41] Research has shown that resistance training after participation in aerobic exercise prevents a return to preintervention blood pressures in hypertensive adolescents.[42] Resistance training also positively impacts lipid profiles,[17,43] fat-free mass as measured by skin fold testing,[15] and self-esteem[44] in preadolescents and adolescents.

Participation in strength training, in addition to proper diet, may positively impact bone acquisition and be beneficial for individuals at high risk for the development of osteopenia or osteoporosis and for optimizing bone health. In a study of Junior Olympics weight lifters, those who participate in strength training have had significant increases in bone mineral density in the

8: The Youth Athlete

lumbar spine and femoral neck in comparison with age-matched control patients.[45]

Program Development

The AAP, the ACSM, the American Orthopaedic Society for Sports Medicine, and the National Strength and Conditioning Association suggest that under proper program design and adult supervision, strength training in children and adolescents is a safe and worthwhile endeavor.

The most appropriate age to enroll a child in a strength training program should be an individual decision based on the child's maturity level, attainment of appropriate developmental milestones, and the type of sports participation. General requirements for readiness would include the desire to participate, the discipline needed to perform resistance training several times a week, and the capacity to listen and the ability to follow directions. Most children will have attained these characteristics and have proper balance and postural control by age 7 or 8 years. The AAP continues to discourage participation in power lifting, bodybuilding, competitive weight lifting, or 1-RM until Tanner stage V has been achieved. Athletes should undergo a preparticipation physical examination before initiation of a strength training program. This examination will identify contraindications to participation, provide the opportunity for anticipatory guidance, and detect any injuries that have not healed.

The program's effectiveness is dependent on its design and progression. The program duration should be a minimum of 8 weeks, each session 20 to 30 minutes in length. The ACSM recommends a minimum frequency of twice per week, with three times per week believed to be the most effective. The program design needs to include the initial weight intensity (amount of weight), the type of resistance (free weights, body weight, machines and/or therabands/balls), the desired volume (sets × repetitions), exercise selection and order, and amount of rest between sets. Exercises should include the core musculature and all major muscle groups, with the initial program including between six to eight exercises. The exercises should incorporate both single joint and multijoint exercises throughout the full range of motion. The emphasis should be on proper technique and form, rather than the amount of weight or the number of repetitions completed. Varying any component directly impacts the effectiveness and results of the program. For example, shortening the rest periods between sets increases the aerobic component of the program. Increases in weight intensity should be introduced slowly in increments of 5% to 10%. The program should incorporate a proper 10-minute warm-up and cool down. The program itself should be diversified over time to prevent boredom and to optimize performance. Progression can be achieved by increasing the weight, number of sets, exercises, and/or training sessions.

Summary

Strength training in youth is a safe and effective way to increase muscular strength and neuromuscular coordination when performed under proper supervision and with a proper program design. The health benefits of participation far outweigh the potential risks. As the number of obese children continues to rise, strength training will be a safe and effective way of promoting physical activity in children and improving their psychological, metabolic, and cardiovascular parameters. Further research is needed to determine its effectiveness in preventing injury and improving sports performance in the preadolescent.

Annotated References

1. American Academy of Pediatrics: Active healthy children: Prevention of childhood obesity through increased physical activity. *Pediatrics* 2005;117:1834-1842.

   This policy statement was developed by the AAP to address the epidemic of inactivity and pediatric obesity. The statement concludes with suggestions on encouraging, monitoring, and advocating increased activity in children.

2. Faigenbaum A, Zaichowsky LD, Gardner DE, Micheli LJ: Anabolic steroid use by male and female middle school students. *Pediatrics* 1998;101:E6.

3. VandenBerg P, Neumark-Sztainer D, Cafri G, Wall M: Steroid use among adolescents: Longitudinal findings from Project EAT. *Pediatrics* 2007;119:476-486.

   This study used data from Project Eat-II (Eating Among Teens) to determine prevalence, persistence, and predictors of anabolic steroid use in middle school and high school students from 1999 to 2004. Prevalence remained stable at approximately 1.5%, with decreasing use with progressing age. Dissatisfaction with weight and inadequate knowledge of nutritional concepts correlated with increased usage.

4. American Academy of Pediatrics: Weight training and weight lifting: Information for the pediatrician. *Phys Sports Med* 1983;11:157-161.

5. US Consumer Product Safety Commission: NEISS Query Results. Available at https://xapps.cpsc.gov/NEISSQuery/performEstimates.do. Accessed May 14, 2008.

6. Byrd R, Pierce K, Rielly L, Brady J: Young weightlifters performance across time. *Sports Biomech* 2003;2: 133-140.

   This case series evaluated the effectiveness and safety of Olympic weight lifting in 11 males and females. Study duration was 22 months. Significant gains in strength were noted per kilogram of body weight, and no injuries were reported.

7. Jones CS, Christensen C, Young M: Weight training injury trends: A 20 year survey. *Phys Sport Med* 2000;28:61-72.

8. Risser WL: Weight-training injuries in children and adolescents. *Am Fam Physician* 1991;44:2104-2110.

9. Mazur LJ, Yetman RJ, Risser WL: Weight-training injuries: Common injuries and preventative methods. *Sports Med* 1993;16:57-63.

10. Malina RM: Weight training in youth-growth, maturation, and safety: An evidence-based review. *Clin J Sport Med* 2006;16:478-487.

    This article is an evidence-based review of 22 resistance training protocols in prepubertal and early pubertal youth. The conclusion made after a review of the literature was that resistance training was effective and not inhibitory toward growth and development and is relatively safe.

11. Lillegard WA, Brown EW, Wilson DJ, et al: Efficacy of strength training in prepubescent to early postpubescent males and females: Effect of gender and maturity. *Pediatr Rehabil* 1997;1:147-157.

12. Rians CB, Weltman A, Cahill BR, et al: Strength training for prepubescent males: Is it safe? *Am J Sports Med* 1987;15:483-489.

13. Sadres E, Eliakim A, Constantini N, et al: The effect of long-term resistance training on anthropometric measures, muscle strength, and self-concept in pre-pubertal boys. *Pediatric Exercise Science* 2001;13:357-372.

14. Ramsay JA, Blimkie CJR, Smith K, et al: Strength training effects in prepubescent boys. *Med Sci Sports Exerc* 1990;22:605-614.

15. Sailors M, Berg K: Comparison of responses to weight training in pubescent boys and men. *J Sports Med Phys Fitness* 1987;27:30-37.

16. Vrijens J: Muscle strength development in the pre- and post-pubescent age, in Borms J, Hebbelinck M, (eds): *Pediatric Work Physiology.* Basel, Switzerland, Karger, 1978, pp 152-158.

17. Weltman A, Janney C, Rians C, Strand K, Katch F: The effects of hydraulic-resistance strength training on serum lipid levels in prepubertal boys. *Am J Dis Child* 1987;141:777-780.

18. Faigenbaum AD, Westcott WL, Micheli LJ, et al: The effect of strength training and detraining on children. *J Strength Cond Res* 1996;10:109-114.

19. Faigenbaum AD, Milliken LA, Loud RL, Burak BT, Doherty CL, Westcott WL: Comparison of 1 and 2 days per week of strength training in children. *Res Q Exerc Sport* 2002;73:416-424.

20. Sewall L, Micheli LJ: Strength training for children. *J Pediatr Orthop* 1986;6:143-146.

21. Christou M, Similios I, Sotiropoulos K, Volaklis K, Pilianidis T, Tokmakidis SP: Effects of resistance training on physical capacities of adolescent soccer players. *J Strength Cond Res* 2006;20:783-791.

    This case-control study used sports-specific testing to evaluate performance with soccer training alone, soccer and resistance training combined, and a control group. The strength component was used twice weekly for 16 weeks. The soccer and resistance training group had significant improvements in maximum bench press, leg press, squat jump, countermovement jumps, and 30-m speed. Soccer technique testing did not improve significantly with resistance training.

22. Faigenbaum AD, Milliken LA, Westcott WL: Maximal strength testing in healthy children. *J Strength Cond Res* 2003;17:162-166.

    This prospective study evaluated the safety of 1-RM in male and female children at ages 6 to 12 years. No injuries occurred in this study under well-controlled supervision using proper form with both upper and lower body weights.

23. American Academy of Pediatrics Council on Sports Medicine and Fitness, McCambridge TM, Stricker PR: Strength training by children and adolescents. *Pediatrics* 2008;121:835-840.

    This policy statement reviews the latest literature and makes recommendations for safe and effective strength training in children and adolescents.

24. Ozmun JC, Mikesky AE, Surburg PR: Neuromuscular adaptations following prepubescent strength training. *Med Sci Sports Exerc* 1994;26:510-514.

25. Peltonen JE, Taimela S, Erkintalo M, Salminen JJ, Oksanen A, Kujala UM: Back extensor and psoas muscle cross sectional area, prior physical training, and trunk muscle strength: A longitudinal study in adolescent girls. *Eur J Appl Physiol Occup Physiol* 1998;77:66-71.

26. Falk B, Mor G: The effects of resistance and martial arts training in 6 to 8 year old boys. *Pediatr Exerc Sci* 1996;108:48-56.

27. Blimkie CJ, Ramsay MJ, Ramsey J, et al: The effects of detraining and maintenance weight training on strength development in prepubertal boys. *Can J Sport Sci* 1989;14:104.

28. Dominguez R: Shoulder pain in age group swimmers, in *Swimming Medicine IV.* Erikkson B, Furberg B, (eds): Baltimore, MD, University Park Press, 1978, pp 105-109.

29. Hejna WF, Rosenberg A, Buturusis DJ, Krieger A: The prevention of sports injuries in high school students through strength training. *Natl Strength Coaches Assoc J* 1982;4:28-31.

8: The Youth Athlete

30. Lephart SM, Abt JP, Sell TC, Nagai T, Myers JB, Irrgang JJ: Neuromuscular and biomechanical characteristic changes in high school athletes: A plyometric versus basic resistance program. *Br J Sports Med* 2005; 39:932-938.

This study evaluated 27 female high school athletes participating in an 8-week plyometric or basic resistance training program. Both groups studied had improved knee extensor isokinetic strength, improved knee and hip flexion angles, and increased activation of the gluteus medius as determined by electromyographic testing.

31. Hewett TE, Meyer GD, Ford KR: Anterior cruciate ligament injuries in female athletes: Part 2. A meta-analysis of neuromuscular interventions aimed at injury prevention. *Am J Sports Med* 2006;34:490-498.

This study evaluated six published interventions toward ACL injury in female athletes. The meta-analysis of these six studies revealed a significant effect on neuromuscular training programs on ACL injury incidence in female athletes.

32. Lenhard RA, Lehnhard HR, Young R, et al: Monitoring injuries on a college soccer team: The effect of strength training. *J Strength Cond Res* 1996;10: 115-119.

33. Hetzler RK, Coop D, Buxton BP, Ho KW, Chai DX, Seichi G: Effects of 12 weeks of strength training on anaerobic power in pre-pubescent male athletes. *J Strength Cond Res* 1997;11:174-181.

34. Hoffman JR, Ratamess NA, Cooper JJ, Kang J, Chilakos A, Faigenbaum AD: Comparison of loaded and unloaded jump squat training on strength/power performance in college football players. *J Strength Cond Res* 2005;19:810-815.

Forty-seven college-age football players were divided into groups to perform eccentric and concentric squat jumps, concentric only squat jumps, and a control group. The groups did not demonstrate significant differences in power, vertical jump height, 40-yd sprint speed, or agility performance.

35. Gorostiaga EM, Izquierdo M, Iturralde P, Ruesta M, Ibanez J: Effect of heavy resistance training on maximal and explosive force production, endurance, and serum hormones in adolescent handball players. *Eur J Appl Phys* 1999;80:485-493.

36. Blanksby B, Gregor J: Anthropometric, strength, and physiological changes in male and female swimmers with progressive resistance training. *Austral J Sport Sci* 1981;1:3-6.

37. Query J, Laubach L: The effects of muscular strength/ endurance training. *Technique* 1992;12:9-11.

38. Steinherz LJ, Sterinherz PG, Tan CT, Heller G, Murphy ML: Cardiac toxicity 4 to 20 years after completing anthracycline therapy. *JAMA* 1991;266:1672-1676.

39. Kaplan NM, Gidding SS, Pickering TG, Wright JT Jr: 36th Bethesda Conference: Systemic hypertension. *J Am Coll Cardiol* 2005;45:1346-1348.

This article summarizes current expert opinion on sports participation in individuals with systemic hypertension.

40. Maron BJ, Ackerman MJ, Nishimura RA, Pyeritz RE, Towbin JA, Udelson JE. Task Force 4: HCM and other cardiomyopathies, mitral valve prolapse, myocarditis, and marfan. *J Am Coll Cardiol* 2005;45:1340-1345.

This article summarizes the current expert opinions regarding sports participation with underlying cardiomyopathy or structural heart defects.

41. Treuth MS, Hunter GR, Pichon C, et al: Fitness and energy expenditure after strength training in obese prepubertal girls. *Med Sci Sports Exerc* 1998;30:1130-1136.

42. Hagberg JM, Ehsani AA, Goldring D, Hernandez A, Sinacore DR, Holloszy JO: Effect of weight training on blood pressure and hemodynamics in hypertensive adolescents. *J Pediatr* 1984;104:147-151.

43. Fripp RR, Hodgson JL: Effect of resistive training on plasma lipid and lipoprotein levels in male adolescents. *J Pediatr* 1987;111:926-931.

44. Faigenbaum AD, Zaichkowsky LD, Westcott WL, et al: Psychological effects of strength training on children. *J Sport Behav* 1997;20:164-175.

45. Conroy BP, Kraemer WJ, Maresh CM, et al: Bone mineral density in elite junior olympic weightlifters. *Med Sci Sports Exerc* 1993;25:1103-1109.

Chapter 41

Throwing Injuries in Young Athletes

W. Ben Kibler, MD   Aaron Sciascia, MS, ATC, NASM-PES, NS

Introduction

Pediatric overhead athletes have a relatively high incidence of shoulder and elbow injuries. In addition to injuries such as dislocations and labral injuries that occur in adults, pediatric overhead athletes experience injuries related to muscular weakness, skeletal immaturity, and maladaptations and are affected by extrinsic factors such as level of competition, intensity of play, duration and frequency of play, and the biomechanical and physiologic demands of each sport. Some studies have suggested that athletes of a young age should have limits on participation in sports such as baseball and tennis based on the potential injury risk to the shoulder and elbow. It has been noted that intensely competitive, young, active athletes can develop deleterious maladaptations in flexibility and strength in areas subjected to repetitive tensile overload. A kinetic chain-based perspective on why upper extremity injuries occur in these patients, a review of known extrinsic and intrinsic factors related to the cause of the injuries, and current evaluation and treatment techniques are necessary to treat these injuries.

The Kinetic Chain

Physiologic muscle activation results in several biomechanical effects that allow efficient local and distal function. The preprogrammed muscle activations result in anticipatory postural adjustments, which position the body to withstand the perturbations to balance created by the forces of kicking, throwing, or running. The anticipatory postural adjustments create proximal stability for distal mobility.

Muscle activations create interactive moments that develop and control forces and loads at joints. Interactive moments are moments at joints that are created by motion and the position of adjacent segments. They are developed in the central body segments and are key to proper force at distal joints and for creating relative bony positions that minimize internal loads at the joint. There are many examples of proximal core activation providing interactive moments that allow efficient distal segment function. They either provide maximal force at the distal end, similar to the cracking of a whip, or they provide precision and stability to the distal end. Maximal shoulder internal rotation force to rotate the arm is developed by the interactive moment developed by trunk rotation. Maximal elbow varus torque to protect against elbow valgus strain is produced by the interactive moment resulting from shoulder internal rotation. Maximal fastball speed is correlated with the interactive moment from the shoulder that stabilizes elbow and shoulder distraction and produces elbow angular velocity. Accuracy of ball throwing is related to the interactive moment at the wrist produced by shoulder movement.

Trunk or leg weakness will change the interactive moments at the shoulder and elbow, increasing the distraction loads and shear stresses. Because of the kinetic chain activation and the interdependence of the body segments, the site of the symptoms (victim) may not be the sole site of alterations (culprit). Without elbow elevation and extension before maximal shoulder rotation, increased tensile loads are seen at the elbow ligaments during arm acceleration. This deleterious situation is familiar to baseball pitching coaches and is called the "dropped elbow," meaning that the elbow is positioned below the level of the shoulder in the acceleration phase; this position is the "kiss of death" for the elbow.

Factors Contributing to Pain and Injury in the Shoulder and Elbow

Baseball Extrinsic Factors

Pain is a frequent presenting symptom in young players, especially pitchers, participating in Little League baseball (ages 9 to 14 years). Studies have estimated that 26 to 35 per 100 youth baseball pitchers in a season are afflicted with some variation of shoulder and/or elbow injury.[1,2] These studies found that self-reported shoulder pain occurred in more than 30% of pitchers, and self-reported elbow pain occurred in more than 25% of pitchers immediately following a game.[1,2]

The dysfunction of the shoulder and elbow in the pediatric overhead athlete appears to be multifactorial.

Major contributors to shoulder and elbow pain in young baseball players are age, height, and weight. According to one study, the risk of elbow pain increased as age and weight increased.[1] As the body increases in mass, the increased force generated will have a potentially negative outcome on the skeletally immature athlete. In the same study, the authors also reported that elbow pain decreased with increased height. However, as elbow pain decreased with height, shoulder pain increased. This finding may indicate that more stress is being placed across the shoulder because of the longer lever (the arm).

The number of pitches thrown in a particular game also could affect the durability of the arm. In one study, the number of pitches thrown in a game and during the season among pitchers ages 9 to 14 years was assessed.[2] The authors found no significant difference between the number of pitches thrown in a game and elbow pain. However, there was a significant difference between increasing pitch counts and shoulder pain. When examining the total number of pitches thrown over a season, both shoulder and elbow pain increased as the pitches thrown increased. Increased elbow pain was associated with throwing more than 600 to 800 pitches per season, whereas increased shoulder pain was associated with throwing more than 800 pitches per season. It appears that the cumulative effect rather than the acute effect may be the most important factor.

The type of pitch thrown is another factor that should be considered. One study found that throwing a curveball requires an increased amount of force and torque at the elbow and shoulder.[3] The forces and torques are similar to throwing a fastball or slider; however, the dramatic difference in mechanics makes the curveball a difficult pitch to master. Similarly, another study showed that young pitchers are 50% more likely to experience shoulder pain by throwing a curveball and 80% more likely to experience elbow pain by throwing a slider.[2]

Baseball Intrinsic Factors

Changes in bone that affect arm rotation have been documented as a result of repetitive throwing in baseball players. Imaging studies have shown that the change in rotation is due to increased retroversion of the humeral head in relation to the shaft.[4] These changes averaged 10° to 15° and are thought to be positive adaptations, allowing the humeral head to externally rotate farther before contacting the posterior glenoid. The magnitude of these changes in rotation cannot progress after epiphyseal closure, and they cannot be modified by flexibility exercises, suggesting that these changes are permanent after skeletal maturity.

Glenohumeral internal rotation deficit (GIRD) is a common factor associated with injury in throwing athletes. GIRD is defined as side-to-side (internal rotation) asymmetry of greater than 25°, an absolute value of less than 25°, or a side-to-side loss of total arc of motion greater than 25°. It is thought to be produced by acquired posterior capsular contracture and/or posterior muscle stiffness and is frequently seen in various types of shoulder injuries. GIRD creates abnormal scapular kinematics because of the windup effect of the arm on the scapula. As the arm is forward flexed, horizontally adducted, and internally rotated in throwing or working, the tight capsule and muscles pull the scapula into a protracted, internally rotated, and anteriorly tilted position that causes downward rotation of the acromion. GIRD also affects glenohumeral kinematics by shifting the humeral center of rotation posterior superiorly in cocking and anterior superiorly in follow-through. The abnormal kinematics have been significantly associated with labral injuries.

There are very few differences between the throwing mechanics of young pitchers and adult pitchers. There is a proximal to distal kinetic chain of activation of the body segments in both groups to propel the arm and ball. However, there are differences in young and adult pitchers in the manner of kinetic chain segment activation. Young pitchers have increased trunk and leading hip rotation velocity from cocking to acceleration compared to adult pitchers. This is probably the result of a decreased capability for lower core force production. This disassociation between the upper and lower trunk rotation produces a tendency to "open up," with the arm trailing behind the body, and may result in increased anterior loads across the shoulder as well as increased medial loads across the elbow.

Tennis Extrinsic Factors

Of all injuries that occur in tennis, 20% to 45% are located in the upper extremity, with the shoulder and elbow the most frequently injured structures. According to survey data from the 1998 United States Tennis Association Boys' (16 to 18 years old) and Girls' (16 years old) National Championships, 25% to 35% of the participants had previous or current shoulder pain, whereas 22% to 25% reported previous or current elbow pain. Of those males who reported shoulder pain, 38% experienced anterior shoulder pain, 30% experienced posterior shoulder pain, and 32% noted both anterior and posterior shoulder pain. Of the females who reported shoulder pain, 56% experienced anterior shoulder pain, 15% experienced posterior shoulder pain, and 31% experienced both anterior and posterior shoulder pain.[5]

Tennis involves high body segment velocities, motions, and loads. Data from adult players show that the elite player must generate 4,000 W of energy (1.2 horsepower) in each serve. The entire body is involved in generating the energy. Trunk rotation velocity is approximately 350°/s, shoulder rotation velocity approaches 1,700°/s, and elbow extension velocity approaches 1,100°/s. These velocities are developed rapidly over 0.4 to 0.6 s, creating large accelerations in the shoulder. The total arc of shoulder internal and external rotation averages 146°. These velocities and accelerations produce ball velocities of 95 to 110 mph in females and 120 to 135 mph in males. There are no comparable data for loads in pediatric athletes, but the forces are quite high as shown by serve velocities approaching 85 mph in females and 105 mph in males.[6]

These loads are frequently applied and with high-energy demands. The elite pediatric tennis player averages 2.3 hours of practice or play per day, 6.1 days per week. Energy expenditure evaluation reveals that the metabolic demands in tennis are 70% alactic anaerobic, 20% lactic anaerobic, and 10% aerobic.[7]

The shoulder is at a high risk of injury in tennis because it faces high loads and forces while maintaining ball and socket kinematics. Loss of ball and socket kinematics, with excessive translation of the glenohumeral joint, may result in labral pathology, including degeneration or tears. Rotator cuff symptoms often occur secondary to glenohumeral instability. Other injuries can include humeral periostitis and bicipital tendinitis. Unlike pediatric baseball injuries, growth plate pathology is not a common occurrence in the shoulder. Acute shoulder injuries are uncommon, however; shoulder dislocations and acromioclavicular separations may occur from direct trauma, such as falling on the shoulder.

Lateral epicondylitis (tennis elbow), medial epicondylitis, and injury to the medial epicondylar growth plate can be seen in skeletally immature tennis players. Lateral epicondylitis occurs more frequently in recreational tennis players than in elite level tennis athletes, particularly in those recreational tennis players with poor backhand mechanics. It has been noted that the frequency of tennis elbow in world-class athletes ranges from 35% to 45%.[8] This frequency is much lower in elite junior athletes. The occurrence of tennis elbow has been associated with equipment-related issues such as incorrect grip size; metal racquets; heavier, stiffer, more tightly strung racquets; and racquets with increased vibration.

The larger core muscles of the body develop the force generated during the service motion. The hip and trunk are responsible for generating 51% of the energy used during tennis actions, whereas the shoulder force production is minimal (13%). Serving in this manner using the ground reaction forces and core activation is known as the push-through style of serving. This is accomplished by flexion of the lower extremity through activation of the knee musculature as well as the rotation of the trunk by the hip and core musculature. The leg muscles show a sequential pattern of activation from the back leg to the front leg, and the activation peaks before ball impact. The push-through serve is characterized by increases in ball velocity because of the longer time it takes to achieve a fully cocked position and the shorter time spent in the acceleration phase of the service motion. The knee flexion and hip counterrotation components are critical links in being able to optimally perform this motion. The push-through serve uses integration of multiple links in the kinetic chain by specific patterns of muscle activation, which reduces the degrees of freedom in the entire kinetic chain.

The push-through mechanism of kinetic chain activation has several advantages for the shoulder. It allows the forces to be developed in the larger core muscles, allowing the shoulder muscles to be maximally activated as stabilizers and compressors. It also provides a proximal stability, which allows maximal distal mobility of the arm and hand. Finally, it allows a stable base for long axis rotation, the coupled shoulder internal rotation/forearm pronation that imparts maximal force to the racquet and ball.

In contrast to the push-through serve, the pull-through serve is less productive. This service style is characterized by a lack of knee flexion and hip counterrotation. The leg muscle activation is not sequenced from back to front but activates at the same time, immediately at or after ball impact. As a result of not performing either action, the athlete must use the trunk muscles to generate the energy necessary for accomplishing the overhead task. In order for the arm to move forward, the nondominant external oblique and rectus abdominis muscles must pull the trunk through the sagittal plane of motion rather than rotate it through the transverse plane. The performance results of the pull-through mechanism include inconsistency in the serve and no topspin on the serve. This mechanism also creates increased load and stress at the distal joints (shoulder and elbow) and increases the risk of injury. Lack of knee flexion results in a 23% increase in shoulder internal rotation load and a 27% increase in elbow valgus load.[9]

Tennis Intrinsic Factors

Evidence has shown that prepubescent athletes, in comparison with postpubescent athletes, have less muscle mass and generate lower amounts of force.[10] Although this decrease in force production can allow the younger athlete to be somewhat resistant to fatigue and produce increased quantities of skill repetition (such as the tennis serve or baseball pitch), the skill being performed is less efficient because of increased but less refined amounts of neuromuscular activation and the smaller muscle mass. Therefore, the younger athlete, who depends on contributions from all kinetic chain segments to perform his or her skill, is susceptible to overuse injury when repeated inefficient motions are performed or there is a deficiency within one or more of the kinetic chain segments. This is often seen in athletes who experience shoulder and elbow pain as a result of poor throwing or serving mechanics or who have kinetic chain deficits such as scapular dysfunction or poor hip control.

As a result of the differences in the physiologic muscle characteristics of younger athletes, there are proximal kinetic chain factors that should be considered. It has been shown that mechanical alterations during the tennis serve and the baseball pitch, such as incomplete

8: The Youth Athlete

knee flexion in cocking or incomplete cocking of the shoulder, create increased loads in the shoulder and elbow as the athlete tries to maintain maximal serve or pitch velocity. In a 2003 study, the effect of altered proximal kinetic chain function on the loads seen at the elbow was evaluated.[11] In studying two groups of Olympic tennis players who developed the same ball speed, the authors found that the group that exhibited knee flexion less than 10° in the cocking phase of the tennis serve increased internal rotation force at the shoulder and the normalized valgus load at the elbow by 21% (6.3% of body weight compared with 5.2%), and that the resulting absolute value, 73.9 Nm, was in the range that has been documented to be above the safe level of repetitive load. These data show that a lack of proximal activation can increase the distal loads for the same force or energy output, thereby placing the upper extremity at risk for an overload injury.

GIRD also is a common maladaptation in pediatric tennis players. This condition appears at an early age and progresses with age and years of play. Current thought recognizes GIRD as a key initiator of a series of biomechanical alterations that lead to altered humeral position in arm rotation that predispose the shoulder and elbow to injury.

Physical Examination

Overuse injuries are seen more often in pediatric overhead athletes than anatomic injuries such as glenoid labrum or rotator cuff injury. Motor control is still developing in these athletes, so mechanical flaws, if neither identified nor corrected, may occur and can cause pain in the shoulder and elbow. The mechanical flaws can lead to the development of compensatory muscle patterns and altered muscle activations between global and local muscles in both upper and lower extremities, which creates an environment for overuse injury. This prevalence of overuse injury requires a thorough clinical evaluation to identify the cause of the symptoms.

It is possible to detect musculoskeletal maladaptations early, before they become deleterious. The musculoskeletal base evaluation should evaluate for local alterations such as instability, muscle injury, and inflexibility and should screen for kinetic chain alterations such as hip rotation inflexibility, lumbar weakness, lack of core stability, and scapular dyskinesis. In clinical practice, these alterations are found 49% to 100% of the time in association with shoulder and elbow injuries.[12]

The examination of the throwing athlete with elbow symptoms should include evaluation of the proximal factors that may influence elbow loading. Specific attention should be paid to evaluation of the shoulder, trunk, and hip/leg. In the patient history, questions should be asked about prior leg or back injury and any shoulder symptoms. A relatively common finding is of previous ankle sprain, especially on the contralateral

(plant foot) side. Also, many athletes will report shoulder pain or decreased function (ball velocity or ball location) before the onset of elbow symptoms.

In the physical examination, assessment of posture while standing can determine the presence of lumbar lordosis, which is common and decreases core trunk stability and anticipatory postural adjustments. Screening evaluation of the hip and leg can be accomplished by the one-leg stability series, which includes the one-leg stance and the one-leg squat. Inability to achieve balance of the trunk over the planted leg directs attention for further evaluation and rehabilitation efforts as part of the treatment. Dynamic trunk strength can be assessed by testing in all of the planes of trunk motion. The patient stands a given distance (usually 3 inches) from a wall. In sagittal plane testing, the patient faces away from the wall and is asked to slowly move his or her body backward, keeping his or her feet flat on the floor, to just barely touch his or her head against the wall. Initially, this can be done with both legs on the ground, then progress to partial weight bearing on each side and ultimately to single-leg standing. Sagittal plane core strength testing creates eccentric activation in the abdominal, the quadriceps, and hip flexor muscles and concentric activation in the hip and spine extensors. Frontal plane testing is done by having the patient stand with one side then the other 3 inches from the wall. While standing on the outside leg, he or she is asked to barely touch his or her inside shoulder to the wall. This test evaluates eccentric strength of the quadratus lumborum, the hip abductors, and some long spinal muscles that are working in the frontal plane. Transverse plane motion is tested by having the patient stand 3 inches from the wall and progress similar to the sagittal plane test from bilateral weight bearing to single-leg stance and alternately touch one shoulder and then the other just barely against the wall. Quality of motion and speed can be assessed. With lesser degrees of core strength, there is a greater breakdown in the ability to maintain single-leg stance and the ability to just barely touch the wall. This test will assess transverse plane motions, which incorporate abdominal muscles, hip rotators, and spine extensors. Therapy can then be instituted based on the muscles and planes of motion that are found to be deficient. Hip range of motion is frequently altered, especially in rotation, and can be evaluated by seated testing of internal/external rotation. Trunk flexibility in flexion/extension and lateral bend also can be evaluated by asking the athlete to bend in these directions.

Scapular dyskinesis can affect shoulder and elbow loads by altering the stable platform for long axis rotation and not allowing full cocking when the scapula is excessively protracted. Scapular assessment can be accomplished by evaluating the resting scapular position and dynamic scapular motion upon arm motion. Alterations of scapular position/motion, termed scapular dyskinesis, are common in association with arm injury and fall into three categories according to the activations,

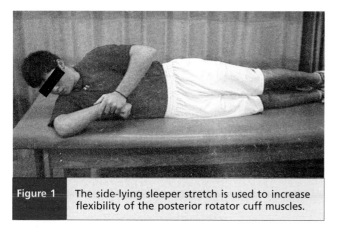

Figure 1   The side-lying sleeper stretch is used to increase flexibility of the posterior rotator cuff muscles.

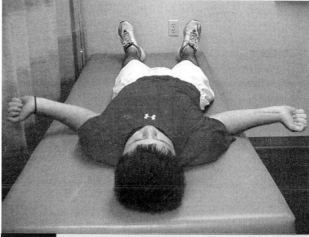

Figure 2   The open book stretch can be implemented into a treatment program to combat tightness in the pectoralis minor muscle. A rolled towel is placed down the length of the spine to accentuate thoracic extension during this stretch.

strength, and flexibilities of the supporting musculature. If one of the three patterns, inferior medial border prominence (type I), medial border prominence (type II), or superior medial border prominence (type III), is present, rehabilitation of the scapular muscles should be included in the treatment. Strengthening and reeducation of the scapular muscles can be achieved through the implementation of exercises that moderately activate the serratus anterior and trapezius muscles. When working optimally, both muscles have been suggested as being critical to functional scapular movement.

The shoulder should be evaluated closely for local injury and because of its important role in elbow force generation through interactive moments and regulation through long axis rotation. Shoulder rotation can be evaluated by stabilizing the scapula and determining the end ranges of glenohumeral motion. Rotator cuff strength should be evaluated, and testing for labral injury and instability should be done.

Treatment

If anatomic injury exists, such as labral pathology or instability, the same principles and protocols used to treat adult athletes can be used. Because most injuries in pediatric athletes are the result of overuse, activity modification and/or rest should include a reduction in the number of pitches thrown per inning or game in baseball or number of matches played per week or tournament in tennis.

Athletic performance is dependent on appropriate functioning of the individual components of the kinetic chain and appropriate coordination of the individual segments. Each segment plays a critical role in helping an individual achieve optimal athletic performance. A typical progression to follow to ensure each segment is optimized is (1) establish core strength and stability; (2) increase flexibility of hip, pelvis, and shoulder muscles; (3) restore scapular kinematics and strength; and (4) strengthen the scapulohumeral muscles (rotator cuff) and thoracohumeral muscles (latissimus dorsi and pectoralis muscles).

Athletes who are not skeletally mature (ages 8 to 18 years) should focus on core strength and stability as well as developing strength and balance in the periscapular musculature before developing global shoulder muscle strength and mass. This group also needs appropriate amounts of rest between training, practices, and competition to allow their bodies time to recover before introducing the next athletic exposure. This group often has deficits in the kinetic chain (weak and tight hip and/or abdominal musculature) and the scapula (strength and stability) in the presence of injury or in decreases in performance. Therefore, this young group of athletes should be able to perform more challenging dynamic kinetic chain-based exercises once the deficits are corrected.

To create a stable base, the rehabilitation protocols start with the primary stabilizing musculature such as the transverse abdominus, the multifidus, and the quadratus lumborum. Because of their direct attachment to the spine and pelvis, they are responsible for the most central portion of the core stability. Exercises include the horizontal side support and isometric trunk rotation. These exercises can be performed by athletes at all levels. This stage of rehabilitation not only restores core function by itself but also is the first stage of extremity rehabilitation.

Flexibility of both the upper and lower extremity can be increased via standard static and/or ballistic stretching. The hamstring, hip flexor, and hip rotator muscle groups should be targeted for the lower extremity, whereas the pectoralis minor and posterior shoulder muscles should be the point of focus. Range-of-motion exercises specific for shoulder rotation should be instituted if GIRD is found. Such exercises would include the passive sleeper or cross body stretches (**Figure 1**) and open book stretches (**Figure 2**).

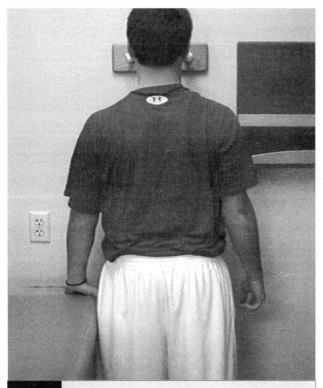

Figure 3   The low row is an isometric exercise that has been found to moderately activate the serratus anterior muscle. The patient is instructed to slide the scapula down toward his or her back pocket.

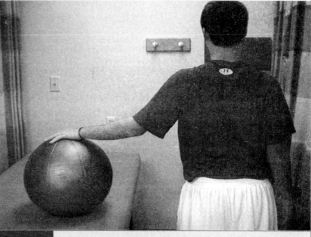

Figure 4   The inferior glide exercise, which focuses on activating the serratus anterior and the lower trapezius muscles, is performed by having the patient actively depress the scapula with the arm in a position of abduction.

Periscapular muscles such as the serratus anterior and the lower trapezius should be a point of focus in early training and rehabilitation. Early training should incorporate the trunk and hip to facilitate the kinetic chain in a proximal to distal sequence of muscle activation. Little stress is placed on the shoulder during the movements of hip and trunk extension combined with scapular retraction. All exercises are started with the feet on the ground and involve hip extension and pelvic control. The patterns of activation are both ipsilateral and contralateral. Diagonal motions involving trunk rotation around a stable leg simulate the normal pattern of throwing. As the shoulder heals and is ready for motion and loading in the intermediate or recovery stage of rehabilitation, the patterns can include arm motion as the final part of the exercise. Specific exercises known as the low row (**Figure 3**) and inferior glide (**Figure 4**) have been shown to activate the serratus and lower trapezius at safe levels of muscle activation.

The scapula serves as the base or platform for the rotator cuff. A properly stabilized scapula allows for optimal rotator cuff activation. A recent study found that rotator cuff strength increased as much as 24% when the scapula was stabilized and retracted.[13] For this reason, the early phases of training should focus on scapular strengthening rather than rotator cuff strengthening. Once the scapula is properly stabilized, more advanced exercises can be incorporated to strengthen the larger global muscles around the shoulder.

Conditioning programs may be developed based on the findings of the musculoskeletal evaluation. Kinetic chain deficits should be addressed before the implementation of routine fitness components. Exercises targeting the scapula and trunk stabilizers as well as stretches aimed at regaining flexibility of tight musculoskeletal structures would be appropriate. The conditioning programs should be as sport specific as possible, periodized to minimize deleterious overloads, and adjusted if the physical examination demonstrates developed deficits. The authors recommend integrating these programs with sport-specific activities, placing greater emphasis on mechanics and skills during the season while addressing strength, power, and weight gains (or losses) during the off season. Musculoskeletal flexibility should be emphasized daily. Proper recovery will take place if the body is given frequent periods of rest. This component of fitness is often overlooked and can lead to injury if not regularly attended to.

Summary

Shoulder and elbow injuries in youth athletes are common and seem to be increasing. The major causative factors can be categorized into growth and development factors, musculoskeletal maladaptations that affect kinetic chain development and regulation of force, technique factors in the throwing or serving motions that increase joint loads, and participation factors that result in too many pitches being thrown during a game in a week, season, or entire year. Evaluation, treatment, and prevention strategies must take each of these factors into account.

Annotated References

1. Lyman S, Fleisig GS, Waterbor JW, et al: Longitudinal study of elbow and shoulder pain in youth baseball pitchers. *Med Sci Sports Exerc* 2001;33:1803-1810.

2. Lyman S, Fleisig GS, Andrews JR, Osinski ED: Effect of pitch type, pitch count, and pitching mechanics on risk of elbow and shoulder pain in youth baseball pitchers. *Am J Sports Med* 2002;30:463-468.

3. Escamilla RF, Fleisig GS, Barrentine SW, Zheng N, Andrews JR: Kinematic comparisons of throwing different types of baseball pitches. *J Appl Biomech* 1998;14:1-23.

4. Crockett HC, Gross LB, Wilk KE, et al: Osseous adaptation and range of motion at the glenohumeral joint in professional baseball pitchers. *Am J Sports Med* 2002;30:20-26.

5. Safran MR, Hutchinson MR, Moss R, Albrandt J: A comparison of injuries in elite boys and girls tennis players. *Transactions of the 9th Annual Meeting of the Society of Tennis Medicine and Science*. Modern BV, Bennekorn, 1999, The Netherlands, vol 4, p 6.

6. Kibler WB: Biomechanical analysis of the shoulder during tennis activities. *Clin Sports Med* 1995;14:79-86.

7. Chandler TJ, Kibler WB (eds): Muscle training in injury prevention, in *Sports Injuries: Principles of Prevention and Care*. London, Blackwell, 1993, pp 252-261.

8. Nirschl RP: The etiology and treatment of tennis elbow. *J Sports Med* 1974;2:308-323.

9. Fleisig GS, Nicholls R, Elliot BC, Escamilla RF: Kinematics used by world class tennis players to produce high-velocity serves. *Sports Biomech* 2003;2:51-64.

   This study examined the service characteristics of Olympic-level tennis players. The authors found that those players who do not have large amounts of knee flexion during the cocking phase of the tennis serve have higher amounts of load at the shoulder and elbow. This evidence demonstrates the need for tennis players to appropriately use the links in the kinetic chain to decrease the risk of injury during a violent biomechanical action such as the tennis serve. Level of evidence: I.

10. Paterson PD, Waters PM: Shoulder injuries in the childhood athlete. *Clin Sports Med* 2000;19:681-692.

11. Elliot BC, Fleisig GS, Nicholl R, Escamilla RF: Technique effects on upper limb loading in the tennis serve. *J Sci Med Sport* 2003;6:76-87.

    This study examined the loads placed on the shoulder and elbow during the tennis serve in male and female Olympic tennis players. The authors found that those players with large amounts of knee flexion during the tennis serve had lesser amounts of torque at the shoulder and elbow.

12. Burkhart SS, Morgan CD, Kibler WB: The disabled throwing shoulder: Spectrum of pathology. Part I: Pathoanatomy and biomechanics. *Arthroscopy* 2003;19:404-420.

    This is a comprehensive review article of the different mechanisms that can cause pathology in the thrower's shoulder. It encompasses biomechanics and pathoanatomy that have been proven on a clinical basis. It presents the "victim versus culprit" approach to evaluating a painful throwing shoulder, disseminating the various causes of injury to help direct treatment toward the cause rather than the symptoms.

13. Kibler WB, Sciascia A, Dome D: Evaluation of apparent and absolute supraspinatus strength in patients with shoulder injury using the scapular retraction test. *Am J Sports Med* 2006;34:1643-1647.

    This study showed that demonstrated rotator cuff weakness is dependent on the position of the scapula during the testing procedure. Both injured and noninjured subjects elicited significant increases in active elevation strength with the scapula in a position of retraction in comparison with a position of resting posture. Level of evidence: I.

8: The Youth Athlete

Section 9

Imaging Update

SECTION EDITOR:

TIMOTHY AVERION-MAHLOCH, MD

Chapter 42

Imaging

Timothy Averion-Mahloch, MD

Introduction

MRI, CT, ultrasound, radiographs, and nuclear medicine all are well-established technologies for diagnosing musculoskeletal disease. MRI has made significant progress in the availability of higher field strength magnets, specifically the 3.0 T magnets, and improved imaging protocols developed by its manufacturers. Larger detector arrays have been developed using CT technology, increasing the number of detectors and improving spatial resolution. Ultrasound has been used most often in academic centers, and newer scanners have improved resolution. The increased prevalence of digital radiology and computed radiology has allowed greater access to the images by more clinicians, has enabled better communication between physicians, and allows variation of window and level settings to optimize both osseous and soft-tissue findings.

The 1.5 T MRI remains the standard of care and has adequate image quality for most musculoskeletal imaging. Although 3.0 T MRI is used most often by clinicians, challenges presented by imaging at this higher field strength include higher specific absorption rate, which is a measure of energy deposition in the patient by the radiofrequency field; the presence of magnetic susceptibility artifacts; and the noise of the gradient field (sound pressure levels in a 3.0 T magnet can be nearly twice those in a 1.5 T magnet). Although image optimization can be improved in some areas, 3.0 T MRI is advantageous over 1.5 T MRI because of its enhanced ability to characterize trabeculation in the bones and better visualization of small structures secondary to improved spatial resolution. In addition to the possible improvements in spatial resolution, 3.0 T MRI also can reduce imaging times in musculoskeletal and other applications. Nevertheless, these improvements in image quality are accompanied by increased energy deposition in the patient, the discomfort of the noisier system, and the significant additional cost of the 3.0 T magnets. Because of the additional cost of the 3.0 T systems and the economic environment of continuously decreasing reimbursements, it is likely that 1.5 T MRI will remain the standard technology for some time.

Multidetector CT also has become increasingly available for clinical use. The thin slice thickness and collimation of the x-ray beam reduces the effects of beam-hardening artifacts, allowing better visualization of orthopaedic hardware and better spatial resolution in both the slice direction and the transverse plane. As a result, the radiation dose to the scanned area is increased but is necessary in some clinical situations, especially in anatomic regions that are less sensitive to radiation, such as the joints.

Imaging of the Shoulder

Direct magnetic resonance arthrography (at 1.5 T) of the shoulder for detecting superior labral anterior and posterior (SLAP) tears has been compared with arthroscopy, the gold standard technique for identifying labral tears. The sensitivity and specificity of direct magnetic resonance arthrography for detecting labral tears was 82% and 98%, respectively. However, the arthrographic and arthroscopic classification (that is, the exact extent and location) of the labral tear was concordant in only 66% of cases. This accentuates the importance of subtle signs of labral tears on magnetic resonance arthrography and the limited value of SLAP tear classification by MRI. Two studies evaluated the performance of MRI for detecting anteroinferior labral injuries such as labroligamentous injuries and Bankart, anterior labroligamentous periosteal sleeve avulsion, Perthes, and glenoid labral articular disruption lesions.[1,2] The sensitivity and specificity of 1.5 T magnetic resonance arthrography for diagnosing these lesions was 88% and 91%, respectively.[3,4] Arthrography in 3.0 T MRI also is accurate for diagnosing labral tears, yielding a sensitivity of 86% to 90% and specificity of 100%. These studies confirm the accuracy of direct magnetic resonance arthrography for detecting labral tears.

Labral tears typically are evaluated using direct magnetic resonance arthrography (MRI after arthrography for injection of diluted gadopentetate dimeglumine into the joint). However, conventional MRI and indirect magnetic resonance arthrography (MRI after intravenous injection of gadopentetate dimeglumine) also have been used for labral evaluation. A study comparing indirect magnetic resonance arthrography with conventional MRI showed no statistical difference in the accuracy of these tests for detecting labral tears (78% to 86% versus 70% to 83%, respectively).[5] Indirect magnetic resonance arthrography was more sensitive but

9: Imaging Update

less specific than conventional MRI for detecting labral tears (sensitivity of 84% to 91% versus 66% to 85%, and specificity of 58% to 71% versus 75% to 83%). Thus, neither of these techniques is as sensitive or specific as direct magnetic resonance arthrography.[5]

The accuracy of ultrasound for diagnosing rotator cuff tears has been evaluated in multiple studies over the years and is correlated with operator experience. Ultrasound done by an experienced radiologist has been as accurate as MRI in the evaluation of full-thickness rotator cuff tears (sensitivity and specificity of 81% to 92% and 94% to 100%, respectively) but is significantly less sensitive for detecting partial-thickness rotator cuff tears when done by similarly trained radiologists (sensitivity and specificity of 13% to 71% and 68% to 100%, respectively).[3] Combined secondary signs of rotator cuff tears (such as cortical irregularity of the greater tuberosity and the presence of joint fluid) yielded a sensitivity of 60% and a specificity of 100%. The inability to visualize the tendon (found in only 24% of patients with full-thickness supraspinatus tears) is 100% specific for a full-thickness tear. New ultrasound techniques using tissue harmonic imaging may improve cuff visualization, but such benefits have not yet been quantified.

MRI has been established as a sensitive and specific imaging modality for evaluating the rotator cuff, with recent studies suggesting diagnoses for specific MRI findings and imaging techniques. One proposed constellation of these findings is internal (posterosuperior) impingement, which includes an articular-sided tear of the supraspinatus or infraspinatus tendon, subcortical cystic changes at the posterior aspect of the greater tuberosity of the humerus, and posterosuperior labral pathology.[4] The use of abduction and external rotation sequences in indirect magnetic resonance arthrography of the shoulder increased sensitivity for the detection of partial-thickness supraspinatus tendon tears. However, the abduction and external rotation images were of no value in detecting full-thickness tears.

Magnetic resonance spectroscopy has been used to measure intramuscular fat content, and its use for evaluating the chronicity and potential for surgical repair of rotator cuff tears is promising. With rotator cuff tears, specifically tears of the supraspinatus tendon, supraspinatus muscle atrophy and fatty infiltration are disproportionate to that of the deltoid. Quantified assessment of supraspinatus muscle atrophy may be more reliable using the deltoid as a control for comparison because fatty infiltration of the muscles increases with age in the uninjured rotator cuff. The lipid content in the supraspinatus muscle was evaluated in asymptomatic patients and in those with partial-thickness, full-thickness, and chronic tears of the supraspinatus tendon.[6] The apparent lipid content of the supraspinatus muscle was measured by proton magnetic resonance spectroscopy as 13.7% in asymptomatic patients, 29.5% in patients with partial-thickness tears, 48.6% in patients with full-thickness tears, and 66.1% in pa-

tients with chronic tears. The relationship of the lipid content within these muscles to the clinical outcome in patients undergoing surgical repair still needs to be studied, but it is possibly a quantifiable measure of the prognosis of attempted surgical repair.

Comprehensive reviews of rotator cuff pathology by both ultrasound and MRI techniques have been published,[7,8] along with a recent study of MRI capsular anatomy and pathology of the rotator cuff interval.[9]

Imaging of the Elbow

MRI is effective for evaluating ligamentous and tendinous structures in the elbow. High-resolution MRI (most easily obtained with a 3.0 T system) has been valuable in the evaluation of a painful, snapping elbow; a thickened synovial fold in the humeroradial joint is a possible cause of symptoms. An anatomic study of the anterior bundle of the ulnar collateral ligament of the elbow showed a variable attachment of the distal insertion. Accordingly, the authors of this study recommend caution in diagnosing a partial detachment of the anterior band of the ulnar collateral ligament because of this variability.[10] Magnetic resonance arthrography may be beneficial to better define suspected partial tears of the ulnar collateral ligament. MRI also is effective in evaluating biceps tendon pathology[11] and the compartmental anatomy of the elbow.[12]

Imaging of the Wrist

MRI is a valuable tool for evaluating the tendons, ligaments, and soft tissues of the wrist and has been shown to be the most sensitive modality for detecting early degenerative changes in the hand and wrist in patients with inflammatory arthritis. These findings include subcortical edema, marginal erosions, synovitis, and inflammatory changes along the tendon sheaths. The detection and characterization of tenosynovitis of the wrist and hand was compared using MRI with and without intravenous contrast. MRI with intravenous contrast was found to be superior to nonenhanced MRI and more accurate in the diagnosis of inflammatory arthritis. The tendons most commonly affected are those of the carpal tunnel, with tenosynovial enhancement more prominent in the flexor tendons than the extensor tendons in patients with inflammatory arthritis.

MRI also is valuable for evaluating soft-tissue masses and injuries. The MRI criteria for distinguishing ganglion cysts from synovitis are presented in **Table 1**. The limitations of MRI for evaluating the wrist also have been evaluated. Routine MRI evaluation of the wrist has been shown to be inadequate to assess articular cartilage in the wrist; sensitivity for detecting cartilage injuries of the articular surfaces of the distal radius, scaphoid, lunate, and triquetrum was found to be 27%, 31%, 41%, and 18%, respectively, and specific-

Table 1

MRI Criteria for Distinguishing Ganglion Cysts From Synovitis

	Shape	Margin	Internal Structure	Enhancement Characteristics	Sensitivity	Specificity
Ganglion cysts	Multilocular	Defined	Septations	Wall	89% to 94%	85% to 95%
Synovitis	Diffuse, crescentic	Diffuse	Heterogeneous internal signal	Diffuse	33%	33%

(Data from Anderson SE, Steinbach LS, Stauffer E, Voegelin E: MRI for differentiating ganglion and synovitis in the chronic painful wrist. Am J Roentgenol 2006;186:812-818.)

ity was 91%, 90%, 75%, and 93%, respectively. High-grade lesions were more reliably found than low-grade lesions.[13]

The comparative effectiveness of MRI and CT for evaluating occult scaphoid fractures has been studied. Multidetector CT is highly accurate in depicting occult cortical fractures but is inferior to MRI in evaluating trabecular injuries, whereas CT is superior to MRI in demonstrating cortical morphology.[14] The efficacy of CT arthrography and MRI (without arthrography) for evaluating interosseous ligament tears has been studied.[15] These modalities were comparable for evaluating palmar and central segment tears of the scapholunate and lunotriquetral ligaments. CT arthrography was slightly more accurate than MRI without arthrography in detecting dorsal segment tears. However, magnetic resonance arthrography was not evaluated in this study.

The efficacy of ultrasound to evaluate wrist pathology is comparable with that of electrodiagnostic evaluation for carpal tunnel syndrome, with a sensitivity of 94% and a specificity of 65%. The use of ultrasound for evaluating the triangular fibrocartilage complex is promising. A small study found seven of eight triangular fibrocartilage complex tears with high-resolution sonography; the presence of these tears was confirmed with MRI.[16] The sonographic character of giant cell tumors of the tendon sheath, which appear as solid, hypoechoic masses with internal vascularity, has been studied.[17]

Imaging of the Hip

Magnetic resonance arthrography showed a sensitivity of 44% and a specificity of 96% for intra-articular bodies in the hip. A study performed by Duke University showed that magnetic resonance arthrography is helpful in diagnosing acetabular labral tears.[18] Conventional MRI with a large field of view (FOV) was 8% sensitive for detecting acetabular labral tears, conventional MRI with a small FOV was 25% sensitive, and magnetic resonance arthrography with a small FOV was 92% sensitive, reflecting the importance of focusing the MRI examination on the hip for optimum diagnostic information. Correlation of magnetic resonance

arthrography and arthroscopy of the hip has shown areas of anatomic variation along the acetabular labrum. The most common anatomic variation is a sublabral sulcus at the posteroinferior aspect of the acetabular labrum, a site remote from the location of most labral tears and identified in 17.4% of hips with arthroscopy and 22.4% of hips with magnetic resonance arthrography.

Conventional radiographs, CT, and MRI all have been used to evaluate cam and pincer femoroacetabular impingement. CT and MRI findings are best characterized by oblique axial imaging and include osteophytic changes, chondral injury, acetabular labral tears, and subcortical edema. The triad of abnormal morphology of the femoral head-neck junction (osteophytic change), anterosuperior cartilage abnormality, and anterosuperior labral abnormality found using magnetic resonance arthrography was seen in 37 of 42 patients with cam-type femoroacetabular impingement.[19]

Sonography has been used to evaluate and treat patients with a painful, snapping hip. Under static imaging, 95% of patients had a normal examination, and a snapping iliopsoas tendon was identified in only 23% of patients with dynamic imaging. However, after injecting anesthetic into the iliopsoas bursa, 73% of these patients had complete or partial pain relief. Sonography can be used to diagnose tendinopathy and tendon tears, bursal fluid, and adjacent soft-tissue masses; to guide peritendinous iliopsoas injections; and to evaluate acute tendon tears.

The efficacy of MRI versus ultrasound for assessing acute and healing hamstring injuries has been evaluated. The sensitivity for detecting acute hamstring injuries is similar for MRI and ultrasound, but the findings on MRI were more sensitive and specific for evaluating healing on follow-up examinations. In addition, the strongest predictor of the clinically required amount of time off from activity by a patient was the longitudinal length of the tear as seen on MRI. Similar results were found for both MRI and ultrasound in the diagnosis of acute injuries to the rectus abdominis and pectoralis muscles. Both modalities also are able to diagnose contracture in the deltoid muscle. However, MRI has been shown to be superior for evaluating chronic injuries and for following the progression of healing.

9: Imaging Update

Imaging of the Knee

MRI remains the most accurate imaging modality for the detection and characterization of meniscal tears. Several associated or secondary findings of meniscal tears have been studied, including the relationship of meniscal tears to meniscal extrusion, the relationship between radial meniscal tears and prior meniscal surgery, and the sensitivity for detecting meniscal fragments. Medial meniscal extrusion has been associated with meniscal pathology. An extrusion of the meniscus of greater than 3 mm (medial to the medial tibial margin) is associated with severe meniscal degeneration, a large meniscal tear, a complex meniscal tear, a large radial meniscal tear, or a tear of the meniscal root. Radial tears of the meniscus are more common in patients following prior meniscal surgery. There was a 32% prevalence of radial meniscal tears in postoperative knees and a 14% prevalence of radial meniscal tears in patients without prior surgery.[20] A study of meniscal tears with fragments displaced into the notch and recess demonstrated that displaced fragments were detected in 41% of meniscal tears during arthroscopy and in 36% of meniscal tears on MRI. The sensitivity and specificity for MRI detection of these displaced fragments was 71% and 98%, respectively, for tears with recess fragments, and 69% and 94%, respectively, for tears with notch fragments.[21]

New technology and techniques for evaluating the meniscus also have been explored. The 3.0 T MRI has an accuracy, sensitivity, and specificity for detecting medial and lateral meniscal tears of 94%, 96%, and 89%, respectively, in the medial meniscus and 94%, 94%, and 94%, respectively, in the lateral meniscus. Kinematic MRI, which may be done with a flexible knee coil in open MRI, has been used to evaluate meniscal tears, positional displacement, and associated findings. Displaced meniscal tears were associated with grade 2 or 3 tears of the ipsilateral collateral ligament in all cases, and nondisplaced meniscal tears were associated with normal ipsilateral collateral ligament tears in 88% of cases.

Increased signal intensity, thickening, and cysts within and adjacent to the anterior cruciate ligament (ACL) are common findings that often are clinically insignificant, and there was no clinical evidence of instability in the patients studied.[22] In addition, cysts within or adjacent to the ACL were found in 35% of patients with thickening and increased internal signal intensity in the ACL.[22]

MRI of the posterolateral corner of the knee was evaluated in a 2007 study.[23] Injuries to the posterolateral corner are not common, but undetected injuries can be a source of chronic instability and pain in the knee and predispose the patient to osteoarthritic changes. The structures of the posterolateral corner sometimes can be seen on MRI examination. The popliteomeniscal fascicles are seen in 60% to 94% of uninjured patients, and the popliteofibular ligament is seen in 8% to 53% of these same patients. The arcuate ligament and fabellofibular ligaments are seen in 10% to 46% and 33% to 48%, respectively, of these patients. Additional findings of a posterolateral corner injury, the Segond fracture, and the arcuate sign (an avulsion of bone from the fibular attachment of the arcuate ligament) also were reviewed. Even without direct visualization of the posterolateral corner structures, edema posterior to the popliteus tendon can indicate an injury to the underlying structures of the posterolateral corner, and MRI is the best tool for the evaluation and characterization of such injuries.[23]

Many techniques and sequence protocols have been explored for articular cartilage evaluation using MRI. The improved signal-to-noise ratio with 3.0 T MRI systems allows greater spatial resolution and contrast resolution. T2 relaxation times demonstrate lengthening (brighter signal on T2 images) in the presence of osteoarthritis. The accuracy of coronal short tau inversion recovery sequences for detecting cartilage contour irregularities is 87% to 94%. In addition, the degree of subcortical marrow edema is associated with more severe cartilage degeneration. Although development of additional and better techniques will continue, MRI is the best imaging method for evaluating degenerative changes in articular cartilage and postsurgical cartilage characterization after abrasion arthroplasty, microfracture, subchondral drilling, autologous chondrocyte implantation, or autologous transplantation of cartilage.[24]

The accuracy of low-field MRI versus high-field MRI has been evaluated to verify the clinical utility of these lower field magnets for imaging of the knee. Despite a lower intrinsic signal in low-field MRI, excellent correlation between the accuracy, sensitivity, and specificity of the detection of meniscal tears and ACL injuries has been shown for 0.2 T and 1.5 T magnets. The accuracy for detecting medial meniscus, lateral meniscus, and ACL tears was 91% to 93%, 88% to 90%, and 93% to 96%, respectively, at 0.2 T. In comparison, the accuracy at 1.5 T was 91% to 94%, 91% to 93%, and 97% to 98%, respectively.[25]

Ultrasound has been used to evaluate bursae and fluid collections about the knee, soft-tissue masses, and superficial tendon and ligament injuries and also has been effective in detecting arthrofibrosis of the knee following total knee arthroplasty. The key findings for arthrofibrosis were synovial thickening and neovascularity. When a thickness cutoff of the synovial membrane of 3 mm is used, sensitivity and specificity for detecting arthrofibrosis are 84% and 82%, respectively. MRI also has been used to assess the normal anatomy and pathology of the posterolateral corner of the knee[26] and anatomy of the PCL and posterior capsule.[27]

Imaging of the Ankle and Foot

Because fractures of the foot are poorly demonstrated on routine radiographs, CT is recommended for characterizing tarsal fractures. In a large study of 388 patients with acute ankle and foot trauma, fractures were identified by CT in 89% of these patients.[28] However, conventional radiography was significantly less sensitive for detecting these fractures. The sensitivity for detecting these fractures by conventional radiography was 87% for calcaneal fractures, 78% for talar fractures, and only 25% to 33% for midfoot fractures. In addition, Lisfranc fracture-dislocation was not detected by conventional radiography in 24% of patients with this injury. The plain film radiographic appearance of calcaneal fractures correlates poorly with the final outcome. Measurements of osseous angles and relationships are not useful in determining the clinical outcome of intraarticular calcaneal fractures. Outcome scores and physical evaluation are more meaningful and statistically unrelated to the conventional radiographic appearance of the fractures.[28]

A study of collegiate basketball players from Duke University demonstrated the potential of MRI to evaluate stress changes in the bone before fracture or onset of pain.[29] Early identification of these stress-related changes in the metatarsals allowed preemptive treatment and thus a more rapid return to activity for these patients. A separate retrospective study of muscular injuries to the calf demonstrates the distribution of these injuries.[30] Half of the injuries are to a single muscle and half are to multiple muscles. The single muscle injuries are evenly split between the medial head of the gastrocnemius and the soleus, with the lateral head of the gastrocnemius only rarely injured in isolation. Of the multiple injuries, 60% included a combination of gastrocnemius and soleus strains.

Spring ligament tears are well demonstrated by MRI. A full-thickness gap in the spring ligament was seen in 79% of patients with tears found at surgery.[31] Increased fluid-sensitive signal was seen in all patients with a spring ligament tear, and other findings include ligament thickening and a wavy appearance. A different study noted that it is common to have a focal lesion detected in MRI of the calcaneus adjacent to the insertion of the cervical and interosseous ligaments.[32] This finding represents a prominent vascular remnant that typically is not related to pathology.

Sonography has been shown to be useful for diagnosing peroneal tendon subluxation. Dynamic sonography detected tendon subluxation in all patients found to have this abnormality at surgery. However, 20% of asymptomatic ankles also showed peroneal tendon subluxation. Sonography also has been used to evaluate the extensor pollicis longus tendon and localize tendon rupture and the location and size of the tendon gap for preoperative planning.

The sensitivity of MRI, CT, and bone scintigraphy for detecting tibial stress fractures has been measured.[33] The sensitivity for detecting stress fractures is 88% for MRI, 42% for CT, and 74% for bone scintigraphy. MRI also was 100% specific for the detection of tibial stress fractures. CT also has been valuable in assessing stress reactions in the bones. In distance runners, CT

detected abnormalities in 100% of patients with symptoms of medial tibia stress syndrome (shin splints). The abnormalities found on CT include osteopenia, cavitation, and striations. However, findings were similar in 16.6% of patients with a painless tibia. The sensitivity and specificity of CT for medial tibia stress syndrome was calculated as 100% and 88.2%, respectively. In a 2004 study,[34] increased marrow signal was noted in the tibia in 43% of asymptomatic college distance runners. This finding stresses the importance of correlation with clinical symptoms. Grading schemes for stress injuries in the bones have been proposed, and there is correlation between the MRI grade and clinical recovery in patients with stress injuries: grade 0 examinations are normal by MRI; grade 1 findings include subtle periosteal edema; grade 2 and 3 stress injuries demonstrate increasing marrow edema and periosteal edema, and a grade 4 stress injury is accompanied by a fracture in the trabeculae. A study of marrow changes in anorexia nervosa demonstrates the difficulty in diagnosing stress fractures in these patients.[35] The signal characteristics are the same as stress fractures, and the first body parts affected typically are the feet.

Summary

MRI, CT, and ultrasound continue to serve as valuable tools for diagnosing sports-related injuries. Improved technology over the past decade not only allows better definition of musculoskeletal pathology but also has enhanced the ability to identify pathology. Continued study of imaging findings has enabled the surgeon to differentiate the specific findings of musculoskeletal injury from incidental findings, resulting in improved sensitivity and specificity of imaging studies.

Annotated References

1. Waldt S, Burkart A, Lange P, Imhoff A, Rummeny E, Woertler K: Diagnostic performance of MR arthrography in the assessment of superior labral anteroposterior lesions of the shoulder. *AJR Am J Roentgenol* 2004; 182:1271-1278.

   This study evaluated the accuracy of magnetic resonance arthrography for detecting labral pathology, using arthroscopy as the gold standard.

2. Waldt S, Burkart A, Lange P, et al: Anterior shoulder instability: Accuracy of MR arthrography in the classification of anteroinferior labroligamentous injuries. *Radiology* 2005;237:578-583.

   This study evaluated the accuracy of magnetic resonance arthrography for the classification of labral pathology, using arthroscopy as the gold standard.

3. McNally E: Ultrasound of the rotator cuff, in McNally E (ed): *Practical Musculoskeletal Ultrasound.* Philadelphia, PA, Elsevier, 2005, pp 55-56.

9: Imaging Update

This book includes a compilation of multiple studies from 1989 through 2002 evaluating the sensitivity and specificity of ultrasound for detecting full-thickness and partial-thickness rotator cuff tears when arthroscopy is used as a gold standard. The studies of full-thickness rotator cuff tears have been fairly consistent since 1994, with sensitivities of 74% to 92% (with one outlier of 100%) and specificities of 91% to 100%. This confirms ultrasound's utility for evaluating full-thickness rotator cuff tears. However, in the three most recent studies assessing ultrasound for the evaluation of partial-thickness rotator cuff tears, sensitivity has been measured at 13% to 71% and specificity at 68% to 100%.

4. Giaroli EL, Major NM, Higgins LD: MRI of internal impingement of the shoulder. *AJR Am J Roentgenol* 2005;185:925-929.

    This study established the triad of undersurface tears of the supraspinatus or infraspinatus tendons, posterosuperior labral pathology, and subcortical cystic change in the greater tuberosity of the humerus as the radiographic criterion of internal impingement. There findings were correlated with the clinical and surgical findings of internal impingement in these patients.

5. Dinauer P, Flemming D, Murphy D, Doukas W: Diagnosis of superior labral lesions: Comparison of noncontrast MRI with indirect arthrography in unexercised shoulders. *Skeletal Radiol* 2007;36:195-204.

    This study quantifies the sensitivity and specificity of MRI of the shoulder for detecting labral tears with and without intravenous injection of gadolinium.

6. Pfirrmann CW, Schmid MR, Zanetti M, Jost B, Gerber C, Hodler J: Assessment of the fat content in supraspinatus muscle with proton MR spectroscopy in asymptomatic volunteers and patients with supraspinatus tendon lesions. *Radiology* 2004;232:709-715.

    The lipid content in the supraspinatus muscle was evaluated for asymptomatic volunteers and for patients with various degrees of tendon tears. The mean lipid content in the supraspinatus muscle was 13.7% in asymptomatic volunteers, 29.5% in patients with partial-thickness tendon tears, 48.6% in patients with full-thickness tendon tears, and 66.1% in patients with chronic full-thickness tendon tears.

7. Moosikasuwan JB, Miller TT, Burke BJ: Rotator cuff tears: Clinical, radiographic, and US findings. *Radiographics* 2005;25:1591-1607.

    Ultrasound and MRI anatomy and pathology in the shoulder are reviewed.

8. Morag Y, Jacobson J, Miller B, De Maeseneer M, Girish G, Jamadar D: MR imaging of rotator cuff injury: What the clinician needs to know. *Radiographics* 2006;26:1045-1065.

    Clinical applications and radiographic requirements for MRI of the shoulder are reviewed.

9. Krief OP: MRI of the rotator interval capsule. *AJR Am J Roentgenol* 2005;184:1490-1494.

    This article describes the anatomic relationships and ra-

diographic appearance of the rotator cuff interval and presents examples of coracohumeral ligament pathology, including thickening, tears, and rupture of the anterior sling.

10. Munshi M, Pretterklieber M, Chung C, et al: Anterior bundle of the ulnar collateral ligament: Evaluation of anatomic relationships by using MR arthrography, and gross anatomic and histologic analysis. *Radiology* 2004; 231:797-803.

    In this anatomic study of the ulnar collateral ligament, cadaver specimens were studied using MRI and dissection.

11. Chew ML, Giuffre BM: Disorders of the distal biceps brachii tendon. *Radiographics* 2005;25:1227-1238.

    This article reviews distal biceps anatomy and pathology.

12. Toomayan GA, Robertson F, Major NM, Brigman BE: Upper extremity compartmental anatomy: Clinical relevance to radiologists. *Skeletal Radiol* 2006;35:195-201.

    This article reviews upper arm anatomy.

13. Anderson SE, Steinbach LS, Stauffer E, Voegelin E: MRI for differentiating ganglion and synovitis in the chronic painful wrist. *AJR Am J Roentgenol* 2006;186:812-818.

    The key for differentiating synovitis from a ganglion cyst in the wrist is the use of intravenous contrast, which demonstrates heterogeneous internal enhancement in synovitis. Without intravenous contrast, these two entities could not be reliably differentiated.

14. Memarsadeghi M, Breitenseher M, Schaefer-Prokop C, et al: Occult scaphoid fractures: Comparison of multidetector CT and MR imaging: Initial experience. *Radiology* 2006;240:169-176.

    Although multidetector CT is highly accurate for detecting occult scaphoid fractures, it is inferior to MRI. In 11 patients, occult scaphoid fracture was correctly diagnosed using MRI; with CT, the correct diagnosis was made in the 8 patients with cortical involvement, thus missing 3 of the 11 fractures. However, MRI depicted the cortical involvement in only two of the eight patients with cortical irregularities. These findings emphasize the usefulness of MRI for detecting occult fractures and the value of CT for fracture characterization.

15. Schmid M, Schertler T, Pfirrmann C, et al: Interosseous ligament tears of the wrist: Comparison of multidetector row CT arthrography and MR imaging. *Radiology* 2005;237:1008-1013.

    This study compared the accuracy of CT arthrography for detecting injuries to the intercarpal ligaments with that of MRI without arthrography. MRI with arthrography was not compared with CT arthrography, so this study did not address the relative accuracy of these two modalities when arthrography was performed prior to each study.

16. Keogh C, Wong A, Wells N, Barbarie J, Cooperberg P: High-resolution sonography of the triangular fibrocartilage: Initial experience and correlation with MRI and

arthroscopic findings. *AJR Am J Roentgenol* 2004;182: 333-336.

The wrists of a small number of patients were studied using ultrasound to investigate the feasibility of using ultrasound to detect triangular fibrocartilage tears. The initial investigation was promising in seven of eight patients.

17. Middleton W, Patel V, Teefey S, Boyer M: Giant cell tumors of the tendon sheath: Analysis of sonographic findings. *AJR Am J Roentgenol* 2004;183:337-339.

This study evaluated the appearance of giant cell tumors in a small number of patients. As with most imaging modalities, the appearance of the giant cell tumors was a solid mass demonstrating increased vascularity. The relative sensitivity of ultrasound for detecting this vascularity versus other modalities was not studied.

18. Toomayan GA, Holman WR, Major NM, Kozlowicz SM, Vail TP: Sensitivity of MR arthrography in the evaluation of acetabular labral tears. *AJR Am J Roentgenol* 2006;186:449-453.

The importance of using both a small imaging FOV and magnetic resonance arthrography of the hip for diagnosing acetabular labral tears was established in this study. Conventional MRI with a large FOV was 8% sensitive for detecting acetabular labral tears. Sensitivity was improved to 25% with a small FOV. The combination of a small FOV and magnetic resonance arthrography yielded a sensitivity of 92% for detecting acetabular labral tears.

19. Kassasjian A, Yoon LS, Belzile E, Connolly SA, Millis MB, Palmer WE: Triad of MR arthrographic findings in patients with cam-type femoroacetabular impingement syndrome. *Radiology* 2005;236:588-592.

A triad of findings was seen in 37 of 42 patients with cam-type femoroacetabular impingement syndrome. This triad includes abnormal morphology of the femoral head-neck junction, an anterosuperior cartilage abnormality, and an anterosuperior acetabular labral abnormality.

20. Magee T, Shapiro M, Williams D: Prevalence of meniscal radial tears of the knee revealed by MRI after surgery. *AJR Am J Roentgenol* 2004;182:931-936.

There is an increased prevalence of radial meniscal tears in patients following prior partial meniscectomy. The postoperative prevalence of radial tears was 32% and 14% in patients with no prior history of meniscal surgery.

21. Vande Berg BC, Malghem J, Poilvache P, Maldague B, Lecouvet FE: Meniscal tears with fragments displaced in notch and recess of knee: MR imaging with arthroscopic comparison. *Radiology* 2005;234:842-850.

In this study, 41% of torn menisci were found to have partially detached meniscal fragments at arthroscopy. The magnetic resonance detection of fragments displaced into the intercondylar notch had a sensitivity and a specificity of 69% and 94%, respectively. The detection of fragments displaced into the meniscal recesses had a sensitivity and specificity of 71% and 98%, re-

spectively. Hence, some of these small fragments may be missed on MRI.

22. Bergin D, Morrison W, Carrino J, Nallamshetty S, Bartolozzi A: Anterior cruciate ligament ganglia and mucoid degeneration: Coexistence and clinical correlation. *AJR Am J Roentgenol* 2004;182:1283-1287.

ACL ganglia and mucoid degeneration were found to coexist in 35% of patients with either of these findings. However, there was no associated ligamentous instability in these patients or the patients with isolated anterior cruciate ganglia or mucoid degeneration.

23. Bolog N, Hodler J: MR imaging of the posterolateral corner of the knee. *Skeletal Radiol* 2007;36:715-728.

This article reviews the anatomy, pathology, and magnetic resonance appearance of the posterolateral corner of the knee. The lateral collateral ligament and popliteus tendon were seen in all patients, and the popliteomeniscal fascicles were seen on MRI in 60% to 94% of patients. However, the fabellofibular ligament was seen only on MRI in 33% to 48% of patients, the popliteofibular ligament was seen only in 8% to 53% of patients, and the arcuate ligament was seen only in 10% to 46% of patients. Injuries to the posterolateral corner must often be judged by associated findings such as edema rather than by direct visualization.

24. Recht MP, Goodwin DW, Winalski CS, White LM: MRI of articular cartilage: Revisiting current status and future directions. *AJR Am J Roentgenol* 2005;185: 899-914.

This article discusses the appearance of articular cartilage on MRI. An important distinction is made between the appearance of degenerative and traumatic cartilage lesions for application to clinical practice. Traumatic cartilage lesions typically demonstrate focal cartilage defects with acutely angled margins. Degenerative cartilage lesions typically demonstrate thinning, fibrillation, and surface irregularity.

25. Cotton A, Delfaut E, Demondion X, et al: MR imaging of the knee at 0.2 and 1.5 T: Correlation with surgery. *AJR Am J Roentgenol* 2000;174:1093-1097.

26. De Maeseneer M, Van Roy P, Shahabpour M, Gosselin R, De Ridder F, Osteaux M: Normal anatomy and pathology of the posterior capsular area of the knee: Findings in cadaveric specimens and patients. *AJR Am J Roentgenol* 2004;182:955-962.

The posterior joint capsule anatomy in the knee is reviewed.

27. De Abreu MR, Kim HJ, Chung CB, et al: Posterior cruciate ligament and normal posterior capsular anatomy: MR imaging of cadaveric knees. *Radiology* 2005;236: 968-973.

The posterior cruciate ligament and posterior joint capsule anatomy in the knee are reviewed.

28. Schepers T, Ginai A, Mulder P, Patka P: Radiographic evaluation of calcaneal fractures: To measure or not to measure. *Skeletal Radiol* 2007;36:847-852.

9: Imaging Update

The evaluation of outcomes after treatment of intra-articular calcaneal fractures traditionally uses three criteria: outcome scores, physical examination, and plain film radiography. However, this study found little correlation between the radiographic findings and the outcome of treatment. CT may be more valuable in the assessment of these fractures, but this has not yet been quantified.

29. Major NM: Role of MRI in prevention of metatarsal stress fractures in collegiate basketball players. *AJR Am J Roentgenol* 2006;186:255-258.

   MRI of the feet showed early stress-related marrow changes in six patients who played NCAA basketball. Treatment was initiated before the development of pain. Pain developed after MRI in three patients. A fracture line as shown on follow-up MRI developed in one of these patients, who missed the rest of the season. The other two patients were treated and missed no playing time because of their stress-related injuries.

30. Koulouris G, Ting A, Jhamb A, Connell D, Kavanagh E: Magnetic resonance imaging findings of injuries to the calf muscle complex. *Skeletal Radiol* 2007;36:921-927.

   This study reviewed the findings of calf muscle injuries with MRI.

31. Toye L, Helms C, Hoffman B, Easley M, Nunley J: MRI of spring ligament tears. *AJR Am J Roentgenol* 2005;184:1475-1480.

   The specific MRI characteristics of injuries to the spring ligament in the foot were evaluated and correlated with direct pathologic and surgical findings.

32. Fleming J, Dodd L, Helms C: Prominent vascular remnants in the calcaneus simulating a lesion of MRI of the ankle: Findings in 67 patients with cadaveric correlation. *AJR Am J Roentgenol* 2005;185:1449-1452.

Increased signal in the calcaneus, adjacent to the sinus tarsus, is often seen on MRI. This study demonstrated that this finding correlates with prominent vascular remnants within the calcaneus, and increased fluid-sensitive signal on MRI is an incidental finding.

33. Gaeta M, Minutoli F, Scribano E, et al : CT and MR imaging of athletes with early tibial stress injuries: Comparison with bone scintigraphy findings and emphasis on cortical abnormalities. *Radiology* 2005;235:553-561.

   This is a quantitative study of the sensitivity of MRI, CT, and nuclear medicine bone scintigraphy for the evaluation of stress fractures of the tibia in athletes.

34. Bergman AG, Fredericson M, Ho C, Matheson GO: Asymptomatic tibial stress reactions: MRI detection and clinical follow-up in distance runners. *AJR Am J Roentgenol* 2004;183:635-638.

   MRI signs of tibial stress reactions were found in 43% of asymptomatic college distance runners. These signs did not correlate with future clinical symptoms of stress fractures. Therefore, it is vital to correlate the MRI findings with the clinical findings in these patients.

35. Tins B, Cassar-Pullicino V: Marrow changes in anorexia nervosa masking the presence of stress fractures on MR imaging. *Skeletal Radiol* 2006;35:857-860.

   Patients with anorexia nervosa can demonstrate marrow signal abnormalities that are identical to those in stress fractures, and these marrow changes are most prominent in the feet. However, stress fractures of the feet, pelvis, and ribs are not uncommon in patients with anorexia nervosa because of extreme osteoporosis and excessive exercise. Edema in the Kager's fat pad also was seen in patients with anorexia nervosa and is a possible indicator of the severity of the disorder. However, this finding does not aid in the differentiation of the marrow changes of anorexia nervosa from stress fractures because these may often coexist.

Index

Page numbers with *f* indicate figures
Page numbers with *t* indicate tables

Index

C

Index

Fracture-dislocations
  in clavicular fractures, 10
  of the elbow, 42
  Lisfranc, 188–190, 439
  of the spine, 295
Fractures
  acetabular, 93, 93*f*
  ACL injuries and, 397
  avulsion (*See* Avulsion fractures)
  Bennett, 69, 70*f*
  bone scans for (*See* Bone scans)
  boxer's, 69, 69*f*
  clavicular, 10–12, 21
  of the elbow, 42–44, 61
  evaluation of, 92–93
  of the fingers, 69, 73
  hip joint injuries and, 91
  intra-articular, 69
  medial, 11
  osteochondral, 42
  proximal humeral, 8–10, 9*f*
  scapular, 10, 11*f*
  of the shoulder, 5 (*See also under* Clavicle)
  stress (*See* Stress fractures)
  treatment for (*See* Closed reduction; Immobilization; Open reduction and internal fixation (ORIF))
  of the wrist, 74–75
Fragment fixation, 61
Freiberg disease, 393
Frontal plane testing, 428
Fungal infections, 365, 373, 375–376
Furuncles, 372
Fusion, 406, 407

G

Gait training, 203, 260, 274, 276
Ganglion cyst, 436, 437*t*
Gastrocnemius tendon, 111, 331, 439
Gastrocnemius-soleus complex, 183, 260
Gastroenteritis, 371
Gastrointestinal infections. *See* Diarrhea; Parasites; Viral infections
Generalized anxiety disorder, 356
Gerdy tubercle, 140, 157, 181
Giant cell tumor, 437
Giardia intestinalis, 370, 371
Giardia lamblia, 371*t*
Glaucoma, 366
Glenohumeral internal rotation deficit (GIRD), 22, 31, 426, 428, 429
Glenohumeral joint/ligament
  avulsion of, 3
  function of, 3
  hyperextension of, 29
  rehabilitation of, 221, 223–224, 223*f*, 224*f*
  rotator cuff tears and, 29
  shoulder impingement syndrome, 340
Gliding mechanism, for tendons, 329
Glucosamine, 157, 166
Glucose, 345
Gluteus maximus, 274

Gluteus medius
  arthroscopic visualization of, 106, 107
  gait and, 274, 275
  repair of, 107
  snapping hip syndrome and, 86
Gluteus medius syndrome, 88, 91
Gluteus minimus
  arthroscopic visualization of, 106, 107
  gait and, 274, 275
  repair of, 107
Glycemic effect, 350
Glyceryl trinitrate patches, 321–322, 321*f*
Glycogen, 345–347, 349, 381
Glycosaminoglycan
  normal tendon and, 307
  in reparative tissue, 308
  synthesis of, 329
  tendinosis and, 309
Golfer's elbow. *See* Medial epicondylitis
Gonococcal conjunctivitis, 366
Graded symptom checklist, 287, 288*t*, 291
Graft fixation, 399. *See also* Fixation
Graft selection, 138, 143
Gram-negative bacteria, 373
Greater trochanter, 86, 87, 102, 107
Greater trochanteric pain syndrome, 88
Greater tuberosity, 10
Groin and pelvis injuries
  adductor strain, 85, 91
  athletic pubalgia, 83–84, 91
  gluteus medius syndrome, 88, 91
  hip pointer, 85–86, 91
  imaging of (*See under the various imaging techniques*)
  osteitis pubis, 85, 91–93
  piriformis syndrome, 87–88, 91
  snapping hip syndrome, 86–87, 87*f*, 437
  stress fractures, 84–85, 84*f*

H

Haglund deformity, 204, 336
Hahn-Steinthal capitellum fracture, 44
Hamstring tendon
  for ACL reconstruction, 135, 248
  autografting with, 135, 308, 398, 399
  core stabilization and, 269
  exercise and, 260
  imaging of, 114–115, 437
  for PCL reconstruction, 141
  spondylolysis and, 404
  strains of, 111
  strengthening of, 252*f*, 420
  stretching of, 114
  for UCL reconstruction, 51
Hamstring-gracilis tendon, 250
Hand. *See also* Finger injuries; Wrist
  arthritis in, 74
  hook of hamate fractures in, 73–74
  pulley ruptures in, 72
Heart murmur, 359*t*
Heat illness
  athletic performance and, 379, 381, 382–383, 383*t*, 412–413, 412*f*
  in children, 379–380, 411–414

classification of, 380–381
  epidemiology of, 379
  exercise and, 379–380, 411
  hyponatremia, 381–382, 414
  managing, 382–383
  pathophysiology of, 379–380
  prevention of, 383–384, 414
  risk factors for, 380–381, 380*f*, 380*t*, 381*t*, 414
  treatment of, 413–414
Heat Illness Symptom Index, 414
Heat tolerance test, 414
Heel pain. *See* Plantar fasciitis
Hemarthrosis, 95–96, 248, 397
Hematologic disorders, 391
Hematomas, 83
Hemolytic anemia, 368
Hepatitis B, 369–370
Hepatomegaly, 368
Herniation, 83, 91, 403
Herniography, 83
Herpes gladiatorum, 365, 366, 374
Herpes rugbiformus, 374
Herpes simplex virus (HSV-1), 374, 375*f*
Herpes zoster, 375
Heuter-Volkmann principle, 75
High-resolution ultrasonography, testing effectiveness of sclerotherapy with, 322, 323*f*, 335–336, 336*f*, 337*f*, 338, 338*f*, 339*f*
High-voltage galvanic electrical stimulation (HVGS), 247, 248
Hill-Sachs lesions, 3
Hip
  arthroscopy of
    central compartment pathology, 103–105
    instrumentation for, 101, 102*f*
    lateral compartment pathology, 106–107
    patient position for, 101–102, 102*f*
    peripheral compartment pathology, 105–106, 105*f*
    portal placement, 101*f*, 103, 106
    rehabilitation after, 273–280, 274*f*, 279*f*
  biomechanics of, 273–275
  core stabilization and, 263
  imaging of, 437 (*See also under the various imaging techniques*)
  impingement test for, 92, 92*f*, 94
  injury to
    classification of, 91
    instability of, 91, 95–97
    intra-articular diagnoses, 93–98
    patient history, 91
    physical examination, 91–92, 92*f*
    radiographic evaluation, 92–93, 92*f*, 93*f*, 94*f*
  neuromuscular control of, 275
  range of motion in, 428
  sources of pain in, 91, 93–94 (*See also under specific hip injuries*)
  strength of, 267
  subluxation of, 94, 96, 97

Index

Index

Index

biomechanics of, 139
complications of, 145
epidemiology of, 140
evaluation of, 140
nonsurgical management for, 140
physical examination for, 140
surgical management for, 140–141, 143, 144f
Posterior drawer test, 4, 140
Posterior instability, 4–5
Posterior olecranon osteophyte excision, 242
Posterior sag sign, 140
Posterior tibial tendon, 204
Posterior tibialis tendinitis, 393
Posterolateral corner injuries, 135, 140, 145, 146f
Posterolateral drawer test, 144
Posterolateral rotatory drawer test, 62–63
Posterolateral rotatory instability (PLRI), 41, 61–64, 145
Posttraumatic stress disorder, 356
Postural stability assessment, 289
Posture, 301, 301t
Pox virus, 375
Prehabilitation. See Preventive exercises
Preparticipation
bracing and, 200
preparticipation physical examination (PPPE), 359–360, 422
strength training and, 421, 422
Preventive exercises, 420–421
Prone push-up test, 63
Proprioceptive control
ACL rehabilitation and, 250–251, 250f, 399
for cervical injuries, 301
during elbow rehabilitation, 232, 235f
lateral ankle sprains and, 200, 201
menisci and, 173
after microfracture, 260
multiple knee ligament injuries and, 143
Prostaglandins, 112, 113, 309
Prostatitis, 365
Proteins, 346–347, 346t, 347t, 349–350
Proteoglycans
in cartilage, 164
in menisci, 173
tendinosis features, 308t
in tendons, 307
vascular remodeling and, 309
Proximal humeral fractures, 8–10
Pseudoclawing, 69
Psychology. See Rehabilitation psychology; Sport psychology
Pubic tubercle, 83
Pulley rupture, 72
Pulmonary embolus, 369
Pulmonary infections. See Bronchitis; Pneumonia
Pulmonary injuries, 10

Q

Q angle, 119–121, 123
Quadriceps muscle
ACL reconstruction and, 247
isometric strength measurement of, 248, 249
rehabilitation of, 260, 261
strength training and injury to, 420
Quadriceps-patellar bone autografting, 141
Quadruped exercise, 265, 265f

R

Radial head/neck fractures, 42–43
Radiculopathy, 300
Radiocapitellar joint, 47, 49, 61
Radiography, 435
for ankle, 438–439
accessory navicular, 204, 205f
flexor hallucis longus tendon, 205–206
impingement syndrome, 208, 210
lateral ankle sprains, 201, 201f, 202f
os trigonum, 209
peroneal tendon subluxation, 206
syndesmotic injuries, 203, 203f
talus injuries, 207, 208f
for elbow
capitellum fractures, 44f
dislocations, 42
fracture-dislocations, 43f
lateral epicondylitis, 64
medial epicondylitis, 47
osteochondritis dissecans, 59–61
posterolateral rotatory instability, 63
UCL injuries, 50
ulnar nerve injuries, 53
for foot, 438–439
os trigonum injuries, 187, 188f
stress fractures, 192–194
tarsometatarsal joint injuries, 189, 190f
turf toe, 191, 191f
for groin/pelvis, 83, 85
for hand/wrist
acute boutonniere deformity, 71, 72f
finger dislocations, 69, 70f, 71f
finger fractures, 69, 70f
hook of hamate fractures, 73
mallet finger, 70
pulley ruptures, 72
Stener lesions, 73
for hip joint, 92–93, 92f, 435
dislocation, 105
femoroacetabular impingement, 92–93, 92f, 93f, 95
loose bodies, 98, 105
for knee
articular cartilage lesions, 156
LCL injuries, 144

meniscal tears, 175–176
multiple knee ligament injuries, 142
PCL injuries, 140
pediatric ACL injuries, 397
PFJ, 120, 121f, 122f
for lower extremity, 181–183, 182t
for muscles, 112, 114
for osteoarthritis, 5, 127–128, 135
for osteochondroses
Freiberg disease, 393
Kienbock disease, 394
Köhler disease, 393, 393f
Legg-Calvé-Perthes disease, 391, 391f, 392
Panner disease, 389, 390f
for shoulder
acromioclavicular joint injuries, 3
clavicular fractures, 12
proximal humeral fractures, 8, 9f
scapular fractures, 10, 11f
for skeletal maturity determination, 398
for spine, 297, 299, 404
Range-of-motion exercises
for ACL rehabilitation, 247, 248, 250, 399
for acromioclavicular joint injuries, 8
for adductor strain, 85
for cervical injuries, 301
for elbow rehabilitation, 229, 230t, 231t, 236
after hip surgery, 275, 276
after microfracture, 260
for multiple knee ligament injuries, 143
for overuse injuries, 429
after posterior olecranon osteophyte excision, 242
after rotator cuff repair, 217, 218–219t, 220
for scapular fractures, 10
after sclerotherapy, 335
for skier's thumb, 73
after SLAP repair, 221, 222t
for trochlear groove defects, 261
for UCL injuries, 50, 240, 242
after ulnar nerve transposition, 242
Recovery nutrition, 349–350
Red eye. See Conjunctivitis
Reduction. See also Open reduction and internal fixation (ORIF)
of acromioclavicular joint injuries, 8
for finger dislocations, 69
of shoulder injuries, 3, 5
Rehabilitation program
for ankle injuries, 200–204
core stabilization and, 264, 269
for elbow injuries
epicondylitis/tendinitis, 236–239, 239t
general guidelines for throwing injuries, 229–236
Little League elbow, 242
medial epicondylitis, 48
posterior olecranon osteophyte excision, 242

Index

Index

Tennis elbow. *See also* Lateral epicondylitis
  exercise treatment of, 314
  glyceryl trinitrate patches and, 322
  sclerotherapy for, 322, 339–340, 340f
Tenocytes
  extracorporeal shock wave therapy and, 322
  function of, 307, 309–310
  metabolism of, 329
  tendinosis features, 308t, 309
Tenolysis, 209
Tenosynovectomy, 206
Tenosynovitis
  detection of, 436
  flexor hallucis longus tendon and, 205
  peroneal, 206
  posterior tibial tendon and, 204
Tenotomy
  for Achilles tendinopathy, 330–331, 331f
  for adductor strain, 85
  for athletic pubalgia, 83
  for Legg-Calvé-Perthes disease, 392
  for patellar tendinopathy, 332
  percutaneous longitudinal, 330
  for tendinopathy, 330
Therapeutic exercise, 309
Therapeutic ultrasound. *See* Ultrasound, in treatment
Thermal capsulorrhaphy, 33. *See also* Capsulorrhaphy
Thermogenesis, 346
Thermoregulation, 411, 414
Thessaly test, 175
Thixotropy, 31
Thomas test, 92
Throat infections. *See* Herpes simplex virus (HSV-1); Streptococcal pharyngitis, group A
Thrombocytopenia, 368
Thrombophilia, 390
Thrower's Ten program, 230t, 232, 233–234f, 242, 243
Throwing injuries
  in adolescent athletes, 59
  nerve injuries, 52–53
  pathomechanics, 31–32, 32t, 47
  prevention of, 33
  rehabilitation for
    for epicondylitis/tendinitis, 236–239, 239t
    general guidelines, 229–236, 230t, 231t
    for Little League elbow, 242
    for posterior olecranon osteophyte excision, 242
    for UCL injuries, 240, 241t, 242
    after UCL reconstruction, 242–243, 244t, 245
    after ulnar nerve transposition, 242, 243t
    for ulnar neuropathy, 240
    for valgus extension overload, 240
  stress exerted in, 47, 48

treatment of, 32–33
  in youth athletes, 33, 425–430
Thumb fractures, 69
Tibial stress fractures, 192–193
Tibialis posterior tendon, 308, 332
Tibiofemoral joint arthrokinematics, 248
Tinea corporis, 376
Tinea cruris, 376
Tinea gladiatorum, 376
Tinea pedis, 373, 375–376
Tinel sign, 53, 185
Torg ratio, 297, 299
Total daily energy expenditure (TDEE), 346
Toxoplasmosis, 368
Traction periostitis, 85
Transepiphyseal surgery, 399
Transesophageal echocardiography, 361
Transient quadriparesis, 295–298
Transient synovitis, 390, 391
Transitional vertebrae, 403
Translation, 264
Transphyseal ACL reconstruction. *See* Complete transphyseal surgery
Transthoracic echocardiography, 361
Transverse friction massage, 236, 238, 313
Transverse plane motion, 428
Trapeziectomy, 74
Trapeziometacarpal joint injuries, 74
Trendelenburg maneuver, 88, 92
Triangular fibrocartilage complex, 75, 75f, 76–77, 76f
Triglycerides, 345, 347
Triquetral body fracture, 74–75
Trochanter, visualization of, 107. *See also* Greater trochanter
Trochanteric bursitis, 91, 92, 107
Trochlear dysplasia, 120–121, 121f, 126
Trochlear groove, 119, 261
Trunk
  flexibility of, 428
  function of, 264
  key muscles for, 264
  muscular action during tennis, 427
  perturbation training, 268
  plank position, 265, 265f
  quadruped position, 265, 265f
  stability training, 269
  strength assessment of, 428
  walking lunge, 267, 267f
TT-TG offset (tibial tubercle to trochlear groove distance), 121–122, 123f, 126
Turf toe, 190–191, 191t
Tympanic membrane rupture, 367
Tzanck test, 374

U

Ulnar collateral ligament (UCL)
  anatomy of, 48
  as elbow stabilizer, 41
  evaluation of, 49–50, 50f
  imaging of, 436
  laxity of, 61

pathomechanics of, 48, 49
  radial head/neck fractures and, 43
  reconstruction of, 42, 51, 51f, 63, 229, 242–243, 244t, 245
  rotatory instability of, 61–64
  skier's thumb and, 73
  treatment of injuries to, 50–52
Ulnar nerve injuries, 52–53
Ulnar nerve transposition, 48, 53, 242, 243t
Ulnar neuritis, 50
Ulnar neuropathy, 48, 53, 236, 240
Ulnar styloid, 74, 398
Ulnocarpal abutment, 75, 75f
Ultrasonography, 50. *See also* High-resolution ultrasonography
Ultrasound, 435
  in diagnosis
    for Achilles tendon, 320
    for athletic pubalgia, 83
    for gluteus medius syndrome, 88
    for hamstring injuries, 437
    for knee imaging, 438
    for Legg-Calvé-Perthes disease, 391
    measuring spleen size, 368
    for meniscal tears, 176
    for osteochondritis dissecans, 59
    for rotator cuff injuries, 27, 436
    for snapping hip syndrome, 86
    for Stener lesions, 73
    for tendinopathy, 309
    for wrist imaging, 436
  MRI and, 436
  in treatment
    for Achilles tendinopathy, 313
    for elbow rehabilitation, 232
    hyperthermia and, 321
    for patellar tendinopathy, 313
    for piriformis syndrome, 88
    for plantar fasciitis, 186
    for stress fractures, 193
    for tendinopathy, 320, 321
    for tendinosis, 236, 238
    for tennis elbow, 314
Upper respiratory tract infections, 365–368
Upright bilateral rowing exercise, 266, 266f

V

Valgus displacement, 61
Valgus extension overload syndrome, 49, 50, 52, 240
Valgus laxity
  in the elbow, 240
  in MCL injuries, 144
  in Panner disease, 389
Valgus stress
  at the elbow, 41, 47–49, 48f, 49f
  osteochondritis dissecans and, 59
  in Panner disease, 389
  throwing injuries and, 425
  UCL injuries and, 240
  ulnar neuropathy and, 240